Evolutionary Medicine *and* Health

NEW PERSPECTIVES

Edited by

Wenda R. Trevathan
New Mexico State University

E. O. Smith
Emory University

James J. McKenna
University of Notre Dame

New York   Oxford
OXFORD UNIVERSITY PRESS
2008

Oxford University Press, Inc., publishes works that further Oxford University's
objective of excellence in research, scholarship, and education.

Oxford   New York
Auckland   Cape Town   Dar es Salaam   Hong Kong   Karachi
Kuala Lumpur   Madrid   Melbourne   Mexico City   Nairobi
New Delhi   Shanghai   Taipei   Toronto

With offices in
Argentina   Austria   Brazil   Chile   Czech Republic   France   Greece
Guatemala   Hungary   Italy   Japan   Poland   Portugal   Singapore
South Korea   Switzerland   Thailand   Turkey   Ukraine   Vietnam

Copyright © 2008 by Oxford University Press, Inc.

Published by Oxford University Press, Inc.
198 Madison Avenue, New York, New York 10016
http://www.oup.com

Oxford is a registered trademark of Oxford University Press

Library of Congress Cataloging-in-Publication Data

Evolutionary medicine and health : new perspectives / [edited by] Wenda R. Trevathan,
E.O. Smith, James J. McKenna.
     p. ; cm.
   Includes bibliographical references and index.
   ISBN 978-0-19-530706-1 (pbk. : alk. paper)—ISBN 978-0-19-530705-4 (hardcover :
alk. paper) 1. Diseases—Causes and theories of causation. 2. Human evolution.
3. Medicine—Philosophy.   I. Trevathan, Wenda. II. Smith, Euclid O. III. McKenna,
James J. (James Joseph), 1948–
   [DNLM: 1. Disease—etiology—Essays. 2. Evolution—Essays. 3. Epidemiologic
Factors—Essays. 4. Humans—Essays. 5. Philosophy, Medical—Essays. QZ 9 E93 2008]
   RB152.E963 2008
   616.001—dc22   2007016223

Printing number: 9 8 7 6 5 4 3 2 1

Printed in the United States of America
on acid-free paper

CONTENTS

Preface   ix
Contributors   xi

PART ONE
Background

1. Introduction and Overview of Evolutionary Medicine
Wenda R. Trevathan, E. O. Smith, and James J. McKenna
1

PART TWO
Politics, Nutrition, and Diet

2. Human Evolution, Diet, and Nutrition: When the Body
Meets the Buffet
*Bethany L. Turner, Kenneth Maes, Jennifer Sweeney, and
George J. Armelagos*
55

3. Diabesity and Darwinian Medicine: The Evolution of an Epidemic
Leslie Sue Lieberman
72

4. To Eat or What Not To Eat, That's the Question: A Critique
of the Official Norwegian Dietary Guidelines
*Iver Mysterud, Dag Viljen Poleszynski, Fedon A. Lindberg, and
Stig A. Bruset*
96

5. Cow's Milk Consumption and Health: An Evolutionary Perspective
Andrea S. Wiley
116

PART THREE
Sex, Reproduction, and Health

6. Not by Bread Alone: The Role of Psychosocial Stress in Age at
First Reproduction and Health Inequalities
James S. Chisholm and David A. Coall
134

7. Early Life Effects on Reproductive Function
Alejandra Núñez–de la Mora and Gillian R. Bentley
149

8. Impaired Reproductive Function in Women in Western and "Westernizing"
Populations: An Evolutionary Approach
Tessa M. Pollard and Nigel Unwin
169

9. Should Women Menstruate? An Evolutionary Perspective on Menstrual-Suppressing
Oral Contraceptives
Lynnette Leidy Sievert
181

10. An Evolutionary Perspective on Premenstrual Syndrome: Implications for
Investigating Infectious Causes of Chronic Disease
Caroline Doyle, Holly A. Swain Ewald, and Paul W. Ewald
196

11. Possible Role of Eclampsia/Preeclampsia in Evolution
of Human Reproduction
*Pierre-Yves Robillard, Gustaaf Dekker, Gérard Chaouat, Jean Chaline,
and Thomas C. Hulsey*
216

PART FOUR
Environments, Normality, and Lifetime Health

12. Breastfeeding and Mother–Infant Sleep Proximity: Implications for Infant Care
Helen Ball and Kristin Klingaman
226

13. Why Words Can Hurt Us: Social Relationships, Stress, and Health
Mark V. Flinn
242

14. Why Are We Vulnerable to Acute Mountain Sickness?
Cynthia M. Beall
259

15. Evolution and Modern Behavioral Problems: The Case of Addiction
Daniel H. Lende
277

16. After Dark: The Evolutionary Ecology of Human Sleep
Carol M. Worthman
291

———

PART FIVE
Chronic Diseases, Old Treatments, and More Misunderstanding

17. Evolutionary Medicine and Obesity: Developmental Adaptive Responses
in Human Body Composition
Jack Baker, Magdalena Hurtado, Osbjorn Pearson, and Troy Jones
314

18. The Developmental Origins of Adult Health: Intergenerational Inertia
in Adaptation and Disease
Christopher W. Kuzawa
325

19. An Evolutionary Perspective on the Causes of Chronic Diseases:
Atherosclerosis as an Illustration
Paul W. Ewald
350

20. Genes, Geographic Ancestry, and Disease Susceptibility: Applications of
Evolutionary Medicine to Clinical Settings
Douglas E. Crews and Linda M. Gerber
368

21. From Ancient Seas to Modern Disease: Evolution and Congestive
Heart Failure
E. Jennifer Weil
382

22. Evolution at the Intersection of Biology and Medicine
Stephen Lewis
399

CONTENTS

23. The Importance of Evolution for Medicine
Randolph M. Nesse
416

Notes 435
References 441
Index 523

PREFACE

We hope our overview in Chapter 1 makes clear that research in the field of evolutionary medicine has expanded tremendously since the publication of *Evolutionary Medicine* in 1999. Admittedly, we present here only a sampling of the array of possible topics. In developing this book, we began by making a list of scholars working in this area, many of whom were contributors to the 1999 volume. We invited original articles and were gratified that so many of our colleagues responded positively. Of this set of potential authors, 40 prepared the 23 chapters included in this volume.

By inviting the work of active researchers in the field, we have perhaps overrepresented "hot item issues," and inevitably there is some conspicuous though appropriate overlap among chapters, especially those pertaining to female reproductive function, in utero developmental processes in relation to future health, and obesity/diabesity and other contemporary human diseases and disorders related to excessive food consumption.

The majority of the contributors (27 of 44) are biological anthropologists. To a great extent, this distribution was influenced by our accessibility to and familiarity with this particular branch of the discipline. But the remainder of the contributors are physicians, biologists, psychologists, and geographers. Further, thanks to the Internet and the ability to send chapters around the world almost instantaneously, the book has diverse international authorship: the contributors are from the United States (28), the United Kingdom (6), Norway (4), France (3), Australia (2), and Switzerland (1).

We have geared this book toward educated generalists and students at the advanced undergraduate and graduate levels in biology, anthropology, and health sciences, including medicine. Our hope is that general readers, scholars of evolutionary medicine, health care practitioners, and students will find it useful in teaching, thinking, and conducting daily work in the health field.

THE EVOLUTIONARY APPROACH

A list of the primary causes of ill health among people worldwide (other than viruses and bacteria) might look something like this: (1) poverty and lack of access to health care, adequate diets, and safe living and working environments; (2) lack of sufficient time, resources, or inclination to adopt healthful lifestyles that are consistent with our evolved biologies; (3) bad advice from so-called health experts (e.g., co-sleeping is dangerous, stopping menstrual periods is good, cow's milk is good for children, PMS is all in your head); and (4) misguided research and applications (e.g., believing that ulcers cannot possibly be virally caused, focusing on single causes of diseases, concluding that dietary supplementation for pregnant women does not improve infant health). Lack of understanding of the effects of evolution on human health would probably not be included in such a list. Yet contributors to this volume leave open the possibility that evolutionary-based medical approaches might well be able to better identify, conceptualize, and counteract some of the underlying causes of poor health and thus help reduce health inequalities. Evolutionary ways of thinking and doing research may lead to new ways of treating and preventing diseases and disorders, potentially saving lives or, at the very least, improving the quality of life for those whose conditions compromise health or lead to early death.

TEACHING THIS TEXT

As careful readers will note, Randolph Nesse's chapter (23, "The Importance of Evolution for Medicine") could work as an introduction to the field or as a conclusion to the volume, providing direction for future research. In particular, Tables 23–4 and 23–5 (pp. 432–433) may prepare students to read critically the chapters that propose testing evolutionary hypotheses about disease. A useful assignment for courses covering evolutionary medicine might be to have students propose evolutionary explanations for diseases, disorders, and health challenges. In this case, Nesse's table is essential, and it may be suitable to have students read his chapter first or at least early in the course, before they begin to work on the assignment. Nesse's chapter also offers helpful suggestions for teaching a course on evolutionary medicine.

We should point out that although some of the contributors to the 1999 volume are the same as those in this volume, all contributions are original, and so the two volumes could be used together in a class without fear of repetition. In fact, the two volumes together, with a total of 41 chapters, provide a good representation of the subject matter and breadth of evolutionary medicine.

WEB ENHANCEMENT

This volume's companion website, www.oup.com/us/evolmed, provides additional information, as indicated by links in selected chapters. It also provides the full reference list, complete with links to source articles, reports, and databases. The website will be updated frequently and is an excellent resource for students, researchers, and others interested in advancements in the field of evolutionary medicine.

ACKNOWLEDGMENTS

We extend our sincere thanks to the following reviewers: John Bock, California State University, Fullerton; Peter Brown, Emory University; Beverly Ann Davenport, University of North Texas; Jan English-Lueck, San Jose State University; Thomas McDade, Northwestern University; Bettina Shell-Duncan, University of Washington; Joan Stevenson, Western Washington University; and Linda van Blerkom, Drew University.

CONTRIBUTORS

George Armelagos, Department of Anthropology, Emory University

Jack Baker, Department of Anthropology and Bureau of Business and Economic Research, University of New Mexico

Helen Ball, Parent–Infant Sleep Lab and Medical Anthropology Research Group, Department of Anthropology, Durham University

Cynthia M. Beall, Department of Anthropology, Case Western Reserve University

Gillian R. Bentley, Department of Anthropology, Durham University

Stig A. Bruset, Lierskogen Legekontor

Jean Chaline, Biogéosciences et Paléobiodiversity et Préhistoire de l'EPHE, Centre des Sciences de la Terre

Gérard Chaouat, Unité Cytokines dans la Relation Materno-Foetale

James S. Chisholm, School of Anatomy and Human Biology, University of Western Australia

David A. Coall, Center for Cognitive and Decision Sciences, Institute of Psychology, University of Basel

Douglas E. Crews, Department of Anthropology and School of Public Health, The Ohio State University

Gustaaf Dekker, Department of Obstetrics and Gynaecology, Lyell McEwin Hospital

Caroline Doyle, Department of Biology, University of Louisville

Holly A. Swain Ewald, Department of Biology, University of Louisville

Paul W. Ewald, Department of Biology, University of Louisville

Mark V. Flinn, Department of Anthropology and Department of Psychological Sciences, University of Missouri

Linda M. Gerber, Department of Public Health, Weill Medical College of Cornell University

Thomas C. Hulsey, Division of Pediatric Epidemiology, Medical University of South Carolina, Children's Hospital

Magdalena Hurtado, Biological Anthropology Program, Department of Anthropology, University of New Mexico

Troy Jones, Department of Geography, University of New Mexico

Kristin Klingaman, Department of Anthropology, Durham University

Chrisopher W. Kuzawa, Department of Anthropology, Northwestern University

Daniel H. Lende, Department of Anthropology, University of Notre Dame

Stephen Lewis, Department of Biological Sciences, University College Chester

Leslie Sue Lieberman, Women's Research Center and Department of Anthropology, University of Central Florida

Fedon A. Lindberg, Lindberg Clinic

Kenneth Maes, Department of Anthropology, Emory University

Iver Mysterud, Department of Biology, University of Oslo

Randolph M. Nesse, Departments of Psychiatry and Psychology, University of Michigan

Alejandra Núñez–de la Mora, Department of Anthropology, Durham University

Osbjorn Pearson, Department of Anthropology, University of New Mexico

Dag Viljen Poleszynski, Bjerklundsvn

Tessa M. Pollard, Department of Anthropology, Durham University

Pierre-Yves Robillard, Neonatology, Centre Hospitalier Sud-Reunion

Lynette Leidy Sievert, Department of Anthropology, University of Massachusetts

Jennifer Sweeney, Department of Anthropology, Emory University

Bethany L. Turner, Department of Anthropology, Emory University

Nigel Unwin, School of Clinical Medical Science and School of Population and Health Science Medical School, University of Newcastle

E. Jennifer Weil, Phoenix Epidemiology and Clinical Research Branch, National Institute of Diabetes and Digestive & Kidney Diseases

Andrea S. Wiley, Program in Anthropology, James Madison University

Carol M. Worthman, Department of Anthropology, Emory University

CHAPTER 1

Introduction and Overview of Evolutionary Medicine

Wenda R. Trevathan, E. O. Smith, and
James J. McKenna

INTRODUCTION

In a recent Doonesbury comic strip, Garry Trudeau depicts a 60-ish man who has just been told by his physician that he has tuberculosis. When he asks about his prognosis, the doc says, "Depends—are you a creationist?" The patient answers, "Yes, but what does that have to do with tuberculosis?" Being a good evolutionary medicine proponent, the physician responds, "A creationist would want to be treated with streptomycin, because that worked *before* the tuberculosis strain had evolved. Since you don't believe in evolution, then streptomycin should work just fine." "But Doc, aren't there newer drugs?" "Sure, there are much better ones for the evolved strains of tuberculosis because they have been "intelligently designed.' "

Indeed, nothing better illustrates the importance of understanding the role of evolution in medicine than the arms race that infectious agents and drugs have undergone in recent years. During World War II penicillin was found to be extremely effective in reducing the number of deaths from wounds and amputations. In the 1950s, virtually all strains of *Staphylococcus* were vulnerable to streptomycin; today none are. The penicillin used today is no different from that used in World War II, but the strains of bacteria have evolved a resistance to the once-lethal drug. Fortunately, medical and pharmaceutical research has, for the most part, been able to keep up with this arms race by building ever more powerful armaments, but three things stand in the way of continuing success: (1) acceleration of the arms race—because the generation length of bacteria is so short and because they multiply so rapidly they can quickly mutate into an antibiotic-resistant strain; (2) misunderstanding, and even rejection, of the theory of evolution by the vast majority of ordinary citizens in developed countries, where most medical research and health care advances take place; and (3) lack of even a cursory understanding of the scientific basis for human evolution by most of the lay public.

1

EVOLUTION OF HUMANS

Humans are members of the order of mammals known as Primates, an order that traces its origins to approximately 60 million years ago. Characteristics that define humans as primates include binocular, stereoscopic vision, color vision, a high degree of manual dexterity, which emphasizes opposability by the thumb and first digit, omnivorous dietary adaptations, a tendency to live in complex social groups, and a reliance on learned behaviors rather than simple genetically determined responses for survival. The anatomical characters clearly demonstrate that we are closely related to other primates, and most authorities consider the chimpanzee to be our closest relative, although there are some dissenting opinions that are beyond the scope of this brief introduction.

The taxonomic family and subfamily that include modern humans, Hominidae (family) and Homininae (subfamily), respectively, have been in existence for 5–7 million years, and our genus, *Homo*, for about 2 million years (see Figure 1-1). Members of the genus *Homo* are distinguished in the tribe Hominini (which includes chimpanzees and us) by habitual bipedalism (walking on two legs), large brains relative to body size, and dependency on material culture (tools and technology). Until about 10,000 years ago, humans lived in small, multiaged social groups of about 20–30 individuals, were nomadic, and relied on hunting and gathering of wild foods.

One of the keys to the evolutionary success of humans and many other primate species is behavioral flexibility and the ability to adapt to a wide variety of environments, foods, and lifestyles. As environments changed, people who were able to adjust and continue to reproduce passed those abilities on to their offspring so that today humans continue to live, survive, and reproduce under a variety of conditions, including high altitudes, toxic levels of environmental pollution, dense urban populations, extremes of cold and heat, and diets that differ widely from those of our ancestors. We have survived in an environment that today is radically different from the one our ancestors inhabited only 500 generations ago. The human environment has changed more in the last 10,000 years, or even in the last 200, than in the entire course of human evolutionary history.

Inferences about ancestral diets, lives, and health come from three sources: (1) the living nonhuman primates, especially our closest living relatives the chimpanzees and bonobos; (2) the fossil record of primates and hominins; and (3) the ethnographic studies

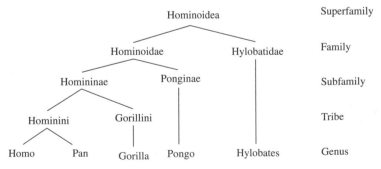

FIGURE 1-1 The hominoid family tree.

of the few remaining populations of hunting and gathering people (e.g., Australian aborigines, Hadza in Tanzania, !Kung of Botswana, Ache of Paraguay, Efé of the Democratic Republic of the Congo, and Agta of the Philippines). Of these three possible sources of data, most of the research discussed in this volume has relied on detailed, ethnographic accounts of the behavior and ecology of living humans. Characteristics reported for contemporary foraging people (hunter-gatherers in the old terminology) include: (1) diets that are composed of from 50 to 80% plant sources; (2) diets that are high in complex carbohydrates and low in saturated fats; (3) high levels of daily activity in search of food, water, and temporary sleeping sites; (4) little to no hypertension and heart disease; (5) near-absence of cancers; and (6) little evidence of psychological and emotional ailments (Eaton, Konner, & Shostak, 1988b). It is tempting to attribute these characteristics to short life expectancies, but more than 8% of the population of most groups studied exceed 60 years of age (Blurton Jones, Hawkes, & O'Connell, 2002). It is true that the exceedingly long lives of many contemporary people is probably of recent origin, but the argument that very few people lived past 50 is unsupported by ethnographic data.

With domestication of plants and animals came numerous changes in human lives, in addition to changes in diet and activity levels. Rather than travel widely foraging for foods, people began to settle in semi-permanent villages where they concentrated their efforts on growing domesticated plants in order to produce sufficient foods to support local families and communities. With increasingly sophisticated agricultural practices came increased population as more people could be supported on the foods grown, fewer died from starvation, and large families became advantageous for working the land. Not only did domestication of plants change the environment, but domestication of animals placed humans in close proximity to a variety of new pathogens, dramatically increasing the risk of infectious disease. It has been estimated that more than 700 microbes known to cause disease in humans were transmitted from animals that we domesticated several thousand years ago (dogs, cats, horses, cattle, goats, sheep, and pigs) (Torrey & Yolken, 2005).[1] In fact, infectious diseases replaced accidents, poisoning, and diseases transmitted by insect bites as the major causes of mortality between the onset of agriculture and industrialization when infectious disease were replaced in developed countries by chronic and noninfectious diseases. These changes in causes of morbidity and mortality have been referred to as "epidemiological transitions," and there is increasing concern that we are now experiencing a third transition whereby infectious diseases are "re-emerging" (Armelagos, Brown, & Turner, 2005).

EVOLUTION, THEORY, AND BELIEF

One of the major stumbling blocks to the use of evolutionary theory in considering human health is the lack of understanding by many people of what constitutes a theory. For many people, a theory is somehow akin to an opinion, as in "I have a theory about boys" or "a theory about girls." or "I have a theory about this or that." In fact, most people do not have real "theories" about much. People have ideas and opinions about how things work, why the weather is what it is, why the opposite sex behaves in the way it does, or why their favorite football team fails to win the big games. These are not theories. A theory is based on repeated observations of a phenomenon that results in an accumulated wisdom and ability to generalize. There is a theory of gravity. We are comfortable saying that gravity is a theory because we have replicated the crucial experiment millions of times and do so every day—we have seen it work with our very eyes. We are comfortable because there have been no exceptions discovered that contradict this theory. In fact, what we have is a law of physics—a phenomenon that is repeatable with exactly the same results every time.

Unfortunately, when it comes to biological phenomena, there is not the level of certainty, of easy observability, and absolute reproducibility found in physics and chemistry. Because biological systems are always changing, albeit in minute ways, there is not the same certainty of outcome. That lack of complete certainty is what makes many people uncomfortable with theories in biology. Somehow, people have assumed that if a phenomenon is not perfectly and infinitely reproducible that it is not a "real" theory. This is simply not the case. Theories are bodies of knowledge that make predictions about natural phenomena. These predictions are just that—predictions, not fortune telling. The variations we see in the outcome of the evolutionary process are evidence that evolution as a process is a fact. It is a process in which we are immersed just as much as the *Streptococcus* bacteria we discussed earlier. Countless numbers of fossils in museums all over the world, as well as the variation in the roses in a garden, are examples of the process of evolution. Evolution is not a theory, it is a fact.

It is interesting to ask why conversations about evolution in Western cultures often involve whether one "believes in" evolution or not. Quite frankly, the phrase "believe in" is an odd one when discussing a scientific concept, or any scientific process. Can you imagine asking someone if she "believes" in gravity? in the change of seasons? in oceans? in the Krebs cycle? In fact, it is odd to think that anyone need "believe" in evolution at all. Evolution is a body of knowledge that is used to make predictions that are either supported or rejected using the scientific method. But perhaps this ubiquitous tendency to ask "Do you believe in evolution?" provides an important clue as to why evolution in the United States, at least, will always be controversial. Many people view evolution as yet another "belief" system, and one that they perceive as conflicting with religious ways of knowing, just as many people believe that they cannot be both Christian and Jewish (i.e., they cannot believe that Jesus was the Son of God *and* that he was just another man). The idea that a belief system is a dichotomous variable permeates much of Western thought. Either you are for us or you are against us is a common way of thinking. This leads many people to the conclusion that they cannot be both Christian and accept and use evolutionary principles to explain behavior and other natural processes. While it is beyond the scope of this book to offer a full and complete account of the views of those who stand in opposition to the use of evolution as a guiding theory in our everyday lives, it is important to understand that those opposed to using evolution as an explanation have very mixed views on the use of evolution in medicine.

BRIEF HISTORY OF EVOLUTION IN MEDICINE

Evolutionary medicine, as presently constituted with its own name and distinct research area, is a very recent phenomenon. George Williams and Randolph Nesse (Nesse & Williams, 1994b; Williams & Nesse, 1991) are often cited as the first to use explicitly the term "Darwinian medicine," which is often used synonymously with "evolut icine" (see Chapters 22 and 23). Although not explicitly referred to as evolut icine, scholars had been "doing" evolutionary medicine for many decades, even if the field did not really achieve professional and public recognition and organization, or its name, until the early 1990s. The publication of the first Williams and Nesse article in the *Quarterly Review of Biology* (Williams & Nesse, 1991) was followed shortly thereafter by a highly publicized American Association for the Advancement of Science (AAAS) symposium in Boston in 1993 entitled "Evolutionary Medicine: Exemplars of An Emerging New Field," organized by two of the three editors of this volume (McKenna and Smith).

From its beginning, evolutionary medicine received widespread public attention. During the week of the 1993 AAAS symposium in Boston, a number of newspapers, including the *Washington Post, Christian Science Monitor, Wall Street Journal, Los Angeles Times, San Francisco Chronicle*, and *Boston Globe*, to name but a few, ran front page stories of the session. AAAS records indicate that almost 500 newspaper and magazine articles were written about the 1993 symposium, exposing about 3.6 million readers worldwide to its content. Many of the authors of the newspaper articles came up with intriguing and thought-provoking titles such as "Evolving Answers" (Anonymous, 1993) in *The Economist*, "Darwin Takes on Mainstream Medicine" (Ezzell, 1993) in the *Journal of NIH Research*, "Diseases That Hark Back to the Stone Age Lifestyle" (Miller, 1993) in the *New Scientist*, "The Flintstone Diagnosis" (Begley, 1993) in *Newsweek*, and "Ancestors May Provide Clinical Answers Say 'Darwinian' Medical Evolutionists" (Goldsmith, 1993) in the *Journal of the American Medical Association*. Quite a reception for a symposium proposal that was initially rejected because the first reviewers had no idea what "evolutionary medicine" meant!

It is important to note that that while the "coming-out party" may have been in 1991, and that while Nesse and Williams may have been the first to talk explicitly about Darwinian medicine, the application of evolutionary thinking to medicine has a long and underappreciated history. As Randolph Nesse notes (Chapter 23), Erasmus Darwin (1731–1802) was one of the first physicians to think explicitly about change in nature and how changes observed in nature might be paralleled in humans, writing in his two-volume work, *Zoonomia, or the Laws of Organic Life* (Darwin, 1796). The work is divided into three parts, with Part 2 entitled "A Catalogue of Diseases Distributed into Natural Classes According to Their Proximate Causes, With Their Subsequent Orders, Genera and Species, and With Their Methods of Cure." So when we refer to Darwinian medicine, we are, in some sense, referring to both Charles Darwin as well as his grandfather.

One of the earliest papers that specifically addressed the place of evolution in medi-cine was by Dudley J. Morton (1884–1960), an orthopedic surgeon and professor of anatomy at Columbia University. In addition to being a physician, Morton was also a scientist and was interested in the evolution of primate feet. In anthropology, he is best known for his collaboration with Professor W. E. Le Gros Clark in developing ideas about human evolution and locomotion. Morton authored a paper published in *Science* in 1926 (Morton, 1926) entitled "The Relation of Evolution to Medicine." In this paper he pointed out that science was a direct producer of new and improved methods of curing and preventing human ailments and disease. He observed that medicine was primarily concerned with the recognition and treatment of that which lies beyond the range of normal human variation. He recognized that understanding what was a true departure from normal, and hence appropriate for clinical intervention, depended directly on knowledge of what constitutes the normal range of human variation and knowledge of what factors maintain normal conditions. He recognized that in order to maintain *normalcy*, medicine had to develop practices that reinforced the natural safeguards the body possessed against forces that would disrupt normalcy. His use of normalcy would likely be problematic today, but the point is clear. In order to understand disease and pathology we have to understand how the body has evolved defenses against possible invasion. He concludes:

> ...all those to whom we owe our important advances in modern medicine are not only fully assured of the fact of evolution, but, in addition, that they are strongly convinced that the scope and rate of our future advances bear a direct ratio with our better understanding of the biological laws which have guided the course of evolution (Morton, 1926, p. 395).

Interestingly, Morton's call for an understanding of the evolutionary basis for human adaptation against disease went largely unheeded by clinicians. However, some particularly visionary medical schools began to recognize the importance of understanding human evolution, and some were prompted to create departments of physical anthropology. In many cases it was within departments of physical anthropology in medical schools that research into human adaptation and disease, as well as adaptations to environmental extremes, was conducted. In the early twentieth century there was interest among a small group of researchers in the questions of how humans adapted and survived in particular environments. People not only survived, but appeared to thrive at high altitude (above 12,000 feet) and in extremes of hot and cold. In addition, and more important from the perspective of evolutionary medicine, was attention paid to human adaptations and associated diseases. In collaboration with geneticists, physical anthropologists began looking for population differences in particular phenotypic characteristics or physiological processes. By the end of World War II there was an accumulating body of evidence of physiological differences in ability to taste certain substances (e.g., phenylthiocarbamide/phenylthiourea, or PTC), the distribution of color blindness, and population variation in hemoglobin (e.g., sickling in red blood cells).

For biologists interested in human adaptation and disease, the relationship between variation in hemoglobin and malaria was a dream come true. Because of its widespread occurrence and its devastating, lethal effects, malaria was of great concern anywhere female *Anopheles* mosquitoes were found. The relationship between human hosts and the *Plasmodium* parasites provided a natural laboratory for the study of human adaptation to disease. In the early 1950s A. C. Allison published a series of papers that suggested that individuals who were heterozygous for the sickle cell gene possessed a relative immunity to the *Plasmodium falciparum* parasite (Allison, 1953, 1954a, b, c; Allison, Ikin, & Mourant, 1954). Allison also demonstrated that natural selection favored individuals with the sickle cell gene in areas with a high prevalence of malaria.

One of the groundbreaking studies of the complex adaptations of humans to mosquitoes, and in turn malaria, was the work of a physical anthropologist, Frank B. Livingstone. Livingstone published a paper in 1958 in which he summarized what was then known about the distribution of the sickle cell gene in human populations (Livingstone, 1958) and recognized that the relationship between mosquitoes, malaria, and humans was a complex one. The major vector of malaria in West Africa is *Anopheles gambiae*. This mosquito is drawn to human habitation and resides in the roofs of thatched huts that are ubiquitous in African villages. *A. gambiae* accounts for a majority of the cases of malaria in West Africa and is able to breed in almost any kind of water, except (1) very shaded water, (2) water with a strong current, (3) brackish water, and (4) very alkaline or polluted water.

For Livingstone the key point was the spread of agriculture and the destruction of large areas of natural vegetation and a concomitant rise in the incidence of malaria. With agriculture there were formed large brightly lit pools that were ideal breeding grounds for *A. gambiae*. Human populations increased dramatically in density and provided an almost continuous supply of hosts for the *Plasmodium* parasite. Finally, by destroying the indigenous forest habitat, humans also destroyed many large mammals that traditionally were the hosts for the parasite. So from an evolutionary perspective, Livingstone was able to account for the high frequencies of the sickle cell gene in populations that had not long been exposed to the malarial parasite. The adoption of a particular farming technique brought about environmental changes that had to be considered in understanding the distribution of sickle-cell disease (Livingstone, 1958).

The significance of Livingstone's work is not in its uniqueness, because numerous similar studies would follow, but in his consideration of the complex interaction between a disease vector, the life history of the parasite, and a costly but effective defense against the parasite, all in the context of human populations. It is this kind of research that physical anthropologists interested in evolution and disease had been conducting long before the dawn of Darwinian medicine.

A few studies on evolution and disease were conducted prior to World War II, but after World War II physical anthropologists along with a few other health scientists began studies on the evolution of human disease in earnest. The early 1990s saw a dramatic increase in the number of papers published with an explicit evolutionary orientation applied to pathology and disease (see Figure 1-2).

The topics and subject matter of evolutionary medicine appear to be of interest not only to a small group of academics, but to the public as well. Science writers are attracted to the field and its content because of the potential relevance to immediate human problems. Swine flu, bird flu, West Nile virus, and mad cow disease, as well as other infectious diseases, are expected to appear in future newspaper headlines. These new and potentially deadly infectious diseases and viruses crossing from animal to human, the epidemics of obesity and asthma, the rise in cardiovascular disease, and the rise in breast and colorectal cancer are all topics of considerable popular interest. In addition to this interest in more "popular" diseases, there is also concern about psychiatric disorders such as depression, attention deficit disorder in children, the causes of sudden infant death syndrome (SIDS), and the benefits of breastfeeding. These are all issues that confront people in the industrialized world every day and are the subjects of coverage in the press.

In spite of this interest, evolutionary medicine has made little impact on clinical research and practice in general (see Chapters 22 and 23). As Lewis notes in Chapter 22, most of the "practitioners" of evolutionary medicine are not clinicians or medical researchers but anthropologists, human biologists, and/or psychologists, as are most of

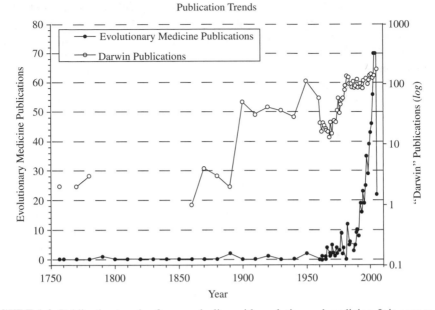

FIGURE 1-2 Publication trends of papers dealing with evolution and medicine. It is easy to see the dramatic increase in published papers in the mid- to late 1990s. Also plotted are the number of papers published over the same period with Darwin or some variant in the title. Data were collected from searches of all major electronic databases (EBSCO, JSTOR, Medline, PubMed, Science Direct, Web of Science). The important point to note is that there was no spike in the Darwin publications at the time when there was a dramatic increase in evolution and medicine papers.

the contributors to this volume. Perhaps the tendency for those not actively involved in clinical medicine and research to write and theorize about evolutionary medicine explains the lack of impact it has had on medicine in general. The lack of widespread, significant impact on the medical profession is understandable (see Chapter 23) for a variety of reasons. Although we have conducted no empirical research to determine the precise reasons for the lack of enthusiasm on the part of clinicians, there are several hypotheses that we might advance. Clinicians have virtually no medical training in evolution. What knowledge they might possess often comes from a few lectures about evolution in their general college biology course. While they might remember something about industrial melanism in the "peppered moth," if prompted, most simply fail to make the connection when it comes to the indiscriminate prescribing of antibiotics for conditions for which the antibiotics will not be effective. It is much easier, and more profitable, to order a battery of diagnostic tests, regardless of the cost/benefit ratio, than to simply adopt a "watchful waiting" view of treatment. Such watchful waiting is, of course, necessary if we are to let the body's own elegantly evolved immune system do what it is designed for. And in no small part, we, the consumers, are to blame. We have been seduced into thinking that any pain, itch, slight swelling, or inflammation is something that must be treated, when, in fact, most of these symptoms are simply the responses of our own immune systems.

On the other hand, changes in medical practice and health-related behaviors proceed as much from consumer input as from medical research itself. (Whether this is a particularly good trend or not is not at issue here.) Consumers are more likely to read or hear the work of anthropologists, human biologists and psychologists than they are the work of medical researchers. This is partially because the medical profession has never felt the need or pressure to offer explanations for the layperson. Like any profession, clinical medicine has a language all its own, and rather than trying to make knowledge more accessible, many clinicians have used technical language to obfuscate issues of real concern. On the other hand, nonclinical researchers have always had to justify what they do to a skeptical public and have been pressured into writing to a nonprofessional audience. Medical consumers are more likely to read *Discover* (and watch the Discovery Channel), *National Geographic*, and *Natural History* than they are to read the *New England Journal of Medicine*, the *Lancet*, or *JAMA*. The net result of this bias is that if evolution has a chance of becoming a part of mainstream medicine, it may come from the insistence of consumers, and not the clinicians.

There have been a few areas where evolutionarily based hypotheses about clinical conditions have been sufficiently empirically tested to be recognized by the clinical medicine community. One striking success story is the work on infant sleep and SIDS (see Chapter 12). Evolutionarily based research on infant sleep has been recognized internationally (UNICEF, WHO, American Academy of Pediatrics, Academy of Breastfeeding Medicine, United States Breastfeeding Committee), and researchers have been invited to contribute to policy formulation and general public health recommendations. Those studying SIDS susceptibility in relationship to sleeping arrangements and feeding methods (breast vs. bottle) have participated in the development of large multinational epidemiological studies, and their input has been responsible for important changes in the orientation and emphasis of these surveys. The work of evolutionarily based researchers has not been integrated into mainstream pediatric medicine smoothly or without tensions; nonetheless, the incorporation of an evolutionary perspective into pediatric medicine is ongoing and widespread (Fleming, Blair, & McKenna, 2006).

The other area that has become increasingly important is the coevolution of host and pathogen in the context of infectious disease and antibiotic drugs. Most physicians today realize that the overprescription of antibiotic drugs as well as poor compliance on the part of patients have contributed to the evolution (most would say development) of strains of bacteria that are virtually resistant to all but the most powerful drugs in our pharmaceutical arsenal. Vancomycin has been characterized as the antimicrobial of last resort and, when used in combination with gentamycin and rifampin, was effective against the "superbugs" until recently, when it was displaced by linezolid (Zyvox™) and the carbapenems (β-lactam antibiotics).

FUNDAMENTALS OF EVOLUTIONARY MEDICINE

A number of fundamental concepts from evolutionary theory underlie and are common to work in this field. No matter how divergent the subjects or topics, several common themes consistently emerge. We assume that most readers of this volume have a general understanding of how the evolutionary process works. Nonetheless, throughout the book authors will introduce or reintroduce basic evolutionary ideas, core concepts, processes, terms, and phrases.

To contextualize a bit, it is important to remember the three basic assumptions of Darwinian evolution. If a trait is to be called Darwinian, it must fulfill these three assumptions. First, for a character or trait to be called Darwinian there must be some phenotypic variation in that character in the population under study. For example, there must be differences in a bacterium's response to a particular antibiotic, some variation in the expression of cardiovascular disease, or the ability of an infant to digest commercial infant formula. Second, some proportion of the phenotypic variation must be the result of an underlying genetic variation. This does not mean that a trait must be under complete genetic control, such as our classic example of the inheritance of a discrete genetic trait like the ability to taste PTC, which is controlled by the presence or absence of a single allele. The ability to taste PTC is a Darwinian trait; it is not the only example. The phenotypic expression of the trait must have some genetic basis, but its phenotypic expression can be profoundly affected by the environment. It turns out that this is very important for the vast majority of human traits that we will consider. For example, individuals may have varying tendencies to express some phenotypic trait, like the ability to digest lactose. In some forms, like kefir or yogurt, lactose may more digestible, but a tall glass of milk is a trigger for extreme gastrointestinal distress for many people (see Chapter 5). Finally, the trait in question must have an effect on fitness—the survival and reproduction of offspring to reproductive maturity. Recall that natural selection operates on individuals who possess traits, behaviors, and characteristics that promote health, survival, and, most importantly, reproductive success over time in a particular environment and gradually eliminates or decreases those traits or characteristics that compromise health or negatively affect reproductive success.

Because health is something that concerns us throughout our entire lives, a number of scholars of evolutionary medicine invoke life history theory as an organizing set of principles to examine how natural selection operates at different stages of the life cycle. Life history theory begins with the premise that there is a finite amount of energy available to an organism for growth, maintenance of life, and reproduction. Allocation of energy to each of these processes represents a series of trade-offs among important aspects of life, such as length of gestation, age at weaning, time spent in growth to adulthood, adult body size, and total life span. Natural selection shapes life history traits, determining which ones will succeed or fail in a given environment. Energy spent in the pursuit of food or mates cannot be used to grow to a larger size, for example. Although some have argued that life history theory may not work in contemporary human populations, it serves as a useful guide for delineating various life cycle phases from the perspective of evolutionary medicine. Thinking in evolutionary terms about life history questions helps us to identify and understand individual decisions about reproduction and patterns of childcare, episodic patterns of growth and development, timing and context for sleep, and susceptibility to certain diseases.

Ultimately, the adaptive value of any particular trait is at least partially determined by the extent to which that trait is congruent, if not complementary, to an overall cluster of functionally related traits—an adaptive suite—of characteristics. Moreover, our evolved physiology ultimately constrains trait variability to a range of "adaptive norms" below or above which life could not be sustained. These limits are the constraints on evolution.

For example, over the course of human evolutionary history there has been increasing pressure for larger and larger brains, but a fundamental constraint or limit on that increase, at least prenatally, is the size of birth canal in an adult female. Although natural selection has "cheated" to an extent, covering the brain in a set of unfused plates, instead of a rigid helmet, allowing humans to be born with brains that are actually too big for the birth canal, there are absolute limits. Our ability to survive at altitude is contingent on the inhalation of oxygen, and for most of us life above 8000 feet is difficult, but there are populations living in the Andes and the Himalayas that survive quite well at that elevation (see Chapter 14). Life, unaided by respiration devices, above 30,000 feet is impossible for humans for any length of time. Populations that have lived at high altitude for generations have adapted to their environment by increases in vital lung capacity, which compensates for the reduced partial pressure of oxygen. These adaptations are true Darwinian traits. Likewise, natural selection ultimately sets limits on our ability to metabolize certain nutrients that are critical for life. Our evolved physiology is designed to accommodate a diet that is drastically different from the typical Western diet. When coupled with a lack of exercise, our chronic consumption of vast quantities of starches (sugars in disguise) and sugars push the capacity of our digestive systems to modulate energy storage with energy consumption leading to a variety of chronic medical conditions (see Chapters 2, 3, 18, and 21).

In a brief overview of Darwinian evolution, it is important to understand *proximate* and *ultimate* causation. This distinction is particularly important for understanding disease. On the one hand we can imagine that the proximate (immediate) cause of a high fever is an infection. In most cases medical practitioners want to treat the proximate cause for the condition, for in doing so they are able to remove unpleasant side effects of the condition. Administration of antiphlogistic (fever-reducing) drugs is a common treatment. However, it has been demonstrated that such treatment rarely reduces the duration or intensity of the infection, although the patient will likely feel better. In fact, an evolutionary perspective suggests that administration of antiphlogistic drugs, except in extreme cases, should be avoided. Humans possess a highly evolved immune system that has many tools to fight off harmful organisms. One of those tools is fever. Fever is a host defense against infection that speeds up certain immunological reactions and reduces the reproduction rate in many pathogens (Kluger, Kozak, Conn, Leon, & Soszynski, 1998). So, in many cases, the treatment of the proximate cause of a condition without an understanding of its ultimate (evolutionary) cause may result in a counterproductive therapy. Certainly this defense (high fever) can exceed an adaptive response (e.g., 105°F in a child), at which point it becomes a defective response that requires intervention. Furthermore, there are some pathogens whose survival and reproduction are enhanced by higher temperatures caused by fever (Ewald, 1994).

Proximate causes denote the more immediate underlying physiological or anatomical factors responsible for a certain expressed behavior or physiological reaction, whereas ultimate causes affect populations and species over much longer spans of time—millions rather than dozens of years. An individual who is gaining excessive weight may ask why, and a polite response might be that the body is absorbing too many calories, which leads to increased fat deposition. A less polite proximate response is: "It's the food, stupid, you're eating too much of it and exercising too little!" The overweight person may be counseled to alter the diet while increasing activity levels. From the standpoint of evolutionary medicine, however, an explanation about the adaptive advantage of being able to store fat during times of excess leading to increased survival and reproductive success in times of scarcity may not be particularly useful or meaningful to a person concerned with looking "fat" or suffering from one of a variety of serious weight-related illnesses like diabetes. In this case, a clinician who focuses on the ultimate or evolutionary explanation (who "practices" evolutionary medicine) will have little or no impact on the patient's health and well-being when compared to the physician who focuses on and treats the proximate causes.

Another example of a defense against some infectious agents is the withdrawal of iron from the bloodstream (Weinberg, 1978). Many pathogens need iron for their own survival, so if insufficient iron is available, the health of the pathogen is compromised. When a patient presents with classic symptoms of anemia, some clinicians see this defense as a defect and prescribe increased iron intake in the form of pills, diet, or injections. Unfortunately, the administration of exogenous iron produces exactly the opposite effect from that which is desired, and the patient often gets worse. There is some concern that the common practice of encouraging higher iron intake in pregnant women maybe contraindicated in those who are also infected by HIV, in that the iron may worsen the infection (Weinberg, Friis, Boelaert, & Weinberg, 2001).

In sum, we need to keep in mind several important ideas: (1) the three basic assumptions of Darwinian evolution must be met for a trait to evolve; (2) life history theory gives us an important perspective for understanding the adaptive value of traits, with traits being advantageous at one stage of life and deleterious or even lethal at another; and (3) that differences exist between proximate and ultimate causation. With these ideas in mind, we turn to a review of the areas in medicine in which a Darwinian perspective has been applied with some success.

INFECTIOUS DISEASE

The pattern of human variation seen today is due in no small part to infectious agents to which our ancestors were exposed, especially since the origins of sedentary agriculture approximately 10,000 years ago. It is no surprise then that the coevolution of humans and pathogens is the area of evolutionary medicine most accepted by the clinical and medical research communities, but this is also the area in which, for an infected individual, the proximate and ultimate processes may come in conflict. For example, consider that for many years, physicians prescribed antibiotics for common ailments such as colds and ear infections in response to demands from patients who were concerned that their ailments could develop into something more serious. As a result, antibiotic-resistant viruses and bacteria have evolved to the point that some are nearly untreatable with current therapies. Although overuse of antibiotics has a negative impact on individual's health in that it compromises a person's ability to respond to other infectious agents, to the person who is ill it seems important to use antibiotics to ward off more serious problems that may develop in the short term.

Immune System

The primary mechanism employed by most vertebrates for responding to invading bacteria, viruses, and helminthes is the immune system. Most significant are immunoglobulins (IgM, IgG, IgA, IgD, and IgE), T-cell receptors, and major histocompatibility complex

(MHC) proteins, also known as the human leukocyte antigen (HLA) complex in humans (Knapp, 2002). Immunoglobins are Y-shaped proteins used by the immune system to identify and neutralize infectious agents like bacteria and viruses. The different types of immunoglobins have evolved to deal with different types of antigens, which are proteins that produce an immune response. IgA is found in areas containing mucus (gastrointestinal tract, respiratory tract, urogenital tract) and prevents colonization of mucosal areas by pathogens. IgD functions mainly as an antigen receptor on B cells. B cells are produced in bone marrow and are referred to as antibody factories. They secrete antibodies that paint microbes, allowing phagocytes (killer cells) to find the microbes more easily. IgE binds to allergens and triggers histamine release from mast cells and also provides protection from helminthes. IgM is expressed on the surface of B cells and is also secreted in a form that has a high affinity for eliminating pathogens in the early stages of B-cell-mediated immunity (before the production of sufficient IgG). T-cell receptors are molecules that are found on the surfaces of T lymphocytes (T cells) and are responsible for recognizing antigens bound to major histocompatibility complex (MHC) molecules. The human leukocyte antigen is the name of a group of genes in the MHC complex region on human chromosome 6 that encodes antigen-presenting protein. The HLA polymorphism is so diverse that it is theoretically possible for every individual to have a unique combination of alleles (Knapp, 2002), enabling our bodies to detect self cells from nonself cells. Infectious diseases are believed to account for the extreme diversity of alleles at this locus, again with the heterozygous form believed to be more resistant. Diseases that may be associated with the HLA polymorphism include leprosy, tuberculosis, malaria, hepatitis B, leishmaniasis, and meningitis (Hill & Motulsky, 1999).

The human genome has evolved a number of defenses against the malaria parasite, such as the sickle cell allele reviewed above. Some scholars have suggested that malaria has been the single biggest killer of humans throughout history, and it has been described as "the strongest known selective pressure in the recent history of the human genome" (Kwiatkowski, 2005, p.171). In addition to sickle cell, malaria appears to be responsible for the distribution of a number of other genetic "disorders" such as glucose 6-phosphate dehydrogenase (G6PD) deficiency, thalassemia, and several hemoglobin variants. All of these alleles cause health problems and even death in some circumstances, but they also confer advantages in the face of chronic malaria infection. Malaria remains high on the list of causes of death throughout the world today, killing as many as 2.7 million people annually (Centers for Disease Control and Prevention, 2004a).

The relationship between infectious disease and genetic polymorphisms has been well known for several decades, but only recently has evolution been integrated into this research. With the addition of evolutionary theory to epidemiology, populations that may be vulnerable to disease outbreaks can be identified and appropriate measures taken. Understanding how genetic resistance to disease has evolved may also lead to discoveries of genotypes that respond differentially to HIV (Samson et al., 1996) or treatments for AIDS, which, in turn, may lead to more effective drugs or vaccines. Furthermore, there is evidence that some polymorphisms that are adaptive in response to infectious diseases may turn out to be maladaptive in certain environments, with certain diets, and with aging, and may lead to greater susceptibility to degenerative or chronic diseases later in life (Hill et al., 1999). Data from the Human Genome Project (HGP) can be used by evolutionary medicine researchers to increase understanding of the origin and distribution of genetic polymorphisms related to infectious and noninfectious diseases.

The role of selection in the development of immune function in the individual throughout the life course is another promising area of research (McDade & Worthman, 1999). Because reproductive rates of most pathogens are so fast and generation lengths so short, long-lived human hosts are at a disadvantage when it comes to the usual work of natural selection on genomes. The response has been that selection has shaped immune systems to develop based on individual experience (e.g., exposure in infancy and early childhood to a variety of pathogens to which immunity develops), "creating a facultative experienced-based system that, on the level of ontogeny, evolves itself" (McDade & Worthman, 1999, p. 715). The lymphatic system develops in response to exposure to varying pathogens, enabling the individual to survive in a specific disease environment. Because of the variation in immune function that results, there is no such thing as a "normal" developmental process, and "culture can interfere in potentially destructive ways when immune defenses are not fully developed" (McDade & Worthman, 1999, p. 715), as with overprotection from pathogen exposure that occurs with using antibacterials in day-to-day activities.

Vaccines and Viruses

As noted previously, in the most developed nations infectious diseases are not a major source of mortality. Improved diet and hygiene (McKeown, 1998), rather than direct medical interventions, have dramatically lowered the life-threatening aspects of infectious disease. Vaccinations, particularly of children, have reduced the incidence of a number of diseases, and smallpox seems to have been completely eliminated as a threat to human health. In fact, diseases that are vulnerable to vaccination are apparently not evolving resistance in the same way as seen with antibiotics (McLean, 1999). This does not mean that viruses cannot evolve such resistance in the future. For example, nucleotide changes in the virus that causes measles have been reported, and there is some evidence that the cessation of vaccination for smallpox may make us vulnerable to related pathogens such as monkeypox, a disease that may have moved into the niche formerly occupied by smallpox (Bangham et al., 1999; McLean, 1999).

Vaccine development is an area that could benefit from an evolutionary approach (Read et al., 1999). The logic of vaccines is to infect a person, typically a child, with a mild strain of the virus, following which immunity typically develops for all strains, including the dangerous ones. This is the procedure used for vaccines for most "childhood" diseases. In areas where vaccines are not available, exposure to mild strains of a virus triggers an immune response that typically works as a good substitute. For example, people who were born before measles vaccines were developed often contracted a mild strain of the virus and became ill, but in the process developed immunity to more virulent strains of the virus. A vaccine designed to kill all strains of a virus may not be the best strategy—better, perhaps, would be the development a vaccine against only the most virulent strains or those likely to evolve virulence, leaving behind mild forms that could "... be used like a free live vaccine that will protect those who are not vaccinated and those who develop insufficient immunity to the administered vaccine" (Read et al., 1999, p. 213). In this way, coexistence of humans and relatively mild pathogens may be better, in the long run, than efforts to eradicate all strains, a strategy that could backfire and lead to the most virulent forms "escaping" drug intervention. In fact, there is evidence that exposure to mild forms of measles, as well as immunization against measles, may provide protection against other pathogens (Aaby, 1995), presumably via stimulation of the immune system. This suggests that total eradication campaigns such as those with smallpox and polio may be ill advised when considered from the standpoint of evolutionary theory because there is always the possibility that defenses against the most hearty (virulent) strains will not be activated by exposure to mild variants, leaving individuals vulnerable to the more virulent strains.

Antibiotic Resistance

When Europeans colonized Africa in the twentieth century, malaria was one of the most dreaded diseases. Quinine, a naturally occurring substance extracted from the bark of the South American cinchona tree, was found to be an effective treatment. Over time drugs used to treat malaria have changed repeatedly as the protozoa have evolved resistance to quinine, chloriquine, primiquine, and mefloquine, among others (Newton & White, 1999). There is some concern that drug development is failing to keep up with pathogen evolution and that preventing exposure to the mosquitoes (or killing them with DDT, as has been recently suggested) may be the best way to curb the spread of this dread disease. And as noted in the Doonesbury comic strip discussed at the beginning of this chapter, tuberculosis is another disease that is evolving drug resistance and that has re-emerged as a feared disease in industrialized nations.

Not only are antibiotics administered to humans of concern, but widespread use of antibiotics in agriculture and animal husbandry (including fish farming) have also contributed to the emergence of drug-resistant strains of pathogens (Bangham et al., 1999). In fact, about half of all antibiotics produced are used in agriculture and animal husbandry (Bangham et al., 1999). Other factors that contribute to the evolution of resistance include failure of patients to follow through on drug regimens. Alexander Fleming, in his Nobel Prize acceptance speech, noted the danger of drug resistance: "It is not difficult to make microbes resistant to penicillin by exposing them to concentrations not sufficient to kill them, and the same thing has occasionally happened in the body.... Moral: If you use penicillin, use enough" (Fleming, 1945, p.11). The failure to kill all the pathogens in the body is usually the result of patients stopping medication when they "feel better." In the case of children, parents often expect that physicians will prescribe antibiotics no matter what the cause of the symptoms may be. Recent studies have shown that doctors prescribe antibiotics about 56% of the time if they perceive that parents expect them and only about 12% if they feel the parents do not expect them (Centers for Disease Control and Prevention, 2003).

A more recent contributor to pathogen resistance is air travel, particularly international travel. A pathogen can leave Bangkok, Thailand, and in no more than a day be in New York City. Such changes in environments open up the possibility of infection to a world of unprepared hosts. Increased urbanization and attendant crowding are also circumstances that enhance transmission, but more recently, crowding seen in refugee camps in the Darfur region of Sudan has produced similar results. Poverty, in general, leads to transmission of pathogens, as well, largely through the lack of public sanitation and clean drinking water. Increased understanding of the evolutionary process will help address some of these factors, but clearly drug resistance is complicated by socio-cultural factors that evolutionary medicine cannot address alone.

Is there a way out of this arms race whereby pathogens develop greater virulence in response to ever more powerful antimicrobials? For a long time, it was assumed that pathogens, most specifically parasites, would evolve toward benign existence rather than increased virulence because their own survival is dependent on the health and survival of the host (Read et al., 1999). This view was based on a false understanding of the evolutionary process and assumed that mutual benefit (and survival) for host and parasite was the "goal." A more accurate view of host parasite evolution involves analysis of trade-offs for both the host and the parasite. Natural selection will favor organisms that have the greatest reproductive success. Parasites and hosts are designed to maximize their reproductive success, and in doing so one of these competitors will lose.

From the preceding discussion one might conclude that modern medicine is hastening the evolution of pathogens toward increasingly virulent strains. However, there is nothing inherent in the evolutionary process that moves it in one direction or the other, from less to greater lethality, or the reverse. In fact, one of the greatest potentials for thwarting future disease outbreaks is the possibility of reversing the evolutionary process so that pathogens evolve toward less dangerous forms that can coexist with human hosts or forms that may even be beneficial to human hosts (Read et al., 1999). Ewald has referred to this as "domesticating" pathogens (Ewald, 1994). To some extent this has already happened with diphtheria, which has apparently evolved toward less virulence in association with vaccination (Read et al., 1999).

Turning the evolutionary process around may be our best tool for reducing the virulence of pathogens. The problem is that pathogens have a very short generation length and are capable of an extremely rapid evolutionary response to environment change. Where attempts have been made to develop a targeted vaccine, as with HIV, efforts have proved ineffective, and, even worse, by using ineffective vaccines, resistance is enhanced (Ewald, 1999a) and there is no end in sight to this process. Development of a totally successful flu vaccine is also unlikely because vaccines must be developed well in advance of the outbreak based on the best guess of which strains will be most successful in the upcoming flu season. Ewald has proposed that our best hope comes from harnessing evolutionary processes to "mold HIV and other sexually transmitted pathogens into milder forms" (Ewald, 1999a). And who knows what else is lurking out there that may be as devastating as AIDS? Medical interventions that are capable of responding to the processes of disease emergence and evolution are much more likely to be successful in the long run than those that target specific disease variants and their manifestations. But this requires a very sophisticated understanding of the evolutionary process on the part of medical researchers.

Pathogens and Phylogenies

Another important tool from evolutionary biology that has been useful in health-related research is constructing evolutionary relationships (phylogenies) among strains of viruses to assess origins and patterns of distribution. For example, HIV has been traced to multiple central African primate populations, with evidence that it may have entered human populations on more than one occasion. Worldwide geographic maps of the distribution of the various strains of HIV may lead to development of vaccines and treatments that are tailored to specific populations (Holmes, 1999). For example, in some parts of the world injecting drug users tend to be infected with a different strain of HIV than those infected via heterosexual contact (Holmes, 1999) . To use the terminology of evolutionary theory, strains of HIV that are maintained by natural selection show different phylogenies from those maintained by genetic drift (Holmes, 1999). Understanding evolutionary relationships among strains of viruses and among pathogens in general may reveal factors that contribute to their spread and increased virulence (Read et al., 1999) and offer possibilities for control of specific pathogens.

Recent work on unraveling the genomes of humans and chimpanzees has revealed evolutionary relationships and suggested possible reasons for some of the differences in not only development, but also susceptibility to diseases. For example, sialic acid is a sugar molecule on cell surfaces that serves as a binding site for organisms that cause diseases such as cholera, malaria, and some forms of influenza. Interestingly, analysis of the genetics of sialic acid in humans and chimpanzees reveals that they differ by a single oxygen atom (Muchmore, Diaz, & Varki, 1998). The differences in this single gene complex may explain why humans are susceptible to diseases like cholera and malaria, whereas chimpanzees are not, and it may be protective against others of which we are not aware (Varki, 2001). It may also explain why malaria has become such a scourge in the past several thousand years (Martin, Rayner, Gagneux, Barnwell, & Varki, 2005). Because the chimpanzee version of the gene is found in all other mammals studied, it has been suggested that the human version, with its associated disease susceptibilities (or protections), is the derived form. Discovery of this tiny genetic difference may lead to new treatments for infectious diseases to which humans, and not chimpanzees, are susceptible. There are other implications for chronic diseases like cancers and even brain evolution that are beyond the scope of this discussion but are reviewed in Varki (2001). When we say that chimps and humans differ by only a small fraction of their genes or DNA, this does not mean that this seemingly small difference does not have a huge impact on health, just as it apparently does on development.

NUTRITION

That diets of most people in industrialized nations are radically different from the diets of our ancestors is one of the most well-known observations from evolutionary medicine. Human nutritional requirements were shaped by the foods that were consumed during the 5–7 million years of hominin evolution. In the past 10,000 years, many new foods have been introduced into human diets with the domestication of plants and animals. The results of dietary and other behavioral changes brought about by the origin of agriculture have been positive in many ways, but the consequences for human health have not always been so sanguine. Among the reasons for dramatic increases in diseases and disorders such as type 2 diabetes, atherosclerosis, hypertension, some cancers, diverticular diseases, and osteoporosis is the fact that our evolved bodies are "mismatched" with the foods we eat today and the levels of energy expended in our daily lives (Eaton & Konner, 1985b; Eaton, Eaton, III, & Konner, 1999; Eaton, Konner, & Shostak, 1988b; Eaton, Shostak, & Konner, 1988). Chapters 2, 3, and 4 in this volume provide extensive reviews of the hypothesized ancestral diets and the evidence supporting the proposal that many contemporary health problems result from this discordance (but see Strassmann & Dunbar, 1999). In general, the major differences in preagricultural and contemporary diets are seen in percent of calories from fats, protein, and carbohydrates and in intake of sodium, calcium, ascorbic acid (vitamin C), and cholesterol (see Figure 1-3).

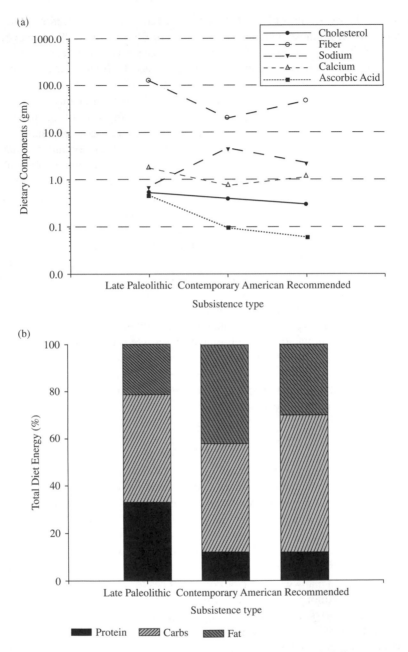

FIGURE 1-3 Late Paleolithic, contemporary American, and recommended dietary composition: a) composition of five components of diet (cholesterol, fiber, sodium, calcium, and ascorbic acid); b) the percent energy intake from protein, carbohydrates, and fats. (From Eaton, Shostak, & Konner, 1988, p. 84.)

Before humans began producing rather than gathering foods, edible components of grasses were consumed rarely and in small quantities; today they comprise more than half of the calories and protein consumed by humans throughout the world (Cordain, 1999). Plants have always made up a substantial part of human diets, but the concentration of food sources in a single family (Gramineae) is relatively recent in human evolutionary history. Furthermore, not only are we consuming considerably more grains than our ancestors, most of the actual cereal-based foods we eat are highly processed and refined so that the more complex carbohydrates of our ancestors' diets have been replaced by highly refined simple sugars. Much of the evidence suggests that the recent changes in food-processing techniques have resulted in declining health for most individuals (see Chapter 2), but if we look at the population level, the production and consumption of cereal grains is the only way to support the world's people. It has been estimated that the number of humans that could be supported on the earth (i.e., the carrying capacity) if they were dependent only on wild resources is approximately 5 million. If this estimate is true we have exceeded the carrying capacity of the earth over three orders of magnitude (1000-fold). It is only through domestication of plants and animals and increased reliance on cereal grains that such population expansion could have occurred.

However, there is a downside to increased grain consumption, especially for populations that have recently begun to depend on wheat as the "staff of life." Diets high in cereal grain lack important vitamins (e.g., vitamins A and C), minerals (e.g., calcium), amino acids (e.g., lysine and methionine), and fatty acids (e.g., linolenic acid) but include antinutrients (e.g., α-amylase and protease inhibitors) that interfere with absorption of other nutrients (Cordain, 1999). Moreover, there is increasing evidence that a number of chronic health problems (e.g., multiple sclerosis, rheumatoid arthritis, celiac disease, and type 1 diabetes) may be due to excessive cereal consumption. In fact, it is possible to map the spread of wheat-based agriculture throughout the world by mapping the prevalence of celiac (gluten intolerance) disease (Simoons, 1981).

Although animal food sources, including insects, have been consumed by humans for thousands of generations, the types of animal products consumed by most people today are much higher in fat than those consumed in the past. The change in the types of animals consumed has important consequences for obesity, heart disease, and cancers. In general the meat of domesticated animals has much higher fat content, than wild animals (see Figure 1-4).

Many of the chapters in this volume reflect the great concern about increasing rates of obesity and type 2 diabetes in many contemporary populations (see Chapters 2, 3, 4, 7, and 8). Because these topics are covered extensively in chapters that follow, they will not be reviewed here. It is absolutely clear, however, that dietary changes are among the best examples of the discordance between ancestral bodies and contemporary lifestyles resulting in a variety of cardiovascular diseases, cancers, and type 2 diabetes.

In summary, the now-familiar refrain that our diets today are different in quality and quantity from those of our ancestors and that the "mismatch" between today's diet and human evolved nutritional needs has negative health consequences has resonated with Western consumers who struggle with weight control, high blood pressure, and diabetes (see Chapter 3). Can "returning to a Paleolithic diet" improve human health? Certainly many contemporary authors of best-selling books on diet and health argue that this is the case, as illustrated by the titles they have chosen: *The Origin Diet: How Eating Like Our*

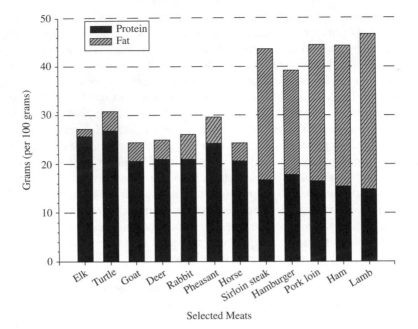

FIGURE 1-4 Fat and protein content of selected wild and domestic meats. (From Eaton, Shostak, & Konner, 1988, p. 108.)

Stone Age Ancestors Will Maximize Your Health (Somer, 2001); *Health Secrets of the Stone Age: What We Can Learn from Deep in Prehistory to Become Leaner, Livelier, and Longer-Lived* (Goscienski, 2005); and *The Paleo Diet: Lose Weight and Get Healthy by Eating the Food You Were Designed to Eat* (Cordain, 2002). However, as noted above, the current world population size is only possible because of the production and consumption of cereal grains. In order for humans to return to Paleolithic food-consumption patterns there would have to be a dramatic reduction in world population, an unlikely scenario, at least voluntarily. Popular authors, like those listed above, argue that by adopting some aspects of ancestral diets (lower fat, more complex carbohydrates, lower sodium, frequent small meals) and lifestyles (more exercise, less alcohol, no smoking, lower stress), we will feel better, live longer, and lose weight. As noted by Turner and her colleagues in Chapter 3, however, many of these popular approaches to incorporating an evolutionary perspective into diet and lifestyle management greatly oversimplify the problem.

HUMAN REPRODUCTIVE HEALTH

Just as contemporary diets are mismatched with evolved nutritional requirements, numerous aspects of contemporary reproductive behavior are mismatched with the reproductive lives of our ancestors, resulting in potential consequences for health, particularly of women. Perhaps the most familiar example is the fewer number of menstrual cycles experienced by ancestral females when compared to modernday Western females. Given that most of their reproductive years were spent in pregnancy and lactation, it has been estimated that ancestral women had only 100–150 menstrual cycles in their lifetimes (see Figure 1-5). Compare this with the 350–400 cycles experienced by a Western woman using birth control who has two or fewer pregnancies and nurses her infant only a few months, if at all. Women's reproductive physiology may not be well adapted to the routine monthly fluctuations of ovarian hormones, particularly estrogen and progesterone, that are associated with the typical menstrual cycle. Perhaps Roger Short put it best: "Since natural selection has always operated in the past to maximize reproductive potential, women are physiologically ill-adapted to spend the greater part of their reproductive lives in the non-pregnant state" (Short, 1976, p. 3), i.e., "having an endless succession of menstrual cycles" (Short, 1976, p.21). Perhaps women's bodies were not "designed" to be exposed to 400 or more monthly surges and falls in estrogen, with the associated effects on cell turnover rates and hormonally sensitive tissue.

It seems likely that these episodic surges in estrogen have an impact on women's health. The most probable impact, as proposed by several scholars (Eaton & Eaton, III, 1999; Eaton, Pike, Short, Lee, Trussell, Hatcher, Wood, Worthman, Blurton Jones, Konner, et al., 1994) is on the estrogen-related cancers of the breast, uterus, and ovaries. Although comparative rates are difficult to obtain, the rate of breast cancer for industrialized nations, where birth control is practiced and childbearing is limited and deferred, is considerably higher than for less developed nations and may be as high as 100 times the rate for women who are not using contraception and are spending the bulk of their reproductive lives pregnant or nursing with sufficient frequency to induce lactational amenorrhea (Eaton, S. et al., 1994). For these women, the hormonal milieus to which they are most commonly exposed are high progesterone levels, rather than high estrogen levels. Furthermore, there is evidence that not only do Western women experience more frequent fluctuation in ovarian hormones, but the absolute levels during each cycle are higher in Western women than in women in less industrialized societies (see Chapters 7 and 8).

The mismatch between evolved dietary needs and modern diets seems somewhat easy to resolve, at least in theory, if not in practice. Few would argue that there is a downside

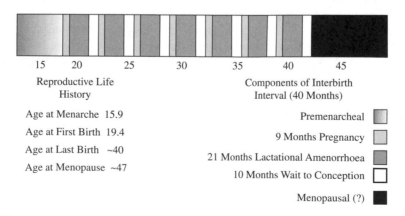

FIGURE 1-5 Hypothetical reproductive history of a female forager. (From Worthman, Smith, & Weil, 1992.)

to reducing fat intake (but see Chapter 4), increasing consumption of complex (rather than simple) carbohydrates, and increasing exercise. Trying to bring women's physiology back in line with ancestral conditions is not as easy to effect, however, because it involves altering reproductive patterns and interfering with hormones. To wit, there are very few popular books written about ways of reducing breast cancer rates by "returning to" reproductive patterns of our ancestors. The point has not been missed by the popular imagination, however, and web sites have sprung up advocating ways of altering menstrual patterns to more closely mimic the hormonal milieus of ancestral women (see Chapter 9). More importantly, pharmaceutical companies have taken note and now are marketing oral contraceptives that not only suppress ovulation, but also suppress menstruation, more closely mimicking the ancestral condition.

Pregnancy

A number of aspects of pregnancy have been subjected to analysis from the perspective of evolutionary medicine, including nausea of pregnancy (commonly called "morning sickness" in the United States), early fetal loss, and eclampsia and preeclampsia. Nausea of pregnancy is an example of a health problem that benefits from questioning whether it is a defense or a defect. Because it can be so debilitating to a woman early in pregnancy, medical approaches in the past sought ways of reducing or eliminating nausea of early pregnancy. A particularly tragic effort to "solve" the problem of morning sickness was the use of thalidomide in the 1950s, resulting in the birth of approximately 12,000 deformed babies and the spontaneous abortion of untold others.

Rather than a problem that has to be fixed, nausea during the first trimester may be a defense, having evolved as a protection against toxins and teratogens that could harm the developing embryo (Profet, 1992). The proximate explanation for nausea and food aversions is likely hormonal (specifically hCG and estradiol, which rise early in pregnancy), but the ultimate explanation may be that women who found potentially harmful food components aversive may have protected their first trimester fetuses from developmental damage, leading to greater reproductive success. Hence, the predisposition toward first trimester nausea could have evolved as a strategy for fetal protection. Certainly there are limits to the adaptive value of nausea and vomiting early in pregnancy. Severe and prolonged nausea results in dehydration and weight loss such that hospitalization is required or death may ensue (Furneaux, Langley-Evans, & Langley-Evans, 2001; Flaxman & Sherman, 2000). This hypothesis, known as the embryo protection hypothesis, has been criticized by some researchers noting that it is based largely on observations of well-nourished women, and that there are potentially severe nutritional consequences among women who were inadequately nourished before pregnancy (Pike, 2000).

It has been estimated that many conceptions are lost before implantation, and 10–20% of those implanted are lost in the first trimester (Haig, 1999). If maximizing reproductive success is how the game of evolution is won, then how can there be benefits to early pregnancy loss? For humans, early pregnancy loss may actually be adaptive under certain circumstances. Quality of offspring overrides quantity because of the huge investment made by women and couples in each pregnancy and the subsequent years of parenting. At the most basic level an evolutionary perspective argues that gestating, giving birth to, nursing, and raising an offspring that is not healthy and capable of reproducing would be "wasted" energy, energy that could be better allocated to future offspring who are healthier and more likely to reproduce. This is a straightforward resource-allocation problem from the perspective of life history theory. Indeed, most of the pregnancies lost in the first trimester have been found to have chromosomal abnormalities (Haig, 1999; Peacock, 1990). In many cases, however, reproductive failure is seen as pathological by clinicians and preventing it is an overriding goal for physicians, women, and couples, rather than as a solution to an evolutionary mistake. This is a clear example of where medicine and evolution might be at odds (Peacock, 1990). While artificial insemination has solved fertility problems for many couples, it is possible that in some cases this is not a solution that should be attempted.

The fetus is sometimes referred to as a graft, and, just as a skin graft often fails, it should not be surprising that the fetal graft sometimes fails, given that mothers and fetuses share, on average, only about 50% of their genes. From an evolutionary perspective it is useful to consider pregnancy an example of parent–infant conflict in that the interests of the mother do not always coincide with the interests of the fetus (Haig, 1999). Sometimes it may be in the mother's best interest to abort a pregnancy that interferes with her own health or the health of her current and future offspring, but it is clearly in the interest of the fetus to maintain the pregnancy, no matter how bad the situation is. Consequently, we would predict that fetuses have evolved strategies to minimize pregnancy loss and hence maximize their fitness. Likewise, mothers should have evolved strategies to detect risky fetuses and act accordingly.

Once the pregnancy survives the first trimester, the termination rate declines appreciably (Haig, 1999), but the potential for maternal–fetal conflict continues, especially in competition for nutrients. From a public health perspective one would predict that if the mother experiences severe undernutrition or malnutrition during pregnancy, the uterine environment for the fetus would be compromised and miscarriage would result. Surprisingly, this prediction is not often borne out: women give birth even under severe food restrictions such as occur with famine and war (see Chapters 7, 8, and 18). Some interpret this to mean that the fetus has ways of prolonging the pregnancy, even if there are negative consequences for maternal health. Of course, just because a fetus survives pregnancy and birth does not mean that its health is not compromised by in utero nutritional stress. Such babies are often born small for gestational age (SGA) due to intrauterine growth retardation (IUGR), and there is increasing evidence that nutritional stress in pregnancy has lifelong effects on health (Adair, Kuzawa, & Borja, 2001; Barker, 1995, 1997; Kuzawa, 2005; see also Chapter 18).

Clinical conditions of pregnancy that result from maternal–fetal competition for nutrients include gestational diabetes and eclampsia/preeclampsia. These conditions benefit from consideration from an evolutionary perspective. For both gestational diabetes and eclampsia, changes in maternal physiology designed to increase delivery of oxygen and nutrients to the fetus become so extreme as to become pathological and usually warrant medical treatment. For a woman without diabetes, blood glucose levels rise after a meal and return to normal levels when counteracted by insulin. During late-stage pregnancy, however, both glucose and insulin levels remain elevated for a longer time after a meal to benefit the fetus. This as an example of the fetal interests working against the maternal interests as the fetus works to obtain more and more glucose at the expense of the mother's health. Elevated glucose levels in mothers can result in hypoglycemia for mothers, but also result in some compromise in fetal health. Not surprisingly, glucose elevation is also associated with excess nutrient intake in pregnancy and is more common in developed countries. Women who develop gestational diabetes often give birth to large infants who are themselves predisposed to developing diabetes later in life (Power & Tardif, 2005). This suggests that there is likely an optimal level of nutritional intake during pregnancy, and too much or too little food can cause pregnancy complications and lifelong health problems for both mother and infant. Thus, we have an example of stabilizing selection, whereby extremes in food intake result in reduced reproductive success.

A major complication of pregnancy worldwide, found both in developing and developed countries, is preeclampsia and its more severe form, eclampsia. Preeclampsia is associated with hypertension in the mother and is estimated to occur in as many as 10% of births. It is also a common cause of premature birth, because the only "cure" is delivery of the fetus and placenta. If the pregnancy is not interrupted, the mother will experience damage to the kidney, liver, and brain, and if it proceeds to eclampsia, maternal convulsions may result. Furthermore, even though the short-term effects may be improved with delivery, there is evidence that there may be lifelong effects on maternal health (Redman & Sargent, 2005). Unfortunately, there is no animal model for preeclampsia, which has inhibited research on causation and potential interventions. It has been argued that preeclampsia/eclampsia is related to the evolution of increased cranial capacity in *Homo sapiens* and derives from the very deep invasion of the placenta into maternal tissue necessary for adequate oxygen exchange for fetal brain development (Robillard, Chaline, Chaouat, & Hulsey, 2003; Robillard, Dekker, & Hulsey, 1999, 2002; see also Chapter 11).

Preeclampsia is usually restricted to first pregnancies, and ways of reducing the incidence of it have been suggested using evolutionary theory and relating the disorders to other aspects of human reproductive ecology, including the frequency of nonovulatory sexual activity, concealed ovulation, prohibitions of incest, rarity of polyandry, and relatively low fertility rate (see Chapter 11). Although there are other interpretations and recommendations for treatment of preeclampsia (Bdolah et al., 2004; Levine et al., 2006; Signore et al., 2006; Venkatesha et al., 2006), the evolutionary medicine perspective holds promise with its somewhat simple recommendation that pregnancy be delayed until after several months of sexual activity, preventing what is not just a disease of first pregnancy, but a "couple disease" associated with exposure to novel sperm (see Chapter 11). Delaying pregnancy for a few months gives the woman's immunological system time to adjust to the man's antigens, decreasing the likelihood that her system will challenge the fetal "allograft" in the early months of pregnancy.

Childbirth

With the origin of bipedalism in our ancestors 5–7 million years ago came alterations in the pattern of childbirth. Birth is not an easy process for most monkeys and the lesser apes, given the close correspondence between the size of the neonatal head and the maternal bony pelvis (see Figure 1-6). Great Apes are the notable exceptions, with humans having a pelvic inlet that is smaller than the head of the neonate.[2] Bipedalism placed even greater constraints on the birth process through alteration of the dimensions and shape of the pelvic entrance and exit. These anatomical changes can help explain a behavioral

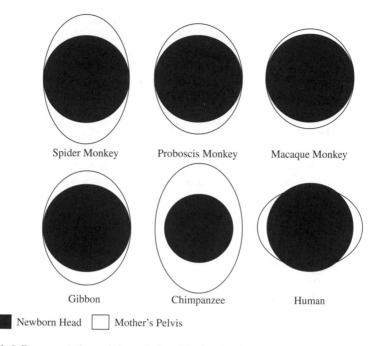

Spider Monkey   Proboscis Monkey   Macaque Monkey

Gibbon   Chimpanzee   Human

■ Newborn Head   □ Mother's Pelvis

FIGURE 1-6 Representation of the relationship in size between the average diameters of the pelvic inlet of adult females and the average head length and width of newborns of the same species (all diagrams reduced to the same pelvic inlet width). (Adapted from Schultz, 1969, p. 154.)

characteristic of human birth: the tendency for mothers to seek assistance at the time of labor and delivery (Trevathan, 1987, 1999). For most primates and most mammals, birth is a solitary event and parturient females typically seek isolation rather than companionship. For humans, the practice of seeking companionship at birth is found in almost all cultures. While it is possible for women to give birth unattended, Trevathan and Rosenberg have argued that throughout human evolutionary history, those females who sought assistance at birth had more surviving offspring than those who delivered their infants alone (Rosenberg, 1992; Rosenberg & Trevathan, 1996, 2002; Trevathan, 1987, 1999). Even a small difference in mortality and morbidity rates over several hundred generations could account for the near-universal practice of accompanied birth.

Women in the past probably did not seek companionship because of a conscious awareness that assistance would reduce mortality; rather, they likely felt more anxiety and uncertainty about labor and delivery and sought companionship for emotional support (Trevathan, 1999). For thousands of years the emotional needs of women at birth have been met by friends and relatives, most likely women, who possessed no particular skills in midwifery, but who cared about the woman and her newborn and were able, by their mere presence, to reduce emotional stresses that could interfere with labor and delivery. Today, most births in industrialized nations take place in hospitals accompanied by personnel unknown to the laboring woman. In many cases her emotional needs are not met, resulting in a view that fear and anxiety in labor are "defects" that need to be dealt with medically (with pain-relieving drugs, for example), rather than "defenses" that once motivated women to seek companionship and assistance at delivery, thereby reducing morbidity and mortality.

If efficiency at bipedal walking were the only constraint in the evolution of the human pelvis, it would likely not be the shape we see in modern as well as fossil humans. However, another constraint was imposed on the evolving human pelvis, and that was an upper limit on the size of the neonatal head that could pass through at birth. This put the birth process in direct opposition to selection for increased brain size in human evolution. Apparently the only way for the opposing trends of reducing size of the pelvic opening for bipedal efficiency and increasing size of the brain to continue was for more and more brain development to occur after birth. The result is that human babies today are born with only about 25% of their brain growth completed. This means that a lot of the motor systems necessary for independent function have not yet developed so that the human infant is much more altricial (i.e., less developed) at birth and more dependent on others than are the infants of most monkey and ape species. The other anatomical accommodation for this pressure for larger and larger brains at birth was the lack of fusion of the bony plates that make up the skull. During the birth process the skull can actually be compressed and deformed to allow passage through the birth canal.

Infancy

One of the areas of human biology where evolutionary medicine has made particularly significant impact is human infancy. There are a variety of reasons why this is so, not the least of which is that we were all infants at one time. This is not as silly as it sounds. The ubiquity of childhood is something with which everyone can identify; even if he or she is not a parent, everyone was once an infant.

Given the selective forces that appear to have constrained prenatal processes, including, but not limited to, the biology of birth and fetal sensitivity to the quality of the environments into which it is to be born (see Chapters 2, 8, and 18), the lack of evolutionary constraints on what parents actually do with and for their infants is remarkable. The specific forms of fundamental caregiving activities exhibited today such as feeding, sleeping arrangements, patterns of social affiliation, communication, and parent–infant attachment, appear to vary significantly from the ancestral economic, social, and physical conditions that might have produced them. One would expect, given an evolutionary perspective, that with so much at stake (i.e., the energy and resources invested in mating, conception, gestation and, parturition), natural selection would have designed a "universal" pattern of childcare. Based on cross-cultural ethnographic data, this seems, in fact, not to be the case.

Among the Efé of the Democratic Republic of the Congo, infants are almost continuously attached to mothers and are allowed to nurse frequently, but infants are also passed around to caregivers other than the mother who live in kin-based extended families. Mothers in horticultural groups in East Africa recruit their oldest daughters as babysitters for their infants, while mothers work in the fields. Economically disadvantaged Brazilian mothers provide care for their infants, but seem to withhold the strongest attachment emotions because of the high probability of infant death. Japanese mothers sleep apart from their husbands with their infants and attempt to minimize the stimulation and excitement of the infants. In traditional Russian families infants are tightly swaddled in blankets, making them easy to handle and restricting their movements. Navajo infants are bound to cradle boards, where they can be easily carried on mother's back (Konner, 1991a).

Human infants are the end product of an evolutionary process that has designed them so that there is the maximum probability that mothers will respond to them. Infants who were slightly less attractive and enticing to mothers would have been ever so slightly less likely to survive. The net result was intense selection for a suite of characteristics that would elicit maximal responsiveness in mothers. While human infants are born to mothers who lack a rigidly programmed set of maternal behaviors, natural selection has favored certain behaviors in infants and certain physiological responses in mothers that increase the likelihood of infants successfully obtaining a meal. The appearance of infants and the concomitant response in mothers makes it likely that infants will be picked up and held. Once that happens, infants have a programmed set of behaviors that guides them towards the nipple. Infant rooting reflex results in the location of the nipple where infants lock on and begin sucking. The ability to suckle and breathe at the same time is particularly advantageous for infants, but is lost in the course of development.[3] For mothers, there is certainly a learning component to breastfeeding (Helsing, 1976; Reeve, Gull, Johnson, Hunter, & Streather, 2004). However, once the basics are mastered, maternal physiology takes over. The initial rise in cortisol subsides, and oxytocin levels begin to rise. Maternal blood pressure decreases, and as oxytocin levels continue to rise, mothers experience a kind of calm. Once nursing begins mothers are transformed in ways that will serve the infant's needs and concomitantly increase her fitness. Under past evolutionary conditions maternal physiology takes over and the episodic endocrine and behavioral changes that occur in mothers and their responses to their infants occur with little fanfare.

However, this bond between mother and infant is not immutable. Parents in all cultures are highly susceptible to local cultural assumptions and practices about infant health and well-being. This responsiveness to cultural proscriptions makes sense in so far as the culture is a reliable source of knowledge about infant care. From an evolutionary perspective, such cultural information should have been selected for its reliability and its fidelity. Unfortunately, in modern Western society this is not always the case. Conflicting cultural values come into play in influencing parental decisions to accept or reject popular ideas about childcare, even when these cultural values are not consistent either with parental emotions and/or the ever-changing experientially based caregiving patterns that seem to make their babies happy.

Culture is so powerful that for at least half a century urban Western women were "fooled" by their cultures into thinking that artificial milk and synthetic formulas were either as good as or better than the species-specific milk their own bodies produced. A major epidemiological study of over 8900 infants followed from birth to one year of age, including 1204 infants who died between 28 days and a year from causes other than congenital anomaly and/or tumors, was conducted to determine the effects on the risk of postnatal death of breastfeeding. Overall, researchers concluded that infants who were ever breastfed had 0.79 times risk of the never-breastfed children for dying in the postnatal period. This means that if all infants born in the United States were breastfed after leaving the hospital, approximately 720 postneonatal deaths could be prevented (Chen & Rogan, 2004) For thousands of generations mothers breastfed their infants, and only in the last century was this tried-and-true childrearing strategy called into question. Not unexpectedly, from an evolutionary perspective, Western mothers have incurred significant costs for following such advice in the form of increased incidence of reproductive cancers (breast, endometrial, or ovarian). Culture has dictated practices that altered human female reproductive physiology in unexpected and even dangerous ways (see Chapter 8).

Breastfeeding is not the only behavior that Western industrialized cultures have attempted to discourage or define as unnecessary. Mothers and infants have slept together for thousands of generations and in much of the world still do so today. Along with the push toward formula feeding in the last century there was pressure for mothers not to sleep with their babies, as well as to distance themselves from their infants at night. Such suggestions are in direct opposition to fundamentally normal and evolutionarily adaptive behaviors and have been based not on empirical scientific studies, but on Western cultural values and ideology. Moreover, the notion that it is important for 2-month-old infants to develop "independence" has became embedded within basic paradigms of pediatric medicine that guide infant care recommendations (McKenna & McDade, 2005). To tell non-Western mothers that infants should be placed alone, in an enclosed pen, in a darkened room, and allowed to cry themselves to sleep would not only be met with astonishment, but would be characterized as child abuse in much of the world.

In addition to solitary sleeping and formula feeding, Westerners fully accepted the advice of Dr. Benjamin M. Spock (1903–1998), who published *The Common Sense Book of Baby and Child Care* (Spock, 1946), a book that by 1998 had sold more than 50 million copies and had been translated into 39 languages. Spock has been considered by many to be overly permissive and indulgent because he advocated that parents be more flexible and affectionate toward their children, but when viewed from an evolutionary perspective he may not seem quite so indulgent. Spock adopted a behaviorist theory of child development that we might call the spoiling theory of development. We should not acquiesce to the every wish of the child lest we spoil the child and produce an adult that is improperly socialized. This idea took hold in Western childrearing practices, particularly around sleep in infancy. Spock advised in the 7th edition of his *Baby and Child Care* book that parents should "...put the baby to bed at a reasonable hour, say good night affectionately but firmly, walk out of the room and don't go back. Most babies have developed this pattern of crying furiously for 20 or 30 minutes the first night, and then they see that nothing happens, they suddenly fall asleep! The second night the crying is apt to last only 10 minutes. The third night there is usually not any at all..." (Spock & Parker, 1998, p.210). Interestingly, in the most recent edition (Spock & Needlman, 2004) this idea has been modified and now suggests that infants can sleep in a room by themselves and if they are placed in a crib to sleep it should be done before the infant goes to sleep. While this is certainly a modified version of Spock's original advice, old ideas die hard. "Steel yourself, go through your bedtime routine, and then after saying goodnight, don't go back in no matter how much you baby cries. Your baby's cries may become more and more desperate as time drags on, but if you can bear it, she will eventually wear herself out or give up and fall asleep" (Larson & Osborn, 1997, p. 228–229)

The point here is that an evolutionary perspective on childrearing has influenced pediatricians to rethink some of the advice that had traditionally been given to parents. For example, it is widely accepted that solitary sleeping infants should not be placed on their stomachs for sleeping. Infants who sleep on their stomachs have diminished nighttime arousal, which promotes artificially prolonged, uninterrupted deep stage sleep among infants. While this may be desirable from a parent's perspective, infants in this sleeping position risk oxygen desaturation, especially when they sleep on soft mattresses, increasing their chances of dying from SIDS (Mosko et al. 1997, 1998). Unfortunately for infant well-being, face-down or prone solitary infant sleep is the most arousal-resistant type of sleep. Under more evolutionarily consistent sleep settings, infants rely on externally based arousals induced by their cosleeping mothers so that their sleep remains more often than not in Stage 1 or 2 (Mosko, Richard, McKenna, Drummond, & Mukai, 1997). In these states, if internal breathing control errors occur, a quick awakening is more likely than if the infant is sleeping solitarily, face-down on its stomach. Frequent waking permits the expulsion of accumulating CO_2, which, while positive in low doses (CO_2 stimulates the breathing reflex), can become fatal if excessive, such as when a baby sleeps face-down into a pillow or soft mattress.

The importance of an evolutionary consideration of patterns of breastfeeding and sleeping has only recently begun to be appreciated. Through the efforts of a number of researchers (Babcock, 1999; Ball, 2002, 2003; Ball, Hooker, & Kelly, 1999; Ball & Panter-Brick, 2001; McKenna, 1986, 2000; McKenna et al., 1993; McKenna & Gartner, 2000; McKenna & Mosko, 2001; see also Chapter 12) public health policy makers are regularly utilizing scientific data on infant sleep patterns in the formation of guidelines. This is clearly an area where the application of an evolutionary perspective has been enormously valuable in dramatically reducing the number of infant deaths due to SIDS.

Childhood

Compared with research in pregnancy and infancy, evolutionary medicine seems to have paid less attention to childhood—the period between weaning and puberty. But there are a number of examples of ways in which childhood health can benefit from evolutionary considerations. The timing of weaning is a topic that evokes discourse that entwines both cultural ideologies and biological processes, and the two may not always be complementary. Among chimpanzees and most human foraging cultures that have been studied, 3–4 years seems to be the typical period of infant breastfeeding, and, perhaps related to that, it is a commonly reported birth interval in great apes and human foraging groups. Some suggest that it is the frequency of nursing bouts by which breast-feeding maintains a 3- to 4-year birth interval. For example, among the !Kung of Botswana and Namibia, mothers were found to nurse their infant more than four times per hour for approximately 2 minutes with a mean interval between bouts of approximately 13 minutes (Konner & Worthman, 1980). This frequent nursing results in elevated levels of 17 β-estradial and progesterone and is implicated in the inhibition of ovulation. Others argue that the long interbirth intervals are due to maternal nutritional shortages. Age, nutritional status, energy balance, diet, and exercise are all factors that have been associated with variation in ovarian function (Ellison, 1990). But although there is a great deal of debate about what factors are primary in maintaining a 3- to 4-year birth interval, suffice it to say that nursing plays an important role.

Has evolution and natural selection favored a time at which mammals should wean their offspring? It would seem that there should be some optimum time for weaning since there is a point when parents should get on with the business of having additional offspring and existing offspring are sufficiently developed to be able to acquire food on their own (Trivers, 1972, 1974). Dettwyler (1995) has examined a number of life history variables to determine what she calls the "natural age of weaning" for humans. For example, if you consider that larger animals tend to nurse their infants longer relative to gestation length than smaller animals (e.g., for gorillas and chimpanzees the ratio of nursing to gestation length is 6:1), the expected weaning age for humans is 4.5 years. In another study of growth and development in nonhuman primates, Smith (1991) surveyed 21 species of monkeys and apes and found that weaning occurs at the time of eruption of the first molars, which would be about 6 years in humans (Smith, 1991). In a comparative study of weaning and maternal investment in primates, ungulates, and pinnipeds, when a neonate has grown to four times its birth weight it is weaned. For humans living in a developed country this would mean that a 7.5-lb. infant should be weaned at around 3 years of age (Lee, Majluf, & Gordon, 1991). For those of us in cultures where breast-feeding, if it occurs at all, often lasts less than one year, breastfeeding until age 3–6 years may seem excessive, but for people in parts of the world where access to appropriate and healthful infant foods is limited, nursing for several years (with supplementation from other sources) may mean the difference between a healthy and a sickly child.

Weaning is not the end of parental care, of course. For humans, as well as some other mammals (chimpanzees, bonobos, killer whales, vampire bats, cotton-tops tamarins, lion tamarins, wild dogs) food sharing after weaning is a well-documented behavior (Blurton Jones, 1987; Burrows, Hofer, & East, 1995; de Waal, 1989; de Waal, Luttrell, & Canfield, 1993; Ekman & Rosander, 1992; Feistner & Price, 1990; Hiraiwa-Hasegawa, 1990; Hoelzel, 1991; Hohmann & Fruth, 1993; McGrew & Feistner, 1992; Nishida & Turner, 1996; Price & Feistner, 1993; Silk, 1978; Wilkinson, 1984). However, the food sharing and provisioning that occur in humans is more highly developed and extends for a longer period than in other species that share food (Lancaster & Lancaster, 1983). In the course of human evolution it is possible that provisioning children between weaning and puberty may have doubled or even tripled the number of offspring that survived to adulthood. This long period of extended childcare by older children and adults probably enhanced the time for learning technological and social skills, also contributing to greater survival and reproductive success. Thus, the costs of extensive parental care were outweighed in human evolutionary history by the benefits of greater reproductive success for the recipient offspring.

The major causes of childhood death worldwide are infectious diseases exacerbated by poor nutrition. Pellitier, Frongillo, Schroeder, & Habicht (1995) estimate that about 70% of deaths of children from birth to age 4 years are due to diarrhea, respiratory infections, malaria, and diseases for which immunizations are available, and that as many as 83% of these deaths are indirectly attributable to malnutrition, even in a mild to moderate form. Consider that respiratory infections are a leading cause of death for children, and yet for most of us in developed nations they are merely nuisances. Rarely do we worry that the common cold will kill us or our children. It is notable that the leading causes of deaths of children in developed nations such as the United States and Western Europe are not typically related to malnutrition and include, for children under 5 years of age, accidents followed by preterm births. In the remainder of the world acute respiratory infection followed closely by diarrheal diseases and preterm births were the major sources of mortality (World Health Organization, 2005c) (see Figure 1-7). (Sadly, homicide is ranked fourth on the list of leading causes of death of children under 5 years in the

Unites States.) Furthermore, being born with low birth weight, itself often due to maternal malnutrition, accounts for almost half of the deaths from diarrhea, pneumonia, and malaria (Black, Morris & Bryce, 2003).

Malnutrition affects health and development in a number of ways short of death. As discussed above for intrauterine growth retardation (see also Chapter 18), small adult stature and even compromised brain development are often the outcomes of nutritional deprivation in childhood. It is notable that the first 5 years of life are the period of most rapid brain growth, and most negative effects are irreversible (Bogin, 1998). One of the negative impacts on child health in this early period is competition from other family members, especially younger siblings. An evolutionary perspective suggests that with birth intervals of 4–5 years, as was likely common in the past, nutritional competition among infants was not as big a problem as it is today, where babies may be spaced only a year or two apart. In general, mortality rates for infants and children increase when birth intervals decrease (Panter-Brick, 1998).

Malnutrition and infection are synergistic—one state makes the other worse (Pellitier et al., 1995). As noted above, malnutrition and poor health in utero and in childhood are commonly associated with lower adult stature. There is evidence that overall lowered

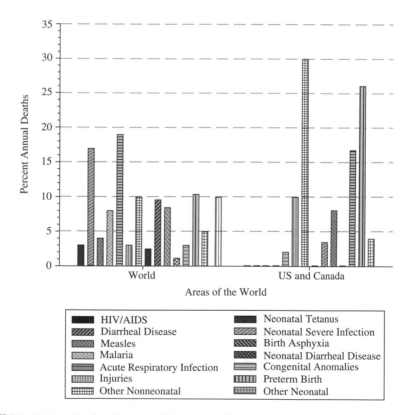

FIGURE 1-7 Mortality data by cause of death for children under 5 years of age including specific sources of mortality for children less than 1 year of age. (From World Health Organization, 2005a.)

immune response may be more directly responsible for slowed growth than nutritional intake itself (Shell-Duncan, 1993). Furthermore, compromised immunocompetence and low food intake also lead to decreased activity levels, themselves linked to chronic diseases throughout the life span.

The effects of psychosocial stress beginning in utero on child health and well-being are explored most directly here in a number of ways and for different purposes by Kuwaza (Chapter 18), Chisholm and Coall (Chapter 6), Núñez de la Mora and Bentley (Chapter 7), and Baker et al. (Chapter 17). Flinn and his colleagues (Chapter 13) studied the stress response in children, by way of measuring levels of salivary cortisol, taking note that cortisol spikes can be correlated with periods of illness. Interestingly (and perhaps predictably, based on the importance of the mother for child health, as discussed above), children who live with their mothers and other close kin have lower cortisol responses to stress than children who live with nonkin or more distant kin, and thus, fewer illness episodes. Even short-term absences of mothers or fathers seemed to have a negative effect on child health among the Caribbean children studied by Flinn.

At one point it was believed that small adult stature under circumstances of low resource availability was adaptive in that small adults would need fewer resources and would fare better under chronically stressful conditions (Seckler, 1982). In fact, a great deal of public policy was based on this "small but healthy" hypothesis, but a broader perspective indicates that small body size also means small organs, less ability to perform work, and lower reproductive success (Martorell, 1989), all of which mean "not healthy" from evolutionary and life span perspectives (especially see Chapters 17 and 18).

Although much of this section has emphasized poor health and causes of child mortality, it is important to note that millions of children survive quite well, even under fairly dire circumstances. In the parts of the world where several million children die every year from diarrhea and respiratory infections, there are also children who had the same levels of infection but did not die—they had social, physical, and behavioral abilities to cope and recover from the illnesses, either on their own or with help from close kin (Panter-Brick, 1998). Imagine two families living in poverty in sub-Saharan Africa in which the toddlers develop severe diarrhea from dirty drinking water—in one family the children die, in the other they live to grow to maturity and have children. In this case, resistance to the effects of diarrhea is a beneficial characteristic, but is it a Darwinian characteristic? Possibly. It is unlikely that there is a diarrhea-resistant gene, but the surviving toddler may have had a slightly stronger immune system, which allowed our survivor to endure severe diarrheal dehydration a bit better. In addition, our survivor's mother might have been slightly better at getting water or our survivor was a member of a family with a tent with good shade. So what is the point? Our survivor's slightly better immune system was the critical factor in survival when coupled with a more favorable local environment. So in this case it is natural selection operating on our toddlers, favoring the one that was best able to endure the consequences of drinking polluted water. Diarrhea in this instance is the "agent of natural selection" that selected against the children (and their genes) in one family and favored the children (and their genes) in the other.

There are circumstances under which a mother may consciously or unconsciously neglect her child so that it dies. While maternal neglect, benign or not, seems abhorrent to most Westerners, in fact, there are some situations where it makes perfect sense from an evolutionary perspective (Hrdy, 1999). For example, when poverty is so grinding that the chances of continued survival are slim (Scheper-Hughes, 1991), it is in the mother's best interest to be indifferent toward the welfare of a child.[4] This has been seen as evidence against a "maternal instinct" to protect her children at all costs, but an evolutionary perspective suggests that under extreme conditions, it makes sense to "cut your losses" and try again to reproduce later when circumstances for raising a child may be improved. The inclusion of a consideration of future survivorship has implications for public health policy. An emphasis on child immunizations in the context of extreme poverty and malnutrition may be nothing more than prolonging life so that immunized children are able to survive so that they may die later of malnutrition (Dettwyler, 1994). Children who are well nourished and otherwise healthy are usually able to survive bouts of childhood diseases, even without immunization.

Just as there is variation in what is considered optimal and even "normal" infant care (discussed above), there is variation in what is considered "appropriate" child care. For example, in many cultures children begin to contribute economically to the household at very young ages and their contributions are usually very important for family survival. In addition to taking care of younger siblings and relatives, children are recruited to do manual labor in direct support of the household. In many Western nations, however, there are laws against child labor, and the years from infancy to puberty are seen as the time for play and education, not for helping the adults of the family "make a living." In fact, play is seen as critical for normal child development in many cultures, whereas its importance is de-emphasized or ignored in others (Panter-Brick, 1998).

The emphasis on education for children is also highly variable worldwide. One bit of information added by the evolutionary perspective, especially considering evidence from hunter-gatherer populations, is that playing and learning in groups segregated by age is novel in the course of human evolution—most children, until formal schooling changed the rules, spent their childhood in multiaged groups, a setting that is superior for acquiring social skills than age-segregated classrooms (Konner, 1991b). Others have suggested that learning by instruction (as in formal schooling) may not be as effective as learning by observation and doing, the method with the longest association with childhood in our species (Levine, 1998). These are examples of ways in which an evolutionary medicine perspective can help assess intellectual development in children.

There is a relationship between child-rearing practices and infant and child mortality rates (Levine, 1998). Levine argues that generally, and on a universal level, parenting goals can be described in terms of a hierarchy of successive goals to which parents direct their efforts and resources, although the extent of parental resources may prevent parents from achieving any of them. Infant survivorship is the first goal, followed by educating children either formally or informally to become self-sufficient; and, finally, if the first two goals are achieved, parents aim to foster in their children values and ideologies expressed through various societal rituals that affirm their own high status and the validity of the cultural system of which they are a part, therein assuring intergenerational cultural continuities. As regards the process by which the third goal is achieved, for example, only where mortality has been greatly reduced can parents "afford" to spend time and resources on nonutilitarian or non–survival-related activities such as dance, music, theater, and soccer.

Where mortality has been greatly reduced, as in developed nations, environmental causes of developmental disorders are often alleviated, allowing genetic causes to be exposed. This means that genetic contributions are often overestimated and that policies have "...elevated the relative genetic contribution to [child development problems]... and given public salience to genetic problems" (Levine, 1998, p. 125). Thus, in industrialized nations, we have learning disabilities, dyslexia, hyperactivity (attention deficit disorder [ADD] and attention deficit-hyperactivity disorder [ADHD]), and other behavioral problems that would have been unremarkable in the past environments of childhood (Worthman and Kuzara, 2005). For developing nations to take their cue from developed nations in dealing with these genetic diseases of childhood may actually be counterproductive. Resources spent on research into the genetic causes of childhood diseases could be better utilized to raise the standard of living of the poorest of the poor through direct subsidy.

This is not to say that genetic contributions to child development should be ignored. Indeed, there are a number of success stories (Richards, 1998), such as the discovery that a diet low in the amino acid phenylalanine, if implemented early in life, can ward off the dangerous and debilitating disease phenylketonuria (PKU), which causes neurological damage and mental retardation when not treated. Thousands of children have been saved from this disease because of routine genetic testing of newborns that is done in most developed nations, including every state in the United States.

The incidence and prevalence of childhood asthma appear to be increasing in many parts of the world, including industrialized societies such as the United States and the nations of Western Europe, reaching a level that leads some to refer to it as a "worldwide childhood asthma epidemic" (Hurtado, Hurtado, Sapien, & Hill, 1999, p. 104). Unfortunately, most of the treatments that have been developed after years of clinical and pharmacological research are effective only for symptom relief and fail to get at the underlying causes of this potentially debilitating disease. Hurtado and colleagues suggest that an evolutionary perspective may help address the underlying causes of childhood asthma. Given the large number of people in the world with the asthma phenotype, evolutionary theory suggests that the asthma phenotype confers an adaptive advantage now or in the past (i.e., the phenotype and underlying genotype were positively selected over the course of human evolution). In modern environments, the asthma phenotype develops in the context of exposure to indoor allergens (e.g., dust mites, pet dander) and relatively low exposure to endo- and ecto-parasites, especially helminths. Where there is a high prevalence of helminths, there is a low prevalence of asthma, and vice versa (Barnes, Armelagos, & Morreale, 1999). It appears that the immunoglobulin-E (Ig-E) response is triggered by exposure to helminths and exhausts the immune response so that it is relatively unaffected by exposure to allergens like pollen and dust mites. When the helminths are eliminated from the environment, the immune system is free to react, even overreact, to allergens. Thus, what appears to be a defect may be an example of a defense against parasitic infections that were more common in the evolutionary past and likely increased with animal domestication (Barnes, Armelagos, & Morreale, 1999). Now this unbridled IgE response has become a defect in environments that are low in parasites and high in "modern" conveniences like mattresses, rugs, blankets, and insulated homes. Hurtado and colleagues add parental care practices and socioeconomic challenges to the evolutionary perspective on childhood asthma and suggest ways in which public health measures may be developed to deal with this complex issue (Hurtado et al., 1999).

One characteristic of human reproduction that has changed remarkably is the significant decrease in the age of onset of menarche in recent generations. This decrease in the age at menarche has been referred to as a "secular trend" (see Figure 1-8) and has been recorded in developed nations. The most often cited causes of this secular trend—better nutrition, more protein and calories in infancy, and improvements in health care—are generally assumed to be signs of well-being. It is not clear that lowered age of menarche is actually an improvement in health, since it appears also to be related to mental health problems in adolescence (Kaltiala-Heino, Martunnen, Rantanen, & Rimpelä, 2003), increased risk for metabolic syndrome X[5] (Frontini, Srinivasan, & Berenson, 2003), and increased rates of some reproductive cancers (Eaton et al., 1994).

What does the decreasing age of menarche say about childhood, particularly in girls? Childhood is often defined as that period between weaning and puberty, but given the variation in age of each of these markers, how can it be a defined life cycle phase? Is an 11-year-old girl who has reached menarche no longer a child? And is a 15-year-old who has not yet reached menarche a child, while her peers who have are "adolescents"?

Puberty is fairly well-defined biological event for most mammals and simply refers to the onset of reproductive function. Perhaps unique to humans, the period following puberty is marked by an accelerated rate of skeletal growth that is referred to as the "adolescent growth spurt" (Bogin & Smith, 1996; Krogman, 1972; Tanner, 1962, 1990; Tanner & Taylor, 1965). Human females have a fairly long period of "adolescent sterility"[6] following menarche when most, if not all, menstrual cycles are nonovulatory. This period

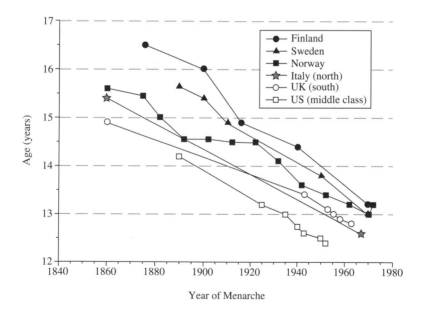

FIGURE 1-8 Secular trends in age at menarche for selected European countries and the United States. (Adapted from Tanner, 1990, p. 160.)

between the appearance of secondary sexual characteristics (enlarged breasts in girls, pubic and axillary hair in both girls and boys) and completion of growth is usually defined as adolescence in humans (Golub, 2000). However, what we are really talking about is puberty, a "universal physiological process" (Worthman, 1998, p. 29), which occurs over time as the body goes through the process of maturing. Adolescence is a cultural construct, and in much the same way as infancy, cultures define the period of adolescence and use it to shape the child into the adult that best fits with the cultural ideal (Worthman, 1998). Thus, adolescence may be seen as a short (or even nonexistent) period or relatively long, depending on how it is defined by a culture. In Western cultures where adolescence may last 10 years (from menarche at age 11 to the age at which alcohol can be legally purchased in the United States and formal education is usually terminated), this long period may be necessary for acquiring the social, intellectual, and technological skills to function as an adult. It should be noted, however, that in some cultures attainment of adult status depends on very specific biological (e.g., birth of the first child) or cultural (e.g., circumcision, marriage) events that may be independent of developmental processes.

Mortality is fairly low during adolescence in most human populations, but this is the time when many emotional (e.g., eating disorders, risk taking behavior) and physical (e.g., obesity, early pregnancy, poor diet) health problems emerge, especially in Western populations (Golub, 2000). It is also a time during which endocrine systems and other physiological processes develop in ways that have a significant effect on later adult health (Worthman, 1999). In fact, just as intrauterine (see Chapter 18) and infant environments have impacts on adult health, so too does the environment of adolescence, with all of these life cycle phases themselves interrelated in their impact on health (Worthman, 1999a, b; see also Chapter 6).

Although we have emphasized the gradual decline in maturation observed in the last century, there is within every population a great range of variation. An important lesson from evolutionary medicine and life history theory is that maturation is sensitive to local environmental situations (including, but not limited to, diet, health care, and parental care practices) and that a textbook-based concept of "normal" adolescence will work only for a small range of the variation observed and primarily what is experienced in the developed world (Worthman, 1999b). As with so many arguments made in this volume, public health measures must look beyond the Western concept of "normal" maturation and "normal" adolescence. Public health policy makers also need to consider the sociopolitical and socioeconomic contexts of developmental problems and intervene at the appropriate level to bring about systemic improvements in health (Chisholm, 1993; see also Chapter 6). "The close associations among resource allocation, pubertal timing, adult competence, and human health make equity in access to resources for child health and development a priority for preventive medicine" (Worthman, 1999, p.154). Improvement in health at all levels requires greater attention to social context than has been given in the past.

CHRONIC DISEASE

Chronic disease is the major source of mortality worldwide, except in sub-Saharan Africa, where infectious disease is the primary cause of death. Worldwide nearly 6 out of

10 deaths (or nearly 35 billion people) are the result of a chronic disease (World Health Organization, 2005c) each year. In the United States it is even worse. Seven of every 10 Americans who die each year, or more than 1.7 million people, will die of a chronic disease (Hoyert, Heron, Murphy, & Kung, 2006) (see Figures 1-9 and 1-10). If there is any area of medicine where an evolutionary perspective might be helpful, it would seem that addressing problems associated with chronic disease should be at the top of the list. It is precisely because humans have developed a robust immunological defense system that works well for short-term problems like infectious disease, but remains highly vulnerable to the slow steady progression of chronic disorders, that an evolutionary perspective might be of help. The prolonged course of illness and disability from chronic diseases like diabetes and arthritis results in extended pain and suffering and decreased quality of life for billions of people worldwide.

There are numerous proximate causes of chronic disease (e.g., obesity, diabetes mellitus, atherosclerosis, hypertension, cancer), but the evolutionary basis for many chronic diseases is poorly understood. The rise of evolutionary medicine has helped place chronic disease in a context where meaningful new therapeutic interventions can be considered. Certainly physicians have been concerned with chronic disease for a long time, but the recommendations for treatment were largely no more than "quick fixes" to the long-term problem. Attention to the evolutionary importance of nutrition and activity as risk factors for chronic disease became apparent in the 1980s, well before the dawn of evolutionary medicine (Eaton & Konner, 1985; Eaton, Konner, & Shostak, 1988a). The general hypothesis that guided this early research was the discordance between the Western diet and the diet of our Paleolithic ancestors (Eaton & Eaton III, 1999b). These differences, not only in diet, but in lifestyle as well, are the underlying cause of many of the chronic diseases that plague modern humans. The research on nutrition and

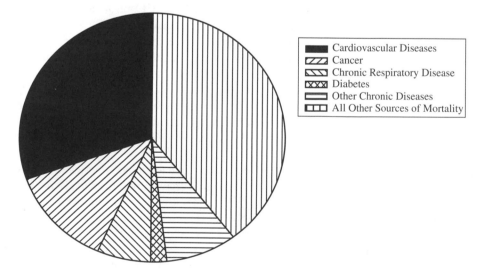

FIGURE 1-9 Causes of mortality worldwide. Data are for 2005. (From World Health Organization, 2005a.)

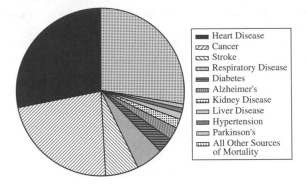

FIGURE 1-10 Causes of mortality in the United States. Data are for 2003. (From Hoyert et al., 2006.)

evolutionary medicine has already been reviewed earlier in this chapter, so here we will confine our discussion to studies of chronic disease.

Exercise

One of the questions that has arisen from the studies of the consequences of modern Western diets and human health concerns the role of exercise in chronic disease. The beneficial effects of exercise on a variety of aspects of health and well-being, not just reduction of chronic disease, have been well documented (Blair, LaMonte, & Nichaman, 2004; NIH Consensus Development Panel on Physical Activity and Cardiovascular Health, 1996; Pate et al., 1995), and considerable effort has been made to make recommended guidelines easily accessible (Centers for Disease Control and Prevention, 2006c). Physical activity recommendations are that adults should: (1) engage in moderate-intensity physical activities (e.g., brisk walking, bicycling, vacuuming, gardening, or anything else that causes small increases in breathing or heart rate) for at least 30 minutes on 5 or more days of the week; or (2) engage in vigorous-intensity physical activity 3 or more days per week for 20 minutes or more per occasion (Centers for Disease Control and Prevention, 2006c). It has been noted, however, that these recommendations may be insufficient to prevent weight gain in some individuals, who will need additional exercise or caloric restriction to minimize the probability of further weight gain (Blair, LaMonte, & Nichaman, 2004).

In spite of the "user friendliness" of these recommendations, Americans are still plagued by a sedentary lifestyle. According to the most recent report from the Centers for Disease Control and Prevention, less than half the adult population surveyed engaged in the recommended level of physical activity, while approximately 35% reported engaging in insufficient levels of physical activity, and 15% of the population reported engaging in less than 10 minutes per week of moderate to vigorous lifestyle activities (Pate et al., 1995). Imagine a Pleistocene ancestor who only engaged in the recommended

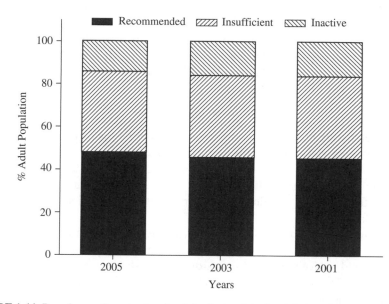

FIGURE 1-11 Prevalence of varying levels of physical activity in adult Americans. Recommended physical activity is defined as moderate-intensity activities in a usual week (i.e., brisk walking, bicycling, vacuuming, gardening, or anything else that causes small increases in breathing or heart rate) for at least 30 minutes per day, or anything else that causes large increases in breathing or heart rate for at least 20 minutes per day, at least 3 days per week. Insufficient physical activity is defined as doing more than 10 minutes total per week of moderate- to vigorous-intensity lifestyle activities (i.e., household, transportation, or leisure-time activity), but less than the recommended level of activity. Inactive is defined as less than 10 minutes total per week of moderate- to vigorous-intensity lifestyle activities (i.e., household, transportation, or leisure-time activity). (From Centers for Disease Control and Prevention, 2006b.)

level of activity. It is not likely that this level of activity would be sufficient to acquire and maintain adequate resources and would enjoy very low reproductive success (see Figure 1-11).

Furthermore, there is considerable evidence that incorporating physical activity into one's life early on is at least one component in lifetime physical fitness. Like their parents, children today are surprisingly sedentary, and in many cases schools are not encouraging physical activity. In a survey of high school students, researchers found that slightly more than half (55.7%) of students were enrolled in a physical education class. Less than one third of those students (28.4%) attended a physical education class daily, and when attending a physical education class, less than 40% (39.2%) were active, that is, exercising or playing sports for more than 20 minutes (Centers for Disease Control and Prevention, 2004b). It is clear from this and numerous other studies that most Americans, young and old, engage in significantly lower levels of physical activity than is recommended—much less than in the recent past, and almost none when compared to our Pleistocene ancestors (Eaton & Eaton, III, 2003).

Our culture has altered not only our dietary patterns, but our activity patterns as well, in ways that are likely to contribute to rise in mortality from chronic disease. While evolutionary medicine has not developed a panacea for this lack of physical activity, it has put the behavior of modern humans living in Western society in context.

Cardiovascular Disease

Diet and exercise are both strongly implicated in the occurrence of cardiovascular disease. Heart disease and stroke are the most common of the cardiovascular diseases and account for about 40% of annual deaths. Almost one fourth of the American population has some form of heart disease. It is important to remember that much of what has been reviewed in the section on nutrition is directly relevant to an evolutionary perspective on cardiovascular disease.

The two major risk factors associated with all cardiovascular diseases are hypertension and serum cholesterol levels. By reducing blood pressure and serum cholesterol Americans could reduce mortality from cardiovascular diseases by 25% and the overall death rate by 13% (Centers for Disease Control and Prevention, 2005a). But what does a view from evolutionary medicine have to see in this case? It should be clear from the preceding discussions that our diet and lifestyle are discordant with our evolved physiology, and this discordance is a major contributing factor to chronic diseases in general, and cardiovascular disease in particular. Evolutionary medicine has been concerned with cardiovascular disease largely from the perspective of prevention and has not focused on the evolutionary adaptations of our cardiovascular systems and how a greater understanding of those adaptations might provide new insights.

Congestive heart disease is one major exception (see Chapter 21). Congestive heart failure (CHF) is often the end stage of cardiac disease. Half the patients who are diagnosed with CHF will die within 5 years, and one in five will die within one year (National Heart Lung and Blood Institute, 1996). CHF is a condition where the heart is unable to pump enough blood to the body's organs. It results from narrowed arteries that supply blood to the heart (coronary artery disease), scar tissue from a past heart attack (myocardial infarction) that interferes with the heart muscle, hypertension, primary diseases of the heart (cardiomyopathy), congenital heart defects, as well as infection of the heart valves or the heart muscle itself (endocarditis or myocarditis). Blood flows out of the heart, but blood returning to the heart backs up, causing accumulation in the tissues. Swelling (edema) in the legs and ankles most often results. Fluid also accumulates in the lungs, and the kidneys are not able to dispose of sodium and water. The sequelae of events associated with CHF is well known to clinicians, but without an understanding of why these events occurred in a particular way. In fact, CHF may not necessarily be a pathological condition and may actually be a defense against blood and fluid loss. That CHF is actually the result of natural selection is considered by Weil (Chapter 21) and is an excellent example of how an evolutionary perspective can change a perceived defect into defense under certain environmental conditions. This new way of conceiving of CHF may lead to new and novel treatments for this major contributor of cardiovascular disease mortality. An understanding of why CHF progresses in a particular way will not quickly offer a magic bullet cure, but by conceiving of diseases from this perspective we can hope to stimulate further research.

Cancer

After cardiovascular disease, cancer is the second leading source of mortality in the United States. Of course, it is impossible to talk about cancer without considering the variety of types of cancers, the array of environmental factors and lifestyle choices, and the genetic factors that affect its prevalence. Epidemiologists generally consider risk factors that are either intrinsic to the individual (age, sex, genetic history) or extrinsic (infections, tobacco use, diet and nutrition, occupational exposure, environmental pollutants). Evolutionary medicine has something to say about both types of cancer risk factor. The intrinsic risk factors are certainly modified by evolution. The risk of most types of cancers increases with age, and certain cancers occur only in one sex due to differences in anatomy. There are some ethnic differences in cancer risk, with genetic inheritance accounting for about 4% of all cancers.

It is clear in Table 1-1 that there are significant differences in the incidence rates of cancers depending on ethnicity. The difficulty, of course, is to tease out the proportion of these differences that are due to genetic factors and/or environmental factors. Given the current state of knowledge, it is unwise to categorically assign certain ethnic groups high-risk status for particular cancers, but the genetic basis for cancers certainly warrants further research (see Chapter 20). There are many factors that contribute to these ethnic differences in cancer incidence, including, but not limited to access to health care, poverty, poor diet, lack of exercise, tobacco use, lifestyle, occupation, as well as some proportion of genetic differences among human populations. Unfortunately, these are questions that have not yet been pursued systematically by many evolutionary medicine researchers. There is some interest among clinicians in the high incidence of hypertension seen in American blacks and the low incidence of certain cancers among Asian and Pacific Islanders, but a discussion of this problem is beyond the scope of this chapter.

We know that inheritance of mutant genes accounts for a proportion of the cancers seen today. Even if there is not a gene for a specific cancer, we know that there is a genetic component. One of the most famous cases is Napoleon Bonaparte. The French have always suspected that the English killed Napoleon by poisoning, but it is much more likely that it was cancer. Napoleon ordered that upon his death an autopsy be performed so that the cause of his death could be immediately confirmed. The determination of the cause of his death was for the benefit of his son, so that he might be able to avoid the disease. The autopsy was conducted by Napoleon's personal physician, Francesco Antommarchi, a Corsican aided by a Scottish army surgeon, Archibald Arnott. Even

TABLE 1-1 Cancer Rates for Men and Women in the United States

Women	Rate[a]	Men	Rate
Breast	124.9	Lung	161.2
Lung	38.0	Prostate	86.4
Colorectal	38.3	Colorectal	61.3

[a] *Rate per 100,000 persons.*
Source: Centers for Disease Control and Prevention, 2006a, b.

though several British military surgeons and physicians were in attendance, they were under strict instructions from Napoleon that they were not to touch his body. The autopsy was unequivocal on the cause of death as stomach cancer. In addition, Napoleon's father, his grandfather, one brother, and three sisters died from stomach cancer (Greaves, 2000).

As discussed in the previous section on human reproduction and evolutionary medicine, women's reproductive cancers have benefited from an evolutionary perspective. Breast cancer is a major concern for women all over the world, but much more so for women in the developed world. One of the primary contributors to the high incidence of breast cancer is the pattern of reproduction common in the developed world. Early menarche, delayed first birth, little if any breastfeeding, and reduced number of pregnancies and births have all been identified as key factors in the incidence of reproductive cancers, and in particular breast cancer (Eaton & Eaton, III, 1999a; Eaton et al., 1994).

Cancer is a chronic disease that is not confined to the developed world, but the risk of getting cancer is greater in the developed world, whereas cancers in the developing world are more often fatal. Only 19% of the world population lives in developed countries, but 46% of the new cancer cases occur there. Interestingly, the probability of dying from cancer is not very different in the developed world when compared to the developing world. The types of cancers most frequently presented are different for developed when compared to developing countries (see Table 1-2). This is not surprising when we consider the effects of poverty on lifestyle and the modification of risk factors.

TABLE 1-2 Age-Adjusted Rate for Cancer by Type and Ethnicity, 1999–2002

	White	Black	Asian and Pacific Islanders	Other
All sites combined	471.7	480.6	289.4	1510.2
Brain and nervous system	7.1	3.9	3.5	12.0
Breast, cervical, & uterine	87.9	82.2	53.5	240.3
Colorectal	53.7	59.7	39.0	138.7
Esophagus	4.8	7.1	2.3	9.9
Gallbladder	1.1	1.4	1.5	3.3
Kidney	12.8	13.0	5.3	32.8
Larynx	4.2	6.3	1.4	9.5
Leukemia	12.3	9.3	6.8	39.8
Liver	3.9	6.0	13.3	12.8
Lung	70.2	74.6	37.4	107.3
Skin	17.2	0.9	1.2	104.2
Myeloma	4.9	10.3	3.0	16.7
Non-Hodgkin's lymphoma	19.2	13.3	12.4	57.1
Oral and pharynx	10.2	11.0	7.6	30.8
Ovary	7.7	5.7	5.2	15.3
Pancreas	10.8	14.3	8.1	18.0
Prostate	68.3	97.4	35.4	456.3
Stomach	6.6	12.4	14.1	18.3
Thyroid	7.7	4.6	7.8	22.9
Bladder	22.8	11.2	8.6	60.7

Source: Centers for Disease Control and Prevention, 2006b.

While these data do not directly address the evolutionary question of why there is this geographical dispersion of type of cancers, it is tempting to speculate that as Western culture spreads and many of its features are adopted by people on a worldwide basis, we will continue to see a rise in cancer prevalence due to the modifiable lifestyle risk factors. Of course, the compelling question is what can be done about the spread of Western culture? It is tempting to throw up one's hands and say nothing. We are too far down the road of globalization to halt the exportation of both the positive and the negative aspects of Western culture.

From an evolutionary perspective it is tempting to see cancer as an inevitable consequence of intrinsic evolutionary penalty for two essential characteristics of all living organisms. First, tissue stem cells have the capacity for sustained proliferation and regeneration, as well as a lymphatic system for migration and dispersal. Second, there are mechanisms for shuffling genes and recombination as well as a lack of complete fidelity in DNA copying and repair. While there are multiple physiological systems that have evolved to limit the lifetime risks of these two characteristics, sometimes these protective systems break down. These breakdowns in protection can occur early on in fetal development and give rise to pediatric cancers, but more likely they occur in old age. The average risk of a 25-year-old man dying of cancer by his thirtieth birthday is 50 times less than a man who is 65 reaching his seventieth birthday (Greaves, 2000).

Greaves (2000) has made the observation that for 90% of the cancers, the major risk factors are not our genetic inheritance, but human social engineering, where each of us exercises deliberate and informed choice under normal circumstances. By our own errors we are subjected to repeated and chronic toxic insults that result in proliferative and oxidative stress on tissues, an increased frequency of mutations, and direct damage to DNA. We have taken the basic machinery that is mildly error prone and have significantly ratcheted up the risk for each individual of getting cancer. As we have said so many times before, cancer is another one of those complex chronic diseases that has been present in humans for thousands of generations, but has in recent times markedly increased in prevalence in the population.

While women's cancers have received much attention, men's cancers have not. The leading cause of cancer death among men is lung cancer, followed by prostate cancer (see Table 1-3). Prostate cancer is a common form of cancer and is fast becoming the most commonly diagnosed type of cancer; it will likely soon overtake lung cancer as the leading cause of death in men (Centers for Disease Control and Prevention, 2006d). Current treatments for prostate cancer are crude, feminizing, and not particularly effective. Some 30% of men over 50 have clinically silent prostate cancer, and 50% of men over 80 are affected. So the message is that most men, if they live long enough, will develop prostate cancer, but its potential lethal consequences are preempted by other more acute causes of death.

What are the causes of prostate cancer, and can an evolutionary perspective help us understand this disease? In the United States the primary cause has been thought to be environmental or occupational toxins, but the evidence that has been assembled is very weak. Diet could also play a part, in particular excess caloric intake and reduced energy expenditures, but the mechanisms are unclear at best. Other candidate explanations include high levels of insulin-like growth factor-1 (IGF-1), more cell division, less cell

TABLE 1-3 Cancer Prevalence in Developed and Developing Countries

Developed > Developing	Approximately equal	Developed < Developing
	Lung	
Colorectal		
Breast		
Prostate		
		Stomach
Bladder		
	non-Hodgkin's lymphoma	
Kidney		
Pancreas		
		Leukemia
		Liver
	Ovary	
		Oral cavity
		Cervix/Uteri
		Esophagus

Source: Mackay, Jemal, Lee, & Parkin, 2006.

death and hence more cells, more oxidative stress, and greater risk to labile DNA (Greaves, 2000).

A more reasonable explanation first requires an understanding of the physiological function of the prostate, which is to lubricate and facilitate sperm flow and fertilization. The prostate is dependent on a supply of testosterone. Relative to other male mammals, human males have enormous prostates. The only other animals that can claim a comparably sized prostate are dogs (*Canis familiaris*), and they are the only other mammal that experiences an appreciable rate of prostate cancer. The possible function for such large prostates in humans could be related to our mating system. While there are other mildly polygynous mammals today, the degree of polygyny may have been greater in our evolutionary past. Males who were capable of mating often and producing healthy robust sperm could well have had a slight competitive advantage over less well-endowed males. While there is a decrease in testosterone production with age in males, it is nothing like the decline in estrogen production with age in females. Consequently, while the constant bombardment of target-sensitive tissue in males is one factor that allows males to produce viable sperm quite late in life, there is a cost, and that is the likelihood of developing prostate cancer (Greaves, 2000). Again, while this evolutionary explanation does not offer a cure for prostate cancer, it does put this disease in an evolutionary perspective and suggests that it is the outcome of varying selective pressures at different life stages. It is this kind of evolutionary thinking that may produce new and novel treatments for this disease.

While the link between lifestyle and other cancers seems plausible and is based on good scientific evidence, no cancer is more the direct outcome of the discordance between our evolved physiology and our current lifestyle than are lung and throat cancer due to smoking. The relationship between smoking and lung cancer is so well accepted in most developed countries that it does not bear repeating here.

The interesting question is how humans could have begun indulging in a behavior that is so unnatural, initially unpleasant, and clearly learned. The earliest records of smoking are depictions in Mayan art from 2000 years ago. By all accounts Mayans were the originators of the practice, but it became common among many Native American cultures. Tobacco was introduced to England in 1564 by the crew of the *Jesus of Lubeck*, a slave trader captained by Sir John Hawkings (1532–1595). It did not take long for tobacco to make an impact on English society. Inhaled smoke has a long and distinguished history found in many cultures. Perfumed smoke and incense have been used in ceremonies dating back to Greek and Roman times. Pliny recommended that a cure for obstinate coughs was inhaling smoke drawn through a reed (Greaves, 2000).

It did not take long for an elaborate culture to develop around smoking in Europe. While a number of different plants were smoked, one had particular appeal for its powerful narcotic properties. Jean Nicot (1530–1600) was the French ambassador to Lisbon from 1559 to 1561, and upon his return to Paris he brought tobacco plants with him. Tobacco was an instant hit with the affluent and powerful and quickly spread across Europe. The plant is called *Nicotiana tabacum*, and the psychoactive substance nicotine, in his honor (Greaves, 2000). Sailors from European countries succeeded admirably in spreading the use of the tobacco plant around the world. Interestingly, during the Thirty Years War (1618–1648) involving most of the major European continental powers, the Napoleonic Wars (1799–1815), and the Crimean War (1854–1856), smoking was encouraged by commanders, likely because of the narcotic properties of tobacco that blunted fear and hunger. In fact, During World War I tobacco products were included in military rations (Greaves, 2000).

The point of this little historical digression is to demonstrate the power that a narcotic like nicotine has over human behavior. Smoking has worldwide health implications, and the relationship between smoking and lung cancer is widely accepted (Doll & Hill, 1950). In addition to the lungs, smoking increases the risk of cancers in esophagus, larynx, tongue, salivary glands, lips, mouth, pharynx, urinary bladder, kidneys, cervix, breast, pancreas, and colon. In developed countries smoking accounts for approximately 80% of all lung cancers (World Health Organization, 2005a). Tobacco kills more people worldwide than AIDS, legal drugs, illegal drugs, road accidents, homicide, and suicide combined. Today tobacco kills more men in developing countries (1.8 million) than in developed countries (1.6 million), and soon tobacco-related deaths of women in developing countries (0.3 million) will equal the deaths among women in developed countries (0.5 million). Trends in mortality from tobacco show an unabated trend in both the developed and developing world (Mackay & Erikson, 2002) (see Figure 1-12).

So what does this have to do with evolutionary medicine? The reason that smoking is so pervasive and cessation is so difficult is that nicotine is addictive. As one researcher put it, "If it were not for nicotine in tobacco smoke, people would be little more inclined to smoke than they are to blow bubbles" (Jarvis, 2004, p. 279). If a greater understanding of the evolutionary basis for addiction as well as the exact mode of action of psychoactive drugs, including nicotine, were obtained, there would be a significant increase in the likelihood that some effective therapeutic intervention might be discovered. By reducing the number of people addicted to nicotine, a significant savings in lost lives and productivity could be achieved on a worldwide basis.

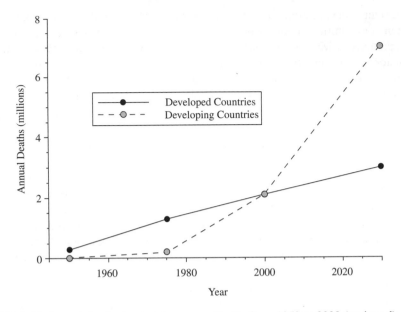

FIGURE 1-12 Annual deaths due to tobacco worldwide from 1950 to 2030 (projected). (From Mackay & Erikson, 2002.)

PSYCHIATRIC DISORDERS

Mental illness is a problem that has been understudied, underdiagnosed, and under-treated on a worldwide basis. It is estimated that 450 million people worldwide are affected by mental, neurological, or behavioral problems at any time. Mental illness is common to all countries, and individuals who suffer from mental illness are subject to social isolation, poor quality of life, and increased mortality. Twenty-five percent of patients visiting a health service worldwide have at least one mental, neurological, or behavioral disorder, but most of these disorders are neither diagnosed nor treated. Mental illness affects and is affected by many chronic diseases such as cancer, cardiovascular disease, diabetes, and HIV/AIDS. Worldwide almost 900,000 people die of suicide every year (World Health Organization, 2005b). Certainly if there is another area where an evolutionary perspective might be helpful, psychiatric disorders is one.

The application of evolutionary theory to psychiatry and the treatment of mental illness has shown great promise and enthusiasm among some clinicians (Nesse, 1984). Mental disorders are different from other kinds of medical problems. While some are caused by primary neural anomalies, many like addiction and mood disorders are often difficult to diagnose and even more difficult to treat. Dysregulated emotions such as anxiety and depression are very common. Mental disorders are widespread, affecting about half of the U.S. population according to some estimates (Nesse, 2006). Additionally con-founding the problem is the fact that about 15% of the population accounts for over half of the diagnoses. People who suffer from anxiety are likely to also be depressed, drug users are likely to be depressed or suffer from bipolar disorder, while people suffering from schizophrenia or obsessive-compulsive disorder or an eating disorder are also likely to suffer from depression or anxiety disorders. Comorbidity is a real problem when dealing with mental illness (Nesse, 2006).

There are at least two broad perspectives on dealing with mental disorders that are common in the psychiatric community. One is the medical model that was a part of the emergence of psychiatry after World War II. The emphasis in the medical model of mental illness is the discovery of a particular neurophysiological basis for a disorder. Along with research into the physiology of mental illness, clinicians became increasingly concerned about accurately defining symptoms of particular conditions and delineating boundaries. While this enterprise increases the precision of discussion of mental disorders among professionals, it also has the added benefit of fitting into the overall diagnostic schema of clinical medicine in general and the rise in importance of insurance companies in orchestrating clinical care. On the other hand, in the 1980s a few psychiatrists began to entertain the possibility that what were considered mental disorders by some could actually be defenses that were shaped and molded by natural selection. Could a mental disorder actually be an individual's way of warding off fitness-reducing events and situations? Alternatively, could some of the mental illnesses actually be the result of selection for other factors that resulted in design compromises? Is it possible that some of the mental illnesses faced by humans today are actually the product of selection for different characteristics that have greater fitness-enhancing properties and these mental illnesses are just the price that we pay for success in other areas?

Possibly because psychiatry found Freudian psychology and Watsonian behaviorism of limited utility in treating a variety of modern psychiatric disorders, clinicians have been willing to accept, at least partially, the tenets of evolutionary theory when applied to treating mental illness. One of the first comprehensive attempts at application of evolutionary theory to mental disorders was a review of how psychotherapy could profit from a greater understanding of the evolution of humans (Glantz, 1987; Glantz & Moehl, 2000; Glantz & Pearce, 1989). One of the areas highlighted in the theories about the evolution of behavior is the importance of reciprocity. Glantz and colleagues recognized that a considerable amount of psychopathology on the individual level had directly to do with emotions and motivations surrounding a lack or a failure of individuals to act in a reciprocal manner. Many people come into therapy without a correct understanding of their emotional rights and duties, their obligations to others, and the obligations of others to them. The whole notion of giving and receiving was shown to be a fundamental aspect of many social relationships that was poorly understood by one or both of the parties.

Why is reciprocity so important in social relations? The answer to that question comes from an understanding of the evolution of social behavior in a more general sense. Briefly, organisms from cockroaches to pine tress to humans are programmed to act in a manner that will maximize their own lifetime reproductive success. In a sense that means that we must act selfishly, and that is the cause for a significant proportion of human interactions. During the course of human evolution, however, there were individuals who would, in addition to acting selfishly, act altruistically to aid a nongenetic relative. Helping kin can actually be seen as selfish behavior because in a sense you are acting to benefit the proportion of your genetic material you and a relative share because of inheritance from a common ancestor. Aiding a potential reproductive competitor is a big deal, and it is one that has concerned evolutionary theorists since Darwin. The important point here is that it only makes sense to do so if there is some guarantee that your act will be reciprocated. It is easy to imagine the power of cooperative behavior in almost every aspect of life and how individuals who solved this fundamental evolutionary dilemma would enjoy an enormous advantage over those who only acted selfishly. Indeed, humans have evolved elaborate psychological mechanisms to insure that we act reciprocally, and one of the most important is guilt as well as social pressure exerted from peers. In short, an understanding of the evolutionary importance of reciprocity gave psychotherapists new techniques to deal with breakdowns in many human social relationships.

There are three broad categories of mental problems (Nesse, 2006): (1) ones that arise from primary brain abnormalities and have a high heritability (e.g., schizophrenia, autism, obsessive-compulsive disorder, bipolar disorder); (2) ones that arise from emotional and behavioral dysregulation (e.g., depression, anxiety, addiction); and (3) affective states that are aversive or socially unacceptable, but nonetheless may be fitness enhancing.

Mood Disorders

At the top of any list of mood disorders, and by inference emotional disorders, is depression. It is hardly worth citing any prevalence data on depression because it has become so common in the United States. During a 1-year period slightly over 20 million adults or about 9.5% of the population suffer from a depressive illness (National Institute of Mental Health, 2006). While at first blush it might not seem that depression should be anything more than a minor annoyance, the truth is far different. Depression has been linked to a variety of chronic diseases (e.g., cardiovascular disease, cancer, Parkinson's disease, and hormonal disorders), and when accompanied by depression any of these chronic disorders is exacerbated.

Depression is found in both men and women, but has different underlying causes. Women are roughly twice as likely as men to experience depression. While hormonal changes associated with the menstrual cycle (see Chapter 10), pregnancy, childbirth, and menopause are known to effect the incidence of depression in women, there are many aspects of our culture that also seem to be contributing risk factors (work in and out of the home, single parenthood, and caring for aging parents).

For men depression manifests itself differently than in women. Depression is associated with an increased risk of cardiovascular disease in both men and women, but men suffer a higher mortality rate (Ferketich, Schwartzbaum, Frid, & Moeschberger, 2000). Depression in men is often masked by alcohol or drugs or by the socially accepted practice of working excessively long hours. Men are less willing to seek help for depression than are women, and it is more difficult to recognize and diagnose in them. In both sexes, severe depression is marked by disruption of sleep patterns. Depressed patients report under different circumstances both an inability to sleep as well as an inability to stay awake. What constitutes a normal sleep pattern for Westerners would be 8 hours of uninterrupted sleep. Worthman (Chapter 16) alerts to the likelihood that sleep is more complicated than it seems, and ideas of what constitutes normal sleep may be founded on little more than convenience and not on any biological reality.

Given that depression, in its most severe form, can lead to suicide and in less severe manifestations to social isolation and diminished quality of life, how could such a disorder have ever arisen in the population in the first place? Depression is nothing new to the human condition. Hippocrates wrote about melancholia, and from his descriptions it is reasonably certain that he was referring to the condition that we know today as depression. For the Greeks, melancholia was due to the excess accumulation of black bile.[7] Depression has been recognized in religion (Valley of the Shadow of Death, Psalms 23:4), art (self-portrait of Frida Kahlo), literature (King Lear), and music (American blues), and so has long been a part of the human experience. While clinicians have made attempts to define depression, evolutionary biologist Robert Sapolsky said it best. Depression is a "... genetic/neurochemical disorder requiring a strong environmental trigger whose characteristic manifestation is an inability to appreciate sunsets" (Sapolsky, 1994, p. 197).

An evolutionary perspective on depression asks why such a psychological condition would have arisen when it is associated with so many costs and is so widespread? One possibility is that depression is an adaptive response to defeat and a mediator of social conflict (Price, Sloman, Gardner, Gilbert, & Rohde, 1994; Stevens & Price, 1996). Rather than challenge a competitor to whom you have already lost, it may be that a reduction in activities and a decrease in social interactions is the most adaptive response. Acceptance of defeat has the unanticipated side effect of intensifying social hierarchies and actually promotes an overall reduction in aggressive behavior. Rather than conceive of depression as mental illness, in the evolutionary context it might be viewed as a biopsychosocial adaptation.

Another possibility is that depression signals the loss of resources that are an important part of reproductive success (Nesse, 1991, 2000; Nesse & Williams, 1994a). Depression may be the signal that causes an individual to stop engaging in the behavior that brought about the loss. For example, abandoning a failed relationship certainly results in depression, and there are certainly times that depression may make an individual less likely to abandon an enterprise in which they are heavily invested. Depression and low mood may, however, cause individuals to stop investment in endeavors with a low probability of payoff.

While an evolutionary perspective does not provide a cure for depression or low mood, it does alert us to the range of mood that is part of normal human experience and suggests strategies for elevating mood that are consistent with our overall fitness-maximizing strategies. The question that arises from this view of depression is: Should all depression be treated? As with most such questions, the answer is: It depends. For people who suffer debilitating depression that significantly impairs their health and quality of life, the answer is a resounding yes. However, an evolutionary perspective alerts us to the possibility that depression may serve as an adaptive warning light that signals to us that we should change something that we are doing. For those types of situation and episodic conditions, treatment may not be warranted.

Anxiety is another emotion that is often viewed as a defect. Some people experience excessive anxiety and worry that persists for long periods of time. The anxiety is described as "free floating" and is not triggered by a specific event, unlike phobias, discussed below. People who experience anxiety disorders worry about the everyday aspects of life, many of which are beyond their control. Twitching muscles, dry mouth, clammy hands, sweating, nausea, diarrhea, and frequent urination are typical symptoms. Elevation of anxiety triggers a cascade of physiological responses in the immune system, as well as in other systems. The activation of the immune system under certain circumstances could have real fitness advantages. Like other systems, our immune system seeks homeostasis. Too much activation leads to autoimmune disorders, and too little results in immune deficiencies. Too much or too little anxiety can be fitness reducing.

"Flight or fight" is the classic response to fear-producing situations and is characterized by sweating, increase in heart rate, increase in respiration rate, increase in blood glucose levels, and the release of epinephrine, as first described scientifically nearly 100 years ago (Cannon, 1914). Of course this response is fitness enhancing in the short run, but we also know that the physiological processes that are incited by the response in long-term health consequences are not positive. On the other hand, too little anxiety does not typically result in a visit to a physician requesting anxiety-inducing drugs, but these individuals can often be found in emergency rooms, standing in a courtroom, or in jail.

Phobic disorders are a classic example of emotions that have been favored by natural selection. Notice that we did not say that the phobic disorders have been favored by natural selection because those responses are extreme manifestations of an adaptive response. In the course of human evolution it is likely that those individuals who were particularly alert or tended to avoid dangerous situations might have enjoyed an evolutionary advantage over those less vigilant or with a slightly blunted sense of danger. While there are certain costs associated with anxiety (e.g., wear and tear on tissues and organs, depletion of hormonal reserves, etc.), there are great advantages to avoiding being eaten. The "smoke detector" principle of the evolution of anxiety suggests that the cost of a few false alarms is significantly less than a positive alarm that goes undetected or ignored (Nesse, 2001; Nesse & Klaas, 1994; Nesse & Williams, 1994a). If these ideas have any merit, that knot in your stomach when entertaining the idea of climbing a tall ladder, or riding the elevator to the top of the Empire State Building, or being slid into a metal cylinder for an MRI exam is the result of natural selection. Carried to an extreme, any of these responses can be debilitating and significantly reduce quality of life, but if experienced acutely under appropriate circumstances, they would be fitness enhancing.[8] Interestingly, here is another example of discordance between our biology and our culture. If we were really in tune with our environment, we would be inherently afraid of guns, knives, electrical outlets, greasy hamburgers, and cars.

Schizophrenia

Schizophrenia is a mental disorder that has been diagnosed in cultures around the world and has an estimated lifetime prevalence of 0.55% (Goldner et al., 2002) with high variation from country to country. The incidence of schizophrenia of 7.5–16.3 cases per year per 100,000 population gives some idea of the variation. It is characterized by impairment in perception or expression of reality as well as social dysfunction. Patients suffer from delusions, auditory hallucinations, and disorganized thinking. Schizophrenics experience significantly lower fitness (0.7) than nonaffected individuals (Feierman, 1982), and the phenotypic population frequency is difficult to explain exclusively on the basis of mutations.

An evolutionary theory of schizophrenia starts from the perspective that the condition is or was favored by selection and is adaptive. The important point here is that psychiatry has recognized the genetic component of schizophrenia and is attempting to explain its persistence in modern populations. There have been a number of theories to explain schizophrenia from an evolutionary perspective. Some have suggested that schizophrenia is the outcome of uncontrolled fluctuations of glycemic levels in the brain coupled with insulin resistance (Holden, 1995; Holden & Mooney, 1994). Schizophrenia has also been connected to celiac disease. Individuals affected with celiac disease have an alteration in gut permeability in which the gut may lose its ability to block exogenous psychosis-causing substances, and circulating levels of these substances lead to schizophrenia and other mental conditions (Wei & Hemmings, 2005). Another suggestion relates the disorder to an extreme variation of hemispheric specialization and the evolution of language due to a single mutation located on the homologous regions of the sex chromosomes (Crow, 1995). Another possibility is that schizophrenia is a consequence of intense selective pressures for higher intelligence or verbal abilities in our evolutionary past. In some sense, schizophrenics are the result of intense selection and demonstrate that the costs for such cognitive advances may be individuals with particular mental vulnerabilities (Nesse, 2006). None of these, nor many other hypotheses have been proven, and so we are still left with a disease that is experienced by people living in the developing and developed worlds and results in individuals who are not fully functioning members of society and experience a reduced quality of life.

Addiction

The problem of addiction is a major area of mental health that demands serious attention and can likely be informed by an understanding of evolutionary theory. Approximately 1.2 billion people worldwide are addicted to nicotine, about 70 million are addicted to alcohol, and 5 million inject illicit drugs (World Health Organization, 2001b). If these estimates are even close to reality, that means that about one person out of three is addicted to some type of psychoactive substance. The costs in lives, lost productivity, and quality of life of such a mental illness is difficult to quantify, and attempts to do so produce numbers that are far beyond the abilities of most to comprehend. What can an evolutionary perspective provide?

If we can generate any effective treatment for the abuse of psychoactive substances, it will require an understanding of not only the neurophysiology of addiction and the proximate causal (e.g., environmental, social, familial) circumstances, but also why humans have such a high vulnerability to psychoactive drugs. A search for a particular gene for a susceptibility to drug abuse is a promising area. It is unlikely that a particular gene will be found because drug abuse and dependence are a complex set of genetic disorders that lack a simple pattern of Mendelian inheritance. Much more likely are the discoveries of gene complexes with relatively small effects that play a role in mediating drug–environment interactions.

Psychoactive drug use has a long history in human evolution. Fermented fruits are likely to have played a role in early hominin foraging strategies (Dudley, 2000, 2002, 2004) to the extent that they were a signal for edible resources. The widespread use of psychoactive substances in human evolution has been argued to be a byproduct of selective pressures for increased brain size and cognitive abilities (Smith, 1999). Only in recent times have humans been exposed to sufficient quantities of psychoactive drugs and in sufficient concentrations that use would be a problem. In the past, consumption of naturally fermenting fruit and the consumption of psychoactive plants was such an infrequent event that it would likely not have been behaviorally disruptive to the individual or to the members of a small close-knit social group. On the other hand, with the improvement in the technology of fermentation and certainly with the advent of distillation, psychoactive substances were available in previously unimaginable volumes and concentrations. Long-term consumption of these drugs is perfectly predictable based on the anatomy of the human brain. These substances are not naturally occurring and consequently represent a novel experience for human brains. They are inherently pathogenic because they bypass the evolved systems of emotional and behavioral control (Nesse & Berridge, 1997). Psychoactive drugs provide the brain with false signals of fitness benefits. The hijacking of normal regulatory processes in the brain can result in continued use of drugs that no longer provide pleasure. Sensory mechanisms that control "liking" and "wanting" may be especially susceptible to drug influence (Lende, 2005; Lende & Smith, 2002). Drugs that block negative emotions may actually be blocking evolved defenses, but under some circumstances this use could actually be fitness enhancing (Nesse & Berridge, 1997).

An evolutionary perspective on substance abuse helps us appreciate how difficult it will be to find effective long-term therapeutic techniques and interventions. As a consequence of our highly evolved big brains and elaborate cognitive abilities, we are also the possessors of neural machinery that is easily derailed by the use of novel psychoactive substances. If nothing else, evolutionary medicine should alert us to any claims of the discovery of a "magic bullet" to cure addiction.

ARE WE LESS HEALTHY THAN OUR ANCESTORS?

Much of the writing on evolutionary medicine, including most of the chapters in this volume, has focused on medical problems or "mismatches," with the usual claim that our modern lives are incompatible with our evolved bodies. The inference often drawn from this view is that we are not as healthy as our ancestors were. Of course, this is nonsense. If we look only a life expectancy, certainly there has been great improvement in the past century. How about quality of life? Again, 70-year-olds living in nonimpoverished circumstances in the developed world are, for the most part, far healthier than their counterparts in contemporary poor populations or in the past. Most of us who are fortunate to continue active and productive lives into our seventies and eighties marvel at how much healthier we are than our grandparents were. Clearly, by almost any measure, human health has improved. But does this mean that we are healthier?

"Maybe so and then again, maybe not" is probably the most reasonable answer to the question. We certainly live a lot longer than our ancestors, but is that the only measure of health? We certainly hope not. There is no doubt that the technological advances in medicine have contributed enormously to our ability to diagnose and treat disease. Never before in the course of human history have we been able to restore normal functioning to damaged cardiovascular systems, replace failing organs with new ones, treat a variety of cancers and prolong life, repair limbs lost in battle or in accidents—the list goes on and on. But we can do better. In spite of all of the advances in medicine we have seen since the beginning of the twentieth century, it is striking to note that it took until the last decade of the twentieth century for scientists to recognize the importance of the evolutionary history of the organism they were treating. Even then, an appreciation of the place of evolution in medicine is woefully underappreciated. There are many reasons for this (see Chapters 22 and 23). It is our belief and the belief of the contributors to this volume that only when clinicians and researchers take into account the role of evolution in shaping the organism being treated as well as, in many cases, the organism causing the problem or condition will we achieve something that approaches sustainable health care for all people.

WHAT DOES EVOLUTIONARY MEDICINE HAVE TO OFFER?

Throughout this chapter we have highlighted the contributions that an evolutionary medicine perspective is beginning to make to understanding health and human well-being. Because of its integrative and holistic approach, the field is well suited to drawing together seemingly disparate collections of data and thinking. However, evolutionary medicine has made only a modest impact on clinical medicine. Is changing the way some aspects of clinical medicine are practiced a reasonable or even desirable goal? We think the answer is a qualified yes.

One thing that evolutionary medicine has to offer is the generation of alternative hypotheses for the causation of various conditions. For example, it makes intuitive sense that if a poorly nourished woman receives dietary supplements during pregnancy, her infant's birth weight will increase. An increase in infant birth weight is a desirable outcome because there is a correlation between infant birth weight and reduced mortality. However, supplementation of maternal nutrition to increase birth weight has turned out to be only modestly effective (see Chapter 18). Evolutionarily based research into this seeming paradox suggests that selection has favored buffering mechanisms that enable a woman to respond slowly or not at all to a variety of nutritional changes (both positive and negative) that occur during pregnancy. In other words, the protective/adaptive ability of maternal metabolism to maintain steady supplies of nutrients to the fetus generally works as well whether maternal nutritional intake is increased or decreased. Of course, this does not mean that pregnant women should not be given supplements when necessary, but it does suggest that adaptations that have been successful for generations (i.e., buffering from pregnancy insult due to poor nutrition) may not be very responsive to short-term fixes. Because these nutritional effects are apparently transgenerational, public health measures to improve infant birth weight should likely begin long before pregnancy and should not be judged as success or failure based on data for a single generation. Too often health-related programs are abandoned if positive results are not achieved in a short time. Evolution is typically an extremely slow process. Our expectations of the rapidity of change should be tempered with some knowledge of how evolution works.

SUMMARY

We have attempted to review much of the data concerning evolutionary medicine—in particular material that was unavailable for the precursor to this volume (Trevathan, Smith, and McKenna, 1999). Both in sophistication of theory and in quality of evidence, we feel that the chapters in this volume show a maturation of the field. For the time being evolutionary medicine is likely to remain the province of a relatively small number of specialists working outside of clinical medicine, but we hope that our efforts and others by our colleagues of similar mind will push the awareness and imminent sensibility of an evolutionary approach into larger arenas. To be sure, only time will tell.

CHAPTER 2

Human Evolution, Diet, and Nutrition
When the Body Meets the Buffet

*Bethany L. Turner, Kenneth Maes, Jennifer Sweeney, and
George J. Armelagos*

As Turner and her colleagues argue so effectively here, modern humans are, indeed, omnivores, and, thus, our species has retained what they refer to as "fundamental physiologically mediated tendencies" to seek out and consume a "tremendous variety of foods." Attempting to find an answer to the question why we are so excessive in our eating (when the opportunities present themselves), they use the concept of "mouthsense" to help explain the degree to which understanding human eating patterns requires reference to cultural experiences against the backdrop of biology, which then helps us to appreciate more than ever how much more complex is the understanding of human eating patterns compared with other mammals. It is odd to think, as they point out, that as a species we lack innate knowledge as to what and how to eat. Instead, we must observe others eating in order to learn a "custom" on which our survival has come to depend. Moreover, the authors provide a view of the Paleolithic as regards what we can and cannot learn especially in trying to create a "Paleolithically correct" diet aimed at (so the promises go) restoring proper dietary balances. The critical perspective they leave us salivating over is, given our evolutionary past, how can we best determine (and then properly respond to) the "right proportions of various types of food categories as well as vitamin and mineral constituents." They make us think about how strange, on the one hand, it is that some contemporary people die because they haven't enough food, while many others ("Westerners") die because they have too much, or that some of us make so many poor selections and eat without (it would seem) caring or the ability to arrange reasonable proportions. Turner et al. end their chapter by warning us that there is no quick fix for teaching ourselves and getting ourselves to "eat right," only more choices to make about what we want to believe and feel about food, especially (at least for some of us) while foraging at our local, ever showcasing supermarkets.

INTRODUCTION

Although guidelines for a healthy diet are widely promoted in the United States, a substantial number of Americans do not consume a healthy diet. This has led to health problems including cardiovascular disease, hypertension, type 2 diabetes, obesity, osteoporosis, anemia, poor dental health, malnutrition, and some types of cancer (United States Department of Health and Human Services (HHS) and United States Department of Agriculture (USDA), 2005). In fact, most Americans are far outside the parameters of what is considered a healthy diet. In comparing data from a 2001–2002 National Health and Nutrition Examination Survey (NHANES) to the dietary standards of the current *Dietary Guidelines for Americans 2005*, the U.S. Department of Health and Human Services and the USDA found that American men and women consume far too few fruits, vegetables, whole grains, and dairy products and far too many saturated fats, starches, and refined sugars (HHS, 2005; USDA, 2004). If we as *Homo sapiens*, literally the "wise ones," are so intelligent, why do we make such bad dietary decisions? Based on their 1992 study, Murphy, Rose, Hudes, and Viteri (1992) suggest that the health community needs to better educate Americans about their food choices and engage in research that will effectively influence adults to improve their diets, a sentiment echoed in *Dietary Guidelines for Americans 2005*. However, given the extent of the problem, this nutritional crisis appears to be more than the result of poor education. Nutritional information is readily available to the public and has been since 1916, when the USDA published its first Food Guide. The many incarnations of the food pyramid that provide guidelines for a balanced diet are ubiquitous, and general nutritional information can be found on the packages of most of the items we consume. Even so, dietary health has not improved substantially in the United States (Morrill & Chinn, 2004) despite almost a century of nutrition education. Perhaps it is not the availability of information, but rather the kind of information, that is critical to changing modern American dietary practices. In this chapter we review literature in developmental psychology, neuroscience, nutrition, and anthropology with an explicitly biocultural focus in order to elucidate aspects of human dietary evolution that inform attempts to improve nutritional health in the United States and elsewhere in the industrialized world.

We present an evolutionary approach with a biocultural perspective (Armelagos, 1987) to help us understand the current dietary dilemma. We are living in a time characterized by soaring rates of obesity, heart disease, hypertension, and diabetes, a health crisis shaped in part by patterns of eating forced to keep up with a fast-paced lifestyle. The "time famine" experienced by dual income families in the United States has led to increased consumption of foods prepared away from the home, which are often nutritionally deficient. Foods prepared away from home are higher in calories, total fat per calorie, saturated fat, sodium, and cholesterol, and are lower in dietary fiber, calcium, and iron, than foods prepared and eaten at home (Guthrie, Lin, et al., 2002). Nowadays, families eat together less often, and more than a third of U.S. parents admit to eating more than one fifth of their meals in the car (Gardyn, 2002).

We as a species inhabit the full range of the earth's environments, with concomitant variation in amounts and types of available resources, which demonstrates that human populations can adapt their diet to widely differing ecological niches. In a cultural sense, many of us are adapted to an industrialized world. But nutritionally speaking, it appears that the industrialized world, where various foods are plentiful on an unprecedented scale, is detrimental to our nutritional health. The relative uniqueness of the industrialized world in the grand theater of our evolutionary environments has prompted many to question whether or not humans are still choosing dietary items according to the biological needs and behaviors shaped by natural selection (Eaton, Eaton III, et al., 1997; O'Keefe & Cordain, 2004; Stinson 1992), and the degree to which cultural factors both reflect and override innate, evolved propensities.

In this chapter we discuss human genetic and developmental mechanisms that reflect an evolutionary history of encephalization, dietary generalism, and markedly increased social learning capabilities. These derived traits influence our diet, taste preferences, and nutrition in dynamic and complex ways. We also consider the two-way dynamic between the biology of food choice and cultural systems. This is a fruitful avenue to explore, given that eating is cross-culturally replete with symbolism, ritual, and performance and treated with great importance. We explore the dietary consequences of encephalization; the biology of taste, distaste, and regulatory mechanisms of feeding; aspects of food choice and the omnivore's dilemma; and the intersection of our Paleolithic legacy, evolutionary medicine, and modern lifestyles. To this end, we argue that the adaptive changes that enhanced our use of high-density food, which were important to survival in our early evolutionary history, now represent a dilemma in an environment were there is an overabundance of nutritionally dense foods.

FEEDING A THINKING BRAIN

A biocultural approach to exploring the evolution of our diets calls for consideration of both physiological and behavioral factors in shaping how and why we eat what we eat. However, if the goal is to understand how the human diet is evolutionarily derived, it is insufficient to only look at the human species. The scope of variation in nonhuman primate diets is too broad to address here (the reader is referred to Milton & May, 1976, for more information on primate dietary patterns; Ankel-Simons, 2007; Chapman & Chapman, 1990; Chivers & Hladik, 1980); however, looking at key trends in our hominin lineage allows us to deduce several important evolutionary developments that took place as human feeding behaviors evolved from those of our hominin ancestors.

Among the suite of features unique to the human lineage is a very large brain. In proportion to our overall body size, we have considerably larger brains compared to our closest ape relatives, other primates, and other mammals in general. However, overall brain size is not the only issue here. Dunbar (1998) points out that what is important to human encephalization is the enlargement of the neocortex. The neocortex is a uniquely mammalian feature of the brain associated with social cognition, those aspects of perception, behavior, and memory associated with social interaction. Dunbar argues that in numerous primates and other social mammals, the size of the neocortex is strongly associated with group size and thus the complexity of social interaction. This association leads Dunbar to suggest that group sociality was a *causal* factor in the evolution of larger brains, especially in the human lineage. In other words, the fitness benefits of increased sociality, which depended on larger neocortices, were the selective factors that structured this evolutionary process. But the neocortex did not change alone—other researchers have emphasized that the neocortex belonged to a suite of anatomical and life history traits that evolved together, feeding back on one another (Kaplan, Hill, et al., 2000). The challenge has been to explain and model these evolutionary feedback processes involving brains, bodies, and behaviors. This endeavor has produced important developments in life history theory.

Aiello and Wells (2002) note that among ancient African hominins, *Homo ergaster* (which they equate to early African *Homo erectus*) shows a dramatic increase in overall body size and cranial capacity compared to earlier *Homo habilis* and australopithecines. The authors interpret these anatomical changes as reflecting a substantial change in lifestyle, including such features as increased energy requirements, increased brain size, and delayed maturation. Charnov and Berrigan (1993) argue that an extended juvenile period entails a prolonged period of social learning and cognitive development and emphasize the importance of long juvenile periods among both chimpanzees and humans. Theoretically, the importance comes from the extra investment that is put into social learning and cognitive development, which pays off in the long run by equipping individuals to compete in a selective arena of steadily increasing sociality.

It therefore appears that social skills and cognitive development were "prime movers" in the evolution of increased encephalization as part of an adaptive complex geared toward learning and social cognition. In humans, this is especially apparent: the average human brain is almost five times the size one would expect given the average human body size (Aiello & Wheeler, 1995, p. 200). There is strong evidence that building and maintaining the neural information processing network of a large brain is metabolically costly (Laughlin, de Ruyter van Steveninck, et al., 1998). So where did the extra needed energy come from? Making the question even more complex, Aiello and Wheeler point out a seeming paradox: while human brains consume a substantial amount of energy, humans do not show a corresponding increase in basal metabolic rate (BMR). To resolve the question of how the human lineage has been able to feed their big brains without an increased metabolic output, Aiello and Wheeler propose the expensive tissue hypothesis (ETH) (see also Gibbons, 1998), which posits that the metabolic demands of an expanding brain are balanced by a decrease in another metabolically expensive organ, namely the gut.

This hypothesis is based on the fact that humans not only have larger than expected brains for the average body size but also smaller than expected guts. Based on fossil hominin morphology, Aiello and Wheeler extrapolate this relationship back to the emergence of early *Homo* approximately 2 million years ago. The authors argue that the *only* way these shifts in gut size could have occurred was if there was a substantial change in the diet. A larger gut serves to extract nutrients from low-quality, hard-to-digest foods such as mature leaves and fibrous plants. A shortening of the intestinal tract implies the opposite adaptation: a shift to easily digested, higher quality foods such as fruits, young plants, oil-rich seeds, and animal protein. Milton (1999, 2000) has also pointed out this fundamental association between gut size and dietary quality. Successfully seeking out these higher quality resources would have involved drastically altered, and possibly more complex, foraging strategies (Aiello & Wheeler, 1995, Fig. 5). In turn, these behavior changes imply increased cognitive activity and versatility.

The ETH does not posit diet as a prime mover in brain evolution: in this model, it was not a dietary change that *caused* an expansion in brain size. Rather, diet "permits a relatively small gut and liberates a significant component of BMR for the encephalized brain. No matter what was selecting for encephalization, a relatively large brain could not be achieved without a corresponding increase in dietary quality unless the metabolic rate was correspondingly increased" (Aiello & Wheeler, 1995, p. 211). In this model diet is a "prime releaser" (Aiello, 1997), giving the green light for brain expansion driven by causal factors having to do with fitness benefits of social cognition (Dunbar, 1998), thermoregulation (Falk, 1990), and maternal investment in big-brained, slow-maturing offspring (Hawkes, O'Connell, et al., 1998).

This research demonstrates the centrality of diet in the physiological and behavioral evolution of the human lineage. If we support the metabolic demands of our big, active brains while maintaining other bodily systems by consuming a high-quality diet, a key question follows: How do we obtain those high-quality foods? As discussed above, there are numerous elements of human diets that intertwine physiology and complex cultural behavior. We now turn to exploring these relationships in greater depth as a way to see how and why humans eat what they do, and when (over the life course and over the course of history) these patterns of behavior develop.

DOES BIOLOGY DETERMINE FOOD CHOICE?

Human food selection, especially during very young ages, appears to be controlled by neural regulatory mechanisms that stimulate feelings of hunger and satiety. Rowland, Li, and Morien (1996) model these neural mechanisms according to a cascade of interactions between the medulla, pons, hypothalamus, and limbic forebrain. In this neurological cascade, numerous signal molecules are involved in the stimulation of hunger and feeding, including norepinephrine, neuropeptide Y, galanin, and opioids (Drewnowski, Krahn, et al., 1992; Rowland, Li, et al., 1996), while opoids, as well as other molecules such as serotonin, insulin, satietin, and corticotropin-releasing hormone, simulate feelings of satiety (Rowland, Li, et al., 1996). Often, feelings of hunger and satiety are stimulated well before an individual actually runs out of energy or consumes harmfully excessive amounts of food (Capaldi, 1996; Deutsch, 1987). This suggests greater complexity to physiological regulation of eating than is assumed by earlier homoeostatic models in which an individual's feeding behavior was in direct, immediate response to physiological deprivation or excess, in an attempt to return, nutritionally speaking, to a homeostatic state (Booth, 1987). Conspicuously absent from this suite of signaling molecules, however, are any that specifically limit fat intake (Phillipson, 1997), despite neural and visceral mechanisms limiting intake of dietary protein and carbohydrates (Friedman, 1989; Li & Anderson, 1989; Tordoff, 1989) and other nutrients (Bates, Sharkey, et al., 1998).

Also innate to human eating behavior are competing tendencies towards neophobia (suspicion of new foods as potentially harmful) and novelty (seeking variety in the diet) (Birch & Fisher 1996; Leathwood & Ashley, 1983). These behaviors are mediated by regulatory mechanisms such as sensory-specific satiety, a type of "palate fatigue" whereby preference for a specific food or taste declines as it is eaten, while preference for new foods and tastes remain unaffected (Drewnowski, 1995; Hetherington & Rolls, 1996).

Humans tend to exhibit several inborn taste tendencies influencing their food choices. These are broadly characterized as similarities in "mouthsense," defined as a suite of taste, textural, and odor perceptions that occur when chemical compounds from foods interact with chemoreceptors in taste papillae on the tongue and odor receptors in the olfactory epithelium (Duffy & Bartoshuk 1996; Rozin, in Wysocki & Pelchat 1993). These receptors are distributed throughout the tongue and all recognize five basic tastes: sweet, bitter, sour, salty, and glutamate, or savory *(umami)* (Duffy & Bartoshuk 1996; Chaudhari, Landin, et al., 2000). Taste, textural, and olfactory signals are generated by these receptors and sent to key areas of sensory convergence in the brain, such as the left orbitofrontal cortex (de Araujo, Rolls, et al., 2003).

Facilitated by these neural sensory and regulatory mechanisms, humans exhibit broad but near-universal taste tendencies, including a persistent liking for sweet tastes and a disliking for bitter and sour tastes, and these tendencies are present at or before birth (Anderson, 1995; Blass, Shide, et al., 1989). Genetic variation in sensitivities to certain bitter compounds such as 6-n-propylthiouracil (PROP) and phenylthiocarbamide (PTC) does affect the degree of liking for bitter compounds and other tastes (Bankovi, Forrai, et al., 1993; Ly & Drewnowski, 2001; Yackinous & Guinard, 2001), especially in women after the onset of menarche (Duffy & Bartoshuk 1996). This genetic variation in taste sensitivity shows the potential for genetic mediation of food choice (Capaldi, 1996). Recent research has suggested an innate, inborn liking for glutamate *(umami)* taste, although not necessarily for its intrinsic taste properties but rather for its ability to enhance the palatability of the other four tastes (Beauchamp, Bachmanov, et al., 1998; Bellisle, 1999). Also, numerous studies show that preferences for the taste of sweet foods are significantly enhanced by adding texture from fat (Drewnowski 1989, 1995, 1997). In this sense, there is empirical evidence for what has been popularly called a "sweet tooth." With Drewnowski's research, we can add the term "fat tooth" to our dietary lexicon.

These complex and varied regulatory mechanisms, taste preferences, and behaviors all make sense when viewed in light of human evolutionary history, even those that may seem counterintuitive. The presence of satiety mechanisms for protein and carbohydrate intake, but not fat intake, was likely highly adaptive for much of human history, where human feeding behavior was more closely tied to resource seasonality, the unpredictability of hunting or scavenging, and the paucity of fat found in most plant foods (Phillipson, 1997). Consuming as much fat as is available is detrimental only when fat is constantly abundant, as it is in many modern food systems (Drewnowski, 1997). The presence of anticipatory hunger cues prior to any actual deficiency, and satiety cues prior to detrimentally high intakes, have obvious adaptive benefits in that actual starvation or excessive intake is avoided (Deutsch, 1987).

Understanding the biology of fat in the diet better elucidates its role in the Paleolithic. Speth and Speilman (1983) were among the first to provide an analysis of the cost and benefits of meat consumption. Their study found that during periods of marginal caloric intake, hunters and gatherers are likely to hunt large ungulates. Since these animals are also subsisting on declining resources, their reserves of body fat become depleted, and lean meat becomes a principal source of energy. The use of large quantities of lean meat has nutritional costs, including elevated metabolic rates, higher caloric requirements, and deficiencies in essential fatty acids. In many gathering and hunting societies, taboos prevent pregnant women from eating meat. Speth (1991) speculates that these taboos prevented excessive protein consumption (above 25% of total calories) that could be harmful to the fetus (see Fessler & Navarrete, 2003, for a cognitive explanation for meat taboos). Hunter-gatherers subsequently develop subsistence strategies that increase carbohydrate and/or fat intake. Speth and Spielmann suggest three strategies that can achieve these results: (1) an increase in the selection and procurement of smaller animals with high fat content; (2) storage of fat-and carbohydrate-rich foods; and (3) an exchange of these items with other groups as an alternate way to procure needed food resources. Recent archeological research has revealed how these strategies played out in the late Paleolithic adaptations of human populations (Stiner, 2001; Stiner & Munro, 2002; Stiner, Munro, et al., 1999, 2000).

Proclivities for sweet and sweet–fat combinations and for glutamate taste enhancement are highly adaptive in guiding omnivores to safe (nonpoisonous), macronutrient-dense foods (Anderson, 1995; Yamaguchi and Ninomiya, 2000). Conversely, human newborns display an inborn dislike of bitter and sour tastes, but this dislike appears to be concentration dependent; bitter and sour solutions that are diluted below certain concentrations fail to elicit any response at all (Mennella & Beauchamp, 1998). This behavior makes sense in light of the fact that while many bitter compounds are in fact poisonous, some contain medicinally beneficial phytochemicals when eaten in small amounts (Dillard &German, 2000; Le Coutre, 2003), while vitamin-rich fruits are often sour when unripe (Laska, Scheuber, et al., 2003; Nishida, Ohigashi, et al., 2000). These studies illustrate the benefits of consuming some unpleasant-tasting foods within an adaptive complex in which potentially toxic substances are avoided. Finally, sensory-specific satiety as a physiological facilitator of variety seeking in food choice provides one adaptive mechanism for overcoming neophobia towards unfamiliar resources (Leathwood & Ashley 1983).

The presence of many of these inborn tendencies among rats, chimps, and other omnivores supports arguments that human food choice is indeed a complex suite of adaptive traits reflecting our mammalian evolutionary history (Bellisle, 1999; Nishida, 1989; Ulijaszek, 2002). The key question that remains, however, is how many of these traits are actually genetically "hard-wired"? As will be discussed below, extensive research suggests surprisingly few. Within the past two decades, human food choice has been increasingly conceptualized around the primacy of learning and the near-constant contingencies of environmental and social contexts. Contrary to homeostatic models of food choice in which humans seek out foods based primarily on innate drives (Beidler, 1982), numerous studies of rats (Leathwood & Ashley, 1983), guinea pigs (Hudson & Distel, 1999), and human children (Birch, 1987; Birch & Fisher, 1996) suggest that there is no such thing as the "wisdom of the body" whereby foods are selected in direct response to physiological needs for specific nutrients such as sodium (Beauchamp, 1989) or animal-based protein (Simoons, 1994).

Moreover, while omnivores tend to seek out and express preferences for diets that are balanced in nutrient composition, it seems clear that what is actually mediating this tendency is the association of sensory properties, including taste, odor, texture, irritant qualities, and even color (Clydesdale, 1993) with positive or negative postingestive consequences (Leathwood & Ashley, 1983). In essence, an animal will not seek out a dietary regime that is balanced so much as one that makes it feel good; diets that are deficient in key nutrients such as protein will not be avoided because they are deficient, but rather because the animal suffers the symptoms of malnutrition. These associated taste properties and postingestive consequences may or may not have any relation to the macronutrient and micronutrient properties of the foods themselves (LeMagnen, 1987; Tordoff, 1989). The strengths of these learned associations show in the rapidity, intensity, and duration of aversions to tastes and even food odors that are associated with negative postingestive consequences such as nausea, allergy, anaphylaxis, or gastric distress (Bernstein, 1999). This can occur to the extent that foods or food odors that were once liked can become disgusting if they are associated with nausea or vomiting (Pelchat & Rozin, 1982), whether or not they had any causal role in the associated ill effects.

Even the mechanisms regulating hunger and satiety are shaped by expectations of meal frequency and duration, meal size and importance, to the extent that feelings of hunger and fullness may occur independent of any physiological deprivation or repletion (Capaldi, 1996; Ramsay, Seeley, et al., 1996). Aside from broad similarities in basic taste perception, preferences for and avoidances of specific foods are typically learned within contexts of social interaction. Indeed, animal studies suggest that most omnivores may be incapable of learning how to select adequate diets early in life unless they are able to observe and learn the feeding behaviors of other, often related, conspecifics (Galef, 1989, 1996). Even innate dislikes of irritant or bitter foods, such as chili pepper and black coffee, displayed by nonhuman primates and dogs are overcome without incentive within human-mediated social contexts (Rozin & Kennel, 1983).

The primacy of social learning in food preferences is especially clear in humans, for whom eating is rarely divorced from social and cultural spheres. Numerous studies point to factors like ethnicity (Hudson & Distel, 1999; Rozin, 1996), family experience (Birch, 1987; Rozin & Millman, 1987), and cultural practices (Lupton, 1994; Mela, 1999; Messer, 1986; Simoons, 1994) as more immediately salient to shaping taste preferences and food choices than biological drives or innate tendencies.

Additional research suggests that many highly salient, learned taste associations and resultant eating behaviors are shaped very early in development. Flavors from foods ingested by pregnant women, including garlic, mint, vanilla, carrot, anise, and alcohol, are present in amniotic fluid and breastmilk (Mennella & Beauchamp, 1998; Schaal, Marlier, et al., 2000) in addition to other compounds normally found in breastmilk such as citric, lactic, and pyruvic acids, salts, urea, amino acids, and sugars (Mennella & Beauchamp, 1996). Rather than acting as passive flavor receptacles, fetuses actively retain and associate liked and disliked flavors, even those related to maternal electrolyte depletion (Crystal, Bowen, et al., 1999), in ways that are known to influence postnatal taste preferences and guide feeding behaviors (Barker, 1982). Following birth, infants are exposed to flavors in breastmilk that further shape acceptance of flavors and flavor variety and willingness to try new foods well into childhood (Blass, Shide, et al., 1989; Hudson & Distel, 1999; Wright, 1987). In turn, food exposure and preferences established during critical periods of social learning in childhood have lasting effects on neophobic tendencies, preferences, and choices throughout life (Birch & Fisher, 1996; Casey & Rozin, 1989).

FOOD CHOICE AND THE OMNIVORE'S DILEMMA: A LEGACY OF EVOLUTION

The shift from viewing hard-wired tendencies to learned behaviors as most critical in shaping taste preferences and food choice does not require abandoning the notion that these learned behaviors are adaptive in an evolutionary sense. The omnivorous behavior that characterizes many primates, including humans, is highly adaptive in that it expands a given species' foraging range and accommodates seasonal variation. Reliance on an omnivorous diet, typically a pattern of collecting with some predation and at least rudimentary sharing, likely shaped the dietary patterns of our hominin ancestors and carry over in part to our own diet.

Although taste preferences and aversions are clearly developed through experiential learning, their adaptive significance remains clear. The ability to quickly recognize a harmful substance by taste or odor and permanently retain that association, despite a delay between ingestion and effect, is clearly adaptive to a variety-seeking omnivore. Likewise, the ability to learn substance avoidance through observing the aversions of others is clearly beneficial to an omnivore (Schafe & Bernstein, 1996). The development of preferences based in part on learning from conspecifics cuts a great deal of trial-and-error out of risky food selection (Galef ,1996), thereby enhancing success in consuming the wide variety of safe foods that satisfy human nutrient needs (Armelagos, 1987). As an example, no unequivocal relationship has been found between modern, cross-cultural pregnancy cravings and nutrient appetites, or between prenatal aversions and food toxins (MacClancy, 1992; Pelchat, 1997; Profet, 1992; Rodin, 1989). Nonetheless, there may be some adaptive significance to these preferences and aversions, especially aversions to easily spoiled foods such as meat (Fessler, 2002). In fact, the heightened taste sensitivity alone could serve as an adaptive and protective behavior through increased maternal scrutiny of any and all potential foods during pregnancy.

It seems clear that on an individual basis, humans have a complex suite of physiological mechanisms by which they become familiar with new foods, distinguish "good" versus "bad" in exploring potential food resources, and commit to memory an extensive and dynamic database of food-related information. At the group level, where knowledge, values and experience are exchanged and shared, humans have equally complex cultural toolkits used to better exploit available food resources. Among these toolkits are culturally constructed systems of food acquisition, preparation, and eating known as cuisines. Paul Rozin (1976) suggests that cuisines are cultural inventions that mediate biological nutritional needs within groups that share knowledge and values. The cuisine of a given group is an analyzable system of shared knowledge and values, which exists amidst a social and natural ecology. Researchers can seek to answer questions of, for instance, why certain changes occur in a group's food selection, preparation, and consumption habits (Farb & Armelagos, 1982). Changes in the dietary system can occur differentially in what Elizabeth Rozin (1982) calls the four components of a cuisine: The foods selected from the environment, the manner of preparation, the flavor principles employed, and rules established for eating. Viewed in this way, change in the environment, or change in any of these four components, influences the entire system in interesting feedback loops. Functionally speaking, one role of a cuisine is to balance neophobia and sensory-specific satiety through the incorporation of novel foods in familiar gustatory contexts (Farb & Armelagos, 1980).

Cuisines represent codified, structured, culturally constructed, and socially learned practices that are complex, highly variable, and contingent on available resources. Cuisines are also highly adaptive in that they allow human groups to efficiently manipulate, and sometimes even create, the food resources around them in ways that are attuned to local environmental constraints. For example, the use of milk and ghee but not of beef in some Indian cuisines permits a sustainable use of cows well adapted to India's climatic and economic landscape (Harris, 1978). Another example, widespread and intensive use of spices in many tropical cuisines, may reflect the adaptive use of antimicrobial plant products (Billing & Sherman, 1998) and an adaptive reversal of apparently innate dislikes of bitter tastes (Rozin, Ebert, et al., 1982). Spices also allow what Rozin and Rozin (1981) describe as theme (consistency in flavor) and variation (variety) in food combinations. For example, to an uninitiated palate, the flavor of curry may seem to be a single taste. However, populations who customarily use curry blends in their cuisine vary the spices to provide a different taste, resulting in a multitude of curries that help avoid palate fatigue. In addition to flavor principles, particular processing techniques are nutritionally very useful and sometimes mandatory in avoiding ill effects. These include soaking or cooking to remove toxins from otherwise inedible foods such as bitter manioc (Dufour, 1995), fermenting soy to make it edible while retaining its nutrients (Barnes, 1998), and mixing complementary amino acids through combinations of rice and legumes or lime-processed corn (Farb & Armelagos, 1980; Katz, 1982; Stinson, 1992). The complex suites of rules, techniques, and combinations that characterize the myriad cuisines worldwide clearly represent behavioral adaptations used to maximize the ways in which human populations exploit available resources in the varied environments in which they live.

In sum, there are complex neurological, psychological, and cultural mechanisms by which humans have been able to learn about, associate, manipulate, and create food resources in ways that are highly adaptive. Most of these mechanisms are not hard-wired in the sense that most of them are learned at various points in an individual's life. Within this broad adaptive framework, however, it is possible, and useful, to generalize about the costs and benefits of different subsistence patterns (ways of procuring food) employed by humans throughout our evolutionary history and to use the insights gained to inform our own modern dietary patterns. As we will show, some of the most widespread and popular dietary solutions in the United States attempt to map out lifestyle plans based on the postulated diets of our Neolithic, Paleolithic, and earlier hominin ancestors. A number of these studies follow rigorous scientific methods and have been highly influential in shaping what we know about variety, change, benefits and costs of prehistoric diets. Unfortunately, these scholarly works have been used to create numerous popular publications that claim the same degree of scientific validity. These popular publications have misinterpreted the findings of scientific investigations in evolutionary medicine and have to a large extent ignored our evolutionary history as generalists and omnivores. Molding diets after those of our ancestors is a prime example of the culturally constructed nature of cuisine. While popular diets based on ancestral diets aim to be more adaptive, misinformation and simplification often prevents them from achieving such a goal.

THE SEARCH FOR A TRUE HUMAN DIET

There has in recent decades been a major reinterpretation of human dietary evolution based on reconstructions of dietary patterns during the Paleolithic and Neolithic periods. In the late 1970s, empirical evidence emerged that suggested the transition to agriculture during the Neolithic period brought about significant biological costs, such as stunted growth, increased susceptibility to infectious disease, and increased risk of famine (Cohen & Armelagos, 1984). To theorists at the time, this seemed counterintuitive. Many theorists and the public alike assumed that agriculture, though toilsome, is superior to other modes of production in meeting the nutritional needs of humans on a grand scale. In his influential book, *The Food Crisis in Prehistory*, Cohen (1977) argued that changes at the end of Pleistocene led to larger, more sedentary human populations that soon ran out of their foraged food resources. This supposedly resulted in a nutritional crisis that forced populations to shift to primary food production (i.e., farming), as opposed to foraging, in order to have enough food. This theory led to hypotheses that can be tested in various archaeological contexts throughout the Old and New Worlds. If Cohen's theory was the case, then evidence of nutritional deficiencies such as skeletal lesions or growth disruptions caused by nutritional insults should be apparent in different settings directly *before* local origins of agriculture. In turn, the same kind of evidence would be expected to decline after agriculture was fully implemented (but see Armelagos & Harper 2005). However, the archaeological record did not provide such evidence.

In fact, emerging empirical evidence suggested a decline in health *with* the shift to agriculture. Populations that underwent a subsistence shift to primary food production showed an increase in infectious and nutritional diseases (Cohen, 1989; Cohen and Armelagos, 1984). The rise in infectious disease was predictable, since populations were becoming sedentary, denser, and larger, and these demographic changes would lead to more exposure to pathogens that are more easily transmitted (Armelagos 1990, 1998). Moreover, with the reliance on single grains to provide the bulk of dietary calories and nutrients, groups became more susceptible to famine as the result of blights and droughts in an unpredictable climate from year to year. In addition, rising social inequality with increasing population density and sedentary life increased the potential for nutritional deficiencies in lower, more vulnerable social strata (Armelagos & Brown, 2002).

These bioarchaeological and paleodemographic studies all led to the realization that the transition from hunting and gathering to agriculture during the Neolithic had significant, negative effects on human populations. This in turn led to research, grounded in the emerging field of evolutionary medicine (Williams & Nesse, 1991), that suggested there was much to learn about our American dietary trends by comparing them to those of contemporary hunter-gatherers. In a seminal paper, S. Boyd Eaton and Melvin Konner (1985) championed what they called the Paleolithic diet. Eaton and coworkers used the archaeological record and recent foragers' patterns of subsistence to analyze the nutritional properties of wild game and "uncultivated" vegetable foods. The authors' goal was not to constrain a specific diet or even set of diets that encompassed all human populations throughout our evolutionary history. Rather, they were clear in their objective to outline broad nutritional similarities between widely varied hunter-gatherer diets, such as micronutrient content, amounts and types of fats, proteins and sugars, and fiber content. References to a "Paleolithic average" should therefore be interpreted in terms of general nutritional characteristics, not in terms of actual foodstuffs. Within this framework, Eaton and Konner provided a strong contrast between the "average" preagricultural forager diets, based largely on wide varieties of collected wild plants and hunted lean meat with minimal processing, and the "average" American diet (Eaton & Konner, 1985, Table 5). Modern foragers consume about 55% fewer calories from dietary fat (20% vs. 36%), more than 600% more fiber (100 vs. 15 g/d), and have 55% less body fat on average as measured by skinfolds (9.6 vs. 17 mm) compared to modern Americans. Eaton and coworkers have expanded their database to include more nutritional information on game animals and what they call "wild" vegetables (Eaton, Eaton III, et al., 1997, 1999), including the amounts of fiber (Eaton, 1990), calcium (Eaton and Nelson, 1991), and a host of important micronutrients in these foods. Importantly, Eaton and colleagues emphasize the inertia of biological evolution: in the 10,000 or so years between the shift from hunting and gathering to agriculture, there has been insufficient time for any genetic adaptations to the rapid changes in human diets. Therefore, no matter how much our dietary *behavior* has changed over the past 10 millennia, *biologically* human populations have remained the same. Eaton and colleagues used this disconnect to characterize modern humans as "Stone Agers in the fast lane" (Eaton and Konner, 1986; Eaton, Konner, et al., 1988). Importantly, the authors note that evolved gustatory behaviors, such as strong proclivities for sweet and salty tastes and fatty textures, convey selective benefits to hunter-gatherers. This is because food sources with these characteristics tend to be calorically dense and relatively scarce in environments where game animals are lean, water possibly scarce, and plant foods low in sugars. However, in modern, industrialized food systems where sugars, salts, and fats are in endless, easy supply, these same evolved behaviors can lead to overconsumption, obesity, and metabolic diseases. Humans have only had a regular surplus of food for the past century, yet the effects of this surplus on health are immediately obvious. In 2004, 65% of the adult American population was overweight and obese (Stein & Colditz, 2004) and in 2005, an estimated 30.5% of U.S. adults were clinically obese (Li, Bowerman, et al., 2005).

This increased attention to the disparity between modern and Paleolithic dietary patterns, and the notion that many modern humans are eating against the evolutionary grain, so to speak, led to a more intensive reexamination of both the modern foragers' and modern Americans' diets. Eaton and colleagues' original 1985 article captured the attention of physicians and nutritionists, and the authors (Eaton, Eaton III, et al., 1997) have continually updated the key elements and merits of the diet that patterned the nutrition of our Paleolithic ancestors. Eaton, Shostak, and Konner (1988) expanded their model in *The Paleolithic Prescription*, which provides a program of diet, exercise, and "design for living" that was highly adaptive for Paleolithic populations. In fact, they argue that the dietary characteristics of our remote ancestors may serve as a reference standard for modern human nutrition—"a model for defense against certain 'diseases of civilization'" (Eaton & Konner ,1985, p. 288).

Contrasting with Eaton and Konner's modeled Paleolithic diet is the average American lifestyle. As of 2001, 72% of married Americans with children under 18 were employed outside the home (Jabs & Devine, 2006). Americans today have more stringent time constraints and increasingly purchase prepared foods. While in the 1960s, 65% of the American family food dollar went to grocery stores, in 1997 only 50% did (Park & Capps, 1997). Because both parents work, little time is invested in preparing foods, and as a recent *Time Magazine* article explained, the shared family meal has become a "quaint kind of luxury" (Gibbs, 2006).

Many families believe that long work hours, inflexible schedules, and overtime work leave them without the necessary energy to prepare meals that meet their nutritional ideals. People cope by adopting different food-procurement strategies such as keeping the home stocked with microwavable foods, cooking large meals on Sundays to be reheated throughout the week, or stretching a large pot of soup through several meals by adding ingredients each night (Devine, Conners, et al., 2003; Jabs and Devine 2006). In addition, the American public has demonstrated a desire to spend less time cooking, and the food industry has responded with more prepared foods, takeout meals, and devices such as microwaves, rice cookers, and other options to decrease cooking time. Despite the increasingly limited time spent on preparing meals at home, these meals are likely still more nutritious than counterparts purchased away from home. Families that eat meals together tend to consume less soda and fried foods and far more fruits and vegetables (Gibbs, 2006).

However, another modern food-procurement strategy involves extensive consumption of foods prepared outside of the home. Eating out has increased from 10% of all food expenditure in 1960 to 47% in 1998 (Beale, 2000; Caplan, 1997). Between 1970 and 1990, the typical dual income family increased their annual market work by 600 hours, and this may account for why consumption of food away from home increased from 18% to 32% of total calories between 1977–78 and 1994–96 (Finkelstein, Ruhm, & Kosa, 2005). Since 1985, fast food sales have increased at a faster rate, growing annually at a rate of 6.8% and comprising 34.2% of all food purchased outside the home in 1997 (Jekanowski, 1999). More than a third of U.S. parents say they eat takeout food regularly and one fifth of all meals are consumed in a car (Gardyn, 2002). Foods prepared outside the home, and often chosen for meals eaten "on the run," are usually high in dietary fat, sodium, and calories and low in fruits, vegetables, fiber, calcium, and iron. Because of the time famine dual income families experience, many are consuming more ready-prepared meals, eating fewer family meals at home, and eating more meals away from home, all of which may lead to nutrient deficiencies and negative effects on their health (see Chapter 3).

The modern American lifestyle has wrought changes not only to the diet, but to activity patterns as well, which the *Dietary Guide for Americans 2005* (HHS and USDA, 2005) emphasizes as equally important to overall health. Jeffery and Utter (2003) and Stein and Colditz (2004) found that over the past 20 years, Americans have increasingly used private vehicles for transportation, and there has been a commensurate decline in use of bicycles, public transportation, and walking. Inactive leisure activities involving television viewing, video games, and home computers require decreased amounts of physical activity, and many labor-saving devices such as lawn mowers, television remote controls, and garage door openers have further decreased normal daily activity levels. These two studies also link these sedentary activities to greater weight in children and adults, due either to a corresponding decrease in physical activity or an increase in related food consumption. Stein and Colditz determined that in 2004, 60% of the U.S. population did not participate in regular physical activity and that 25% of the population was almost completely sedentary.

It is not our objective to imply that Paleolithic subsistence is inherently superior to that in industrialized countries such as the United States, nor is it our objective to imply that the modern American diet is wholly unhealthy. The increased capabilities for food production, transport, and storage that characterize industrialized food systems have contributed, in many nations, to a life expectancy of over 70 years, far beyond Eaton and Konner's Paleolithic average. However, the modern American dietary pattern does differ substantially from the diets of our Paleolithic ancestors, as do food-procurement strategies, in that the American diet is based primarily on refined carbohydrates and fats, limited in both nutrient quality and breadth, and requiring almost no physical activity whatsoever to obtain. Reliance on this dietary pattern has increased within the last 50 years, translating our abundance of food into a health crisis.

EVOLUTIONARY MEDICINE AND DIET: *CAVEAT EMPTOR*

Eaton and colleagues provide an intriguing hypothesis that many current health problems, including obesity, diabetes, heart disease, hypertension, and osteoporosis, can be explained at least in part by our deviation from the dietary pattern that characterized much of our evolutionary history. However, the authors also temper their interpretations by cautioning that formal dietary recommendations based on a Paleolithic model are premature, emphasizing that an "awareness of Paleolithic nutritional patterns should generate novel, testable hypotheses grounded in evolutionary theory" (Eaton & Eaton III, 2000, p. 67). This rigorous analytical perspective has been echoed by Cordain, Eaton, Sebastian, et al. (2005), Cordain, Gotshall, Eaton, and Eaton III (1998), Cordain, Watkins, and Mann (2001), and Somer (2001), in attempts to assess and apply the Paleolithic diet to contemporary populations and offer practical dietary solutions (Cordain, 2002; Cordain & Friel, 2005).

With these scholarly studies, however, has come a flood of popular publications, including *NeanderThin: A Cave Man's Guide to Nutrition* (Audette & Gilchrist, 1995), *Nourishing Traditions: The Cookbook That Challenges Politically Correct Nutrition and the Diet Dictocrats* (Fallon & Enig, 1999), *Charley Hunt's Diet Evolution: Eat Fat and Get Fit* (Hunt, Eades, et al., 1999), *Health Secrets of the Stone Age* (Goscienski, 2003), and *Metabolic Man: Ten Thousand Years from Eden* (Wharton, 2001). These authors do not engage in the level of research that characterizes the work of Eaton and coworkers, Cordain and associates, and Somers. Instead, they have relied on the on catchy titles and promotional materials.

These popular books show that, unfortunately, evolutionary medicine has spawned for-profit dietary prescriptions that are scientifically vacuous and theoretically sterile (Armelagos, 2004). A prime example of this phenomenon is the book *Eat Right 4 Your Type* (D'Adamo & Whitney, 1996). In this book, the authors present individualized diet plans based on a person's ABO blood type, customizing diets to different ABO blood groups that they claim represent separate trajectories in the course of human evolution. For example, they argue that blood type O is the earliest to have evolved and dates back to the origin of Cro-Magnon populations, and that type O populations were and still can be characterized as optimal meat eaters. Conversely, blood type A populations were originally cultivators who emerged about 25,000–50,000 years ago and have a evolved a sensitive digestive tract that is best adapted to a vegetarian diet. Blood type B reflects the evolution of nomadic ancestors who migrated out of Africa to Europe, Asia, and the Americas about 15,000– 10,000 years ago, and individuals with type B blood are advised to include dairy products in their diet. The AB blood type first appeared about 1500 A.D. through the recent intermingling of various groups, and type AB individuals are advised to eat a blend of the type A and type B diets.

In examining D'Adamo and Whitney's evolutionary scenario, it is difficult to find a single fact that can be used to support their arguments about the typological nature of blood groups or the relationship of the blood groups to diet. In fact, studies of ABO blood type distribution across human populations have found strong associations to infectious disease prevalence, *not* to dietary needs. Aho et al. (1980) predict differential suscepti-bility to influenza according to blood type, while Koda et al. (2001) suggest that the frequencies of alleles coding for different blood types are shaped by natural selection. Seymour et al. (2003) are even more specific, modeling the distribution of the ABO blood system according to distinct selective pressures from bacterial and viral pathogens. The distribution of ABO blood types in populations therefore reflects disease risk, not subsistence pattern. Nonetheless, D'Adamo and Whitney present their "evolutionary" argument for the ABO diet types as established science and have convinced readers of its validity. *Eat Right 4 Your Type* has been so successful (over a million copies have been sold and it has been translated to into 40 languages) that D'Adamo and Whitney have published companion books, such as *Cook Right 4 Your Type* (1998) and *Live Right 4 Your Type* (2001). When advice such as this is sold as evolutionary medicine, it surely has an impact on popular perceptions of the paradigm. Those readers that recognize these books as scientific nonsense could not only reject it, but also reject evolutionary medicine and the evolutionary paradigm altogether. Or worse, they will have bought into a perversion of evolutionary medicine that is built on assumptions and "facts" that have no scientific basis (see Armelagos, 2004).

ASSESSING THE EVOLUTION OF HUMAN DIETS

At this point we can revisit a key question, namely: Why do we in the modern world make such unhealthy dietary choices? We know that part of what makes human food choice so adaptive is that it is highly varied and that much of it is contingent on external influence and learning. As a species, humans are able to eat an incredible variety of resources; through processing techniques we can even turn poisonous plants into nutritious foods, and through cuisines we can create endless resource combinations. We also know that there are a few tendencies, such as a preference for sweet tastes and fatty textures, that appear to be inborn and lifelong, and that in our modern world where sugars and fats are consistently abundant, these inborn tendencies can create harmful effects on our health. Similarly, we know that for much of our evolutionary history, human populations had diets that, however varied, were very different from the prepared foods that make up the base of our modern diets. How can we use this knowledge to address the modern nutritional crisis, while avoiding the pitfalls of bogus "evolution-ary" diets?

Perhaps one way is not to focus on just the types of foods, but the *variety* of foods in our diets. Perhaps we should view the capacities for negotiating and shaping our gusta-tory environment as more significant in an evolutionary sense than hard-wired tendencies such as our sweet tooth or fat tooth (Ramsay, Seeley, et al., 1996). In this sense, the Paleolithic diet becomes significant not only for its high fiber content and paucity of sugars, but also for its wider breadth: Cordain, Brand Miller, Eaton, et al. (2000) note that modern hunter-gatherer populations, who are often relegated to marginalized lands, utilize varying percentages of over 100 food resources each. In the modern world, it seems that there are more choices than ever in what to eat, but the vast majority of foods in the American diet are different combinations of the same few ingredients, such as corn, sugar, and animal fat. Sidney Mintz (1996, p. 118) cites the USDA's list of 10 major sources of calories in the United States as "whole and lowfat milk; white bread, white flour, rolls, and buns; soft drinks, margarine and sugar; and ground beef and American cheese," while the Food and Agriculture Organization (FAO) reports that over the past 30 years American intake of oils and sugars has doubled (FAO/Earthscan 2003). In 1996, the average American ate 152 pounds of caloric sweeteners per year (USDA, 1998). This reliance on a few staple foods is potentially as significant to our poor dietary health as the staples themselves.

What may then be maladaptive about dietary habits in the modern world is not the excessive consumption of calorically dense foods but a dramatic narrowing of dietary breadth; the causal arrow is not drawn just to innate proclivities run amok but to another innate capacity, that of extreme omnivory, suppressed. The gustatory plasticity and generalist subsistence strategies displayed by humans was and is well suited to varied and fluctuating environments, which human populations have faced throughout their evolutionary history (Colson, 1979; Eaton, Eaton III, et al., 1997, 2002; Nestle, 1999; Nishida, 1989; Ulijaszek, 2002). What may be selected, therefore, is hard-wired flexibility in various capacities for learning food preferences during early development (Barker, 1982; Hudson & Distel, 1999; Mennella & Beauchamp, 1996) and through social interaction (Galef, 1996; Ramsay, Seeley, et al., 1996; Rozin, 1982, 1996; Nestle, Wing, et al., 1998). This hypothesis fits well with more general models that show the selective benefits of phenotypic and behavioral plasticity during human evolution (Potts, 1998) and omnivory in general (Galef, 1989; Rodman, 2002).

It should be noted that a handful of population-level adaptations have arisen in response to limited food resources, including the ability to digest lactose into adulthood (Simoons, 1982), although some, such as favism, are as much in response to endemic disease as to food resources (Stinson, 1992). Overall, however, we argue that to habituate and socialize one's taste preferences to a narrow range of foods, thereby winnowing one's diet to a few processed macronutrients to the near exclusion of dietary variety, is what makes modern food choices so maladaptive. The modern American diet, with its reliance on fast food, processed fats, and carbohydrates, and marginal inclusion of unprocessed plant foods, could therefore be seen as not only too fatty and too loaded with "carbs" but also entirely too narrow.

Adding to this problem is the plethora of diet plans centered on weight loss or weight management through dietary restriction. Americans perceive restrictive diets to be the most effective, turning to books that advise cutting out all flour and sugar (Gott & Donovan, 2006) or eating disproportionate quantities of rice (Gurkin Rosati & Rosati, 2006), grapefruits and cider vinegar (Dunford, 2002), or cabbage soup (Danbrot, 2004). However, if we look at humans as omnivores who evolved to learn about, manipulate, and consume a wide array of resources, the shortcoming of these diets is immediately obvious: there is no dietary variety. Our emphasis on breadth as a critical component of a healthy diet underscores the potentially substantial role that dietary monotony, through the prodigious marketing efforts of the modern food industry, has on derailing long-term health. Assessments of modern diet plans would benefit from critical scrutiny based on our evolutionary history of consuming widely varied food resources.

CONCLUSION

We have provided a number of biocultural avenues for understanding the dilemma of what many consider the dietary crisis in the United States. The ways in which food and the body interact provide some key pieces to the puzzle of why we eat what we eat. Our physiology and phylogenetic history have developed complex interactions with food, made even more complex by our capacity to learn about and manipulate food resources. As we have shown, biological checks and balances are easily manipulated or overridden by social and cultural factors, in this case with deleterious health effects. Our reliance on high-density foods, relatively scarce for much of our evolutionary history, can easily be made maladaptive in an industrial food system that provides such foods in unprecedented abundance. As important, our reliance on substantial dietary breadth has become distorted in a modern food system, our diets paradoxically limited by our reliance on thousands of prepared foods made from a few high-density ingredients.

It is therefore clear that an evolutionary and biocultural perspective is of critical importance when exploring the causes of and solutions to the growing dietary crisis in the United States. Examining the mechanisms of human feeding behavior while elucidating the evolutionary events that have shaped them allows us to better understand how our modern eating habits fit in, or not, to the rest of our evolutionary history. Ultimately, quick-fix diet fads, especially those that claim a basis in evolutionary medicine, must be replaced in popular publication with rigorous scientific research and sound biocultural models if the epidemics of diabetes, obesity, and other health problems are to be effectively addressed. Contextualizing human diets and human food choice within an evolutionary, interdisciplinary, and biocultural framework is, as we hope to have shown here, the most powerful way to understand and alter our modern dietary patterns to achieve better health.

CHAPTER 3

Diabesity and Darwinian Medicine
The Evolution of an Epidemic

Leslie Sue Lieberman

Lieberman's eclectic and comprehensive review of the metabolism of eating and the ecology of factors surrounding eating, including why we eat as we eat, what we eat, and why so much at each setting, is remarkable for its depth and range. Integrating proximate and ultimate explanations, she traverses across the many different disciplines, illuminating an evolutionary point of view on diabesity and the neuroendocrinology and physiology of eating, carbohydrate metabolism, and fat storage. Yet she also addresses the range of emotional factors and learned processes that explain why it is apparently so difficult for our species to get the proper proportions of food down to more optimal levels, especially in industrialized nations. She talks of the role of novelty, our need for companionship, the way friendship affects eating, as well as mood, and discusses the meaning of food during rituals and cere- monies, all of which "seduces" omnivores to eat often, even if we are less hungry than our actual behavior might suggest. She discusses the texture and colors of food and shows why, from a psychological point of view, the old expression "Your eyes are bigger than your stomach" is really true, as humans are not capable (see also Chapter 2) of judging more optimal portions using internal hunger cues. Finally, she points out the many ways in which cooking has augmented our intellectual capacities by incorporating tools needed to harvest food and how cooking expands our dietary breadth by killing poten- tial pathogens such as parasites. Her chapter is a bountiful feast, full of all consuming tidbits of knowledge!

INTRODUCTION

Comparative and evolutionary perspectives provide lenses through which to view the growing pandemic of the co-occurring conditions of obesity and type 2 diabetes. The conditions are linked because type 2 diabetes results from metabolic processes associated with obesity. "Diabesity," first proposed in 1980, has been used by a number of researchers (Astrup & Finer, 2000; Daly, 1994; James, 2005; Zimmet, Alberti, & Shaw, 2001).

The underlying assumption is that the diabesity pandemic is the result of a mismatch of Stone Age genotypes adapted to environments with fluctuating food availability and high energy demands and contemporary Space Age lifestyles with abundant food and low energy costs (Broadhurst, 1997; Chakravarthy & Booth, 2004; Eaton, Strassman, Neese, Elwald, Williams, et al., 2002; Neel, 1962) (see also Chapters 2, 4, 8, and 18). These ancient cognitive, behavioral, and physiological genotypes and phenotypes adapted to feast and famine and exercise and rest cycles persist today in evolutionary novel obesogenic environments (Boon, Stroebe, Schut, & Jensen, 1998; Booth, Pinkston, & Poston 2005; Brownell & Horgan, 2003; Cordain, Gotshall, Eaton, & Eaton, 1998; Hill & Peters, 1998; Liebman, 1999; Lieberman, 2006; Nestle, 2003; Speakman, 2004; Wansink, 2004a, b, c). Obesogenic landscapes coupled with our metabolic efficiency have created a perverse normalcy of excessive weight gain (Bray, 1987; Brownell and Hogan, 2003; Kuzawa, 1998; Nestle, 2003; Popkin, 2001; Rolls, 2003; Speakman, 2004; Spurlock, 2005).

This chapter examines the nexus of human biology and behavior and characteristics of contemporary environments that are conducive to obesity and type 2 diabetes. A Darwinian medical perspective is used to suggest approaches that differ from current cognitive–behavioral interventions to stem the growing pandemic of diabesity and its adverse health outcomes.

Definitions and Diagnostic Criteria

Diabetes is a group of metabolic diseases characterized by high blood sugar or hyperglycemia. Type 1 diabetes, previously called insulin-dependent diabetes or juvenile diabetes, is an autoimmune disease with usual onset in childhood. It affects about 5% of all individuals with diabetes. Type 2 diabetes, previously called non–insulin-dependent or adult-onset diabetes, usually occurs in adults who are obese but has been increasing among overweight children and adolescents. It affects approximately 90% of all individuals with diabetes. The remaining 5% of individuals with diabetes include women with gestational diabetes caused by metabolic alterations in pregnancy and people with diabetes caused by genetic abnormalities, infectious diseases, and trauma (American Diabetes Association, 2004a; Centers for Disease Control, 2005b). The focus of this chapter is type 2 diabetes.

Diagnostic Criteria for Diabetes

Chronic hyperglycemia or a high blood sugar level is the defining hallmark of diabetes. It can result from defects in pancreatic insulin secretion and/or insufficient insulin action in muscle or adipose (fat) tissue. The American Diabetes Association (2004a, b) defines type 2 diabetes as a random glucose $\geq$ 200 mg/dl (11.1 mmol/l) or a fasting plasma glucose $\geq$ 100 mg/dl (5.6 mmol/l) or a 2-hour oral glucose tolerance test with a plasma glucose $\geq$ 200 mg/dl (11.1 mmol/l). Individuals with diabetes may have the following symptoms: frequent urination, hunger, thirst, weight loss, blurred vision, and skin itchiness, among others (American Diabetes Association, 2004a). Insulin levels may be high, low, or normal. Neurological and vascular damage can occur throughout the body, leading to kidney failure, blindness, and lower limb amputations (Zimmet, Alberti, & Shaw, 2001). Diabetes currently affects more than 20 million American adults (American Diabetes Association, 2004a, b; 2006). More than 85% of individuals with type 2 diabetes are significantly overweight, obese, or have a recent history of obesity (American Diabetes Association, 2004; Centers for Disease Control, 2002).

Diagnostic Criteria for Obesity

Obesity is the primary risk factor for type 2 diabetes and related conditions such as metabolic syndrome, syndrome X, insulin resistance metabolic syndrome, and impaired glucose tolerance. All these conditions are characterized by elevated insulin and glucose levels. Medically, obesity is defined as an excess amount of body fat (National Institute of Diabetes, Digestive and Kidney Diseases, 2001), but body fat is rarely measured by clinicians or researchers. The diagnosis of obesity is based on standard values for waist circumference, hip/waist circumference ratio, body weight for age, sex, and height, and body mass index $[(BMI) = wt (kg)/ ht (m^2)]$. BMI is widely used in epidemiological and clinical research. BMI has the following classification system: underweight (less than 18.5), normal weight (18.5–24.9), overweight (25–29.9), obese class 1 (30–34.9), obese class 2 (35–39.9), and morbid obesity (40 and greater). The BMI classification system applies to both males and females (National Institute of Diabetes, Digestive and Kidney Diseases, 2001).

In addition to total body fat, the distribution of fat in the body is involved in the regulation of energy use and risk for chronic diseases (Bouchard & Johnson, 1988; Bray, Bouchard, & James, 1998). A centripetal distribution of fat (i.e., apple shape) is indicated by a large waist circumference and large stores of fat in the abdominal viscera. Visceral fat confers a greater risk for cardiovascular disease and type 2 diabetes than large deposits of fat on the hips and thighs (i.e., pear shape) (Bouchard & Johnson, 1988; Bray, Bouchard, & James, 1998).

There are a number of ways of measuring body fat. Skinfold (fatfold) measurements are taken at standardize sites on the body (e.g., mid-upper arm over the triceps muscle, medial mid-thigh) and used in population-, age-, and sex-specific equations to estimate total body fat. Other techniques that measure body fatness, such as dual-energy X-ray absorptiometry (DEXA), underwater or hydrostatic weighing, bioelectrical impedance, near infrared interactance, computed tomography (CT), magnetic resonance imaging (MRI), and ultrasound, require expensive equipment, are time consuming, and are rarely used in public health contexts (Heymsfield, Lohman, Wang, & Going, 2005; University of Georgia, 1998).

In summary, type 2 diabetes and related conditions, (for example, metabolic syndrome) are defined by high levels of blood glucose (i.e., hyperglycemia). In contrast to the direct measures of blood glucose, obesity or an excess amount of body fat is inferred from physical measurements of body size and mass, such as height and weight. Because body composition is not measured, BMI classification may not accurately reflect fat stores for women with low bone mass or males with high muscle mass. However, BMIs of 30 or greater are used worldwide to define obesity and report its prevalence (Figure 3-1).

Male and Female Obesity Levels

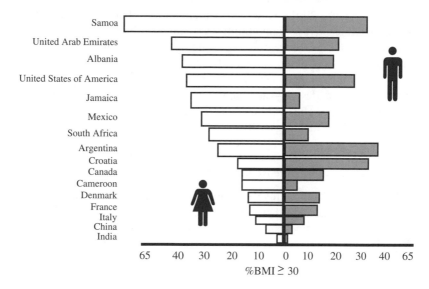

FIGURE 3-1 Prevalence of obesity in selected countries. (From International Obesity Task Force 2006 www.itof.org. Figures from late 1990s to 2002.)

METABOLIC MECHANISMS REGULATING OBESITY AND DIABETES

Humans have a complex physiological system used to maintain energy balance. Hormonal and neurological mechanisms control appetite (i.e., hunger and satiety), food consumption, and energy and nutrient storage in organs and tissues (Wynne, Stanley, McGowan, & Bloom, 2005). There are multiple pathways with significant redundancy that favor both a drive to eat and a low sensitivity to satiety (Melanson, 2004; Wynne, Stanley, McGowan, & Bloom, et al. 2005). Additionally, humans have an extraordinary ability to store fat, a good ability to store proteins, and, with moderate physical activity, a daily turnover of carbohydrate stores (Bray, 1987). Natural selection has favored fat storage and metabolic thriftiness in infants, children, and pregnant and lactating women, especially when energy intakes are low and/or energy demands are high due to illness burden, growth and development, pregnancy, and lactation (Kuzawa, 1998; Lieberman, 2003; Neel, 1962, 1999a, b; see also Chapter 18).

Energy balance is closely regulated despite huge variations in daily food intake and energy expenditure (Bray, 1987; Bray, et al. 1989). Bray calculated that the "average" nonobese, adult American male consumes approximately 1 million kcal a year. With only a 10% alteration in either energy intake or expenditure, the result can be a 30-lb.

(13.6-kg) weight gain in a single year. Even a tiny surfeit of 5 kcal a day can result in a 24-lb. (11-kg) weight gain over a 40-year time span (Bray, 1987). During most of human history changes in caloric intake or activity levels compensated for these small surfeits (Jenike, 2001; Leonard, 2001). However, contemporary urban and suburban environments provide few incentives or opportunities to maintain a "normal" body weight so that populations around the world are now experiencing unprecedented increases in obesity (Brownell & Horgan, 2003; International Obesity Task Force, 2004).

Contemporary environments are providing the means—high food availability and low-energy-expenditure lifestyle—and evolution has provided the mechanisms of efficient energy storage and metabolic thriftiness that are driving the diabesity pandemic (Eaton, Eaton, & Konner, 1999, Lieberman, 2006).

The Regulation of Appetite

The regulation of food intake involves physical factors (e.g., gastric distension and emptying), gut enzymes and other peptides (e.g., amylase, cholecystokinin, ghrelin), neuropeptides (e.g., dopamine, neuropeptide Y (NPY), pancreatic peptide (PP) and hormones (e.g., insulin, glucagon, leptin, ghrelin). Table 3-1 presents the key peptides and hormones involved in the internal or endogenous control of appetite. Neuropeptides are chemicals that are found in the brain that aid in communication among neurons (Wikipedia, 2006b). Hormones are chemical substances that are produced by organs and tissues and secreted into the blood. They influence the activities, including metabolism, of other organs and tissues (Wikipedia, 2006a).

TABLE 3-1 Internal (Endogenous) Appetite Control

Hormone or neuropeptide	Source	Effect on appetite
Enhances appetite		
Neuropetide Y (NPY)	Hypothalmus	↑
Agouti-related peptide (AG RP)	Hypothalmus	↑
Orexin	Hypothalmus, stomach, intestine, pancreas	↑
Dopamine	Hypothalmus, central nervous system	↑
Resistin	Adipocytes	↑
Ghrelin	Stomach, intestine	↑
Depresses appetite		
Insulin	Pancreas	↓
Pro-opimelanocortin (POMC)	Hypothalmus	↓
Cocaine & amphetamine regulated Transcriptase (CART)	Hypothalmus	↓
Endocanabinoids	Hypothalmus	↓
Leptin	Adipocytes, stomach, placenta	↓
Adiponectin	Adipocytes	↓
PP-fold peptides PYY, PP, NPY	Intestine, pancreas (PP)	↓
Cholecystokinin (CCK)	Intestine	↓
Proglucagon, GLP-1, OXM	Pancreas, intestine, central nervous system	↓

Source: Wynne et al., 2005.

Insulin is a hormone essential in regulating carbohydrate and fat metabolism by facilitating energy storage in cells (Porte, Baskin, & Schwartz, 2002). It is produced by the pancreas and secreted in response to eating and the concentration of glucose in the blood. Insulin levels reflect the sensitivity of muscle and adipose tissue to the insulin-mediated transport of glucose into cells. This sensitivity is determined to a large extent by the total amount of body fat, and particularly, the amount of visceral or abdominal fat. This fat is more metabolically active than fat located in other parts of the body (Wynne et al., 2005). When adipose tissue cells (i.e., adipocytes) fill with triglycerides and fatty acids, they become resistant to the transport of glucose, causing a rise in blood levels of glucose (i.e., hyperglycemia) that trigger a rise in insulin secretion. If the high insulin levels are unable to reduce blood glucose concentrations to normal levels, then individuals are considered to have insulin resistance or "prediabetes" (ADA, 2004b). Although insulin primarily regulates carbohydrate metabolism, it also has roles in increasing fat storage and decreasing the breakdown of muscle protein to make glucose (Wynne et al., 2005). If glucose or its stored form, glycogen, are not used for fuel, then fat is oxidized or "burned" for fuel and ketones are produced. Using ketones to meet energy demands prevents the muscle protein from being used to meet energy needs and preserves muscles that are needed for foraging and other activities. Ketones also decrease hunger and elevate mood (Cahill and Veech, 2003).

Insulin receptors are widely distributed in the brain. Insulin has a direct effect on the hypothalamus and acts to decrease food intake and body weight. However, experiments with administration of insulin causes a drop in blood glucose levels, which stimulates eating (Nicolaidis & Rowland, 1976). When this occurs, the counterregulatory hormone glucagon is produced by the pancreas and facilitates the release of energy stored as glycogen in the liver. This results in a rise in blood sugar to re-establish glucose homeostasis (Wynne et al., 2005). Insulin responses linking peripheral sensitivity to the central nervous system are mediated by interactions with other hormones and neurotransmitters (e.g., leptin, NPY) (Wynne et al., 2005).

The hypothalamus has both hunger and satiety centers that influence feeding behaviors. Specific hypothalamic nuclei are the targets of neuropetides and hormones (Wynne et al., 2005). These peptides are involved in energy homeostasis but also have pleiotropic or other effects. For example, the hypothalamic peptide pro-opiomelanocortin (POMC) is decreased by fasting and increased in the presence of leptin, a hormone secreted by adipocytes (fat cells). Mutations in the POMC gene or abnormalities in processing POMC result in early onset obesity, adrenal insufficiency, and red hair in humans (Wynne et al., 2005).

Eating activates many central nervous system neuropeptides that create pleasant sensations and act as endogenous rewards. These peptides include dopamine, endocannabinoids, and serotonin (Wynne, et al., 2005). Other hormones and neuropeptides produced by the stomach, intestines, adipocytes, pancreas, and other organs respond to eating and influence these reward pathways (Wynne et al., 2005). For example, leptin has a direct influence on the hypothalamic reward pathways (Fulton, Woodside, & Shizgal, 2000).

The links between obesity and diabetes involve the balance of several adipocyte signaling proteins or neuropeptides, including leptin, adiponectin, and resistin. After a meal, adipocytes release leptin, which acts on the appetite-control center activating the pro-opiomelanocortin (POMC) and cocaine and amphetamine regulated transcript (CART) neurons in the hypothalamus and creating a state of satiety or "fullness." People (may) stop eating. Mice lacking the gene for leptin production or lacking leptin receptors overeat and become obese. When leptin-deficient mice are given leptin, they eat less and lose weight (Halaas et al., 1995). However, mice and rats are more sensitive to leptin deficiency that promotes weight gain than they are to high levels of leptin that decrease appetite and promote weight loss (Levin & Dunn-Meynell, 2002). This imbalance in leptin sensitivity may reflect selection for high sensitivity in dietary environments of unstable or inadequate food availability and a diminished regulatory role for leptin in environments of food abundance (Wynne et al., 2005). Although leptin was the basis for the development of antiobesity drugs, the administration of leptin has not been an effective approach to appetite control or weight loss in humans (Wynne et al., 2005).

Adiponectin is produced by the adipocytes in response to food restriction and weight loss in laboratory rodents and humans (Hu, Liange, & Spiegelman, 1996). It decreases insulin resistance and increases muscle cell metabolism (Wynne et al., 2005). If adipocytes fail to produce adiponectin, a decreasing adipocyte sensitivity to feeding and energy intake could lead to overconsumption of food and obesity. Because some overweight diabetic patients are deficient in adiponectin, it has become a new target for development of obesity drugs to boost adiponectin levels (Wynne et al., 2005).

Resistin is a recently identified adipocyte peptide that decreases insulin resistance and promotes fat storage. Levels of resistin, unlike adiponectin, increase with obesity and decrease with weight loss (Ahima, Qi, & Singhal, 2006). Drugs that decrease resistin also increase adiponectin. Researchers are actively seeking other adipocyte peptides.

The gastrointestinal (GI) tract also produces many neuropeptides that respond to energy homeostasis by regulating hunger and satiety. (Table 3-1) Ghrelin is a protein that acts in the hypothalamus to stimulate appetite. It is produced primarily by the stomach in response to fasting, and levels decrease after eating (Cummings et al., 2001). In humans, ghrelin levels, like leptin, are high in the morning and low at night, which is appropriate for diurnally active humans (Cummings et al., 2001). Some obese individuals have low ghrelin levels or demonstrate a slow response in the decline of ghrelin levels with eating. Therefore, they continue to eat increasing their risk of excessive calorie intake and obesity (Wynne et al., 2005).

Other GI track neuropeptides include the PP-fold peptides (PYY, PP, NPY) secreted by cells in the intestine and pancreas. These peptides, like ghrelin, decrease rapidly after eating and produce satiety by acting in the hypothalamus. Some obese humans have low levels of PYY and a slow response to food intake (Arosio et al., 2003; Challis et al., 2003). Rodents and humans given PYY and PP reduce their food intake, lose weight, and improve their control of glucose levels (Challis et al., 2003). However, acute stress has been shown to override the satiety effects of PYY (Wynne et al., 2005).

Cholecystokinin (CCK) and the proglucogon products (GLP-1, OXM) are hormones produced primarily in the intestine and released in response to eating. They increase satiety and decrease food intake (Wynne et al., 2005). CCK stimulates the release of enzymes from the pancreas and gallbladder, increases intestinal motility, slows gastric emptying, and decreases food intake (Wynne et al., 2005). CCK is also found in the brain, where it acts as a neurotransmitter involved in the regulation of reward behavior, memory, anxiety, and satiety (Crawley & Corwin, 1994). CCK and GLP-1 normalized blood glucose levels when administered to people with diabetes (Nauck et al., 1993). Administration of OXM reduces ghrelin levels (Cohen et al., 2003)

In summary, food intake and metabolism are regulated by complex interactions of many peptides produced by and acting in the central nervous system, GI tract, and other organs. Because the prime regulatory mechanisms are sensitive to hunger and relatively insensitivity to satiety, eating is favored over restricted food intake. This makes evolutionary sense in environments with fluctuating and uncertain food supplies. The regulatory system promotes eating when you can, eating as much as you can, and storage of energy for times when food is not available. The identification of adipocyte hormones and neuropeptides and the elucidation of their mechanisms of action on appetite provide helpful insights into the development of new therapeutic products and molecular and cellular targets that have an evolutionary basis rooted in dietary constraints present throughout most of hominin evolution (Lee & DeVore, 1968; Ungar & Teaford, 2002).

Other Biological Factors Implicated in the Etiology of Diabesity

In addition to the endocrine and GI systems involved in diabesity, recent research has found that obese individuals suffer chronic, systemic low-grade inflammation. Adipocytes secrete a number of different cytokines (e.g., interleukin-6, tumor necrosis factor-α), which are a class of proteins that promote inflammation (Lee and Pratley, 2005). Moreover, obesity increases the number of macrophages (i.e., immune cells associated with inflammation that engulf and digest cellular debris) in adipose tissue. Both cytokines and macrophages increase with psychosocial stress (Black, 2006). Cellular inflammation and chronic activation of the immune system subsequently lead to obesity, insulin resistance, and type 2 diabetes (Lee and Pratley, 2005). Reducing fat stores decreases the inflammatory response and reduces insulin resistance (Black, 2006).

Cutting-edge research points to intestinal microorganisms or microflora, which are implicated in obesity because of their heightened ability to extract calories from food, particularly polysaccharides (i.e., sugars found in plant foods). Some bacteria also enhance fat deposition (Backhed, Ding, Wang, Hooper, Koh, et al., 2004; Ley, Blackhed, Turnbaugh, Lozupone, Knight, et al., 2005). Experiments with mice demonstrate that the presence of Firmicute bacteria in the gut is correlated with obesity and insulin resistance (Backhed et al., 2004; Henig, 2006; Ley et al., 2005). If research on humans confirms this association, then gut microorganisms will present a new target for therapeutic interventions (Backhed et al., 2004; Henig, 2006).

COGNITIVE AND BEHAVIORAL REGULATION
OF APPETITE AND EATING

Appetite and food intake are regulated not only by biological factors but also by psychological states (e.g., depression, anxiety) (Boon et al., 1998; Polivy & Herman, 2006), social contacts (Wansink, 2004b), beliefs (Rozin, 2000, 2005) cultural practices and habits (Kittler & Sucher, 2004), hedonics (e.g., taste) (Drewnowski, 1997; Johns & Keen, 1985), and atmospherics (e.g., lighting, music) (Wansink, 2004a, b). Vision, olfaction, taste of edible stimuli, and even thinking about food initiate the cephalic phase of digestion with the secretion of saliva, gastric acid, gastrointestinal hormones, and pancreatic enzymes (Katschinski, 2000).

Although individuals voluntarily diet to lose weight for health and esthetic reasons, both experimental and naturalistic observations document that humans are very stressed by voluntary food restriction when food is available (Polivy & Herman, 2006; Rogers, 1999). When individuals do restrict food, they rebound with overconsumption and "yo-yo" between weight loss and regain (de Lauzon-Guillain et al., 2006; Hill, 2004; Polivy & Herman, 2006). Cognitive control of eating is a demanding task, especially in environments with persistent cues to eat. These stimuli (for example, the sight and smell of food) lead to the disinhibition of eating behaviors in which people lose control, "go off their diets," and sometimes develop disordered eating patterns (e.g., binging and purging) (Hill, 2004; Rogers, 1999; Polivy & Herman, 2006). Polivy and Herman (2006) argue that restrained eating and chronic dieting are behaviors that defy our evolutionary heritage and that restrained eating or "calorie conservation" makes evolutionary sense only when food is in limited supply. Self-control when the food supply is limited may be helped by the tendency to decrease intake when there is limited variety (i.e., sensory-specific satiety) (Raynor & Epstein, 2001). Our evolutionary history reflects food deprivation by necessity and not by choice so that when food is available humans are biologically and psychologically prepared to eat. Polivy and Herman conclude that dieting in obesogenic environments is a "recipe for overeating and distress" (2006, p. 34).

Psychosocial distress increases cortisol, a hormone that raises blood sugar levels and increases the storage of abdominal fat (Melanson, 2004). Researchers have begun to examine the role of stress in populations with high rates of obesity and diabetes. For example, diabesity has been linked to stress-inducing historical, social, and economic circumstances reflecting discrimination and health disparities among indigenous peoples, including Native Americans (Ferrier and Lang, 2006). Many good examples of historical trauma, genocidal and ethnic "cleansing" campaigns, and blaming-the-victim policies and practices are documented in *Indigenous Peoples and Diabetes. Contemporary Empowerment and Wellness*, edited by Ferrier and Lang (2006).

Stress is related to a rise in the number of people with sleep deprivation and sleeping disorders (Keith et al., 2006). Short habitual sleep duration (e.g., 5 hours vs. 8 hours per night) is associated with reduced leptin and elevated ghrelin levels (Taheri, Lin, Austin, Young, & Mignot, 2004). People with shorter sleep duration have higher BMIs due to increased appetite and energy intake (Keith et al., 2006). They also suffer a higher prevalence of sleep apnea (i.e., temporary cessation of breathing), wake frequently during the night, and are fatigued with low activity levels during the day (Keith et al., 2006).

Other Behavioral and Lifestyle Factors Contributing to Diabesity

Other behavioral factors may be contributing to the diabesity pandemic. Keith and colleagues (2006) have generated a long list of potential contributors. These include the declining number of people who are smoking tobacco. Smoking suppresses appetite, reduces food intake, and increases metabolism, thereby reducing the risk of obesity. Temperature regulation of microenvironments (e.g., air-conditioned cars) reduces energy expenditures needed to maintain comfortable body temperatures. Pharmaceutical use has increased, and some drugs are linked to weight gain (e.g., injected insulin, antipsychotic drugs). Endocrine disruptors (e.g., insecticides, herbicides, detergents, resins, plasticizers) that may alter fat metabolism are found in food and water.

In addition, there are a number of recent demographic trends that may be contributing to the pandemic. For example, there is an increase in weight with age, and people are living longer. With declining birth rates in many countries, the middle and older age segments of populations are increasing relative to the younger component (Popkin, 1994, 2004). An increasing percentage of the U.S. population is comprised of obesity-tolerant ethnic groups who value larger body sizes (Brown & Konner, 1987; Kittler & Sucher, 2004). People choose mates who look like themselves (i.e., positive assortative mating) so that large-bodied people marry other large-bodied people, providing a potential genetic and social basis for increases in the proportion of the population who are large-bodied and/or obese (Keith et al., 2006). The etiology of the diabesity pandemic is clearly multifactorial.

EVOLUTIONARY MECHANISMS, THRIFTY GENOTYPES, AND PHENOTYPES IN OBESOGENIC ENVIRONMENTS

Although this chapter focuses on the contemporary environment, it is important to review the theoretical underpinnings of the current ideas about the deleterious nature of genotypic thriftiness. Geneticist J. V. Neel proposed a thrifty genotype for glucose utilization among Native Americans as an evolutionary explanation for the high prevalence of type 2 diabetes seen in those populations (see Chapters 4, 17, 18, and 19; Neel, 1962, 1999a, b). He hypothesized that a feast-and-famine existence conferred a selective advantage and increased reproductive fitness for those individuals who had the ability to release insulin quickly, to thriftily store energy during times of food abundance, and to efficiently utilize energy deposits during dietary deprivation. Shifts to modern lifestyles rendered a once adaptive genotype detrimental, leading to obesity and type 2 diabetes (Neel, 1962, 1999a, b).

Many authors have expanded on the thrifty gene hypothesis for other populations with additional selective pressures: cold stress from water and long oceangoing voyages for Pacific Islanders, extreme cold stress for Eskimo and Aleut populations, and high seasonal energy demands under conditions of slavery for African Americans (Lieberman, 2003). In conclusion, the thrifty genotype hypothesis does not fit well for all cases, but it raises the possibility of a well-supported genetic explanation for the proneness to obesity and the high prevalence of type 2 diabetes for many populations. In addition, other microevolutionary processes (e.g., founder effects for island populations) and recent dietary and lifestyle changes have helped to increase the prevalence of "diabesity."

Thrifty Phenotypes and Prenatal Programming

Alternatively, David Barker has proposed thrifty phenotypes that develop through processes of prenatal "programming" in response to conditions such as high circulating glucose levels and nutrient deficiencies in the uterine environment (Barker, 1998a, b, 1999, 2004, 2006). During pregnancy nutrient supply and demand vary depending on a number of factors: maternal body composition, maternal dietary intake, placental blood flow, and the fetal genotype (Barker, 1998a, 2004; de Moura & Passos, 2005; Kuzawa, 2005, see also Chapter 18). Many researchers have substantiated that low birth weight and/or small body size or thinness in full-term infants are associated with an increased risk for obesity, type 2 diabetes, insulin resistance or metabolic syndrome, increased blood pressure, coronary heart disease, hypertension, and stroke when coupled with moderate to high weight gains in infancy, childhood, and later in life (Barker, 1998b, 2004, 2006; de Moura & Passos, 2005, Hales & Barker, 2001, Kuzawa, 2004, 2005; Plagemann, 2006). These associations have been established in populations around the world including British men (Hales et al., 1991; Baker 1998a, b), Asian Indians (Yajnik, 2004; Yajnik et al., 1995), Filipino children (Kuzawa, 2004), Chinese infants (Jie et al., 2000), Native Americans (Hanson, Imperatore, Bennett, & Knowler, 2002), and Mexican Americans (Valdez et al., 1994).

Barker postulates that low-birth-weight babies have metabolically thrifty mechanisms for fat storage and reduced rates of glucose oxidation in insulin-sensitive target tissues (Barker 1999, 2005; Barker et al., 1993; Yajnik, 2004; Yajnik et al., 1995). Adverse uterine environments alter many hormones involved in energy homeostasis, including leptin and cortisol. In addition, catabolic steroids rise with undernutrition, limiting lean body mass. In contrast, high-birth-weight infants or exposure in utero to excess glucose levels in diabetic mothers may preferentially decrease (i.e., downregulate) their sensitivity to glucose, predisposing them to insulin resistance, metabolic syndrome, obesity, and type 2 diabetes (Kuzawa, 1998). Barker calls for preconception, prenatal, and early life interventions to limit later life chronic diseases (Barker, 1998a, 2005). These preventive interventions would affect intergenerational health outcomes.

Thrifty Energy Cycles and Physical Activity

Chakravarthy and colleagues (Booth et al., 2002; Chakravartthy and Booth, 2004) argue that the combination of continuous food abundance and physical inactivity disrupts the evolutionarily programmed biochemical cycles that were adaptive for the feast/famine and physical activity/rest cycles of past lifeways. They view sedentary lifestyles and the reduction in energy expenditure as key conditions leading to a disruption of normal cycling of carbohydrate and fat stores, thus altering the insulin sensitivity of muscle and adipose tissues and production and use of metabolic regulatory peptides. Obesity and diabetes are referred to as "inactivity-mediated diseases," where neither glycogen stores in muscle (about 900 kcal) nor tryglycerides stored in adipose tissue (about 120,000 kcal) are routinely expended (Chakravarthy and Booth, 2004). Sedentary lifestyles result in an "unabated storage of fuel without the stimulus for its utilization" (Chakravarthy and Booth, 2004, p. 10).

Data from many sources support an argument that more attention should be paid to the overall reduction in energy expenditure and the frequency and intensity of activity in the etiology of diabesity (Campbell & Cajigal, 2001; Cordain et al., 1998; Jenike, 2001; Leonard, 2001). For example, endurance-trained athletes used as a proxy for hunting and foraging populations exhibit very efficient use of triglycerides or fatty acids for energy and use muscle glycogen sparingly, improving the potential for survival (Booth et al., 2002; Chakravarthy and Booth, 2004). Conversely, bed rest is associated with increases in plasma glucose, insulin resistance, and poor use of energy stores.

Exercise increases skeletal muscle mitochondria, which enhance cellular metabolism and insulin sensitivity. There is a low prevalence of type 2 diabetes in contemporary populations with economies demanding high levels of physical activity such as hunting and foraging, horticulture, and pastoralism (Diamond, 2003). Even the extremely high caloric intake of U.S. lumberjacks (4500–8000 kcal/day) balanced by energy expenditures results in an average BMI of only 25.5 (Lehtonen & Viikari, 1978). In summary, some researchers make a strong case for physical activity as a "core catalyst" to regulate the physiology of energy balance and call for an increased focus on physical-activity interventions to control the pandemic of diabesity (Chakravarthy and Booth, 2004; Eaton & Eaton, 2003; Eaton et al., 2002).

THE SCOPE OF THE PROBLEM: GLOBAL OBESITY PREVALENCE

The epidemic of overweight and obesity has now reached more than 1.6 billion persons, and in the United States two thirds of adults are overweight or obese, with some segments of the adult population reaching a nearly 80% prevalence (Kuczmarski, Flegal, Campbell, & Johnson, 1994; World Health Organization, 2006). The prevalence of overweight and obesity among adults and children has grown threefold or more since 1980 in many developed and developing countries (International Obesity Task Force, 2004; Kuczmarski et al., 1994; Lobstein, Baur, Uauy, & International Association for the Study of Obesity [IASO], 2004; Wild, Roglic, Green, Sicree, & King, 2004). In some small island populations, for example, the Samoans of the South Pacific, 75% are obese. In other countries such as China and India, where obesity rates are low (1–5%), the number of obese individuals is high because the populations are very large (International Obesity Task Force, 2004; WHO, 2000a, b). These countries have a growing public health burden from obesity and continue to cope with segments of the population that are underweight and undernourished (Popkin, 1994, 2004) (see Figure 3-1).

The U.S. National Health and Nutrition Examination Surveys (NHANES) showed a 40% increase in the number of overweight adults and 100% increase in the number of obese adults in the 25-year period between the 1976–80 and the 1999–2002 surveys (Flegal, Carroll, Ogden, & Johnson, 2002). Recent estimates are that more than two thirds of children 10 years of age and older who are obese will remain obese as adults (Magarey, Daniels, Boulton, & Cockington, 2003).

The obese also are getting fatter. The fastest growing group in the United States are the morbidly obese, whose BMI is ≥50. There are 9 million U.S. adults who are at least 100 lb. (45 kg) overweight (Hedley et al., 2004; Anonymous, 2005).

In 2000 the World Health Organization estimated that there were 22 million overweight children and adolescents worldwide, representing a remarkable increase in obesity within the last decade. A more recent estimate classifies 20 million children age 5 years and younger as overweight (World Health Organization, 2006). A number of studies indicate that 15–30% of children in developed countries are overweight (de Onis & Blossner, 2000; Lobstein et al., 2004) and more boys than girls are overweight (Hedley et al., 2004). Kim and colleagues documented a 73% increased in overweight babies in the United States in the period 1980–2001 (Kim et al., 2006). The prevalence of overweight and obesity is higher among Hispanic/Latino and African American/black compared to non-Hispanic white youth (Hedley et al., 2004; Kim et al., 2006). There are no geographic regions untouched by the pandemic of overweight and obesity (Bellenger & Bray, 2005; Ford, Giles, & Deitz, 2002; Popkin, 1994, 2001, 2004; Popkin & Gordon-Larson, 2004, Martorell, Khan, Hughes, & Gummer-Strawn, 2000).

THE SCOPE OF THE PROBLEM: DIABETES GLOBAL PREVALENCE

In 2003 the worldwide estimate for the number of adults with type 2 diabetes was 194 million compared to 135 million in 1995 and 30 million in 1985 (Figure 3-2). The projected global estimate for 2025 is 333 million (International Diabetes Federation, 2003) and for 2030 it is 366 million adults with diabetes (Wild et al., 2005). Wild and colleagues estimate that from 2000 to 2030 the worldwide population of adults will increase 37% but the percentage change in the number of adults with diabetes will be 114% (Figure 3-2). The *Diabetes Atlas 2003* contains estimates of diabetes prevalence for 212 countries within the seven regions of the International Diabetes Federation (International Diabetes Federation, 2003). The lowest regional prevalence (1.2%) is in sub-Saharan Africa, and the highest regional prevalence estimates are in the eastern Mediterranean, Middle East, and North America (7.8%). Many small island populations have the highest prevalence

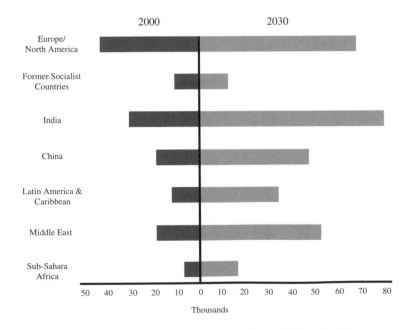

FIGURE 3-2 Worldwide prevalence of type 2 diabetes. (From Wild et al., 2004.)

estimates of type 2 diabetes, for example: Mauritius (15%), Barbados (13.2%), and Tonga (11.5%) (International Diabetes Federation, 2001, 2003). Currently India, China, and the United States account for nearly half of the world's population with type 2 diabetes (International Diabetes Federation, 2003).

Countries and regions with the greatest increases in diabetes prevalence are undergoing rapid demographic, lifestyle, and nutritional transitions characterized by increases in the number of people over 65 years of age, the proportion of the population living in urban areas, and increased access to prepared foods and public transportation (Drewnowski & Popkin 1997; IASO International Obesity Task Force, 2004; Popkin 2001; 2004; Popkin & Larson, 2004; Wild et al., 2005).

The United States in 2005 had an estimated 20.8 million individuals with diabetes (Centers for Disease Control, 2005b). There is wide variation in the estimated prevalence among ethnic groups within the United States: 15.1% American Indians/Alaskan natives, 13.3% non-Hispanic blacks, 10.2% Hispanic/Latino Americans, and 8.7% non-Hispanic whites (Centers for Disease Control, 2005b; International Diabetes Federation, 2003; Mokdad et al., 2000, 2001). Type 2 diabetes is increasing rapidly among overweight and obese children, especially among children from populations with a high prevalence of adults with diabetes. Six million (25%) U.S. children are overweight or obese, and one quarter of this group are estimated to have impaired glucose tolerance or "prediabetes" (Miller, Rosenbloom, & Silverstein, 2004). Eighty-five percent of children with type 2 diabetes were overweight or obese at the time of diagnosis (Young & Rosenbloom, 1998). These diabesity trends are expected to continue because contemporary environments are conducive to a surfeit of calories and fat stores. These aspects of our obesogenic environment are explored in the remainder of this chapter.

CHARACTERISTICS OF THE DIETARY OBESOGENIC ENVIRONMENT

There are a number of aspects of contemporary environments and lifestyles that predispose humans to excessive fat storage and type 2 diabetes. Some of the physiological/metabolic and cognitive/behavioral factors have been described previously in this chapter. The remainder of this chapter will focus on the dietary environment and food-related behaviors. The hallmarks of global dietary modernization are increased energy intake with processed energy-dense foods, increased quantity, and increased ingestion frequency. These dietary changes are coupled with behaviors that reduce energy expenditure. For example, television viewing is a low-energy-expenditure activity (i.e., couch potato), and it is frequently associated with increases in energy intake (e.g., potato chips) (Wansink, 2004a).

CONTEMPORARY DIETS: MACRO- AND MICRONUTRIENTS

S. Boyd Eaton and colleagues have extensively researched and written about Paleolithic diets and their relationship to contemporary diets and health outcomes (Eaton et al., 2002, Eaton & Eaton, 1999; Eaton, Shostak, & Konner, 1988). They note that there is very little in common between Paleolithic diets composed primarily of wild plant and animal foods and contemporary diets. Although geographic variability was high, Paleolithic diets were generally lower in fat and considerably higher in fiber than diets today. The fats in Paleolithic diets were primarily long-chain polyunsaturated fatty acids. Carbohydrates were chiefly from fruits (e.g., berries, figs) and vegetables (e.g., squashes, tubers) and consumed with little processing. In contrast, for most contemporary populations, macronutrients and calories are from processed grains, fatty domesticated animals, high-fat dairy products, and refined sugars. Contemporary, globalized diets are "fat rich and fiber poor" (Drewnowski & Popkin, 1997; Lieberman, 2003; Popkin, 2001).

Carbohydrate foods in contemporary diets are processed and refined. They often have high glycemic indexes. The glycemic index is a measure of the metabolic impact of a food or meal and the resulting increase in insulin and plasma glucose concentrations (Foster-Powell, Holt, & Brand-Miller, 2002). The enhanced insulin response promotes the storage of energy and increased adiposity. Globalized fast food meals often have a high glycemic load. They are a combination of low bulk, fiber-poor starches, fatty or oily foods (e.g., French fries), and highly sugared drinks. High fructose corn syrup used to sweeten both foods and beverages does not produce a quick insulin release so people do not experience satiation and may continue to eat for a longer period of time, increasing their intake of calories (Melanson, 2004).

Food-processing technologies are used to produce foods that have desirable characteristics, including sweet taste and smooth or crunchy textures. Fat produces a smooth texture at room temperature (e.g., butter) and when it is cold (e.g., ice cream). When fat

TABLE 3-2 Food Qualities and Atmospherics

Food Qualities and Serving Characteristics

    Variety (color, taste, shape)
    Attractiveness (shape, color, arrangement)
    Amount (large serving sizes, stockpiles)
    Presentation (jumbled rather than in discrete piles)

Environmental (Exogenous) Appetite Control Increasing Food Intake

    Containers & Serving Dishes (large containers, dishes and bowls; short; wide
      glasses, visible food)

Atmospherics

    Eating effort (low effort-fingers, forks, bit sizes, shelled nuts, easy-open packaging)
    Music (slow prolongs eating, fast increases rate of eating)
    Aromas (initially pleasant increases eating)
    Comfortable seating (increases eating time)
    Low lighting (disinhibits and increases eating time)
    Number of people (the number of people eating at a table is positively correlated
      with the amount of food consumed per person)
    Eating norms (people conform to expectations and observations of others)
    Distractions (TV, games, conversation, other distractions)

Source: Wansink, 2004.

is subjected to high temperatures, it produces a crunchy texture (e.g., French fries, fried chicken) (Drewnowski, 1997; Spurlock, 2005). In addition to taste and texture, food technology has produced foods with high energy and nutrient density and low bulk, facilitating increased consumption. In addition, there are many other characteristics of food that compel people to overeat (e.g., variety, portion size) and characteristics of the obesogenic environment that promote eating (e.g., food advertisements in print and electronic media, low lighting in restaurants, bulk purchases, and stockpiling) (Wansink, 2004a, b) (see Table 3-2).

GLOBALIZATION OF FOODS: ENORMOUS VARIETY

The globalization of diets has increased local dietary diversity, which is an important factor increasing consumption (Rolls et al., 1981; Wansink, 2004b, c). As big-brained omnivores we enjoy and seek dietary variety to balance our nutrient requirements. For example, people eat more at buffets that often have an enormous variety of foods (Schacter & Rodin, 1974; Wansink, 2004b).

Humans seek variety in their food even when taste is not varied. In a series of experiments with jelly beans, people given a bowl with jelly beans of six different colors ate about 60% more than those given a bowl with jelly beans of only four colors, even though both bowls had the same number of jelly beans and all the colors tasted the same. In another experiment people were presented with jelly beans either in piles separated by color or as a mixed assortment. People ate an average of 13 jelly beans if they were separated by color but 22 jelly beans (69% more) if colors were mixed (Wansink, 2004c). Further experiments with M&M's® candies corroborated these findings. People given the bowl with 10 colors ate 91 versus 64 (43% more) than those given 7 colors (Wansink, 2004a, b).

Successful fast food chains have capitalized on these findings. Offering small alterations in the basic hamburger, for example, increases consumption in both experimental and naturalistic settings (Schlosser, 2001; Wansink, 2004a). Fast food giants such as McDonald's® have responded to the obesity epidemic and the popularity of low-carbohydrate diets by adding salads and other healthful options to their menus, thereby increasing choices and profits (Brownell & Horgan, 2003; Buckley, 2004; Nestle, 2003; Schlosser, 2001). McDonald's also has menu items that are specific to national tastes. For example, there is the Prosperity Burger in Malaysia, a Kampong Burger in Singapore, and Pizza McPuffs in India. The strategy is to produce a cuisine with novel fusions of food items and spice appealing to local tastes.

In addition, unique and appealing names and descriptions of foods are positively related to increased consumption. How many ways can you say "chocolate cake"? For example, people more frequently selected and ate "Belgian Black Forest Double Chocolate Cake" than "Chocolate Cake," although the items were identical (Wansink, 2004c). Hundreds of new food items are added to the market place each year. In 2004, 948 new reduced-sugar products were introduced into the U.S. marketplace (Spurlock, 2005). In addition to product variety, the globalized food market has variety in product sizes and a penchant to supersize.

GLOBALIZATION OF FOOD: SUPERSIZING

For fast foods, supersized portions are more profitable, consumers expect them, and they get more food for their money (Spurlock, 2005). Food costs associated with supersizing are low relative to the costs of advertising, packaging, and labor (Brownell & Horgan, 2003; Nestle, 2003; Spurlock, 2005). Research has demonstrated that portion size and perceived portion size are powerful determinants of how much a person eats (Diliberti, Bordi, Conklin, Roe, & Rolls, 2004; Rolls, 2003; Wansink, 2004a, b;Young and Nestle, 1995).

Often packaging connotes a unit size that is expected to be one serving. A single packaged large muffin appears to be a single serving, but the label informs the consumer that the 660 kcal muffin is really three servings (Nestle, 2003). The USDA portion sizes are often only one eighth to one fourth of the sizes served in fast food and other restaurants. For example, a USDA standard soft drink is 8 ounces (100 kcal), but many restaurants routinely serve 32 ounces (400 kcal), and it is often part of a supersized "meal deal" (Anonymous, 2005). Another example is cooked pasta, with official serving sizes ranging from 1/2 cup (USDA) to 1 cup (U.S. Food and Drug Administration), whereas restaurant servings averages 2.6–3.3 cups (Young and Nestle, 2003). Hamburgers are supersized and loaded with energy-dense fatty extras like cheese and bacon and "special sauces." One recent U.S. trend has been an increase in average size and caloric content of appetizers. Examples include fried mozzarella sticks (830 kcal), spicy chicken wings often called "buffalo wings" (1000 kcal), and fried onion rings with dipping sauce (2130 kcal) (Jacobson & Hurley, 2002).

A large body of research exists on portion size that demonstrates that individuals miscalculate portion sizes for all types of foods (Godwin, Chambers, & Cleveland, 2004; Rolls, 2003; Wansink 2004c; Wansink & van Ittersum, 2003; Young & Nestle, 2003). People routinely select sizes that they consider normative that are larger than the USDA "standard" sizes. Even with the aid of measuring devices, the ability of young adults to estimate correct portion sizes is poor. Using photographs of foods to teach portion sizes did not significantly improve the ability to estimate correct sizes (Furbisher and Maxwell, 2003). Furthermore, experience does not insure accurate assessment of portion sizes. Bartenders misjudged and poured 26% more alcohol into short, wide glasses compared to tall, narrow glasses (Wansink, 2004b; Wansink & van Ittersum, 2003). Teaching portion sizes using common objects or the human body as a guide may be helpful; for example, a deck of cards as the equivalent of 3.5 oz of meat, a tennis ball the size of one-half cup, and the tip of the thumb the equivalent of one teaspoon are common examples. Cross-cultural and ethnic differences on culturally salient "common" measures have not been well researched or developed.

When individuals choose larger portion sizes, they consume more (Rolls, 2003; Young and Nestle, 2003). In a movie theater people given large buckets of popcorn ate 50% more than those given smaller buckets. When both groups were asked to estimate the amount or the calories they had eaten, there were no significant differences in their reported estimates. In an M&M candy experiment, people who were given 1-lb. bags of M&M's ate 120 M&M's, compared to people given a 1/2 lb. bag, who ate 63 M&M's while they watched a videotape. The researchers suggest that the size of the package or portion gives people a perceptual consumption cue as to what is "normal" or acceptable regardless of what they actually consume (Grier and Rozin, 2006; Wansink, 1996;

Wansink & van Ittersum, 2003). In another experiment nutrition experts using smaller spoons and bowls consumed less than half the amount of ice cream as those using the larger utensils and bowls. The two groups did not report a significant difference in estimated intake (Wansink, van Ittersum, & Painter, 2006).

Additionally, people who buy food in large quantities or bulk also eat more of those foods than if they buy them in smaller units (Wansink, 2004b). Experiments that alter the caloric density without changing portion sizes (Rolls, 2003) indicate that humans miscalculate food portion sizes and appear to be insensitive to the amount of food consumed and its caloric density (Melanson, 2004; Wansink, 2004c).

From an evolutionary perspective the lack of sensitivity to internal cues of satiation, defined as the inhibition of hunger and appetite within meals, may have been advantageous so that eating continued when food was available in feast and famine conditions. Furthermore, there may have been little selective advantage to be able to accurately and precisely judge portion sizes because the natural environment already constrained the size and amount of available food (Jenike, 2001; Ulijaszek & Strickland, 1993; Ungar and Teaford, 2002). The paradox of relying on visual cues, but being a poor judge of portion size and how much one can eat is exemplified by common saying and aphorisms. In English this is *"Your eyes are bigger than your stomach"*; in Spanish *"Come con las ojos"* (You eat with your eyes); and in German *"Die Augen sind grösser als der Magen"* (Your eyes are bigger than your stomach).

Furthermore, judging portion sizes and consumption volume is confounded by consuming food that you do not see or only partially see. For example, people who acquire food from a fast food drive-in window will eat in their cars and do not see the full contents of their purchase as they consume the food from the bag or container. Bags, boxes, and canisters of fast foods and snacks are packaged in ways that preclude viewing the contents (Wansink, 2004a), and some foods are heated in microwave ovens and eaten directly from their containers.

Additionally, people are distracted by a wide range of stimuli and will continue to eat until food is consumed or until an environmental cue, such as the end of a television program, signals that it is time to stop eating (Wansink, 2004b). Obesogenic environments provide both the cues and the resources that apparently decouple physiological factors such as hunger and satiety from the amount and timing of food ingestion (Melanson, 2004). In sum, people do not see what they are eating, misjudge portion sizes, are susceptible to labeling tricks, are insensitive to the amount of food they ingest, and are distracted or multitask during consumption. All of these factors foster overconsumption and diabesity (Wansink, 2004b).

GLOBALIZATION OF FOOD: UBIQUITOUS VISUAL FOOD STIMULI

Although much has been written about the roles of gustation (i.e., taste) and olfaction (i.e., smell) in food selection and eating behaviors (Drewnowski 1997; Johns & Keen, 1985), relatively little has been written about the evolution and role of primate vision as the primary sense used to promote food and negotiate the current obesogenic environment. Two features of primate vision are particularly important: binocular vision allowing depth perception and color vision (Cartmill, 1974; Conroy, 1990; Jolly, 1985). This primate legacy of binocular or stereoscopic vision aided hominins relying on depth perception to locate geographical landmarks, track, trap, and hunt game (Lee and DeVore, 1968; Winterhalder and Smith, 1981). R. H. Post (1962) postulated that color vision conferred a selective advantage to human hunters and foragers because they could see prey more readily.

Modern environments are filled with an array of visual stimuli of actual food items, their representations in media, and universally recognized iconic images and logos (e.g., McDonald's Golden Arches). These images transcend cultural and linguistic boundaries and easily identify sources of food. The visual appeal is purposeful and effective because vision is the primary primate mode of perception (Jones, Martin, & Pilbeam, 1992). Visual stimuli and just thinking about food initiate the cephalic phase of digestion (Katschinski, 2000).

These stimuli signal learned messages about the nutritional and physiological effects of particular foods. For primates, initial signals are often visual rather than olfactory, with color as a primary salient property (Dominey & Lucas 2001, 2004; Post, 1965). Color changes in ripening vegetables and fruits signal sensory changes, for example, increased aroma, increased sweetness, softer texture, reduction in toxins (e.g., lectins, phenols), and presence of other biologically active substances (e.g., plant estrogens, vitamins) (Dominy & Lucas, 2004; Vorobyev, 2004; Wolf, 2002). Leaf maturity is also signaled by color change from reddish to green and used by folivorous primate species to select edible leaves. Young leaves often contain more protein and micronutrients, lower levels of toxins, and less fiber than older leaves (Dominy & Lucas, 2001, 2004). Color changes may also signal potential physiological consequences such as the production and/ or release of insulin and increased thermogenesis (LeBlanc, 2000). In turn, these metabolic responses to eating may promote further eating behaviors, initiate activity, and facilitate growth and development, all of which have evolutionary implications for survival (Chakravarthy & Booth, 2004; Cordain et al., 1998; Jenike, 2001; Ulijaszek & Strickland, 1993).

Humans also use color changes to signal when food is cooked. For example, vegetables, if sautéed, will retain their color but with continued cooking become dull, and red meats are "browned" to retain moisture and flavor. Some foods (e.g., lobsters) change color on cooking. Applying heat and observing color changes (e.g., rare vs. well-cooked meat) can indicate that pathogenic bacteria (e.g., *Escherichia coli*), other microorganisms, and parasites (e.g., *Trichinella spiralis*) have been killed. Food that is spoiling often changes color (e.g., browning of lettuce leaves). Food technology is used to enhance and retain natural colors in fruits, vegetables, fish, and meat (Fellows, 2000). Color is often used to enhance the serving of food, and cooks from around the world are encouraged to prepare attractive food service that incorporates consideration of color (Rombauer and Becker, 1997). Cookbooks often have beautiful color illustrations of food dishes and serving suggestions along with recipes.

Humans are attracted to colorful foods. For example, Mars "color-refreshed" M&M's by adding blue and holiday colors (e.g., pastels for Easter), potato and vegetable chips are available in many colors, and children like brightly colored soft drinks such as Kool-Aid®. Supermarkets display fruits and vegetables in colorful arrangements often appealing to the eye rather than the nose because they are wrapped or in refrigerated displays. Americans talk about the importance of taste and aroma as variables used in the selection of fruits and vegetables, but they often select fresh produce based on color, size, shape, and blemish-free appearance (Lieberman, unpublished data; Nestle, 2003).

Food images are ubiquitous in obesogenic environments and stimulate purchases and eating (Brownell & Horgan, 2003; Spurlock, 2005; Wansink, 2004a, b). Restaurants display plastic food models, and menus with colorful pictures are common throughout the world. Restaurant take-out windows place colorful food pictures on marquees near ordering stations. Full-color food ads in magazines and newspapers, billboards, and hand fliers are also common.

Colorful television and computer Internet ads for foods are abundant, especially advertisements aimed at children. In 2004 $13 billion of an approximately $144 billion fast food advertising budget was spent on food advertising aimed at children in the United States (Spurlock, 2005, p. 307). Seventy percent of U.S. children age 6–8 years in one poll thought that fast food was healthier than home-prepared food (Story & French, 2004), and 73% of Pakistani children thought that soft drinks were a healthy choice for frequent consumption (Rachagan, 2004).

In the United States children watched an average of 20,000–40,000 TV commercials per year and 11–19 food commercials per hour on Saturday mornings (Story & French, 2004). Based on a six-nation study in Asia, children in the Philippines and Malaysia watched 20 minutes of advertising per hour. Forty to 75% of the commercials on television programming for Asian children were for food and beverages often high in sugar, fat, and salt (Rachagan, 2004). Children develop brand loyalty at an early age and frequently influence family purchases via "pester power" to the extent that they request particular products and brands (Rachagan, 2004). Multinational food companies have begun to exploit other technologies that accommodate visual advertising including, cell phones, iPods, MP3 players, digital video discs, and corporate-sponsored web sites (Kaiser Family Foundation, 2006).

GLOBALIZATION OF FOOD: FORAGING, EATING, AND REDUCED ENERGY EXPENDITURE

The abundant visual cues in contemporary environments facilitate successful foraging and efficient exploitation. These environments present evolutionarily novel opportunities to forage for highly reliable and abundant energy-dense foods with low energy expenditures (Lieberman, 2006). The application of foraging theory provides insights into why humans have become so "successful" in optimizing their energy intakes and producing a diabesity pandemic. Foraging theory, a component of behavioral ecology, uses cost/benefit models to predict food-related behaviors, prey (including plants)–predator interactions, and characteristics of the environment (Mann, 2004; Winterhalder & Smith, 1981). Most cost/benefit models use energy as the currency. Ultimately the goal is to link the costs and benefits to reproductive success (Illius, Tolkamp, & Yearsley, 2002; Drewnowski & Popkin, 1997; Popkin, 2004; Popkin & Gordon-Larsen, 2004; Winterhalder & Smith, 1981).

The costs of obtaining foods have all drastically diminished with dietary globalization. Urban environments have abundant food patches: in homes (pantries, refrigerators, freezers), school cafeterias, movie theaters, kiosks, street vendors, convenience stores, shopping malls, supermarkets, gas stations, and restaurants. McDonald's, has more than 31,000 stores worldwide (McDonalds, 2006; Spurlock, 2005), Subway® 22,000 (Subway, 2006), Pizza Hut® 20,000 (Pizza Hut, 2006), and Kentucky Fried Chicken® (KFC) 12,000 (Kentucky Fried Chicken, 2006). Many of these fast food franchises are found in more than 100 countries.

A number of studies have demonstrated a relationship between geographical density of fast food restaurants and obesity rates (Drewnowski & Spector, 2004). Within low-income neighborhoods in the United States there are more fast food restaurants, fewer supermarkets, and fewer opportunities for safe exercising compared to higher income neighborhoods (Booth et al., 2005; Maddock, 2004). In Chicago the median distance between any school and the nearest fast food restaurant was 520 m and 78% of schools had a fast food restaurant within 800 m. Children can walk to these "food patches" in about 5–10 minutes (Austin et al., 2006). Accessible and well-advertised food patches reduce search and travel times and, hence, time and human energy expended in these activities. Urban and suburban areas provide the convenience of having food delivered to your home or worksite, thereby reducing search and travel to zero.

An array of food patches (e.g., school cafeterias, fast food restaurants, gas station convenience stores, supermarkets, etc.) provide high-calorie, nutrient-dense, and inexpensive food. There is appealing variety, and the food requires little preparation prior to consumption. There are no issues of diminishing returns in exploiting these patches because the supply of food is limitless. Only purchasing power and satiety are limitations. Drewnowski and Spector (2004) demonstrated that individuals with limited incomes purchase energy-dense fast foods that provide more calories per dollar than expensive less energy-dense fruits and vegetables. The marginal value theorem predicts this purchasing behavior because people are expected to maximize their rate of return in calories given their investment in time, energy, and money (Sinervo, 1997). Although eating fast food optimizes energy intake per unit cost, it can lead to poor nutritional balance (Drewnowski, 2004).

Americans increasingly value convenience and low time and energy investments in food preparation (Rozin, 2005). In a recent survey, 34% of Americans indicated that they preferred to "dine out" or have a meal catered in their home even for holiday meals at Thanksgiving and Christmas (Hales, 2005). Americans consume a large proportion of their meals away from home. On an average day in 2004, 40% of American adults were eating in restaurants. Food consumed in restaurants requires little time or energy spent on acquisition, preparation, cooking, service, or cleaning up after the meal. Restaurants are attractive and create atmospheres that are conducive to eating with lighting, aromas, comfortable seating, distractions, and high food salience (Wansink, 2004) (see Table 3-2).

In addition to low-energy-cost access to food, industrialized nations are modern marvels of human energy-saving lifestyles created by technology, the built environment, daily habits, and cultural values (Lieberman, 2006). Appealing to the human inclination for energy conservation, contemporary environments reduce human energy expenditure with motorized mobility (e.g., cars, buses, elevators, moving sidewalks) and wireless and remote control devices (e.g., cell or mobile phones, garage and TV remote controls) (Cordain et al.,1998; Rozin, 2005). For example, the number of hours of sedentary activities such as watching TV and DVDs and playing videogames are positively corre-lated with weight gain for both children (Dennison et al., 2002; Rachagan, 2004) and adults (Leonard, 2001; Stroebele & de Castro, 2004; Wyatt, Peters, Reed, Barry, & Hill, 2005). The Kaiser Family Foundation has been documenting children's television and computer viewing behavior and program content for a number of years (1999, 2003, 2005, 2006). Children 2–18 years of age watched or used media nearly 6.5 hours per day, with 81% reporting daily television watching (Rideout, Roberts, & Ulla, 2005). Television watching both reduces energy expenditure and increases energy intake, con-tributing in both ways to the net energy surfeit and diabesity (Rachagan, 2004). For every hour of TV watched the obesity percentage rose by 6% in children (America's Obesity Crisis, 2004). Because television remote controls and cordless and cellular phones are widely available, people no longer get up from chairs to change channels or answer the telephone. We continue to reduce the small amounts of energy spent as part of our daily routines, and these cumulative changes in lifestyle contribute to the global diabesity pan-demic (Rozin, 2005; Wyatt et al., 2005).

DIABESITY AND DARWINIAN MEDICINE

The current pandemic of obesity and type 2 diabetes is the result of very rapid changes in lifestyles that have capitalized on millennia of evolutionary selective pressures favoring physiological patterns, nutritional requirements, and cognitive and behavioral repertoires adapted to environments with fluctuations in food availability and periodic high energy expenditures (Lieberman, 2003, 2006). Humans have evolved a complex system of adi-pose, gut, and pancreatic hormones, enzymes, and neurotransmitters that respond to food intake and signal the hypothalamus to regulate appetite and influence various organs and tissues to metabolize or store energy (Chakravarthy & Booth, 2004; Neel, 1962). These regulatory mechanisms are more sensitive to hunger than satiety, and humans respond to food characteristics (i.e., variety, large portion sizes) and characteristics of the dietary environment (i.e., abundant food patches, convenience, pleasant eating environments) with increases in food consumption (Wansink, 2004b).

Cognitive/behavioral approaches to slow the growing diabesity pandemic have not been successful in managing it. For example, billions of dollars have been and continue to be spent on weight-reduction diets, special foods, books, over-the-counter remedies, exercise and health club memberships, and nutritional counseling (Jeffcoat & Bakker, 2005). We are a nation of dieters. In the United States dieting to reduce body weight is the most common approach, but numerous studies document that restricted eating is not an evolutionary adaptive strategy (Polivy & Herman, 2006). Annually, 44% of woman and 29% of men in the United States are dieting (Friedman, 2003). If people lose weight, 95% regain the weight, often exceeding their baseline weight when they initiated dieting (Ikeda et al., 2005). We are losing the "war" on obesity and diabetes because the strategies are ineffective in obesogenic environments (Friedman, 2003; Spiegel & Nabel, 2006).

Eaton and colleagues (2002) have called for "evolutionary health promotion" that takes into account issues of both health and disease, based on adopting a conceptual framework that interprets contemporary human conditions in light of our evolutionary past (Eaton et al., 2002; Speakman, 2004). The approaches that Eaton and colleagues (2002) suggest in *Preventive Medicine* alert physicians to the evolutionary context in which once adaptive genotypes and phenotypes become mismatched with contemporary lifestyles—Stone Age genes in Space Age environments (Eaton et al., 2002). Based on the data presented in this chapter, their strategies do not appear to go far enough in suggesting a closer look at physiological/metabolic and cognitive/behavioral regulatory mechanisms. They suggest conventional approaches that require dietary restraint and motivation to increase activity. Current approaches focusing on behavioral interventions are contrary to what we know about human cognition, behavior, and physiology that drive eating behavior and fat storage in obesogenic environments. Interventions to reduce psychosocial stress and increase sleep duration may be more amenable to change than behaviors associated with eating (Keith et al., 2006).

As noted previously, one approach to preventing, controlling, and reversing the undesirable sequelea of diabesity is to develop new pharmaceuticals that operate at the molecular level opposing or enhancing the effects of gut and adipose tissue peptides, hormones, and neurotransmitters on the appetite-control nuclei in the hypothalamus. Some rodent experiments have been promising, and new drugs are being developed (Wynne et al., 2005). Thus far, antiobesity drugs have either not proved effective (e.g., leptin) or they have had serious side effects (e.g., PhenFen and pulmonary hypertension) (Bray et al., 1998; Wynne et al., 2005). A novel approach to decreasing diabesity is to develop drugs that interfere with the inflammatory response and restore insulin sensitivity (Lee and Pratley, 2005). Primary prevention and pharmacological therapies targeting molecular changes are most likely the approaches that will have some impact on the diabesity pandemic.

The only long-term successful approach to sustained weight loss has been surgery (i.e., gastric bypass, stomach stapling), which carries a number of health risks (e.g., rupture of the stomach) (Pear, 2006). An estimated 200,000 surgeries were performed in 2006 (Centers for Disease Control, 2005b; Pear, 2006).

An intergenerational approach would focus on maternal health and the intrauterine environment in the prevention of low-birth-weight babies, who are at increased risk for the development of diabesity (Barker, 1998a, b, 2004, 2005). Ideally the interventions would occur preconception and continue throughout the pregnancy. This primary prevention approach has the potential for a large impact on the diabesity pandemic because it would alter fetal metabolic programming.

Finally, there are alterations in the food supply, such as smaller portion sizes served in restaurants, foods packaged in smaller units, and the elimination of soda and candy from schools. These changes would be more acceptable if portion sizes were made to appear larger, for example, by serving them on smaller plates (Wansink, 2004b, c). Alterations in the eating environment to reduce the salience of food cues (e.g., fewer food commercials on television) and increasing attention to eating by eliminating distractions and multitasking have the potential to curb eating and reduce the risk for diabesity (Wansink, 2004a, b). If the decline in tobacco use can be used as an example, then broad policy and legal interventions might prove effective in changing behaviors associated with eating and physical activity. For example, in December 2006 the Board of Health of New York City passed a ban on trans fat use in restaurants that would go into effect in 2008 (MSNBC News Service, 2006).

CONCLUSION

Evolution has honed human proclivities for eating large portions of food and physiological capacities for energy storage that, when coupled with modern lifestyles that include energy-dense food abundance and energy-saving conveniences, promotes weight gain, obesity, and type 2 diabetes. Predictions are that the worldwide pandemic of diabesity will continue to escalate over the next few decades, with the majority of new cases in India and China. An evolutionary medical approach would de-emphasize alterations in food intake or dieting and refocus efforts on early life prevention and pharmaceutical intervention.

CHAPTER 4

To Eat or What Not to Eat, That's the Question

A Critique of the Official Norwegian Dietary Guidelines

Iver Mysterud, Dag Viljen Poleszynski,
Fedon A. Lindberg, and Stig A. Bruset

That "microcultural factors" pertinent to understanding (if not predicting) the negative impact that dietary recommendations will have on different families living under different circumstances in different regions in Norway is a cornerstone of the argument and research reported by Mysterud and his colleagues. In their critique of the official Norwegian Diet Guidelines, the authors suggest that, if followed precisely, the guidelines will contribute to the very problem of increasing rates of obesity and diabetes they are trying to solve. From one region to another, the authors point out, a reduction in the consumption of fat has not as might be expected led to a reduction in weight-related diseases; the authors do not believe that a lack of physical exercise is a factor, either. Rather, they argue that more attention needs to be placed on assessing individual metabolic processes and the interactions among consumed foods and how these factors distinguish individual dietary effects with respect to weight gain. The emergence of starches and processed sugars as a predominant part of the diet seems to be the cause of obesity in Norway, all the while fish remains heavily represented in the diet. They suggest that attention to more of a specieswide diet is critical, especially to individual differences. Most important, they insist that supposedly scientific-based, governmental dietary guidelines should never be, as is the case in Norway (they contend), influenced by "market considerations." Although their focus is Norway, the reader could substitute any number of countries (e.g., Great Britain, Canada, the United States) and see some of the same factors they discuss.

The diet of our remote ancestors may be a reference standard for modern human nutrition and a model for defense against certain "diseases of civilization."

S. Boyd Eaton and Melvin Konner, 1985

INTRODUCTION

Chronic diseases are the major cause of morbidity and mortality in modern, affluent societies, Norway being no exception, and the prevalence seems to be increasing. Spokesmen from the nutrition authorities nevertheless claim that Norwegians in general are in good health (Kaare Norum/Christian Drevon, personal communication), attributing this to, among others factors, the official dietary policies that have been promulgated during the past few decades. However, one Norwegian newspaper summarized the estimated number of chronic problems and diseases in 1999[1] and found 9 million diagnoses distributed among 4.5 million inhabitants (Table 4–1 on webpage), more than two per adult person. Although the figures are 8 years old, they illustrate our point: the populations of industrially advanced countries are often fraught with preventable diseases that were virtually unknown in hunter and gather societies. Based on these data it seems unreasonable to conclude that we are an exceptionally healthy society, as spokesmen from the nutrition authorities do. In this light it is informative that Norwegians spent NOK 16.2 billion (about US$ 2.5 billion) on various medications in 2006.[2]

The Norwegian health care system is over 400 years old (Moseng, 2003, Schiøtz, 2003). During the first phase of institutionalized health care, the primary emphasis was on ridding the cities of pests and implementing hygienic measures. The widespread initiation of better personal hygiene and public sewage systems, combined with a significant reduction in poverty, changed the face of health care in Norway. During the last century, with the advent of antibiotics and other drugs, the health care system shifted its focus to treating illnesses and symptoms. The focus was to treat illness once it occurred (i.e., a "downstream" system), rather than on preventing illness (an "upstream" system) (Poleszynski, 2001). In our view, this historic shift away from a preventive to a symptomatic treatment strategy has been detrimental to public health. Although prevention could keep people healthy, the implementation of such a strategy requires not only having good models for explaining what causes these diseases, but also understanding how diseases may be treated once they have manifested themselves. To this end we find an evolutionary perspective fruitful, as this gives a basis for comparing people's health before the agricultural (Neolithic) revolution started some 10,000 years ago, with the current conditions. People in traditional societies were generally not often afflicted with chronic diseases like cancer, cardiovascular disease, type 2 diabetes, high blood pressure, osteoporosis, and autoimmune diseases (Cohen, 1989; Crawford & Marsh, 1989; Goldsmith, 1999; Johansson, 2001; Lindeberg, 1994; Lindeberg, Berntorp, Carlsson, Eliasson, & Marckmann, 1997; Lindeberg & Lundh, 1993; Lindeberg, Nilsson-Ehle, Terént, Vessby, & Scherstén, 1994; Lindeberg, Nilsson-Ehle, & Vessby, 1996; Lindeberg & Vessby, 1995; McCarrison, 1963; Price, 1970; Stefansson, 1960). The relatively short average life expectancy in many Neolithic populations, compared with present-day populations, has been ascribed to a higher level of traumatic events, such as occasional starvation, vagaries of the weather, violent encounters with other tribes, accidents, infections, and contact with poisonous insects and dangerous animals. The harsh realities of life not only led to a high involuntary infant mortality rate, but also to infanticide and selective homicide of handicapped and elderly who were unable to provide for themselves (McKeown, 1991).

In many respects, modern humans seem less healthy than our ancestors, based on the prevalence of chronic disease. This seems a paradox in light of the fact that we have access to more scientific knowledge about how to avoid disease and remain healthy than at any time in history, as well as more scientific data on healthy diets, on the benefits of regular exercise, and on a healthy lifestyle in general. Life expectancy in developed countries since the Neolithic has been increasing in leaps and bounds, in particular during the last few centuries, with the virtual elimination of abject poverty and starvation, improved living standards, educational level, and public and personal hygiene. Such measures have, at least until recent decades, in most countries more than compensated for the increased prevalence of unhealthy diets and lifestyles. This is shown by a general increase in life expectancy in most industrialized countries. Another factor that has prolonged life into old age is our willingness to care for the elderly and spend huge resources on keeping them alive by treating chronic diseases and performing life-saving medical interventions, even if it does not necessarily mean that they are enjoying good health. Nutritional adequacy is a prerequisite for good health from the womb to the grave, and Western governments decided after World War II that public health would be well served by teaching people how to compose healthy diets for all phases of life. Of several options available, the official guidelines were based on nutritional research performed by established institutions arguing that if everybody were secured a minimum level of nutrients, many deficiency diseases could be avoided. In contrast with this, we argue that the official guidelines *in themselves* constitute part of the health problem in our time because they contribute to creating many of the very problems that they are intended to solve. We will illustrate this by focusing on the official recommendations for healthy eating in the Nordic countries in general and on Norway in particular. It is our contention that, among other problems, the guidelines developed by Norwegian authorities ignore or pay little attention to (1) evolutionary arguments and research, (2) experiences of indigenous/traditional peoples, (3) biochemical, metabolic, and hormonal effects of foods, (4) differing bioavailability of nutrients in various foods, (5) the variability of individual needs in large groups with special requirements, and (6) the difference between average nutrient requirement to prevent deficiencies and the optimal nutrient intake needed to achieve the highest possible level of health.

NORWEGIAN DIETARY RECOMMENDATIONS

The official dietary recommendations were formulated after World War II based on wartime considerations of adequate nutrition. Norway based its recommendations on international and U.S. guidelines coordinated with the other Nordic countries (Eeg-Larsen, 1971). In 1968 medical societies in Denmark, Finland, Norway, and Sweden issued their first joint statement on "Medical Aspects of the Diet in the Nordic Countries." The first official Nordic Nutrition Recommendations (NNR) were issued in 1980, with subsequent editions published in 1989, 1996, and 2004 (Alexander, Andersen, Aro, Becker, Fogelholm, Lyhne, Meltzer, Pedersen, Pedersen, & Þúrsdúttir, 2004 [hereafter referred to as the NNR, 2004]). Although these guidelines were developed for the Nordic population, they are very similar to the U.S.Recommended Dietary Allowance (RDA) guidelines. The expressed goal of these guidelines is provide adequacy, *not* to *maximize health* for each individual by showing them how they may ingest the level of nutrients that gives the best possible health (an *optimal* intake; point 6 above) (NNR, 2004, p. 11). Neither is it a goal to *eliminate* diseases caused by suboptimal or unbalanced nutrient intakes, but to *reduce the risk* of their occurrence. The combined effect of just reducing the risk of occurrence of diet-associated disease, coupled with a low ambition in terms of health goals, makes it possible to maintain harmony between commercial interests in the food-processing industry and official health policies, as well as to perpetuate the dominance of a symptom-oriented medicine in the public health care system. Although not explicitly stated, the NNR thus serves as a justification for maintaining status quo in health, agriculture, industry and trade. This means that the guidelines are based on politics rather than of science (Scientific Committee on Food, 2000).

RENEWED INTEREST IN HEALTH

Norwegians have experienced a renewed and increasing interest in healthy eating during the last decade, but the concomitant behavioral changes have been limited to the upper echelons of society. Although an evolutionary perspective on nutrition was first published for a general audience in Norway in the mid-1990s (Bruset & Henriksen, 1996), the general public has only become actively engaged in the topic during the last 5 years. This popular interest has been fueled by translated versions of the "Zone" books by Barry Sears (Sears, 1999, 2001, 2002, 2003; Sears & Lawren, 1995, 2000), *Eat Right for Your Type* by Peter J. D'Adamo (D'Adamo & Whitney, 1996, 1999), the Atkins low-carbohydrate diet (Atkins, 1992, 2001), as well as two books in Norwegian based on a diet with a reduced glycemic load (i.e., having a negligible effect on blood sugar) combined with aspects of a Paleolithic and a "Mediterranean diet," but with a lower carbohydrate and higher protein content than the traditional Cretan diet (Lindberg, 2001, 2002). All of these books have become bestsellers in Norway, in particular the latter two. The authors of these books have in common that they recommend foods that are consistent with our evolutionary heritage, i.e., foods containing more protein and fat and fewer carbohydrates, particularly refined ones, than the official dietary goals. They also recommend keeping the glycemic index and glycemic load (Foster-Powell, Holt, & Brand-Miller, 2002; Jenkins, Wolever, Taylor, Barker, Fielden, Baldwin, Bowling, Newman, Jenkins, & Goff, 1981) as low as possible in each meal. The most controversial issue has been the claim that neither wheat (and other high glycemic processed grains), potatoes, or cow's milk are optimal foodstuffs for humans (in the sense of securing the best possible health), while a general consensus has emerged that refined sugars should be kept relatively low, i.e., at a maximum of 10% of total dietary energy (henceforth, E%) (NNR, 2004). This limit seems to be set arbitrarily, because there is no doubt that a sugar intake of 10 E% is much higher than was found in the diet of our Paleolithic ancestors throughout evolution, as well as in the diets of modern-day hunter-gatherers and early Neolithic populations.

EVOLUTIONARY ARGUMENTS AND RESEARCH

Official guidelines have ignored evolutionary approaches to diet and medicine, and official "experts" have dismissed or downplayed such approaches when setting dietary standards. Evolutionary approaches to medicine (Nesse & Williams, 1994; Stearns 1999; Trevathan, Smith, & McKenna 1999; Williams & Nesse, 1991) and diet (Cordain, 2002; Cordain, Brand Miller, Eaton, Mann, Holt, & Speth, 2000; Cordain, Eaton, Mann, & Hill, 2002; Eaton, Eaton III, & Konner, 1997, 1999) give important clues to understanding how our body was designed by natural selection in order to increase survival and repro-duction in ancestral environments, as well as what types of foods we have been selected to ingest. Since the appearance of behaviorally modern humans (Cro-Magnon) some 50,000 years ago, and even more so since the agricultural revolution 10,000 years ago, culture has evolved much more rapidly than the human genome (Armelagos, Goodman, & Jacobs, 1991; Boehm, 1978; Rosenberg & Rosenberg, 1990). One result has been an ever-greater discrepancy between the way we live and eat and the lifestyle to which our genome was originally adapted. Evolutionary evidence indicates that this discordance fosters the diseases of civilization or chronic degenerative diseases, those that cause the most morbidity and mortality in contemporary nations (Eaton, Cordain, & Lindeberg, 2002; Eaton & Konner, 1985; Eaton, Konner, & Shostak, 1988; Eaton, Strassmann, Nesse, Neel, Ewald, Williams, Weder, Eaton III, Lindeberg, Konner, Mysterud, & Cordain, 2002). An evolutionary approach to nutrition and lifestyle in general represents a new paradigm for understanding chronic degenerative diseases but, surprisingly, is totally ignored in the official recommendations for healthy eating in Norway.

Paleolithic Diet

The diets of our Paleolithic ancestors varied considerably due to differences in geogra-phy, local climate, and the impact of global ice age periods. However, a common charac-teristic of their diets was an exclusive reliance on wild and nonprocessed meat, fish, fowl, eggs, vegetables, fruits, berries, nuts and roots, and even insects. The average food energy requirement during the Paleolithic was estimated to be approximately 40% higher than the requirement of an average office worker today (Cordain, Gotshall, & Eaton, 1997; Cordain, Gotshall, Eaton, & Eaton III, 1998). The food was more nutritious (more nutri-ents per energy unit) and protein rich and less energy dense. Paleolithic hunters and gath-erers ingested fewer carbohydrates than we do, with an estimated intake range of 2–5 to 40 E%, and the carbohydrate sources had a low glycemic and insulin index (i.e., they elicited more stable blood sugar and insulin responses after meals) (Holt, Brand Miller, & Petocz, 1997). According to a growing body of literature, many of our ancestors had a relatively high fiber intake (inversely related to the meals' fat content) and an ample intake of phytochemicals from vegetables, berries, roots, nuts, and fruits (Burkitt & Eaton, 1989; Cordain, Brand Miller, Eaton, Mann, Holt, & Speth, 2000; Eaton, 1992; Eaton & Eaton III, 1999; Eaton, Eaton III, & Konner, 1997; Eaton & Konner, 1985; Eaton, Konner, & Shostak, 1988; Eaton & Nelson, 1991). The intake of fatty acids was based on natural, unprocessed fats of high quality, and not on partially hydrogenated fatty acids, or heated and refined oils and fats, as may be found in modern diets. The variation in fat intake for our ancestors was considerable and varied from 20 to 85 E%, while at the same time their intake of long-chain polyunsaturated ω-3 fatty acids (C20–C22) was considerably higher than in the modern populations. Our ancestors had a much lower ω-6:ω-3 ratio, commonly as low as 1–2:1 (Eaton, Eaton III, & Konner, 1997; Eaton, Eaton III, Sinclair, Cordain, & Mann, 1998; Skjervold, 1992), compared with 10:1 (Eaton, 1992, Eaton, Eaton III, & Konner, 1999) and even as high as 40–50:1 in certain "junk food" diets in the United States (Hunninghake, 2005). Researchers suggest that Norwegian ω-6:ω-3 ratio is slightly better than the United States at perhaps 6–7:1 (Solvoll, Lund-Larsen, Søyland, Sandstad, & Drevon, 1993). Research indicates that a ratio lower than 3:1 results in fewest long-term disease vulnerabilities (Hunninghake, 2005; Simopoulos, 1999).

On the other hand, Paleolithic people *did not* ingest cow's milk or any other type of milk postweaning, cereal grains, table salt (NaCl), white sugar, potatoes, industrially processed and refined grains, pesticide residues, radioactive material in food from nuclear fallout, artificial/synthetic food additives and sweeteners, or genetically modified food. This is expanded in webnote 4–1.

Are Modern Humans Genetically Adapted to Agricultural Diets?

Why has natural selection not weeded out those individuals who are most vulnerable to the "diseases of civilization"? There are a number of factors that offer insight into this question.

1. The rate of evolutionary change is sufficiently slow, and too little time has passed, perhaps 400–500 generations since the rise of agriculture, for great genetic differences to be present between modern humans and our Paleolithic ancestors. Agriculture arose at almost the same time in the Middle East and in Asia 10,000 years ago. However, it took several thousand years before people in other parts of the world changed their subsistence patterns to sedentary agriculture. In Scandinavia farming only started about 5500 years ago (Cordain, 1999), and it was not until several thousand years later that grains became a staple food in Norway. This translates to between 220 and 275 generations (given generation times of 25 and 20 years, respectively) for northern Europeans to become adapted to cereal grains, or approximately half of the number of generations for the first farmers in the Middle East and Asia from the onset of agriculture. Given sufficient selection pressure, this many generations afford ample opportunity for significant genetic changes to take place. However, this does not seem to have been the case, something that may be explained by points 2 and 3 below.

2. The chronic degenerative diseases have affected people too late in life to have been effectively eliminated by natural selection. Even though the current trend is that obesity and type 2 diabetes afflict people at ever-lower ages (Duncan, 2006; see also Chapter 3), this is a recent phenomenon. Previously, such diseases mostly afflicted people at the ages of 50–60 and above (Cleave, 1975; National Research Council, 1989). At such ages, most people have already reproduced and copied their genes—which are adapted to a Paleolithic lifestyle and diet—to the next generation (Neel, 1999).

3. Such diseases are thought to involve too many genes for natural selection to eliminate them. It has been argued that chronic diseases are influenced by many genes

(Neel, 1999). Unlike diseases caused by defects in single genes, selection will take much longer when several genes are involved (Neel, 1999).

4. Turning to agricultural practices, there are several reasons why these have not created conditions that could have eliminated these degenerative chronic diseases. Since the onset of agriculture, grains have never been eaten exclusively, and they have always been part of a mixed diet, so the isolated effects of a high-grain intake would not be easy to detect. In earlier times, whole grains or larger parts of the grains (the endosperm, bran, germ) were utilized, so that far more of the nutrients were ingested. In addition, there is an essential quality difference between freshly milled flour from traditional stone mills and flour that is industrially ground in modern steel roller mills and used after a longer storage time (Campbell, Hauser, & Hill, 1991; Hall, 1976). Finally, most cultures have developed food-conservation techniques (e.g. sprouting and fermentation) that make grains better suited as human food than when these techniques are not used. Such techniques have been part of our cultural evolution to increase food digestibility and palatability, spurring us to compete successfully with other organisms over grains and other plant foods (Johns, 1990; Katz, 1987, 1990). Although processing grains has improved the quality of meals, this process also has slowed down the genetic adaptation to such foods.

For the reasons stated above it is unlikely that evolution since the agricultural revolution systematically could have affected the human gene pool in ways that would have altered the susceptibility to type 2 diabetes, atherosclerosis, cancer, osteoporosis, and other common modern chronic illnesses. Such diseases seem to be a result of the fact that our genome still remains largely adapted to a Paleolithic existence (Tattersall, 1998). This is particularly the case for people in Nordic countries, where the agricultural revolution first gained foothold 5000–6000 years after its onset in the Middle East (Mikkelsen, 1979). The recentness of grain dependency may be an important explanation of why these countries are located at the world peak when it comes to autoimmune and inflammatory diseases like type 1 diabetes, multiple sclerosis, rheumatoid arthritis, childhood asthma, and allergies. (Hunninghake, 2005), which in many instances may be caused by a high and daily intake of wheat and other cereal grains.

The arguments above should not be taken to imply that agriculture is the only factor that has influenced our susceptibility to diseases of civilization (Strassmann & Dunbar, 1999). Nor should they be taken to imply that no evolutionary change could have occurred since the rise of agriculture. Biochemical variations between different human populations could influence how individuals react to environmental factors like diet and lifestyle (Weatherall, 1995; Williams, 1998). Hunter and gatherer societies are often used as a reference point for what a Paleolithic diet might have looked like, but, in fact, modern hunter/gatherers may not be genetically representative of *all* humans (Kelly, 1995). In theory, some people may have changed genetically since the agricultural revolution. For example, subsistence farmers who have been growing and eating wheat and other cereal grains for many generations may have gradually adapted to them (Lutz, 1995, 1998). The same may be true for rice and cow's milk as well (Børresen, 1994a, b). Cultures being dependent upon certain foods for survival for a number of generations may have developed a tolerance or increased metabolic efficiency to those foods, and those who tolerated them best left the most descendants. This is the case in some pastoral human populations that use milk from cows and other milk-producing large animals. Populations with a long dependence on milk and milk products generally have a high proportion with the ability to digest lactose due to the presence of lactase type II enzyme (Caucasians, some African tribes) (Bloom & Sherman, 2005; Durham, 1991; Patterson, 2000; Simoons, 1969; Swallow, 2003) (see Chapter 5), a feature that is not present either in Asian populations or in indigenous Amerindians.

The association between heavy reliance on a particular food and genetic adaptations to that food is also seen in the spread of domestication of grains and the ability to digest gluten. In accordance with such a hypothesis, there is a close negative statistical correlation between the frequency of celiac disease (gluten intolerance) and a marker gene (HLA-B8) that mirrors the spread of agriculture.[3] There is less celiac disease in the Middle East, but increasing frequencies as one moves west- and northwards (Cordain, 1999; McNicholl, Egan-Mitchell, Stevens, Phelan, McKenna, Fottrell, & McCarthy, 1981; Simoons, 1981). As we would expect, populations that were the last to embrace the agricultural revolution would have the highest frequency of celiac disease. This seems to be the case for Ireland and Nordic countries, where the frequencies of celiac disease are higher than in populations from southern Europe and the Middle East (Cronin & Shanahan, 2001; Mäki, Mustalahti, Kokkonen, Kulmala, Haapalahti, Karttunen, Ilonen, Laurila, Dahlbom, Hansson, Höpfl, & Knip, 2003).

The extent of variation among subgroups of modern populations when it comes to tolerance for agricultural foods (particularly cereal grains) is not known.[4] Even if future research proves that certain populations may tolerate agricultural foods better than others, we are left with compelling theoretical and empirical evidence of our lack of adaptations to modern cereal grains, refined sugar, and carbohydrate-based diet and lifestyle.

What We Are Adapted to Eat

The populations of northern Europe in particular are in the rather unique situation, compared with most world populations, of having a large proportion of the adult population adapted to lactose (cow's milk), since most of them have retained an ample production of the enzyme lactase in the digestive system even in old age (Patterson, 2000, p. 1060). Nordic populations are also well adapted to a large intake of fish and crustaceans and, with such foods, a relatively large intake of long-chain ω-3 fatty acids (Bates, 1987). Due to the northern latitude and relatively short exposure to UVB radiation from the sun, cod liver oil has been an important deterrent against vitamin D deficiency and has been used as a food supplement since the eighteenth century. In addition to fish and crustaceans, a significant part of long-chain fatty acids has also been recovered from tissue of large game (moose, reindeer) that is found in large numbers in Finland, Sweden, and Norway. Such animals have historically been an important food source. Nordic countries have only been inhabited for a maximum of 12,000 years, and the agricultural revolution came many thousands of years later than in the Middle East and southern Europe. Therefore, their populations are less well adapted to agriculture than these populations. As mentioned, the Nordics adopted a diet dominated by grains as late as during the last few hundred years (Grøn, 1984). Logically, we are therefore compelled to investigate what kind of diet we are better adapted to.

THE HISTORICAL EXPERIENCE OF
INDIGENOUS/TRADITIONAL PEOPLES

An important part of an evolutionary approach to the "diseases of civilization" is to examine the health of the people before the rise of agriculture as well as the industrial revolution. This is the second topic ignored by the official guidelines. It is not our intention to present the past as any kind of idyllic era or paradise without problems (see, e.g., Diamond, 1997a; Edgerton, 1992; Keeley, 1996; Low, 1996; Ridley, 1996; Shermer, 1997 to the contrary). Our ancestors certainly faced hardships, reducing their life expectancy and increasing their morbidity and mortality. We are happy not to have to cope with intermittent starvation, attack by predators, parasites, fatal infections, deadly insect and snake bites, etc. However, there is no doubt that certain aspects of our ancestors' lives were better than today, particularly with respect to mental and physical health, stamina, and general well-being: A number of researchers, explorers, missionaries, and others who during the past centuries were in contact with people leading a "traditional" lifestyle have independently observed that these populations seemed to be virtually free from modern diseases and health problems like cancer, cardiovascular disease, type 2 diabetes, arthritis, psoriasis, dental caries, and even acne (Crawford & Marsh, 1989; Goldsmith, 1999; McCarrison, 1963; Price, 1970; Stefansson, 1960). This is, for example, the case for the !Kung San people of the Kalahari desert (see Cohen, 1989, for review). Another well-documented example is adult Melanesians on Kitava Island in the Trobriand Islands. Here the Swedish physician Staffan Lindeberg and coworkers thoroughly documented a seemingly absence of cardiovascular disease (stroke and heart attack) in a group of humans who were little influenced by modern Western diets (Lindeberg, 1994; Lindeberg, Berntorp, Carlsson, Eliasson, & Marckmann, 1997; Lindeberg & Lundh, 1993; Lindeberg, Nilsson-Ehle, Terént, Vessby, & Scherstén, 1994; Lindeberg, Nilsson-Ehle, & Vessby, 1996; Lindeberg & Vessby, 1995). Moreover, osteoporosis was found to be totally absent on the nearby island Kiriwina (Johansson, 2001). Among non-Westernized populations like the Yanomamö Indians in Brazil and Venezuela, blood pressures increase from the first to the second decade but, in contrast to industrialized populations, do not systematically increase during subsequent years of life (Oliver, Cohen, & Neel, 1975). It seems that many chronic diseases, common in modern societies, have been more or less absent in populations that have not adapted modern agricultural practices and crops. However, such diseases have a tendency to appear as soon as such humans change their environment and adopt a modern Western-type lifestyle (Cleave, 1975; Price, 1970).

The transition in people's health with the advent of the agricultural revolution is studied in fields like evolutionary biology and paleopathology (Aufderheide & Rodríguez-Martín, 1998). In most parts of the world, the diet of hunters and gatherers has been based on animal proteins and fat found in meat, fowl, fish, crustaceans, etc. (Cordain, Brand Miller, Eaton, Mann, Holt, & Speth, 2000), with the addition of some vegetable material in times of shortage. When grain was substituted for meat as the dominant part of the diet, a reduction in stature and a number of health problems gradually emerged (Aufderheide & Rodríguez-Martín, 1998; Cohen, 1987, 1989; Cohen & Armelagos, 1984; Cordain, 1999; Larsen, 1995, 2000; Ortner & Aufderheide, 1991) (see Chapter 2 and webnote 4–2).

At the beginning of the agricultural revolution, populations relied on grasses of marginal nutritional value. Even if agricultural practices gradually were refined and adapted to local conditions, it is likely that many humans became ill or functioned more poorly as a direct consequence of eating such foods (Cordain, 1999). Since our genetic makeup in this regard appears to have changed little during the relatively short time period since human populations began to eat cereal grains (Eaton, Strassmann, Nesse, Neel, Ewald, Williams, Weder, Eaton III, Lindeberg, Konner, Mysterud, & Cordain, 2002), it is reasonable to conclude that this (i.e., humans functioning suboptimally) is still true, particularly whenever grains constitute a large part of the diet. This is in fact the case for ethnic Norwegians/Nordic peoples, since they are among the populations of Europe where the agricultural revolution started the latest (5500 B.P.) (Cordain, 1999). In addition, almost 1000 years passed after the first use of grains until the agricultural revolution gained foothold (Mikkelsen, 1979). Alternatively, it can be argued that to a certain extent, human culture has compensated for some of the deficits: Improved agricultural practices, selective crop breeding, and technique of preparation have certainly improved.

BIOCHEMICAL, METABOLIC, AND HORMONAL EFFECTS OF FOODS

A third problem with the recommended Norwegian guidelines is that they do not take into account the varying metabolic and hormonal effects of food. Long-chain fatty acids are precursors for pro- and anti-inflammatory eicosanoids, high-glycemic foods increase circulating insulin, adrenalin, and cortisol levels, and high-protein foods stimulate pancreatic glucagon excretion. Therefore, the macronutrient composition of meals has a profound influence on our hormone status (Allan & Lutz, 2000; Sears, 1997; Sears & Lawren, 1995). These and many other hormonal effects of foods are important for health because they are related to, among others, obesity, blood pressure, heart disease, and cancer. This is briefly discussed in a recent report by Norwegian experts (Norwegian Nutrition Council [NNC], 2000) but is not reflected in the official guidelines.

DIFFERING BIOAVAILABILITY OF NUTRIENTS IN VARIOUS FOODS

The fourth aspect that the official guidelines ignore is the fact that foods differ considerably in biological availability (bioavailability) of nutrients. For example, even if cereal grains contain iron and zinc, these minerals are not easily absorbed by the digestive system. The same is true of magnesium and iron absorption from cow's milk. On the other hand, meat contains bioavailable nutrients like iron and zinc, fruits and vegetables contain a host of well-absorbed antioxidants, and nuts in addition contain balanced macronutrients (Rimestad, Borgejordet, Vesterhus, Sygnestveit, Bjørge Løken, Trygg, Pollestad, Lund-Larsen, Omholt Jensen, & Nordbotten, 2001; USDA Nutrient Data Base, 2005[5]). By implication, "natural" and unrefined foods, such as were eaten before the advent of agriculture, are in principle more conducive to human health than grains and potatoes, especially in processed form, since they contain many more essential nutrients (Halton,

Willett, Liu, Manson, Stampfer, & Hu, 2006; Willett, 2006). In addition, these nutrients are more bioavailable to the human body, reflecting our adaptation to Paleolithic diets during millennia in the past.

VARIABILITY OF INDIVIDUAL NEEDS IN LARGE GROUPS WITH SPECIAL REQUIREMENTS

The fifth topic that the official guidelines ignore is the fact that various individuals for genetic reasons need different amounts of nutrients to avoid disease in modern environments. The guidelines do not seem to take into account the important concept of genetic polymorphism and therefore offer the same recommended daily intakes of vitamins and minerals to everybody, in spite of the fact that genetic variations may cause differences in the needs for a number of nutrients of 1:100–1000 (Ames, Elson-Schwab, & Silver, 2002; Williams, 1987, 1998). Furthermore, a significant part of the world's population tolerate well neither gluten/gliadin (not only celiac), nor the effect of exorphins[6] in general or cow's milk (lactose, caseomorphins) (webnote 4–3).

PREVENTION OF DEFICIENCIES VERSUS OPTIMAL NUTRIENT INTAKE

The sixth ignored topic is that food supplements, in addition to healthy foods, may be necessary for modern humans to achieve the best possible health. It is imperative to emphasize the difference between the average nutrient requirement to prevent deficiencies and the optimal nutrient intake needed to achieve the highest level of health possible.

A basic tenant in orthomolecular medicine (Pauling, 1968) is to supply each individual with optimal levels of nutrients in order to "live longer and feel better" (Marinacci, 1995; Pauling, 1986). That the need for specific nutrients varies between individuals (Ames, Elson-Schwab, & Silver, 2002), is not even considered in the Nordic guidelines (NNR, 2004), where the word "optimal" is missing in the index. The idea here is that "good health" will reign if only the "requirements" are met, and no attempt is made to find out if higher intakes may have a potential for leading to better health. We exemplify the importance of an optimal nutrient intake by focusing on vitamin D (see webnote 4–4).

THE BIG CONTROVERSIES IN NORWAY

Unfortunately, knowledge from academic disciplines like evolutionary biology and paleopathology has not been considered relevant by those designated as experts in formulating official guidelines for healthy living for the Nordic populations. Neither is this the case for guidelines developed elsewhere. The facts concerning the prehistoric and historical health problems encountered with the introduction of "new foods" are completely ignored by the very authorities who—according to governmental directives—are responsible for issuing dietary recommendations.

Official guidelines have urged Norwegians to eat bread and cereal grains, potatoes, cow's milk, and margarine for decades. Perhaps the primary reason for such advice is that

Norwegians developed a tradition for eating exactly such foods (with the exception of margarine) during recent centuries based on their availability and the lack of other foods. However, Norwegians have also had a tradition for ingesting more animal fat than today,[7] but authorities nevertheless actively recommend a reduced intake. We argue that such short-term traditions should not be a relevant guide for dietary recommendations, whether they are based on the consumption of more bread and potatoes or of less fat.

Cereal grains, cow's milk, and margarine are typically highly processed before consumption and are often eaten at the expense of foods that can be eaten directly without or with minimal processing (eggs, nuts, seeds, avocado). Refined and industrially processed foods are typically stripped of important nutrients, which contributes to a lower intake of vitamins and trace minerals (Hall, 1976). The practice of adding back some of the vitamins does not make such products "enriched," even if major health benefits have been registered after the recent addition of folate in the United States (Hall, 1976; Hoffer, 2005).

Let us in the following focus on problems with cereal grains, potatoes, and a high-carbohydrate and low-fat diet.

Problematic Cereal Grains

Leading nutritionists in Norway claim that humans are well adapted to cereal grains and recommend eating more bread and grains/cereals, but offer no evidence that this would be more beneficial to health than eating in accordance with a Paleolithic diet. This view of the beneficial qualities of a cereal diet totally ignores the evolutionary arguments showing that grains can be a problematic food for many humans, particularly when eaten frequently and in large amounts, potentially displacing other foodstuffs for which humans are better adapted (Cordain, 1999). Processed cereal grains are energy dense, and a high consumption displaces effectively the intake of nonstarchy, low-glycemic vegetables. Since humans have relatively small stomachs, increasing both the intake of energy-dense and satiating bread, potatoes, rice, and pasta and nonstarchy vegetables is simply impossible.

A number of problems associated with recommending cereal grains as a staple food to the whole population are frequently ignored: (1) Grains contain a large percentage of easily digestible starches (60–70%); (2) grains like wheat and corn generally contain *lectins* that can function as *"insulin mimics;"* (3) grains have an *unfavorable nutrient content*; (4) the *biological availability* (bioavailability) of certain vitamins and minerals in cereal grains is low; (5) grains contain several defense chemicals or *antinutrients* that function to prevent them from being eaten by insects and animals; (6) grains contain a high level of the storage protein *gluten*, which is linked to a number of chronic diseases; and (7) historically, wet conditions have proven to be a problem with *mycotoxins* in grains. This is expanded upon in webnote 4–5.

For the above reasons consumption of significant amounts of cereal grains may not be healthy for many people, even if some people may tolerate a higher intake of whole grains in spite of their levels of antinutrients like phytates and lectins. An argument could be made for consumption of white flour, since it in fact contains fewer antinutrients. However, white flour contains very few nutrients and is highly glycemic and insulinogenic. Therefore, consumption of foods made with white flour or with refined flour several times a day is not advised (Hall, 1976). A possible strategy would be to prepare the bread in such a way that antinutrients are neutralized or eliminated at the same time as the fat and protein content is increased.[8]

Problems with Potatoes

A high intake of potatoes also seems unwise. During the last few decades consumption of potatoes has been reduced due to a decrease of intake of boiled potatoes, while the intake of potato chips and French fries has surged dramatically (i.e., acryl amide, peroxidized and trans fatty acids). Boiled potatoes have been in part replaced by rice, pasta, and other foods made with refined flours. A recommendation to increase potato consumption would, apart from increasing the total glycemic load of the diet, most likely increase the intake of fried potatoes and other processed potatoes and increase levels of easily peroxidized polyunsaturated fats that most nutrition experts agree are detrimental.

A more sensible approach, given today's obesity problem and high availability of food, would be to advise eating more nonstarchy vegetables, e.g., cruciferous vegetables like broccoli, cauliflower, Brussels sprouts, cabbage, watercress, bok choy, turnip greens, mustard greens and collard greens, radishes, turnips, kohlrabi, as well as vegetables in the onion family. Besides supplying more vitamins and fiber than refined grains and potatoes, most vegetables have a very low or negligible glycemic load. However, one problem involved in eating large quantities of vegetables is the volume they require in the stomach. Vegetables are bulkier and less energy dense than starchy (bread, potatoes) and fatty foods, and increased consumption of the latter displaces vegetables from the diet. Since the average intake of total fat in Norwegian diets is now reduced to as little as 30–35% of total energy (after several decades of low-fat recommendations), it seems that the best advice to improve the diet would be to reduce the intake of sugar and starchy foods. Consumption of healthy fats, i.e., natural, unprocessed fats and oils, should be encouraged, since these have never been proven causal in any major disease (e.g., Ravnskov, 2000). In fact, ω-3 and ω-6 fatty acids, as well as 8–10 amino acids, are absolutely essential for good health. In contrast, high glycemic carbohydrates are not essential, since the body is able to produce all the glucose it needs from other macronutrients (such as amino acids and glycerol). A growing body of research has demonstrated that even saturated fatty acids from cow's milk are protective of cardiovascular disease (Biong, Veierød, Ringstad, Thelle, & Pedersen, 2006; Elwood, Pickering, Hughes, Fehily, & Ness, 2004; Skjervold, 1992) as well as other illnesses like cancer (Parodi, 1997; Parodi, 2004).

Some nutritionists in Norway recommend eating more potatoes, arguing that they are rich in fiber and vitamin C. However, many vegetables, such as broccoli and cabbage, are more nutrient rich than potatoes (see Table 4–2 on webpage). We conclude that reducing the intake of sucrose, potatoes, and cereal grain products and increasing the intake of vegetables is the most sensible recommendation for good nutrition in Norway.

Problems with a High-Carbohydrate and Low-Fat Diet

In a recent report by Norwegian experts (NNC, 2000), it is stated that carbohydrates are not transformed into fat in the human body, a statement that clearly is incorrect (Aas, Kase, Solberg, Jensen, & Rustan, 2004; McDevitt, Bott, Harding, Coward, Bluck, & Prentice, 2001; Minehira, Bettschart, Vidal, Di Vetta, Rey, Schneiter, & Tappy, 2003;

Quistorff & Grunnet, 2003; Schwarz, Linfoot, Dare, & Aghajanian, 2003). Carbohydrates consumed in excess of energy needs are transformed into long-chain saturated fatty acids in the body (Quistorff & Grunnet, 2003).

Following the argument of NNR 2004, saturated fatty acids would not be dangerous if synthesized from glycemic carbohydrates like potatoes and bread, which are highly recommended. Because long-chain saturated fatty acids found in food are the same as those synthesized from carbohydrates, it is argued that saturated fats as such are not dangerous and unhealthy. If they were, a logical conclusion would be to avoid all excess glycemic carbohydrates, because they are substrates for the synthesis of endogenous saturated fatty acids.

Another argument that speaks against the idea that saturated fats found in animal fat are detrimental to health is that all animal fats (included fatty fish) consist of a great number of different fatty acids, including saturated fatty acids of short and long chains (Cordain, 2006; Enig, 2000). Because hominins have eaten animal fats for millions of years, our lineage must be adapted to a great variety of fatty acids, saturates included.

In NNR 2004, Nordic nutrition authorities recommend a higher intake of foods rich in starch and a lower intake of foods high in sugar and fats. At the same time, they also recommend a reduction in energy density. However, starch-rich foods are quite energy *dense* (Rimestad, Borgejordet, Vesterhus, Sygnestveit, Bjørge Løken, Trygg, Pollestad, Lund-Larsen, Omholt Jensen, & Nordbotten, 2001) when compared to nonstarchy vegetables and most fruits and berries. Paradoxically, the literature to which the authorities sometimes refer (NNC, 2000) shows that an increase in the fat intake from 18 to 40 E% does not seem to significantly influence whether or not a given person becomes overweight (Willett, 1998b). A number of traditional peoples in good health (Masai, Samburu, Inuit) regularly eat diets consisting of 60–80 E% as fats, a large part of which constitutes saturated fatty acids (see Ravnskov, 2000, for overview; Biss, Ho, Mikkelson, Lewis, & Taylor, 1971; Mann & Shaffer, 1966; Mann, Shaffer, Anderson, & Sandstead, 1964; Mann, Shaffer, & Rich, 1965; Mann, Spoerry, Gray, & Jarashow, 1972; McCormick & Elmore-Meegan, 1992; Shaper, 1962) and low in glycemic carbohydrate. In addition, a number of clinical trials demonstrate that diets with a low carbohydrate and a high fat and/or protein content actually have highly beneficial effects on a number of common diseases, including obesity and heart/cardiovascular disease (Abbasi, McLaughlin, Lamendola, Kim, Tanaka, Wang, Nakajima, & Reaven, 2000; Brehm, Seeley, Daniels, & D'Alessio, 2003; Foster, Wyatt, Hill, McGuckin, Brill, Mohammed, Szapary, Rader, Edman, & Klein, 2003; Jeppesen, Schaaf, Jones, Zhou, Chen, & Reaven, 1997; McLaughlin, Abbasi, Lamendola, Yeni-Komshian, & Reaven, 2000; Reaven, 2005; Samaha, Iqbal, Seshadri, Chicano, Daily, McGrory, Williams, Williams, Gracely & Stern, 2003; Sharman, Kraemer, Love, Avery, Gómez, Scheett, & Volek, 2002; Westman, Yancy, Edman, Tomlin, & Perkins, 2002; see also Kopp, 2006). This does not mean that a high-fat diet should be followed by the population as a whole, as some diet experts, physicians, and experienced laypersons advise (Donaldson, 1961; Kwasniewski, 1999, 2000; MacKarness, 1958; Pennington, 1953a, b; Skaldeman, 2005; Westman, Yancy, & Humphreys, 2006). However, it is inappropriate not to note that several population groups and possibly several millions of individuals all over the world have enjoyed good health with a fat intake of up to 75–80 E% and have done so for millennia (Banting, 1864; Brillat-Savarin, 1995 (1st ed. 1825); McClellan, 1930; McClellan & Du Bois, 1930; Stefansson, 1937, 1946, 1960; Tolstoi, 1929).

In diets supplying the same amount of energy, there is no reason to favor high-glycemic carbohydrates at the expense of natural fats, and there are no proven benefits in connection with weight reduction (Astrup, Toubro, Raben, & Skov, 1997; Golay, Allaz, Morel, de Tonnac, Tankova, & Reaven, 1996; Willett, 1998a). This is actually stated in the report from the nutrition authorities (NNC, 2000), but is not reflected in the guidelines.

High-energy-density meals composed of a combination of high-glycemic carbohydrates (starches and sugars) and high fat (often processed and of poor quality) are generally not recommended for sedentary people. The combination of a high insulin level caused by ingested carbohydrates followed by ample amounts of fat may cause rapid weight gain (Ledikwe, Blanck, Kettel Khan, Serdula, Seymour, Tohill, & Rolls, 2006). However, to our knowledge no evidence exists that meals or food products with a high content of, for instance, butter or coconut oil and low-glycemic carbohydrates are detrimental to health.

The real culprits seem to be high-glycemic carbohydrates that are "carriers" of refined fats. By reducing the intake of sugar, flour, and processed potatoes, one automatically reduces the fat intake as well, especially the highly processed fat so common in fried foods. It would be far healthier to replace such high-glycemic carbohydrates with non-starchy vegetables, legumes, nuts, and healthful (unprocessed) fats.

Several studies have shown that there is no linear association between energy intake (both increased and reduced) and weight (Kasper, Thiel, & Ehl, 1973; Keckwick & Pawan, 1956; Olesen & Quaade, 1960). This view is also stated in one report from the authorities (NNC, 2000), but the official guidelines nevertheless advise people to lower their fat intake in order to reduce overweight "in populations with low physical activity and high prevalence of obesity" (NNR 2004, p. 164).

The authorities do not take into account that a high-carbohydrate diet increases the concentration of insulin and triglycerides in the blood—two important markers for heart disease. As such, a diet with a low carbohydrate content, compared with a high-carbohydrate diet supplying the same amount of energy, is more "heart friendly" (Abbasi, McLaughlin, Lamendola, Kim, Tanaka, Wang, Nakajima, & Reaven, 2000; Jeppesen, Schaaf, Jones, Zhou, Chen, & Reaven, 1997; McLaughlin, Abbasi, Lamendola, Yeni-Komshian, & Reaven, 2000).

Furthermore, they do not take into account that diets with a high glycemic load favor oxidation, glycosylation, and insulin resistance (Bell, 2000; Bucala, Cerami, & Vlassara, 1995; Ceriello & Pirisi, 1995; Chen, Azhar, Abbasi, Carantoni, & Reaven, 2000; Marfella, Quagliaro, Nappo, Ceriello, & Giugliano, 2001; Saydah, Miret, Sung, Varas, Gause, & Brancati, 2001). Nor do they discuss the consequences of a high postprandial insulin level caused by such foods, i.e., in promoting cardiovascular disease, inflammation, endothelial dysfunction, hypertension, lipid abnormalities, and increased appetite (Ceriello & Pirisi, 1995; Després, Lamarche, Mauriège, Cantin, Dagenais, Moorjani, & Lupien, 1996; Fontbonne & Eschwège, 1991; Paolisso & Giugliano, 1996; Pyorala, Miettinen, Laakso, & Pyorala, 2000).

Studies have shown that the postulated causal connection between cholesterol, saturated fats, and heart disease does not exist (Ravnskov, 2000). Ten studies, including the Framingham Heart Study, show that there is no significant difference in cholesterol levels between groups with coronary heart disease and healthy subjects (Ravnskov, 2000). The French and Finns have equally high cholesterol levels, but the French have much lower incidence of heart disease (between two thirds and three quarters less, depending on the region of Finland) (Ravnskov, 2000). On several South Pacific islands the populations for millennia probably have eaten large amounts of coconut fat, which contains 90–95% saturated fatty acids. The official view is that such a diet promotes cardiovascular disease. However, these populations enjoy excellent general and cardio-vascular health (Enig & Fallon, 2005; Fife, 2002; Price, 1970; Prior, Davidson, Salmond, & Czochanska, 1981).

Scientific evidence has thus demonstrated that neither saturated fatty acids nor dietary cholesterol is detrimental to health. Saturated fatty acids do not in general raise blood cho-lesterol levels, contrary to what the nutrition authorities have claimed. Cholesterol-rich, nutritious, and healthy foods like eggs were previously advised against. According to NNR 2004 (p. 163), "expert groups, mainly in the USA, have recommended that the cho-lesterol intake in adults should be kept below 300 mg/day." Since the average intake in the Nordic countries is estimated at 250–350 mg/day, "the current recommendation does not set an upper intake level for cholesterol." No reference is made to the fact that cholesterol in foods in general does not cause hypercholesterolemia (Ballesteros, Cabrera, Saucedo, & Fernancez, 2004). Eggs contain high-quality protein, vitamins A and D, many polyun-saturated fatty acids, lecithin, and a number of other important micronutrients.

According to NNR 2004 (p. 13), the diet should contain approximately 5–10 E% of polyunsaturated fatty acids (one third to one sixth of the total energy intake from fats), of which 1 E% should consist of ω-3 fatty acids (ω3). This means that the recommended ω-6:ω-3 ratio is set at 5–10, something that is not in line with our evolutionary heritage (Simopoulos, 1999). Consumption of large quantities of polyunsaturated fats, particu-larly ω-6 fatty acids, which are found in margarines and in most cereal grains and refined oils, increases the ω-6 load and stimulates inflammatory processes by creating an unfa-vorable eicosanoid balance (Hunninghake, 2005; Sears & Lawren, 1995). A high intake of polyunsaturated fats increases the need for antioxidants, since polyunsaturated fatty acids are more easily oxidized than saturated and monounsaturated fatty acids (Halliwell & Gutteridge, 1989; Skjervold, 1992).

Examinations of the fatty acid composition of aortas of patients having died from ischemic heart disease showed that the fats found in the victims' arteries were almost identical in composition to margarines (Biong, Veierød, Ringstad, Thelle, & Pedersen, 2006). In addition to having removed trans fatty acids from margarine in Norway, a wise thing to do would be to replace much of the ω-6-fatty acids from soy oil with some satu-rated fatty acids from coconut or palm kernel oil and monounsaturated fatty acids from rapeseed or olive oil. This would improve the ω-6:ω-3 ratio and thus counteract inflam-matory processes in the body that are involved in chronic diseases.

The authorities simply neglect the criticisms of the ruling nutrition dogma that fat consumption is unhealthy (see, to the contrary: Donaldson, 1961; Enig, 2000; Erasmus, 1993; Kwasniewski, 1999; Pennington, 1953a, b; Sears & Lawren, 1995; Westman, Yancy, & Humphreys, 2006; Yancy, Foy, Chaleckil, Vernon, & Westman, 2005) and that unadul-terated cholesterol may be a cause of cardiovascular disease (see Colpo, 2006; Ravnskov, 2000, 2002, for criticism of this hypothesis).

OBESITY IN NORWAY

The prevalence of obesity has increased the last 30 years, with the situation becoming even worse during the last 5–10 years (Tverdal, 1996), in particular for children (Brundtland,

Liestøl, & Walløe, 1975, 1980; Knudtzon, Waaler, Skjærven, Solberg, & Steen, 1988; Knudtzon, Waaler, Solberg, Grieg, Skjærven, Steen, & Irgens, 1988; Tell & Vellar, 1988; Waaler, 1983; see also Chapter 3). Many analysts expect a corresponding increase in type 2 diabetes (global WHO prognosis: 170 million diabetics at present, 300 million in 2025).[9]

During recent decades dietary fat intake among Norwegians has been reduced to 32 E%, of which 15% consists of saturated fatty acids. Nevertheless, the incidence of obesity and type 2 diabetes has "exploded."

The strong increase in sugar consumption has probably been an important contributing factor in the development of the obesity "epidemic." Since most bioavailable carbohydrates (sugars and starches) are transformed to blood glucose and, when ingested in excess of what the body manages to burn to cover its needs, turn ultimately to body fat, there is in principle no difference between sugary and starchy foods when it comes to the effect on adiposity. Intake of starches (long glucose chains) and refined sugars has increased in Norway concomitantly with the reduced intake of fats (as a result of official recommendations). At the same time, total energy intake has decreased somewhat (NNC, 2000) and the protein intake has remained stable. Reduction in fat intake has not led to less obesity; in fact, its displacement by sugars and starches may in fact have contributed substantially to the obesity epidemic.

Research indicates that more people currently are physically active in their leisure time than 20 years ago. This is stated in the report from the nutrition authorities (NNC, 2000), who also admit that the documentation on how much physical activity in which young people engage is poor (NNC, 2000). Notwithstanding, the authorities conclude that lack of exercise is the major culprit for the obesity epidemic.

It seems reasonable that a lower level of physical activity could be part of the obesity epidemic, but so far the existing data actually contradict this observation. Although there is a clear statistical correlation between physical inactivity and obesity, there is no evidence that physical inactivity is in fact the cause of the increased prevalence of obesity (Petersen, Schnohr, & Sorensen, 2004). A possible explanation may be that the development of obesity due to poor diet leads to inactivity, which in turn starts a vicious circle. Alternatively, it may be that a reduction of fat coupled with an increased intake of high-glycemic carbohydrates has led to an increase the prevalence of type 2 diabetes and obesity (Salmeron, Ascherio, Rimm, Colditz, Spiegelman, Jenkins, Stampfer, Wing, & Willett, 1997; Salmeron, Manson, Stampfer, Colditz, Wing, & Willett, 1997; Westman, Mavropoulos, Yancy, & Volek, 2003; Westman, Yancy, & Humphreys, 2006).

Using Occam's razor, there are most probably other, more important factors behind the obesity epidemic. Our hypothesis is that this in part must be caused by the increased intake of easily digestible high-glycemic carbohydrates from refined sugar and other starchy foods. Since Norwegian authorities for several decades have recommended eating carbohydrates at the expense of fat, while (until recently) at the same time they have not suggested curtailing the consumption of sweet soft drinks, they inadvertently may have contributed to the epidemic of obesity and type 2 diabetes. This is also consistent with the experience of many people who have not managed to keep their weight down in spite of being physically active and for those who have drastically reduced their weight in spite of *not* exercising. One key to understanding weight reduction without an increase in exercise seems to be the suppression of appetite induced by high-fat and/or high-protein foods, one mechanism being the stabilization of blood sugar (Skaldeman, 2005).

Little knowledge exists about the changes in the body composition of the population, i.e., the relative weight of muscles and fat, which is actually more important than mere changes in body weight (Allan & Lutz, 2000; Lutz, 1998). It is likely that the percentage of body fat in the population has increased more than the average body weight due to the current high-carbohydrate diet, given the reduction of manual labor performed.

GENERAL DISCUSSION

We are critical of the current dietary recommendations in Norway for a number of reasons. They are not based on science, but on political, historical, and fiscal considerations. For this reason, a totally different nutrition paradigm is needed. Internationally, we see a gradual change in terms of nutritional recommendations. In the United States and France recommendations seem to be in transition and now allow greater variation in the composition of macronutrients.[10] In contrast, the most recent Nordic guidelines recommend that most people *increase* their consumption of potatoes, bread, and cereal grains, the argument being that the intake of these staple foods has declined during recent decades and that this is undesirable from a health perspective. This advice is offered with no regard for metabolic differences between individuals (Weatherall, 1995; Williams, 1987, 1998), e.g., the low carbohydrate tolerance of large parts of the population (obese, type 2 diabetics, insulin resistant, etc.). It is our view that it is unscientific to give specific, rigid recommendations and expect them to be of benefit to the whole population. The use of Norwegian guideline slogans like "eat more bread and potatoes" or "drink more milk" obviously is based on local food-production policies and tradition, and not on a broad evaluation of the available scientific documentation. Perhaps it may be sensible to recommend "eating as many vegetables as possible" or "eating more fish," but there is no scientific basis for recommending a strict percentage distribution between macronutrients. In fact, following narrow guidelines based on "what Norwegians have traditionally eaten in the recent past" (cereal grains, bread, and potatoes) may negatively affect a large part of the population and at least those who are diabetic and/or overweight/obese.

Another major problem with the official guidelines is that they focus singlemindedly on just one factor at a time. For several decades they focused almost solely on eating "less cholesterol and fats," now being replaced with "exercise more" and, recently, "drink less soft drinks and eat less sugar." Although recommendation to exercise more and to ingest less sucrose may be considered to be science based, nutrition is a far too complex and holistic a science to be presented in such a simplistic and reductionist manner.

One consequence of the recommendation to eat more potatoes may have been that the population not only eats more potato chips and French fries, but also shuns healthful fats. The recommendation to eat more bread may have made people eat more white bread, baguettes, spaghetti, and pizza.[11] This implies that one should not recommend such foods (potatoes, bread) without specifying exactly under what circumstances this might be beneficial and for whom.

Based on extensive literature searches and the clinical experience of two of us (FL and SB) with more than 15,000 patients, we are convinced that any individuals experiencing type 2 diabetes, overweight, hypertension, cancer, or cardiovascular diseases may bene-fit from dietary changes that lower the dietary glycemic load. Most important would be to increase the ingestion of high-quality, i.e., animal proteins and of natural unprocessed oils and fats and to substitute high-glycemic plant foods like grains and sweet fruits with low-glycemic foods like berries, vegetables, nuts, and seeds. For those having developed insulin resistance it is important to substitute high-glycemic carbohydrate foods (sugars and starchy foods) with foods containing natural fats, including cold-pressed olive and rapeseed oils, as well as good sources of ω-3-fatty acids (walnuts, cold-pressed ω-3–rich plant oils, fatty fish, and green leafy vegetables such as purslane), while consuming less ω-6 fatty acids. In sum, this means mimicking the way our Paleolithic ancestors ate.

Our view is that the recommendations by the official Norwegian nutrition authorities are not in agreement with a broad array of scientific data and approaches. It is now time to question how these recommendations came about and to set new standards.[12] There is also a need to investigate which alternative guidelines current recommendations were compared to or tested against. To our knowledge no such comparisons were made; hence the official recommendations cannot be trusted. It is also ironic that some reports from the authorities (NNC, 2000) are in better agreement with scientific data than current recommendations, which clearly are based not on science, but on politics.

Bases for Recommendations

A common and expected reaction to our arguments may be that several of them may not be supported by scientific studies of "gold standard," i.e., prospective, randomized placebo-controlled intervention trials. However, even if nutrition studies in general are not amendable to this design, it is possible to obtain evidence-based knowledge in nutrition science by other means, for instance, by careful observations of individuals or groups over protracted time periods. Such observations may include hard data such as glycosylation of red blood cells (HbA1c), inflammatory markers, blood pressure, or hormone levels.

Compliance is obviously a great problem, and it is not possible to mask foods in such a way that nobody knows what they are eating. One also should beware of the socio-political and economic reality of contemporary research. In the area of nutrition, it is generally problematic to receive funding for carrying out long-term research, since such research does not aim at marketing patented products. The pharmaceutical industry funds most of the clinical medical research in Norway (Poleszynski, 2001) and elsewhere, and it is not in their interest to study effects of nonpatentable approaches like nutritional medicine for two reasons: (1) nonpatentable products yield much smaller profits than patented ones; and (2) a nutritional approach is in direct competition with patented drugs. Furthermore, large food-producing corporations do not usually fund studies on nutrition, one of the reasons being that they are not allowed to market foods with health claims.

Dietary recommendations to the general population should ideally be based on evidence from animal studies, epidemiological studies, evolutionary considerations, studies of prehistoric/historic people and their traditional and new diets, and, last but not least, basic medical research. When all these approaches are taken into consideration, it seems obvious that current dietary recommendations in Norway are not based on the total wealth of scientific information available.

CONCLUSION

The current dietary guidelines contribute to chronic diseases in Norway: they are not based on scientific evidence, and people are poorly advised. Furthermore, the authorities' double message on nutrient intake (i.e., women of reproductive age should take folic acid, and we all should take cod liver oil, but supplements in general are not needed) is confusing to many. Therefore, we are not surprised to see that the population increasingly suffers from a multitude of easily preventable chronic diseases. The logical conclusion for the Norwegian nutrition authorities would be to change their recommendations in accordance with the best available scientific data from a host of approaches, taking into account that the population is by no means homogeneous. The evidence clearly shows that a Paleolithic diet may be optimal for many if not most of us, that nutrient needs vary substantially from individual to individual, and that optimal nutrient intake in many cases is many times greater than the currently recommended "adequacy." If such new guidelines were issued, they could contribute importantly to the struggle for reducing the incidence of chronic disease not only in Nordic countries, but also on a global scale.

ACKNOWLEDGMENTS

We appreciate the comments from Neal Smith and Wenda Trevathan on various earlier drafts and answers from Loren Cordain and Johnny Laupsa-Borge on various requests about specific points. A portion of this paper was presented at the fifteenth annual conference of Human Behavior & Evolution Society (HBES), University of Nebraska, Lincoln, NE, June 4–8, 2003. The first author (IM) was funded by the Norwegian magazine Mat&Helse (www.matoghelse.no) to attend the conference.

CHAPTER 5

Cow's Milk Consumption and Health
An Evolutionary Perspective

Andrea S. Wiley

Wiley provides a step-by-step cultural, historical, and biological overview of worldwide differential adaptations to lactose. She examines through cross-cultural materials and physiological studies the effects of dairying practices on the abilities of geographically diverse people to break down lactose (by way of the enzyme lactase) for easy and proper absorption by the gut. After reading what she has to say, we will no longer be quite so comfortable when someone responds to the widely seen American commercial for milk that begins "Got milk?", especially when the answer is: "Sure, I got milk. Shouldn't everybody?" One of the most useful concepts she illuminates here, which is relevant to all aspects of evolutionary medicine, concerns what George Williams calls "the fallacy of medical normalcy," the idea that if some pattern of behavior or physiological reaction is "normal" or "expectable" among Westernized people, then the medical assumption must be that it is normal, right, desirable, and healthy for everyone. Unfortunately, this is not the case, and no better example makes this point than Wiley's exploration of "lactose impersistence" and the vast majority of the world's peoples who cannot easily (if at all) digest lactose without negative health consequences, and why. She calls the phenomenon of labeling lactose intolerance in the Western medical paradigm a "disorder" rather than as species-wide norm an example of "bio-ethnocentrism." Throughout her chapter she shows that the history of domesticating dairy animals over the millennia "is necessary but not sufficient" for explaining both geographical and cultural variations in lactose persistence.

INTRODUCTION

The consumption of cow's milk among children and adults is an evolutionarily novel behavior. Access to milk in the postweaning period became possible only in populations that domesticated mammals for milk production. The oldest documentation of milking is

116

from Libya, about 5000 B.C. (Davidson, 1999), and milking remained an exclusively Old World practice until Europeans settled in the New World. Only some Old World populations, such as northern Europeans, and pastoralist populations of Africa, Arabia, and Central Asia made extensive use of milk, and they evolved genetic adaptations to do so. Other populations in sub-Saharan Africa, East and Southeast Asia, the Pacific Islands, and the Americas did not consume milk and did not evolve such adaptations. However, consumption by children and adults among populations without such adaptations is becoming more widespread (Wiley, 2007), raising questions about the biological effects of this novel food in populations without a history of drinking milk.

Cow's milk consumption among older children and adults is of importance from an evolutionary perspective for at least three reasons:

1. Milk is a unique food; it is the only food consumed by humans or other mammals that is produced by a given mammalian species for the purpose of being consumed by that species. Milk contains a number of substances that enhance growth, maturation, and provide immunity to local pathogens.

2. Milk contains lactose, a unique disaccharide found nowhere else in nature (Patton, 2004). Lactose requires the pancreatic enzyme lactase to be digested and absorbed in the small intestine. In the vast majority of mammals lactase is produced early in life; then its production ceases around the time of weaning. For humans to continue to digest milk throughout life, they must have mutations in their DNA that allow lactase to continue to be produced; these mutations appear to have become widespread in only northern Europeans and a few herding populations of Africa and Asia.

3. Because this new source of milk derives from bovids (e.g., cows, goats, and sheep), it reflects and supports growth patterns that are quite distinct from those of humans.

This chapter addresses the following questions.

• How do the unique evolutionary histories of different cultures contribute to variation in lactase production and milk-consumption patterns?

• What are the consequences for individuals derived from populations with evolutionary histories that have not included milk consumption but who live in societies in which milk consumption is promoted?

• What are the life history consequences of milk consumption well after the typical age of weaning, especially when the milk derives from a different species? There are several reasons to believe that continued milk consumption might alter early and later life history parameters in ways that have positive and/or negative effects on health.

The material presented in this chapter also challenges what George C. Williams described as the fallacy of "medical normalcy" (Williams, 2000), or what I consider to be "bio-ethnocentrism." Both of these concepts refer to a tendency to consider as "normal" for *Homo sapiens* characteristics that are most common only in certain groups, especially Europeans. One of the contributions of an evolutionary perspective on health and medical practice is to challenge these biases by contributing to the understanding of the nature and evolution of individual and population physiological differences.

GENETICS OF LACTOSE DIGESTION

Lactase is a digestive enzyme that breaks down lactose, a sugar found only in mammalian milks, into its component sugars, glucose and galactose. The latter two sugars can then be absorbed and used for energy. In most mammalian species, lactase production is high at birth and then declines, reaching residual levels around the time of weaning. As a result, adult mammals produce little or no lactase. This decline in lactase activity is under genetic control (Sahi, 1994b) and cannot be induced by continued milk consumption.

There is both individual and population variation in adult lactase activity in *Homo sapiens*. There are populations in which high frequencies of adults continue to produce lactase in adulthood and those in which lactase production declines to low levels by adulthood (Sahi, 1994a). As Table 5-1 shows, high rates of lactase persistence appear only among northern Europeans, herding populations of the Middle East and Arabian Peninsula and sub-Saharan Africa, some South Asians, and descendents of these populations. In other words, most humans follow the ancestral mammalian pattern, in which lactase production ceases around the age of weaning (Bayless & Rosensweig, 1966; Sahi, 1994a). This basic pattern is referred to as *lactase impersistence*, while continuing to produce lactase in adulthood is referred to as *lactase persistence*.

Genealogical studies have found an inheritance pattern for lactase persistence that is consistent with a dominant mode of expression for these alleles (Kretchmer, 1972). The gene for the lactase enzyme is found on chromosome 2 and is not variable across populations in ways that correlate with differences in lactase persistence. However, the genetic regulation of the lactase gene is variable, and the actual mutations associated with lactase persistence have been identified in an area of DNA near the lactase gene (Enattah et al., 2002).[1]

TABLE 5-1 Rates of Lactase Persistence in Human Populations

Population	Estimated prevalence (%)
Northern Europeans	~95
European-derived Americans	~85
Central Europeans	~70–85
Southern Europeans	~20–70
Middle East/North Africa	~30
Sub-Saharan Africa	
herding populations	~80–85
nonherding populations	~10–20
Indians (Indian subcontinent)	
northern	~70
southern	~30–40
Hispanics	~30
Native Americans	~0–38
African Americans	~20
East and Southeast Asians	~0–5
Oceania (non-European)	~15–25

Source: Sahi, 1994a.

EVOLUTION OF LACTASE PERSISTENCE

It is widely accepted that the origins of animal domestication set the stage for selection to favor the ability to digest lactose in adulthood, for without opportunities to consume mammalian milk in adulthood, there would be no advantage to continued production of lactase (Durham, 1991; McCracken, 1971; Simoons, 1978). Indeed, all populations with high rates of lactase persistence have long histories of dairying (Durham, 1991). Given that milk is rich in several nutrients, Simoons (1978, 2001) proposed that individuals with a mutation allowing them to consume milk throughout life would have been healthier and better nourished compared to those without the mutation. Researchers have suggested that a 3–7% fitness advantage would have been sufficient to generate the high frequencies of lactase persistence found in dairy-dependent populations (Flatz, 1987; McCracken, 1971). As Durham (1991) pointed out, however, there are many populations, such as those in the Mediterranean region and North Africa, with long histories of keeping dairy animals that also have low rates of lactase persistence (Simoons, 1981). These groups often make use of fermented milk products (e.g., yogurt, kefir) or cheese, and the process of their production reduces lactose concentrations in the final products. Thus, having a history of dairying is necessary but not sufficient for explaining global variation in lactase persistence, and only populations drinking substantial amounts of unmodified fluid milk would have benefited from the ability to digest lactose.

Is there some advantage to being able to drink fluid milk that does not accrue to those who convert milk to yogurt or cheese? Lactose, which is only found in unmodified milk, can enhance calcium absorption in the small intestine (Flatz & Rotthauwe, 1973; Gueguen & Pointillart, 2000). Vitamin D, which is synthesized in skin cells in the presence of UVB light (although it can also be consumed in fish oils), also functions to absorb calcium in the small intestine. High UVB light conditions exist throughout the year around the equator, but only seasonally at higher latitudes. If an individual does not produce or consume enough vitamin D, lactose can substitute for vitamin D and facilitate calcium absorption. High rates of lactase persistence tend to cluster among populations living at high latitudes, where overall levels of UVB light are lower (Bloom & Sherman, 2005; Durham, 1991). Durham (1991) proposed that when exposure to UVB light is reduced and vitamin D synthesis is likewise diminished, lactose can increase calcium absorption (Flatz & Rotthauwe, 1973). Not everyone is convinced by this hypothesis (see Simoons, 2001), and furthermore, while the vitamin D/lactose/UV light hypothesis may help explain the very high frequencies of lactase persistence among northern Europeans, it has little relevance for understanding lactase persistence in populations at lower latitudes such as the pastoralists of sub-Saharan Africa where exposure to sunlight is much greater. For them there may be other nutritional advantages to adult milk consumption. Fluid milk may be important as a source of hydration, or lactose may serve as an important carbohydrate, a nutrient rare in the diets of groups who only consume the products of their herd animals.

Other evolutionary forces have also contributed to global variation in rates of adult lactase persistence (see webnote 5-1 for a discussion of the link between malaria and lactase persistence). Genetic drift, which typically occurs in small populations, may have been important in reducing diversity in genes associated with lactase activity in non-African populations. There is greater diversity in these genes among contemporary African populations, as there is with other genes. This suggests a greater antiquity and/or larger population size of human populations in Africa and that some of this genetic diversity was lost among populations that migrated out of Africa (Hollox et al., 2000). Gene flow has also played an enormous role in shaping the distribution of lactase persistence among historical and contemporary populations, especially in areas colonized by northern European populations (Flatz, 1987). Collectively, natural selection, gene flow, and genetic drift have generated the current more-or-less continuous distribution in population frequencies of lactase persistence (Sahi, 1994b).

Although most humans are lactase impersistent, following the ancestral mammalian pattern of reduced lactase activity postweaning, dietary and nutrition policies in countries around the world increasingly promote milk consumption, especially for children (World Health Organization, 2004). The Food and Agriculture Organization (FAO) reports that the majority of its member countries have school milk programs, and milk is generally subsidized for students (Griffin, 2004). Most countries with national dietary guidelines now include milk as either a separate food category or as an option among protein-rich foods (Food and Agriculture Organization, n.d.; see also Chapter 4). What are the health consequences of drinking milk for individuals who are lactase impersistent? What is known about the effects of milk consumption on childhood growth, maturation, and long-term health?

LACTOSE INTOLERANCE

The most obvious immediate consequence of drinking milk by individuals who are lactase impersistent is a condition called primary lactose intolerance, which is a cluster of symptoms including nausea, cramping, gas, and diarrhea (Swagerty, Walling, & Klein, 2002). These result from the lactose disaccharide passing undigested through the small intestine into the colon. Water is drawn into the colon, and bacteria partially ferment the sugar. Aside from the obvious discomfort that accompanies these symptoms, they can contribute to maldigestion of other nutrients, especially minerals, in the gastrointestinal tract (Phillips, 1981).

It is well documented that not everyone who is lactase impersistent is also lactose intolerant (see Cheer & Allen, 1997; Suarez, Adshead, Furne, & Levitt, 1998). Some experience no symptoms when they drink milk; others experience all of the above symptoms quite severely. For most, the symptoms of lactose intolerance are dose dependent and most likely to occur when large amounts of fresh milk are consumed. Fermented milk products such as yogurt are less likely to cause symptoms among individuals with lactase impersistence because bacteria partially ferment the lactose and convert some of the glucose into lactic acid (Adolfsson, Meydani, & Russell, 2004). Some bacteria in the gastrointestinal tract produce lactase and further improve lactose digestion and tolerance of milk (Adolfsson et al., 2004). Likewise, cheeses, especially those that are dry and/or aged, have relatively little lactose left after the separation of the curds from the whey and hence cause relatively few symptoms of lactose intolerance (see webnote 5-2 for a discussion of individual variation in lactose intolerance).

Recognition of population variation in lactase has gradually filtered into medical understandings and practice. Up through the 1960s, the general medical understanding was that lactase persistence and hence lactose tolerance were the norm for the species. Bayless and Rosensweig's foundational work (1966, 1967) provided compelling evidence for population variation in physiological responses to milk and overturned notions that lactose tolerance was "normal" for all humans.

Although medical organizations now appear to consider lactase impersistence as modal for the human species, their descriptions of this "condition" nonetheless tend to treat it as the deviant condition. For example, the American Academy of Pediatrics describes lactase impersistence (note *not* lactose intolerance per se) in the following way:

> Late-onset lactase *deficiency* (adult hypolactasia) is a common *disorder.* Approximately 90% of adult American blacks and 60% to 80% of Mexican-Americans, Native American Indians, Asians, and most Middle-Eastern and Mediterranean populations have *abnormal* findings on lactose tolerance tests (American Academy of Pediatrics, 1985, p. 636, emphasis added).

Likewise, lactase impersistence is described by the American College of Gastroenterology as "a *shortage* of the enzyme lactase, which is *normally* produced by the cells that line the small intestine" (American College of Gastroenterology, 2004, p. 1, emphasis added). The various terms used to describe lactase impersistence, such as lactose maldigestion, malabsorption, or lactase deficiency also reflect a continued perception of it as the deviant, rather than the ancestral condition. The term *adult-type hypolactasia* is favored by the leading lactase researcher Timo Sahi (1994b) to describe low levels of lactase activity among adults. However, he dismisses the possibility of using *hyperlactasia* as its counterpart, but given that hypolactasia is the ancestral condition and the norm for the species, individuals with higher lactase activity in adulthood could be properly described as having *hyperlactasia.*

Thus there is still a tendency to treat lactase impersistence, the most common form among humans, as deviant or "abnormal" (Wiley, 2004). This is of concern because milk production and consumption are increasing among populations with no history of milk consumption and among whom the majority of individuals are lactase impersistent (Wiley, 2007). Since the early 1960s, global milk production increased by a factor of 2.4, and the greatest growth in milk production was in Asia, with Thailand, China, and India all reporting more than fivefold increases in production (U.S. Department of Agriculture, 2006). Concurrent with production, there has been tremendous growth in milk consumption in Asian countries since the early 1960s, as shown in Figure 5-1. China leads with a remarkable 15-fold increase. Thailand's increase is about half that, with India, Japan, and the Philippines experiencing a tripling or quadrupling of consumption. More modest, but still marked growth in consumption has occurred in Latin America, especially in Brazil and Peru. Over these same 40 years consumption of milk has not changed or has declined in North America and Europe (all data available from U.S. Department of Agriculture, 2006). China is seen by dairy industries as the country with the greatest market potential for milk, and milk is being widely promoted by the government, in national dietary guidelines, and various health authorities (Chen, 2003a, b). Yet these promotional materials

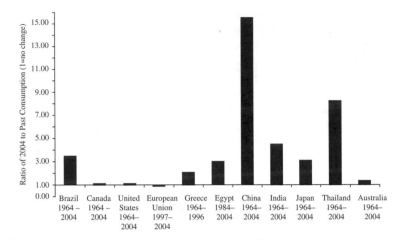

FIGURE 5-1 Global changes in fluid milk consumption: selected countries

rarely mention that over 90% of the population is lactase impersistent and hence a sizable portion of the population is likely to be lactose intolerant. It is notable that the market for yogurt and cheese, rather than fresh milk, is the fastest growing segment of dairy products in China (and also in Japan), and, compared to fresh milk, these are less likely to cause gastrointestinal symptoms (Fuller, Beghin, Hu, & Rozelle, 2004; Schluep Campo & Beghin, 2006).

Beyond problems associated with lactose intolerance that vary across and within populations, it is also important to consider whether cow's milk consumption has other health consequences. If one of milk's functions is to facilitate the growth of nursing mammals, does its consumption beyond the time of weaning result in demonstrable alterations in life history, particularly growth, maturation, or the aging process?

MILK AND GROWTH

In the United States, the idea that cow's milk consumption contributes to child growth can be traced back to the early part of the twentieth century (DuPuis, 2002). This linkage has become a common justification for school milk programs and other governmental programs such as the Special Supplemental Nutrition Program for Women, Infants, and Children (commonly known as WIC) and other efforts to increase consumption, especially among children (U.S. Department of Agriculture, 1990, 2002, 2003). Milk is the only food consumed during mammalian infancy, a period of very rapid growth, so it makes sense that milk should contribute to growth. Milk contains energy, vitamins and minerals, and specific biochemicals that may promote growth. It would seem reasonable that these should collectively support the growth of older children, albeit possibly in a less dramatic way compared to nursing infants.

The positive association between milk consumption and growth in height is widely used in milk advertisements. In the United States, a milk education site announces, "Got Milk? Get Tall" (Milk Processor Education Program, n.d.b). In another advertisement, images of professional basketball players are coupled with milk and statements such as "Hey everybody! Want to grow? About 15% of your height is added during your teen years and milk can help make the most of it" (Milk Processor Education Program, n.d.a). Similar claims are to be found in China, a country recently experiencing tremendous increase in milk consumption. A spokeswoman for one of China's largest dairies contends that consuming more milk will lead to faster growth rates among China's citizens and help make them taller (Chen, 2003b).

The contention that milk consumption should increase height is supported by researchers suggesting that the well-documented increases in average height over the twentieth century in the United States can be attributed to greater milk consumption. For example, Stuart Patton, a well-known physiologist of mammalian lactation writes:

> While many factors have contributed to this increase it is obvious that calcium in the diet would be essential, and that products of the expanding American dairy industry would be the logical source of the calcium enabling this growth... Of course calcium, while essential to increased bone growth and stature, is not the only contribution that milk would be making in this situation. High quality protein and growth-promoting B vitamins and Vitamin D from milk would be other contributing factors (Patton, 2004, p. 115).

There is also a striking parallel in Japan, where Takahashi maintained that milk "seems to be the most effective food for stimulating growth in height.... The short stature of Japanese in the past may be mainly caused by this low calcium diet" (Takahashi, 1966, p. 125). Michael Little and colleagues (Little, Galvin, & Mugambi, 1983; Little & Johnson, 1987) proposed that the relatively tall stature of Turkana pastoralists of Kenya could be attributed to their high protein intake, which derived from a diet based heavily on animal foods such as dairy products. Takahashi's global review of height in relation to ecological factors likewise found that populations with the greatest achieved heights were also those relying heavily on dairy products (Takahashi, 1971).

These statements suggest that it is milk's calcium and protein that are responsible for greater growth in height. While milk does contain substantial amounts of calcium and is also rich in protein, with 8.2 g/cup, there are other constituents of milk that can contribute to growth. First and foremost, milk is a source of calories, although that varies depending on whether it has had some or all of the fat removed. Whole milk has 146 kcal/cup, while nonfat (skim) milk has 86 kcal/cup (245 g) (U.S. Department of Agriculture, 2005). In some countries, such as the United States, fluid milk is fortified with vitamin A (~130 RAE/cup) and vitamin D (99 IU/cup).[2] While any number of milk's constituents may contribute in specific ways to the overall growth process, research to date has focused on calcium and insulin-like growth factor 1 (IGF-1), part of the protein content of milk (see Bonjour et al., 1997; Dibba et al., 2000; Hoppe, Molgaard, Juul, & Michaelsen, 2004; Hoppe, Molgaard, & Michaelsen, 2006; Patton, 2004; Rogers, 2006). It should be noted that in the United States many cows are treated with synthetic bovine growth hormone (rbGH),[3] and this is associated with increased IGF-1 levels in milk (Epstein, 1996; Juskevich & Guyer, 1990). Thus milk is a very complex food, all the more so because of the conditions under which cows are maintained for milk production and the transformations it may undergo in processing, from fat removal to vitamin fortification.

Calcium

Milk contains about 280 mg calcium/cup (U.S. Department of Agriculture, 2005). Calcium is the major component of the inorganic matrix of bone, which gives it strength and resilience (Cameron, 2002), and vitamin D is required to deposit calcium crystals in bone. Thus there is reason to believe that calcium, in association with vitamin D, should be positively related to bone growth in both its density and linear dimensions. However, calcium supplementation studies in Europe (Bonjour et al., 1997; Bonjour, Chevalley, Ammann, Slosman, & Rizzoli, 2001), The Gambia (Dibba et al., 2000), and Hong Kong (Lee et al., 1995, 1994) have found no statistically significant relationship between calcium and growth in height, regardless of whether calcium is supplied as a mineral supplement or as a milk derivative. The studies have found that children supplemented with calcium did not grow more in height than did those in the control groups.

IGF-1

IGF-1 is part of the protein fragment of cow's milk and is structurally similar to insulin (Hoppe et al., 2006). IGF-1 is molecularly identical in bovine and human milk, and levels of IGF-1 are within the same range in human breast milk and cow's milk (including those treated with rbGH) (Juskevich & Guyer, 1990). Recent studies have found that serum levels of IGF-1 increase in response to milk intake (Heaney et al., 1999). There are also positive correlations between IGF-1 levels, milk consumption, and overall animal-source protein intake (Holmes, Pollak, Willett, & Hankinson, 2002). However, it remains unclear as to whether the increase in serum IGF-1 levels is a direct effect of the IGF-1 in milk or if milk stimulates endogenous IGF-1 production (Holmes et al., 2002).

IGF-1 is produced in osteoblasts, which are cells involved in bone growth and remodeling, and it is the most abundant growth factor in bone (Kelly, Cusack, & Cashman, 2003). It increases the uptake of amino acids, which are incorporated into new proteins such as collagen, and it is also involved in calcium and phosphate metabolism (Kelly et al., 2003). In a recent study among well-nourished 8-year-old boys supplemented with either nonfat milk or lean meat for 7 days, serum IGF-1 levels rose significantly more among the milk-supplemented group (Hoppe et al., 2004). Similarly, Hoppe et al. (2004) found that milk intake was positively correlated with both IGF-1 levels and height among 2-year-old boys, as shown in Figure 5-2. More recently a study in the United Kingdom (Rogers, Emmett, Gunnell, Dunger, & Holly, 2006) found a statistically significant positive correlation between milk consumption, leg length, and IGF-1 levels among 7- to 8-year-old boys, but not among girls. These studies suggest that IGF-1, perhaps in conjunction with calcium, is a likely mechanism by which milk contributes to growth in height.

Research on the overall relationship between milk and growth, especially in height, reveals somewhat equivocal results. The classic studies of Orr (1928) and Leighton and Clark (1929) published in *Lancet* were among the earliest work demonstrating a positive effect of milk on height. British school children from urban working class areas were provided with $3/4$–1 pint of whole or skim milk, a biscuit of caloric value equal to that of the skim milk, or no supplement over a 7-month period. Changes in body weight and height were then measured among children aged 5–6, 8–9, and 13 years. Both the whole- and

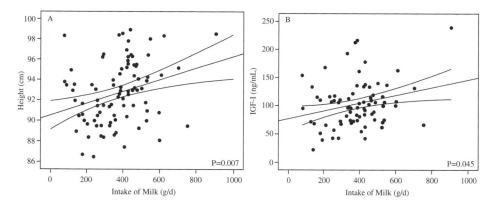

FIGURE 5-2 Height and IGF-1 in relation to milk consumption in 2.5-year-old Danish children. (Reprinted, with permission, from the Annual Review of Nutrition, Volume 26 ©2006 by Annual Reviews www.annualreviews.org; Hoppe, Molgaard, & Michaelsen, 2006.)

skim-milk–supplemented groups grew modestly more than those getting biscuits or no supplement, approximately 0.2–0.4 in. over the 7-month period. Thus milk seemed to have "special" effects on growth above and beyond its caloric value. Subsequent studies of school children in the United Kingdom in the 1970s and 1980s have not shown similar outcomes. Rona and Chinn (1989), Cook et al. (1979), and Baker et al. (1980) reported no consistent positive association between milk provisioning in schools and rates of growth among children age 5–10 years, even when stratified by poverty status and ethnic background. Only Baker et al. (1980) found a very slight increase (2.9 mm) in height among a group of 7- to 8-year-old socioeconomically disadvantaged children provisioned with 190 ml of milk ($n = 281$) compared to the control group ($n = 239$) over 21½ months.

Although there have been several recent supplementation studies designed to test the effect of milk on changes in various aspects of bone biology, including height changes, as Table 5-2 documents, none have demonstrated a positive, statistically significant effect of milk on growth in height. The studies ranged in duration from 1 to 2 years and included girls of European ancestry from ages 6 to 16 years.

Research in less well-nourished and non-Western populations reveals a somewhat different pattern. Lampl et al.(1978) found that Bundi children in New Guinea (age 7–13 years) supplemented with 10 or 20 g of skim milk powder over an 8-month period grew almost twice as much in height as did children who did not receive the supplement (3.3 vs. 1.8 cm). The majority of these children were below the third percentile in height (based on standard of Tanner, Whitehouse, & Takaishi, 1966) at the beginning of the study. In Beijing Du et al. (2004) found statistically significantly positive effects of a school milk intervention program on growth in height among Chinese adolescent girls ($n = 698$, aged 10–12 years at beginning of study, with low baseline milk and calcium intakes) over a 2-year period. The girls who received the supplementation in the original study had been given 330 ml of calcium-fortified milk 5 days a week and grew significantly, but modestly more (0.7 cm) than the unsupplemented group.

A shortcoming of the Chinese study is that the control group was provided with no supplement, so it is impossible to determine whether milk had effects above and beyond

TABLE 5-2 Intervention Studies of Dairy Consumption and Growth in Height in Industrialized Populations

Authors	Study population	Age group (yr)	Sex	Sample Size	Intervention	Duration	Growth Differential Intervention–Control Mean	p-value
Cadogan et al. 1997	Sheffield, UK "White"	mean = 12.2	Female	82	1 pint whole or low-fat milk per day	18 months	0.7 cm	NS
Bonjour et al. 1997	Geneva, Switzerland "Caucasion"	6–9	Female	108	850 mg Ca from milk extract per day	48 weeks	0.4 cm	NS
<880 mg baseline Ca intake							0.6 cm	NS
>880 mg baseline Ca intake							0.0 cm	NS
Bonjour et al. 2001								
1 yr follow up of above							0.7 cm	NS
3–5 yr follow up of above							1.4 cm	NS
Chan et al. 1995	Utah, US "White"	9–13	Female	48	dairy products up to 1200 mg per day	12 months	0.4 cm	NS
Merrilees et al. 2000	New Zealand	15–16	Female	91	dairy products up to 1000 mg per day	24 months	−0.3 cm	NS

its caloric or protein contribution. A study in Kenya compared the growth of 554 school children (mean age = 7.1 years) divided into three groups that were supplemented daily with either a glass of ultrahigh-temperature (UHT) milk, meat, or fat (all with a caloric value of 300 kcal), compared with school children given no supplemental food over a 2-year period. Those who were given milk did not grow significantly more than those given meat or fat or those who were not supplemented at all (Grillenberger et al., 2003). Only the shortest children (those with a baseline height-for-age Z-score below the median) in the supplemented groups grew significantly more (1.3 cm) than those in the control group. However, among these stunted children, those supplemented with milk grew the same amount as those supplemented with nondairy animal foods.

In Japan, Takahashi (1984) concluded that the addition of milk to school lunch programs was the most important factor contributing to the observed increase in height among boys from the 1950s through the 1970s. Similarly, in a more recent study of a large sample ($n = 2766$) of children aged 6–9 years in Malaysia, Chen (1989) reported that the implementation of a school milk program providing 250 ml of milk twice weekly reduced by half the percentage of children who were classified as stunted in height over a 21-month period.[4]

In a recent analysis of the United States Nutrition and Health Examination Survey (NHANES) from 1999 to 2002, Wiley (2005) demonstrated that milk intake (either reported frequency or amount consumed in 24 hours) among 5- to 11-year-olds was not related to height after controlling for age, calories consumed in the past 24 hours, and birth weight. On the other hand, among adolescents age 12–18, when sex, household income, age, and caloric intake were taken into account, individuals reporting greater frequency of milk consumption were significantly taller than those with lower frequency of milk consumption. This effect was small, with each increment of increased frequency (a scale of 0 = never drink milk to 4 = everyday) contributing about 3 mm to height.

In sum, evidence accumulated on the milk–height relationship has not provided strong support for a positive effect of milk on growth (see also the review by Hoppe et al., 2006). It appears that milk may have its most significant effects among children with existing undernutrition or among adolescents. However, few studies have compared milk consumption to supplements of other nutrient-rich foods to ascertain whether milk has "special" growth-enhancing properties that are seen at different periods of growth and development. Most studies are done on children between the ages of 5 and 10 years, but given the relatively rapid growth of adolescents, milk may be able to play a more important role in linear growth after puberty. IGF-1 levels peak around mid-puberty, which corresponds with a rapid rate of growth, and then decline throughout adulthood (Juul et al., 1994). Since milk consumption results in increased serum levels of IGF-1 and IGF-1 levels are already high during this time, milk may be able to have its most potent effects on growth during early adolescence. Thus, despite advertisements and assertions to the contrary, at present it is impossible to say with any certainty that milk has a clear positive effect on height, especially among well-nourished populations.

COW'S MILK CONSUMPTION AND AGE AT MENARCHE

Studies of the relationship between childhood milk consumption and age at menarche have failed to show a consistent effect. The trend toward lower age at menarche over the latter part of the twentieth century has been associated with an increase in consumption of milk and milk products among African Americans (Talpade & Talpade, 2001). Milk may influence age at menarche through a variety of its components. Berkey et al. (2000) and Sanchez et al. (1981) have both reported associations between animal protein intake and lower age menarche, although this result has not been replicated in other studies (Moisan, Meyer, & Gingras, 1990; Petridou et al., 1996). Increased animal fat (Colditz et al., 1987) and calcium intake (Chevalley, Rizzoli, Hans, Ferrari, & Bonjour, 2005) have also been associated with decreased age at menarche and are both related to milk consumption. Chevalley et al. (2005) found a significantly lower menarcheal age among girls supplemented with 850 mg calcium daily for 1 year and that calcium intake was higher among those reaching menarche early (<12.1 years). Recently, milk and dietary calcium were found to have a statistically significant positive effect on weight gain among a cohort of American 9- to 14-year-olds followed for 3 years (Berkey, Rockett, Willett, & Colditz, 2005). The authors determined that the effect was mainly due to the calories in milk. However, other studies of pre- and postmenarcheal girls have found either no relationship between weight gain and milk intake (Phillips et al., 2003) or a significant negative association between milk intake and fatness (Novotny, Daida, Acharya, Grove, & Vogt, 2004). Thus the relationship between milk consumption and age at menarche, if any, is not well understood, and there has been little research on the topic in populations that only recently began consuming cow's milk.

MILK AND LONG-TERM HEALTH CONSEQUENCES

The relationship between cow's milk consumption and child growth and development is important not only for its immediate effects on these processes, but also because patterns of growth and maturation have the potential to influence the risk of later-life diseases, including bone fractures and osteoporosis, various forms of cancer, and cardiovascular disease (CVD). As discussed below, all have been linked to patterns of milk consumption, with both positive and negative impacts on these outcomes.

Osteoporosis

The most frequently cited long-term benefits of childhood cow's milk consumption are its positive effects on bone health and decreased risk of fracture in older adults (see Heaney, 2000; NIH, 1994). However, studies of the relationship between milk consumption and bone density in childhood do not reveal consistent relationships—many find that milk supplementation transiently increases bone density (Bonjour et al., 1997; Cadogan et al., 1997; Chan et al., 1995; Du et al., 2004; Merrilees et al., 2000), or that milk consumption is positively correlated with bone density in observation studies (Black, Williams, Jones, & Goulding, 2002), but other studies do not find this effect (see Heaney, 2000; Lanou, Berkow, & Barnard, 2005; Weinsier & Krumdieck, 2000, for reviews).

Furthermore, among studies finding that milk consumption in childhood had a positive effect on bone mass, the amount of variation explained by dairy foods is extremely small (Weinsier & Krumdieck, 2000). It should be noted that most studies are done on females of European descent and conclusions drawn from these studies may not be applicable to other populations.

The literature on milk consumption and bone health is large and contentious and beyond the scope of this chapter, but there are two points relevant to this discussion. First, osteoporosis, the loss of bone density that often occurs with aging, has come to be seen as a disease with its origins in childhood (Greer & Krebs, 2006; Nicklas, 2003). Because bone loss occurs from the total bone mass an individual has accumulated, the larger the bone mass achieved during growth, the lower (or later) the risk of osteoporosis. Thus, understanding the determinants of child bone density is crucial to understanding this late-life disease. Several studies have shown that milk consumption in childhood is positively correlated with reduced risk of fractures in adulthood (Kalkwarf, Khoury, & Lanphear, 2003; Sandler et al., 1985; Teegarden, Lyle, Proulx, Johnston, & Weaver, 1999), although other studies failed to find evidence of this relationship (Feskanich, Willett, Stampfer, & Colditz, 1997; Lanou et al., 2005; Weinsier & Krumdieck, 2000).

Second, it should also be recognized that other childhood behaviors can have a positive effect on bone density. Several studies have shown that childhood weight-bearing exercise has a strong positive impact on bone density (Anderson, 2001; French, Fulkerson, & Story, 2000; VandenBergh et al., 1995), independent of milk intake. Thus from an intervention standpoint, increasing weight-bearing physical activity among children can offset the later life risk of osteoporosis and bone fracture. Not all interventions need to involve increasing milk intake among children.

Thus claims made about the essential role that milk plays in bone growth should be informed by both replicated scientific studies and an evolutionary perspective, which reveals how other foods and physical activity may have provided for adequate bone health among our ancestors (Eaton & Nelson, 1991). Estimates of Paleolithic calcium intake are high relative to those in the contemporary United States (~1960 mg/day compared to 750 mg/day [Eaton, Eaton III, & Konner, 1999]), and would have been more than sufficient to generate sufficient bone mineralization (although these calcium intakes were not reported for children specifically). Furthermore, children would most likely have been engaging in physical activity sufficient to promote bone mineralization through the remodeling process that occurs when bone is under mechanical load. Children's diets that most closely resemble that of ancestral hunter gatherers (i.e., rich in nongrain plant foods or fish) can contain sufficient calcium in the absence of milk. Engaging in routine physical activity should also promote bone health, in contrast to the sedentary lifestyles of contemporary children, which appears to compromise bone health.

Rationales for U.S. dietary requirements for children that include three servings of milk (or dairy products) per day are based on the fact that most American children do not consume the recommended amount of calcium. In addition, milk and other dairy products contribute more than 70% of the calcium intake in the United States (Goldberg, Folta, & Must, 2002).

Achieving that level of intake without dairy products requires careful attention to selection of foods that naturally contain some calcium and others to which it is added.

Unfortunately, calcium is found in significant amounts in relatively few foods. These foods are not consumed consistently in large amounts by most of the population and tend not to be popular with children (Goldberg et al., 2002, p. 830).

Thus since contemporary children are assumed to dislike the nondairy foods rich in calcium, they should therefore drink lots of milk. But this assumption fails to question whether milk's predominance among available calcium-rich foods is necessarily ideal or whether children's preferences for milk should be encouraged to the exclusion of other calcium-rich nondairy foods.

Another unresolved issue is whether current calcium recommendations are reasonable, or whether they are too high. There is no international consensus on calcium requirements. Even among milk-producing countries, the United States and Canada have much higher recommended amounts than the United Kingdom and the European Union for both children and adults (children: 500–800 vs. 350–550; adolescents: 1300 vs. 800–1000; adults: 800–1200 vs. 700, respectively) (FAO/WHO, 1998). In comparison, daily calcium consumption ranges between 300 and 1000 mg per day around the world (FAO/WHO, 1998). What has come to be known as the "calcium paradox" is the observation that across countries, fracture rates (an index of osteoporosis) are highest in countries with the highest calcium and dairy product intakes and lowest in countries with low intakes (FAO, 2000; Frassetto, Todd, Morris, & Sebastian, 2000; Hegsted, 2001). Within the United States, bone fracture rates are highest among peoples of European descent and lowest among those with African ancestry. This difference is often attributed to population variation in overall bone mass, as African Americans tend to have greater bone mass than those of European descent (Bauer, 1998; Ettinger et al., 1997). Milk intake in childhood does not appear to be linked to adult bone density among African American women, and African American women report lower milk intakes than white women (Opotowsky & Bilezikian, 2003).

Several explanations have been offered for the positive correlation between milk consumption and bone fracture rates across countries. The bone remodeling that contributes to bone resilience derives from complex interrelationships between calcium and vitamin D (among other factors), which is likely to be more abundant given the higher UVB light exposure at lower latitudes, where milk is drunk less commonly (Durham, 1991). Fracture risk is also positively associated with consumption of animal protein across populations, and milk and animal protein intake are generally positively correlated (Frassetto et al., 2000). Further, there are important interactions with physical activity, such that differences in subsistence activities further contribute to this population variation. Thus across populations lactase impersistence and a relative absence of dairy products in the diet do not necessarily contribute to increased risk of osteoporosis. What is also evident, however, is that as populations move to a more Western, industrialized lifestyle (which often includes dairy consumption), the risk of osteoporosis increases (see Lau, Cooper, Wickham, Donnan, & Barker, 1990).

Milk Consumption and Other Chronic Diseases

Milk consumption has been linked to myriad other chronic diseases, including various cancers and cardiovascular disease, increasing the risk of some, decreasing the risk of others (Færgeman, 2003; Heaney, 2000; Moorman & Terry, 2004; Nicklas, 2003). Components of milk that may increase the risk of these multifaceted diseases include saturated fat and IGF-1, while calcium and vitamin D (which is not a natural constituent of milk, but is added to milk in many countries) have been posited as anticarcinogenic (Moorman & Terry, 2004). Whole milk and most cheeses are high in saturated fat, a well-known contributor to cardiovascular disease. Færgeman (2003) observed that countries with the highest rates of cardiovascular disease are those that consume the most dairy products and have the highest frequencies of lactase persistence. As he noted, "the persistence of lactase function is probably a genetic adaptation to easy access to milk of domesticated animals [and] could be a genetic determinant of the acceptability of one major source of animal fat and protein that promotes coronary heart disease" (Færgeman, 2003, p. 62).

Most of the research linking dairy products to cancer has focused on IGF-1. As noted, serum IGF-1 levels rise after milk consumption (Holmes et al., 2002) and IGF-1 both increases cell division and inhibits apoptosis (cell death). These effects have been associated with increased risk of cancers later in life through IGF-1's involvement in the unregulated growth of neoplastic cells, especially in the colon and breast (cf. Ben-Shlomo et al., 2003; Gunnell et al., 2001; Ma et al., 2001; Moorman & Terry, 2004). Furthermore, individuals who are tall during growth and in adulthood have higher IGF-1 levels than those who are shorter (Ben-Shlomo et al., 2003), and height itself is positively associated with cancer risk, perhaps via the IGF-1 mechanism (Gunnell et al., 2001; Rogers et al., 2006). The links among cow's milk consumption, IGF-1, and cancer risk is likely very complex and dependent on numerous other factors, including individual variation in IGF-1 production (Ma et al., 2001). Furthermore, if milk intake in childhood has the capacity to decrease the age at menarche, this could be a route by which milk increases the risk of reproductive cancers, as earlier age at menarche is linked to an increase in breast cancer risk (Berkey, Frazier, Gardner, & Colditz, 1999; Petridou et al., 1996).

There are also data suggesting that cow's milk may reduce the risk of various cancers and cardiovascular disease. Vitamin D downregulates IGF-1 in breast cancer cells and reduces cell proliferation (Giovannucci, 2005). Likewise calcium, which is regulated by vitamin D, stimulates apoptosis. Animal studies suggest that diets deficient in calcium and vitamin D increase the growth and proliferation of breast cells (Lipkin & Newmark, 1999). Strong evidence exists for a protective role of vitamin D and calcium against colorectal cancer (Giovannucci, 2005; Norat & Riboli, 2003). With respect to cardiovascular disease or stroke, intake of dairy products has been found to reduce the risk of hypertension (Massey, 2001; Ruidavets et al., 2006), and milk protein–derived peptides have been shown to lower blood pressure (FitzGerald, Murray, & Walsh, 2004). Dairy product consumption has also been found to be inversely related to risk of type 2 diabetes (Choi, Willett, Stampfer, Rimm, & Hu, 2005; Liu et al., 2005).

CONCLUSION

There are two contrasting perspectives on the impact of milk on health. One suggests that "a diet devoid of dairy products will often be a poor diet, not just in respect to calcium, but for many other nutrients as well" (Heaney, 2000, p. 915). From this view cow's milk consumption is *necessary* for adequate child growth and the achievement of sufficient bone mass. Milk consumption reduces the risk of osteoporosis and other chronic diseases. Milk's benefits derive from its calcium and IGF-1, manufacture of low-fat dairy products, and fortification with vitamin D. The other viewpoint contends that there is no compelling evidence that cow's milk consumption positively influences bone health and that other factors such as physical activity are more important. Further, dairy products may increase the risk of various cancers, especially via the IGF-1 mechanism. There is evidence to support both of these contentions, and at present it is difficult to conclude anything definitive about the effects of cow's milk on life history parameters. Existing evidence shows, however, that there is population variation in milk consumption that correlates with variation in growth, osteoporosis, and cardiovascular disease, suggesting that milk's effects are likely to vary by population and that milk need not be a dietary essential to achieve good health across the lifespan. The existence of the well-described "calcium paradox" and population variation in lactase persistence reveals just how important it is to avoid broad assumptions about the universal benefits of milk in contemporary populations.

Given milk's evolutionary function, it seems odd that milk would not be associated with observable effects on growth or earlier maturation, but these effects, if any, may be invisible when individuals consume a diet high in other sources of calories and protein. Furthermore, growth and maturation are to a large extent under genetic control, as well as being influenced by numerous environmental factors, of which diet is only one. Positive effects of milk on growth may be more visible among populations with marginal nutritional status or among adolescents around the time of the peak growth spurt. If milk does enhance growth among such groups, the effects are not necessarily positive, as acceleration of puberty, rapid growth in childhood, and increases in body mass and height are associated with increased risk of chronic diseases such as reproductive cancers.

Other aspects of human health may also be altered by cow's milk consumption. For example, in the United States cow's milk is not recommended for infants because of its allergenicity and its low iron content (Kleinman, 2004). However, after age 1 year, fluid milk is considered safe, and parents are told they can now give their child cow's milk. Does this message, along with the fact that milk is ubiquitous in grocery stores and affordable compared to formula, encourage parents to terminate breastfeeding (if it has continued for a year already) and convert their child to cow's milk at 12 months? If so, what are the effects on early growth, and how does it alter the growth hormone milieu in ways that have longer term effects? A related question concerns maternal cow's milk consumption during pregnancy, early growth, and the effects on IGF-1 programming. A British study demonstrated that the children of women supplemented with milk during pregnancy who continued to get milk supplements until age 5 years had *lower* circulating IGF-1 levels in adulthood, suggesting that early exposure to IGF-1 through milk might reprogram development of the IGF-1 axis (Ben-Shlomo et al., 2005). Thus much remains to be learned about the life history effects of cow's milk consumption at different points in the life cycle.

An evolutionary perspective on cow's milk consumption concludes that despite the myriad claims about the essential nature of milk in the child and adult human diet, this is not the ancestral condition, and even among populations with genetic adaptations to digest lactose after weaning, the long-term consequences of milk consumption are not exclusively salutary. Milk must be seen within a broader environmental context, one that includes UV light exposure, other components of the diet, including sources of calcium, vitamin D, fat, and protein, as well as patterns of subsistence that shape weight-bearing physical activity. Population genetic characteristics and evolutionary history are also relevant here as both bone mass and lactase persistence vary across populations. While milk is indeed a high-quality animal-source food and can contribute many essential nutrients to the diet (and is certainly superior to soda in terms of the additional nutrients it provides for a similar amount of calories), an evolutionary perspective forces a reconsideration of its privileged place in human diets.

CHAPTER 6

Not by Bread Alone

The Role of Psychosocial Stress in Age at First Reproduction and Health Inequalities

James S. Chisholm and David A. Coall

Chisholm and Coall's description of their work on the effects of psychosocial stress on lowering the age of menarche is a further illustration of Kuzawa's model (see Chapter 18) of how powerful in utero nongenetic effects can be in sensitizing a fetus to the conditions of postnatal risk and uncertainty. Taken together these two (and other) chapters cause us to appreciate even more that the moment of birth is not quite the developmental starting point we once took it to be, but rather, represents a kind of "been there, done that," as least insofar as what a neonate needs to do in order to successfully navigate developmentally the quality of its social and physical conditions. The authors discuss phenotypic markers of mortality risk for fetuses and infants that are initiated by maternal neuroendocrine control systems, processed in the form of mother's subjective experiences and feelings (loss, fear, risk, anxiety), and set in motion a sequence of hypothalamic–pituitary–adrenal (HPA) responses that influence fetal and postnatal development. The types of changes to which the developing child is presensitized potentially facilitate earlier maturity, including age at first intercourse. The interrelationship that in utero events have on later attachment strategies of the neonate and infant reveal many more biosocial continuities between pre- and postnatal events than could have been proposed or imagined just 15 years ago.

The political lesson of twentieth-century Darwinian thinking is, therefore, entirely different from that of nineteenth-century Social Darwinism.... A Darwinian left, understanding the prerequisites for mutual cooperation as well as its benefits, would strive to avoid economic conditions that create outcasts.

Singer, 1999, p 53

Medicine is a social science and politics is nothing but medicine on a grand scale.

Virchow, 1848/1985, p 33

Due in large part to foundational work by Nesse and Williams (1995), Stearns (1999), and Trevathan, Smith, and McKenna (1999), it is becoming accepted that evolutionary theory is useful for understanding human health and disease. In this chapter we build on these foundations by using one of the most dynamic branches of evolutionary theory—life history theory—to better understand health inequalities. We believe that life history theory leads naturally to our focus on two important questions: the determinants of age at first reproduction and the role of inequality in health. In particular, we are concerned with how and why inequality leads to early reproduction and reduces mothers' and children's capability for health and long lives.

LIFE HISTORY THEORY

Life history theory is the study of organism $\times$ environment interactions throughout and across life cycles from an evolutionary perspective. Examples of mammalian life history traits are age at first reproduction, number and size of offspring, interbirth interval, length of parental investment (e.g., nursing), and life span. Central to life history theory is the proposition that in order for organisms to have left descendants, they first had to survive, grow, and develop, and then not only produce offspring but, in the case of long-lived species, particularly mammals, rear them as well. Survival, growth and development, and producing and rearing offspring are the universal and major components of fitness and are forms of work. Doing work requires resources (e.g., energy, nutrients, security, information, time), which sooner or later are always limited. Therefore, natural selection is expected to favor organisms with mechanisms to allocate limited resources preferentially to the particular component (work) of fitness that most increased their ancestors' chances of leaving descendants under similar socioecological conditions. Because selection always favors organisms who leave more descendants (i.e., fitness is always relative), but the resources required for doing the work of leaving descendants are always limited, it is not possible to maximize all the components of fitness simultaneously, and trade-offs are inevitable. For example, if survival is the most pressing adaptive problem, resources will be allocated preferentially to this end, making them unavailable for growth and development or reproduction. Likewise, if the organism has survived to adulthood and producing offspring is its most pressing adaptive problem, the resources allocated preferentially to offspring production will not be available for rearing them (Gadgil and Bossert, 1970).

The most all-encompassing trade-off is that between current and future reproduction. Also known as the "general life history problem" (Schaffer, 1983), the current–future trade-off is a model for predicting an organism's optimal reproductive "strategy" (it need not be conscious) for leaving descendants based on the assumption that there is a trade-off between current and future reproduction. The rationale for this assumption is that beyond some threshold, increased reproduction in the short term (current reproduction) will decrease the number of its descendants in the long term (future reproduction).

This can happen because resources consumed for bearing or rearing offspring in the short term would have resulted in more descendants had they been consumed in the future and/or because current reproduction reduces parents' capability of surviving and thus bearing or rearing future offspring. One important consequence of the general life history problem is that selection is no longer always expected to favor mechanisms that simply maximize number of offspring. This is because consistently producing a small number of high-quality offspring (i.e., with a high probability of survival and reproduction) results in more descendants in the long run than having a larger number of low-quality offspring (i.e., with a low probability of survival or reproduction). And this, in turn, is because producing a small number of high-quality offspring—who are themselves likely to produce a small number of high-quality offspring, who are in turn also likely to produce a small number of high-quality offspring (and so on)—reduces the intergenerational variance in number of offspring. It's an algorithmic fact that increasing x by the multiple y through z iterations (generations) produces a larger number than increasing x through z iterations by a multiple that only averages y through z iterations. To repeat, selection is no longer expected always to favor mechanisms that maximize the production of offspring in the current generation. Instead, it is now expected that under certain circumstances selection will favor mechanisms (adaptations) that have the effect of minimizing intergenerational variance in number of offspring, thereby maximizing long-term fitness or future reproduction (Borgerhoff Mulder, 1992; Charnov, 1993; Gillespie, 1977; Harpending, Draper, & Pennington, 1990; Hill & Kaplan, 1999; Kaplan, 1994; Promislow & Harvey, 1990, 1991; Stearns, 1992).

The circumstances that matter are those of environmental risk and uncertainty, which is how evolutionary ecologists refer in the abstract to threats to an organism's capability to leave descendants (Charnov, 1993; Low, 1978; Seger & Brockmann, 1987; Stearns, 1992). In risky and uncertain environments the quantity, quality, and dependability of resources required for the work of fitness (energy, nutrients, security, time, information) are problematic, so mortality rates are high or unpredictable and the most pressing adaptive problem is to have any descendants at all. Because parents in these environments lack the resources to invest in offspring, their optimal reproductive strategy is to reproduce as early or often as possible. Maximizing offspring quantity (current reproduction) reduces their quality, but since these parents already lack the capability to have much effect on quality, this is just the cost of staying in the evolutionary game. Maximizing offspring quantity maximizes the probability that some will survive and reproduce; any is better than none. It's as if adaptations for trading offspring quality for quantity under conditions of high environmental risk and uncertainty were the phenotypic embodiment of game theory's minimax strategy of minimizing the probability of sustaining the maximum possible loss. This is the "bird in the bush worth none in the hand" or "nothing left to lose" strategy; it is the optimal strategy when the only alternative is lineage extinction or "stepping off a fitness cliff" (Ellison, 1994; Holland, 1992; Keyfitz, 1977).

In safe and predictable environments, on the other hand, the quantity, quality, and dependability of resources are at least adequate, so mortality rates are lower and steadier, survival is not such a pressing problem, and parents can afford to produce a small number of high-quality offspring who are themselves likely to survive and reproduce. Maximizing offspring quality (future reproduction) reduces their number, but since these parents have the capability to maintain or improve offspring quality, this is just the cost of investing in the future. Maximizing offspring quality maximizes the number of descendants in future generations—or the probability of having any descendants after more generations. It's as if adaptations for trading offspring quantity for quality under conditions of low environmental risk and uncertainty were the phenotypic embodiment of game theory's maximin strategy of maximizing the probability of achieving the minimum possible (short-term, one-step-at-a-time) gain, which, as always, is just staying in the evolutionary game. This is the "bird in hand worth two in the bush" strategy; it sets the stage for a slow and steady increase in future fitness by reducing intergenerational variance in number of offspring (Figure 6-1).

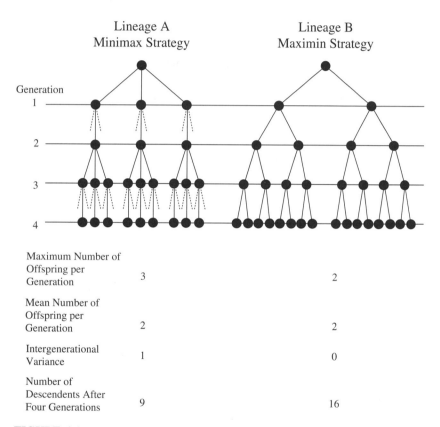

FIGURE 6-1 Schematic representation of the effect of intergenerational variance in number of offspring on number of descendants. Lineage A occupies a risky and uncertain environment and consequently suffers high or unpredictable mortality (dotted lines ending without issue). The optimal strategy for members of Lineage A is to maximize quantity of offspring in each generation (current reproduction), for this minimizes the risk of lineage extinction. Lineage B occupies a safe and predictable environment so all of its offspring survive and reproduce. The optimal strategy for members of Lineage B is to maximize the quality of offspring. Thus, even though Lineage B produces only two offspring per generation (vs. three in Lineage A), their higher quality means that they are more likely to survive and reproduce. Consistently producing a small number of high-quality offspring reduces the intergenerational variance in number of offspring. Over time this results in more descendants (future reproduction) in Lineage B than in Lineage A. This consistency, however, comes at the cost of considerable parental investment, which takes resources away from producing greater numbers of offspring. (Adapted from Chisholm, 1993.)

THE DEVELOPMENT OF REPRODUCTIVE STRATEGIES

There are two main approaches in biology (Stearns, 1982; Tinbergen, 1963). The adaptationist approach is concerned with ultimate explanations of how evolution works and what selection is expected to favor. The mechanist approach is concerned with proximate explanations of how organisms work and how adaptations are realized phenotypically. In order for an organism to develop its theoretically optimal reproductive strategy (life history traits) contingent on local environmental risk and uncertainty, there must be a mechanism whereby information about environmental risk and uncertainty becomes represented in its phenotype to organize the cells, tissues, organs, etc. required to do the theoretically adaptive work proposed. This raises questions about the nature of such information, how it affects reproduction, and how it is incorporated into the phenotype. With regard to the first question, since mortality rates and patterns are determined by environmental risk and uncertainty, they are a good indicator of the local optimal reproductive strategy and information about environmental risk and uncertainty might be expected to represent or index local mortality risk. With regard to the second question, age at sexual maturity is a critical life history trait for it marks the point in the life cycle when organisms have been selected to re-allocate resources from growth to reproduction. Because of the current–future trade-off the timing of age at first reproduction can have major fitness consequences and may constitute the primary target of selection on life history traits (Charnov, 1993; Hill & Hurtado, 1996; Hill & Kaplan, 1999; Promislow & Harvey, 1990, 1991; Stearns, 1992). We might therefore expect information about mortality rates to have an impact on age at first reproduction.

Regarding the third question—how information about mortality rates is incorporated into the phenotype to affect age at first reproduction—the quantity, quality, and dependability of material resources are critical for all organisms. Organisms with inadequate or uncertain material resources (energy, nutrients, antibodies, etc.) are more likely to die. Ellison (1990) thus proposed that the energy imbalance produced by malnutrition or disease in effect provides information about mortality risk that signals metabolic, immune, and endocrine control systems to downregulate reproduction, enabling females to make unconscious "bioassays" of their own health, nutritional status, and growth rates as a means of scaling reproductive effort to the flow of material resources. It makes adaptive sense for organisms with inadequate or uncertain material resources to postpone reproduction—at least until conditions improve—but when they are adequate to reproduce early, for this enables them not only to capitalize quickly on these resources, but also to maximize the probability that their offspring will be born in time to capitalize on them as well (Cole, 1954).

However, it is also known that women with chronically inadequate or uncertain material resources in developing countries often begin childbearing in their teens and go on to have six, eight, or more pregnancies (Alan Guttmacher Institute, 1998; Bongaarts, 1980). Vitzthum (2001) proposed a resolution of this apparent paradox in terms of life history theory and the familiar physiological process of acclimatization. From the perspective of life history theory, ontogeny is the development of reproductive strategies; development itself evolved for reproduction (Bonner, 1965; West-Eberhard, 2003). Because the essential adaptive function of phenotypic plasticity is to maximize the probability of leaving descendants in the environment in which one was born—but these environments may change before maturity—we would not expect age at first reproduction to be determined only by a woman's current energy balance but also her energy balance history. As Vitzthum put it, "a current reproductive 'decision' is dependent on both the *absolute quality* of current conditions and the *relative quality* of these conditions compared to prior conditions and predicted future conditions" (2001, p. 193; original emphasis). Thus, women who have experienced positive energy balance during development acclimatize to these good conditions, in effect "predicting" that they will continue. Should they then encounter a period of negative energy balance, their reproductive systems are downregulated because current conditions do not match those to which they have acclimatized, but which they have "predicted" will continue. Conversely, women who have acclimatized to chronic energy imbalance during development have little reason to "predict" that conditions will improve, and so to maximize their chances of reproducing at all they should reproduce early—even under their chronically marginal conditions and with potential trade-offs in reduced maternal and child health (see later). Again, any offspring, even of low quality, is better than none. (The same adaptationist logic underlies the "fetal origins of adult disease" hypothesis, i.e., that the fetus acclimatizes to conditions in utero, thereby in effect "predicting" the energy balance it will experience after birth. We'll return to this topic later as well.)

Another phenotypic marker of mortality risk, however, is the very experience of risk and uncertainty: the neuroendocrine control systems and subjective feelings associated with activation of the HPA axis by the perception of danger (the causes, correlates, and consequences, including malnutrition and disease, of high or unpredictable mortality rates). Just as malnutrition and disease have been correlated with and are thus predictors of mortality, so too, surely, have feelings of arousal, anxiety, fear, and loss (sadness and depression) been correlated with and are thus predictors of mortality—and, as LeDoux notes, for a very long time: "... amongst vertebrates, the neural system involved in detecting danger and producing defense responses is similarly organized in all species studied. This suggests that evolution long ago figured out how to organize the defense system and has continued to use this organizational blueprint" (1995, p 27; see also Crespi & Denver, 2005).

For humans especially, social relations are always a potential source of danger; the ever-present possibility of competition, aggression, and social exclusion make an adequate quantity, quality, and dependability of social–emotional resources critical. While our survival, growth, and development and ultimate reproduction are always contingent on material resources, they are also always contingent on the empathy and cooperation of others, from whom such blessings flow. This is most especially true for our children because of their extreme and prolonged helplessness—thus selection for the critical role of attachment in buffering them against risk and uncertainty (Bowlby, 1969). Attachment theory and research show that children experience all kinds of environmental risk and uncertainty subjectively as social–emotional insecurity. Their subjective experience of inadequate or uncertain material resources certainly includes hunger, pain, and lethargy, but hunger, pain, and lethargy also activate the HPA axis (McEwen, 1998a; Sapolsky, Romero, & Munck, 2000), producing subjective feelings of insecurity (fear or anxiety), thereby activating the attachment system (Ahnert et al., 2004; Desjarlais et al., 1995; Gunnar, 1998; Gunnar et al., 1996; Gunnar & Donazella, 2002; Kobak, 1999). And when parents are not sufficiently buffered against inadequate or uncertain material or social–emotional resources they are apt to feel anxious and frustrated, and are then less capable of being consistently accepting of and sensitive and responsive to their children (Bowlby, 1973; Conger et al., 1994; McLloyd, 1998; Polan & Hofer, 1999), thereby transducing the impact of their environment on themselves to their offspring.

Human infants also face an inherently greater potential for social–emotional insecurity than other primate infants for several reasons. First, sharing is quintessentially human, while nonhuman primates rarely share. Second, alone among the great apes, human mothers deliver subsequent offspring before the preceding one is nutritionally independent, which means that only human mothers may have to decide which one is the better beneficiary of their limited resources (Kaplan et al., 2000). And alone among primates—except for cooperatively breeding monkeys like the Callitrichidae—human mothers are known occasionally to neglect, reject, or even kill their offspring (Hrdy, 2000, 2005). Finally, we are not only an extremely social species but an extremely intelligent one, with the capability to generate complex mental models of our environments and to manipulate these models so as to predict the future. When our models of the future include images of inadequate or unpredictable material resources, feelings of insecurity are likely to follow.

The distinction between material and social–emotional resources is thus far from absolute. Psychosocial stress (arousal, fear, anxiety, insecurity) consumes energy that might have been better allocated to other functions (Bjorntrop, 1991; Dallman et al., 1995; Susman & Pajer, 2004), leading potentially to faltered growth or nonorganic failure to thrive (Black et al., 1994; Chatoor et al., 1998; Drotar, 1991; Montgomery, Bartley, & Wilkinson, 1997; Rutter et al., 2004; Valenzuela, 1997) or, later, a heightened taste for "comfort foods" and thus obesity (Dallman et al., 2003). Moreover, physical pain and social–emotional pain involve much the same neurobiology (Eisenberger & Lieberman, 2004). As a starting point for disentangling their interactive effects on reproduction, Coall and Chisholm (2003) proposed a response hierarchy model in which fertility evolved to be contingent first on health and nutrition, and then, when these are adequate, on safety or security, as indexed by relative absence of, or means of coping with, the specific kind of environmental risk and uncertainty engendered by high mortality rates leading to short or unpredictable lifespans—i.e., psychosocial stress. Wingfield and Sapolsky (2003) make a similar argument. While acknowledging that reproductive suppression is a common response to acute or prolonged HPA activation, they suggest that the trade-off between survival and reproduction means that selection would favor the capability to reproduce despite such stress whenever the likely alternative was imminent death or other failure to reproduce. We might therefore expect that social–emotional or psychosocial stress would be another phenotypic marker of mortality risk and thus contribute to early reproduction. We summarize below evidence that this is the case for humans and rats (at least with positive energy balance). (For similar evidence in other species see references in Bateson et al., 2004; Kuzawa, 2005; Seger & Brockmann, 1987; Stearns, 1992; West-Eberhard, 2003; Wingfield & Sapolsky, 2003.)

PSYCHOSOCIAL STRESS REDUCES AGE AT FIRST REPRODUCTION

While age at first reproduction is influenced by a multitude of factors, we focus here on age at menarche because it is a precondition for first reproduction yet shows enormous variation, from about 12 years in developed countries to almost 19 in some developing countries (Walker et al., 2006; Worthman, 1999); the range within countries is even greater (Parent et al., 2003). Such a broad reaction norm in such a critical life history trait suggests selection for phenotypic plasticity itself, i.e., selection for the capability for menarche at a wide range of ages, with actual age in this range determined by environmental factors. Given that early menarche is associated with numerous later health problems (see later), a better understanding of these factors might inform efforts at prevention or early intervention. We also focus on age at menarche because it is correlated with another precondition of first reproduction—age at first intercourse (Bingham, Miller, & Adams, 1990; Miller et al., 1998, 2001; Phinney et al., 1990; Sandler, Wilcox, & Horney, 1984; Smith, Udry, & Morris, 1985; Udry, 1979; Udry & Cliquet, 1982; Zabin et al., 1986). Moreover, early psychosocial stress also predicts early first intercourse and first reproduction (Boyer & Fine, 1992; Fiscella et al., 1998; Hillis et al., 2004; Miller et al., 1997; Tubman, Windle, & Windle, 1996; Turner, Runtz, & Galambos, 1999; Wyatt et al., 1999).

Insecure Attachment

More than a score of studies have reported a correlation between early psychosocial stressors and early menarche (recent work includes Bogaert, 2005; Chisholm et al., 2005; Grainger, 2004; the best recent review is Ellis, 2004). Many were inspired by Belsky, Steinberg, and Draper (1991), who first suggested that the attachment process might be an evolved mechanism for the entrainment of alternative reproductive strategies in humans, with insecure attachment histories predisposing men and women to earlier reproduction, more opportunistic and short-term sexual relations, and less consistently sensitive and responsive caretaking. They also made the important prediction that "individuals whose early family experiences are high in stress...should be more likely to undergo pubertal maturation earlier than children whose childhood experiences are more pacific" (1991, p 656). Chisholm (1993, 1999) offered an explicit adaptationist rationale for their mechanist model, noting that the current–future trade-off explained in principle why selection would favor the capability to adjust age at menarche contingent on attachment history. However, focusing as it does on mental constructs like Bowlby's (1969) "internal working models," attachment theory has little to say about the biological mechanisms whereby attachment organization might affect age at menarche. By analogy to Ellison's "bioassay," Chisholm (1993) thus used the term "socioassay" to refer to the psychoneuroendocrine processes whereby psychosocial stress might affect age at menarche in the Belsky et al. attachment model. Socioassays are conceived to assess the outcome of each iteration of the attachment cycle, thereby building the social capital ("connections among individuals" [Putnam, 2000, p. 19]) that the child accumulates during her attachment history. The attachment cycle is the oscillation, repeated many times a day in each of its iterations, between the infant's use of mother as secure base from which to explore and as safe haven to which to return (Chisholm, 1996; Sroufe & Waters, 1977). It is a control system for optimizing the trade-off between using mother as a secure base, which motivates play and exploration and so maximizes growth and development, and safe haven, which motivates return to mother and so maximizes survival. The social capital that the child thus accrues becomes represented phenotypically, not only subjectively, in the internal working models (beliefs and feelings) about herself and mother that she constructs from these social relations, but also objectively, as the neuroendocrine traces of her history of HPA activation (Ahnert et al., 2004; Carter, 2005; Gunnar & Donazella, 2002; Gunnar et al., 1996, 1998; Insel & Young, 2001). If this history has been sufficiently secure (the result of sufficiently consistent, sensitive, and responsive nurturing), her internal working models of self and others will be positive and her HPA axis will have acclimatized to low and infrequent activation and rapid return to baseline levels—in effect "predicting" a secure future; if not, her internal working models will be less positive and her HPA axis will have acclimatized to higher and more frequent activation and slower return to baseline levels—in effect "predicting" an insecure future. This psychoneuroendocrine approach to attachment provides a way to explore the biological mechanisms whereby attachment history might affect age at menarche. Thus, while the human and nonhuman studies discussed below have not measured attachment history, they have measured early psychosocial stress and found that it predicts early maturation. The animal studies have also explored neuroendocrine mechanisms whereby early psychosocial stress may affect maturation.

Early Menarche in Girls Adopted from Developing Countries

Since the first observations by Adolphson and Westphal (1981) and Proos, Hofvander, and Tuvemo (1991), several additional studies have reported that girls adopted from developing into developed countries reach menarche earlier than the average for both their country of origin and their new, host country. In their review of this growing literature, Parent et al. (2003) discuss theory and evidence for several mechanisms that might account for such acceleration. They conclude that "there is no simple and single explanation" (p. 686), but also conclude that the role of genetic factors "is relatively minor and unlikely to explain the variation" (p. 680) and that despite reports that women of low birth weight due to intrauterine growth restriction have early menarche (Adair, 2001; Cooper et al., 1996; Ibanez et al., 1998, 2000; Koziel & Jankowska, 2002), there is no evidence that early menarche in the foreign adopted girls was linked to their birth weight. Likewise, while not ruling out health and nutrition, they note that early menarche has also been observed in girls migrating with their original families and with no evidence of former nutritional deprivation, which "provides further support to the role of factors other than nutrition in relation to the changing environment" (Parent et al., 2003, p. 683).

Even so, Gluckman and Hanson (2006), though citing the Parent et al. review, favor a nutritional explanation in terms of the fetal origins of adult disease hypothesis mentioned above (Barker, 1994; Bateson et al., 2004; 2004; Ellison, 2005a; Gluckman, Hanson, & Spencer, 2005; Gluckman et al., 2005; Hales & Barker, 1992). They seem to believe that these girls must have had low birth weight and then good postnatal health and nutrition, arguing that "the combination of prenatal early life deprivation with childhood nutritional excess, as seen in adopted children [who] migrated from poor to rich countries" (p. 9) is the cause of their early menarche. In their view, because of the girls' presumed intrauterine growth restriction they had low birth weight, and, as a consequence, their growth and development would have been based on the "prediction" that they would encounter similar limited resources postnatally. But having acclimatized to marginal resources prenatally and then been adopted into wealthier countries and encountering relative material abundance instead, they would have matured as early as possible in order to capitalize on their windfall (as Cole, 1954, might have predicted).

This may be so, but in light of theory and evidence discussed above we believe that the role of early psychosocial stress in foreign adopted girls' early menarche should also be considered. If human fertility evolved to be contingent first on health and nutrition, and then, when these are adequate, on safety or security, as indexed by patterns of HPA activation during development (Coall & Chisholm, 2003), the question arises whether these girls acclimatized to poor nutrition in utero and then took advantage of their "unpredicted" postnatal nutritional windfall with early menarche, or acclimatized to psychosocial stress during their early years, "predicted" an insecure future, and had early menarche as a result. One argument in favor of the latter possibility is the emerging consensus that 9 months of gestation is not enough to provide reliable information for the fetus to "predict" its resource flow in the future (Ellison, 2005b; Jones, 2005; Kuzawa, 2005; Worthman & Kuzara, 2005; see also Chapter 18). In fact, 9 months is probably a generous estimate of the amount of time the fetus has to sample its environment and base its "predictions"—as evidenced, for example, by the fact that among women pregnant during the Nazi-imposed Dutch famine winter of 1944–1945 only those exposed during their third trimester gave birth to low-birth-weight infants (Stein & Lumey, 2000; see also Chapter 7, note 1, page 437). If 9 months (still less 3) is inadequate for making a "prediction," then, in this context at least, the concept of fetal "predictions" seems questionable. As Jones (2005) argues, it is not so much that the growth-restricted fetus "predicts" a growth-restricted future, but it simply downregulates growth to conserve the resources it has, in effect sacrificing growth for continued survival, thereby "making the best of a bad start." The adaptationist rationale for this view is the logic of the current–future trade-off: For a growth-restricted fetus, maximizing the probability of its current survival is a more pressing adaptive problem than setting the stage for anything it might or might not encounter in the future. This is the essence of the minimax strategy: minimize the probability of the maximum possible loss (lineage extinction due to death). Downregulating growth in the face of starvation is not an adaptation for "predicting" the future but for survival.

Another reason for considering the role of psychosocial stress in foreign adopted girls' early menarche is that while low birth weight has been correlated with early menarche, the reverse is also true, i.e., not only do women of low birth weight seem to have early menarche, women who have early menarche also seem more likely to deliver low-birth-weight infants (Kirchengast and Hartman, 2000; Scholl et al., 1989). And, as we have seen, a score of studies report that early psychosocial stress is associated with early menarche. On the other hand, whether or not early psychosocial stress is also involved, it may be that the causal arrow points in both directions—i.e., low birth weight contributes to early menarche and early menarche contributes to low birth weight. This two-way causation might be part of the mechanism for Kuzawa's (2005; see also Chapter 18) "intergenerational phenotypic inertia" model of maternal (i.e., nongenetic) effects. Arguing that 9 months of gestation is not enough for the fetus to "predict" its lifetime resource availability, he invokes instead Ounsted and Ounsted's (1968; Ounsted, Scott, & Ounsted, 1986) hypothesis that the nutritional experience of a mother when she was a fetus affects the uterine environment she provides her daughters. (Sons, not having uteruses, are not part of the model.) Citing both human and nonhuman evidence in support, he suggests that each generation provides information to the next, and that this information accumulates over a number of generations, providing a "rolling average" of information about past environments that each female fetus can use to "predict" its future and that the time depth of this information makes it more reliable by discounting seasonal or other short-term fluctuations in the flow of resources (Kuzawa, 2005; see also Chapter 18).

Early Stress Accelerates Maturation in Rats

The clearest evidence that early psychosocial stress also accelerates maturation in other mammals comes from long-term studies of the behavioral neuroendocrinology of rats by Meaney and colleagues (Champagne et al., 2003; Cameron et al., 2005; Meaney, 2001; Meaney & Szyf, 2005). Taking advantage of normal individual differences in maternal behavior in the rat, Meaney's group explores the development of two groups of rat pups, one reared by dams who are one standard deviation above their cohort mean in "licking and grooming" (LG) and "arched-back nursing" (ABN) and the other by dams who are one standard deviation below their cohort mean in LG and ABN. Adult offspring of low LG-ABN mothers are more fearful (increased startle responses, decreased open-field exploration, and longer latencies to eat food in a novel environment), show greater plasma adrenocorticotropic hormone and corticosterone responses to experimental stress, and reduced glucocorticoid negative feedback sensitivity. In other words, their HPA axes are altered, making them more reactive to stress. Most significantly, daughters of low LG-ABN mothers also show earlier vaginal opening—a clear marker of sexual matura- tion. They also show increased sexual receptivity and proceptivity and increased fecund- ability (80% compared to 50% in daughters of high LG-ABN mothers). Moreover, cross-fostering experiments show that all of these differences are due to maternal care- taking behavior, not genetic inheritance. The neuroendocrine mechanism entraining early sexual maturation in the daughters of low LG-ABN mothers involves the effects of HPA activity on the hypothalamic–pituitary–ovarian axis, which controls pubertal devel- opment: greater HPA activity in the daughters of the low LG-ABN mothers causes changes in oxytocin receptors (i.e., gene expression) in areas of the brain that regulate sexual behavior.

INEQUALITY CAUSES PSYCHOSOCIAL STRESS AND SHORTENED LIVES

Recapping briefly, our adaptationist argument is that under conditions of high or unpre- dictable mortality it will generally be adaptive for organisms to maximize current repro- duction, especially by reducing age at first reproduction, for delaying only increases the risk of death without issue. Our mechanist argument is that psychosocial stress indexes or reflects mortality rates and is a proximate cause of early reproduction. We turn now to the issue we raised at the beginning of this chapter: the role of inequality in psychosocial stress and mortality.

While it has always been painfully obvious that absolute poverty is associated with ill health and shortened lives, it is now equally obvious that so too is relative poverty or inequality. The difference between absolute poverty and inequality is the difference between not having enough resources to go around and not having them go around enough. Good social relations constitute social capital (Putnam's "connections among individuals") because they are what make resources go around. Good social relations are assets because they increase the velocity of resources (make them go around faster and farther); poor social relations are liabilities because they inhibit the flow of resources. This is the consensus explanation of the standard finding of research on the relationship between inequality and health: for each step up or down in social or economic hierarchies, there is a corresponding and equivalent step down or up in morbidity and mortality rates. It is unlikely that this ubiquitous "stair-step" pattern is due only to whatever marginal health benefits might flow from the incremental increase in material resources accompanying each upward step, because the pattern is apparent not only when the steps themselves are small, but also when it represents populations in wealthy industrial nations with universal health care. Instead, the evidence suggests that the "stair-step" pattern is largely due to the effects on health and longevity of perceived relative deprivation—the perception that one is "one up" or "one down" on another (Adler et al., 1993; Davey Smith et al., 1990, 1996a, 1996b; Farmer, 2003; Kawachi & Kennedy, 2002; Lynch et al., 2000; Marmot, 2004; Marmot et al., 1991; Marmot & Wilkinson, 1999; Marris, 1991; Sennett & Cobb, 1973; Shorris, 1997; Wilson, 1996; Wilkinson, 1996, 2001, 2005).

Being "one up" or "one down" involves what economists call "positional goods"—i.e., those we value because having them places us in a higher position than those who do not (Hirsch, 1976). Where there is no wealth in any domain, there is no inequality, but as wealth increases above the threshold required for basic survival, people commonly compete for positional goods. This generates hierarchies of power, wealth, or status, depending on the domain of competition. That humans compete for position seems undeniable; all primates have dominance hierarchies, with access to resources largely a function of position in the hierarchy (Boehm, 1999; Sapolsky, 2005). Being "one up" in a hierarchy is widely experienced as good, not only because of priority of access to material resources themselves, but also because of the subjective feeling of security entrained by a history of good access. Security is the interest on social capital. It is freedom from doubt, anxiety, or fear; it is the expectation that one is worthy of good relations with others and that others have good intentions towards oneself. The capability for our experience of social security came with the evolution of the attachment process (Chisholm, 2003). Being "one down" in a hierarchy is widely experienced as bad, not only because of uncertain access to material resources, but also because of the subjective feelings of insecurity entrained by a history of reduced or uncertain access. Inequality is a direct cause of psychosocial stress and shortened lives because overly hierarchical political and economic structures limit the flow of resources so that subordinate individuals and groups don't have enough to go around. Inequality also increases morbidity and mortality indirectly through the neuroendocrine correlates of insecurity. Insecurity results in activation of the HPA axis and release of cortisol; chronic insecurity results in chronic high levels of cortisol. Thus, for example, Flinn et al. (1996; see also Chapter 13) observed significantly higher salivary cortisol levels in children of single mothers without adequate kin support, as did Lupien et al. (2000) in low socioeconomic status (SES) children compared to high, and a significant positive correlation between children's cortisol levels and their mothers' symptoms of depression. In turn, chronic high levels of cortisol increase the risk for many disease conditions, including impaired immune function, coronary heart disease, diabetes, neuronal cell death, and anxiety and depression and consequent increased risk for self-medication with alcohol and drugs, all of which lead to shortened lives (Brunner, 1997; Coe, 1999; McEwen, 1998a; Sapolsky, 1996).

Inequality is thus a significant cause of ill health and shortened lives. But this is a proximate explanation, describing the mechanisms whereby inequality engenders psychosocial stress and how psychosocial stress affects health and longevity. Is there an ultimate, adaptationist explanation for the association between inequality and ill health and short lives?

THE TRADE-OFF BETWEEN SURVIVAL AND REPRODUCTION

Natural selection favors the capability of organisms to leave descendants. When this capability is threatened by high or unpredictable mortality rates, selection is expected to favor mechanisms for minimizing the chance of lineage extinction by reproducing early (health and nutrition permitting). But because resources are always limited, it is not possible to maximize all of the components of fitness simultaneously, and trade-offs are inevitable. From an adaptationist perspective, therefore, the ultimate explanation of the association between inequality and ill health and short lives is this: when the only alternative is lineage extinction, natural selection favors mechanisms for reallocating resources from survival to reproduction—i.e., the capability for making the trade-off between survival and reproduction. According to this view, the numerous maternal and child health problems associated with early menarche or early reproduction are costs of reproduction. The cost of a chance at having any descendants at all (the trade-off between survival and reproduction) is one that both early-reproducing women and their children may have to pay in the form of reduced health or longevity. The costs of early menarche for women include an increased risk for reproductive cancers (Apter, 1996; Eaton et al., 1994; Kelsey, Gammon, & John, 1993; Petridou et al., 1996), obesity and obesity-related disorders (Bjorntrop, 1991; Brindley & Rolland, 1989; Colditz et al., 1987; Cordain, Eades & Eades, 2003; Kirchengast et al., 1998; Garn et al., 1986; Shangold et al., 1989; Solomon & Manson, 1997; Wamala, Wolk, & Orth-Gomer, 1997; Wellens et al., 1992), and depression, drugs, and delinquency (Angold & Worthman, 1993; Angold, Costello, & Worthman, 1998; Bratberg et al., 2005; Caspi & Moffitt, 1991; Graber et al., 1997; Heim et al., 2000; Koff & Rierdan, 1993; Magnusson, Stattin, & Allen, 1985; Ruislova, 1998; Singer et al., 2004). And in addition to the effects of mothers' poor health and shortened lives on their children, because early menarche is associated with low birth weight (Kirchengast and Hartman, 2000; Scholl et al., 1989), and low birth weight is a risk factor for the fetal origins of adult disease (see earlier), the children of early-maturing women may also pay a direct cost.

Allsworth et al. (2005) provide especially clear evidence of the potential cost of early menarche. With data from the Third National Health and Nutrition Examination Survey of 2470 U.S. women, they examined the relationship between age at menarche (early: ≤10 vs. late: >10) and allostatic load (the "wear and tear" an individual accumulates from chronic exposure to stress hormones [McEwen, 1998a, 2005]). After adjusting for age, "race"/ethnicity, education, household poverty, income ratio, smoking, and history of depression, women with high allostatic load scores were more than twice as likely to report early menarche as those with low scores. Allsworth et al. (2005) are the first to describe the relationship between age at menarche and allostatic load but make no attempt to explain it, noting that "[t]his association could have also been observed if an unobserved independent biologic process was associated with both age at menarche and composite allostatic load score" (p. 443). We suggest that this "unobserved process" is the mechanism for making the trade-off between survival and reproduction. When the likely alternative is lineage extinction, selection favors early reproduction. If the cost of early reproduction is reduced health and shortened lives, this is just the cost of continuing the lineage. And because such costs are paid after reproduction, they are invisible to selection anyway.

CONCLUSION: WHY INEQUALITY IS BAD FOR HEALTH

Not all health inequalities are caused by early reproduction, of course, but the logic of the trade-off between survival and reproduction is the logic of the current–future trade-off, which may apply to health inequalities in general. The trade-off between survival and reproduction is a version of the current–future trade-off: it is the sacrifice of future survival for current reproduction. But if an organism has not reached maturity, it is incapable of reproduction, and so is incapable of making this trade-off. Instead, under conditions of risk and uncertainty (causing high or unpredictable mortality), its most pressing adaptive problem is simply to survive and its only option is to sacrifice growth and development (an investment in the future) for short-term (current) survival. By continuing to live it buys time in which conditions may improve. If they do, the organism might then undergo catch-up growth, maturing as quickly as possible in order to capitalize on the improved conditions, just as mature organisms upregulate reproduction when conditions improve. If conditions don't improve, however, sacrificing growth and development endlessly to continue living defeats the ultimate adaptive function of growth and development: preparation for reproduction. Selection therefore could not favor adaptations for survival at the expense of endless failure of growth and development. Instead, selection will favor reduced chances of survival for at least some growth and development, with obvious negative implications for health and longevity. For example, fetal growth restriction does not affect all organ systems equally, but favors those most important for long-term growth and development (notably the brain) over those that are less important (like the kidneys, at the cost of long-term survival due to increased risk for kidney disease [Barker, 2004; Brenner, Garcia, & Anderson, 1988]). And Pike (2005) proposes that preterm birth itself may be due to the growth-restricted fetus sacrificing future survival for a better chance at growth and development outside a growth-restricting uterus. As Jones (2005) put it, these growth-restricted fetuses are "making the best of bad start."

In *Inequality Reexamined* (1992), Sen observes that all ethical theories agree that to have a good society there must be equality of something but disagree about precisely what it is that should be equal. This is a critical question because "the judgment and measurement of inequality is thoroughly dependent on the choice of the variable (income, wealth, happiness, etc.) in terms of which comparisons are made" (Sen, 1992, p. 2). Therefore, because inequality is the source of a great deal of pathology and many shortened lives, the answer quite literally has life and death implications. Sen's answer is "the capability to achieve valuable functionings" (1993, p. 31). His argument is that focusing on human capabilities—what is humanly possible in terms of health, long lives, security, reason, etc.—helps us to clarify the distinction between our means and ends by taking us away from our concern with income, wealth, commodities, rights, opportunities, and so forth, and on to the ends to which they are only means. Building on Sen's work, Nussbaum (1995) conceives of our ends in terms of two thresholds: "... a threshold capability to function beneath which a life will be so impoverished that it will not be human at all; and a somewhat higher threshold, beneath which those characteristic functions are available in such a reduced way that, although we judge the form of life a human one, we will not think it a *good* human life" (1995, p. 81, original emphasis). From the perspective of life history theory, Nussbaum's two capability thresholds look like the trade-off between current and future reproduction; ultimately, inequality is bad for health because it keeps people from rising above these thresholds (Chisholm, 1999). Political planning should therefore aim at the target of minimizing the number of people who are capable only of survival (the first threshold: the minimax strategy of avoiding lineage extinction) and maximizing the number of people who are capable of a good human life (the second threshold: the maximin strategy of investing in the future).

    Acknowledgements. This research was supported in part by an Australian Postgraduate Award and the Swiss National Science Foundation (SNSF) project no.51A240–104890.

CHAPTER 7

Early Life Effects on Reproductive Function

Alejandra Núñez–de la Mora and Gillian R. Bentley

Here Núñez–de la Mora and Bentley demonstrate with remarkable clarity that development itself as well as development toward either positive or negative health outcomes later in life hardly begin postnatally. Rather, explanations of health must be explored beginning with the nutritional and pathogenic environment to which mothers and even grandmothers are exposed. For example, being born small for gestational age (SGA) can set in motion a chain of developmental events that, depending on the stability or lack of stability of resources, increase the risk of breast cancer later in life. The authors show how and why variations in ovarian function involving higher or lower levels of reproductive steroids differ across populations (Central Africans vs. Nepalese vs. Bostonians). They also show, based on their studies of Bangladeshi women in London, how variations in ovarian function can differ and fluctuate depending on changing nutrient and caloric availability and amount of time and energy diverted from reproductive effort to fighting disease. It is clear that developmental risks, at different times in a woman's life cycle, including the mechanisms that precipitate rapid growth and maturation, can create a cascade of responses that may be adaptive in the short term but potentially dangerous in the long run. This is a reality that altogether too many migrant women living in Western countries find out the hard way, by acquiring the same vulnerabilities to cancer, for example, that their more affluent Westerners know all too well.

INTRODUCTION

For the past two decades, innovative methods for monitoring ovarian function have encouraged detailed studies of human reproductive function among genetically, culturally, and ecologically diverse populations in field settings. Research by reproductive ecologists has established that levels of ovarian function, measured as average profiles of salivary progesterone and estradiol, differ considerably within and between individuals and populations (Ellison, Lipson, et al., 1993; Ellison, Panter-Brick, Lipson, & O'Rourke, 1993). Age and acute energetic factors, such as immune challenges, nutritional and/or energetic expenditure, whether voluntarily imposed or ecologically determined, are

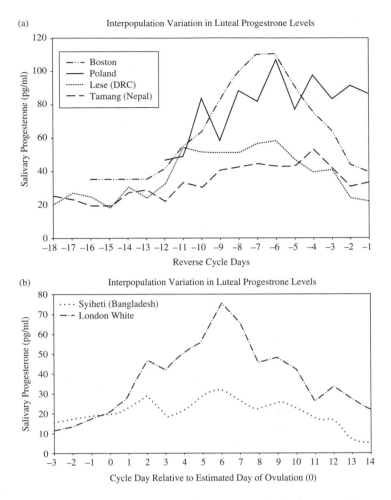

FIGURE 7-1 Interpopulation variation in luteal progesterone levels. Average salivary profiles for women from six populations analyzed by similar radioimmunassay techniques but in two different laboratories that yield slightly different values for steroid hormones. Luteal progesterone data were aligned according to reverse cycle day in panel (a) but according to estimated day of ovulation in panel (b). (a: P. T. Ellison's laboratory at Harvard University; b: R. T. Chatterton's laboratory at Northwestern University). (a) Middle-class Boston women ($n = 126$), Lese horticulturalists from Democratic Republic of Congo (DRC) (formerly Zaire) ($n = 47$), Tamang agropastoralists from Nepal ($n = 45$), and Polish farmers ($n = 20$). (b) Middle-class Bangladeshi ($n = 39$) and London white women ($n = 45$). (Data reprinted with permission from Peter T. Ellison [Boston, DRC], Grazyna Jasienska [Poland], Catherine Panter-Brick [Nepal]. Data for Bangladeshi and London women from Núñez-de la Mora, 2005.)

responsible for some of this variance. How interpopulation variation in ovarian function arises and what its functional significance may be remains poorly understood.

In the first part of the chapter, contrasts are drawn between the clinical and evolutionary viewpoints concerning how to interpret the observed variation in levels of ovarian hormones. A working hypothesis for the origin of this variation is also developed. In particular, the discussion focuses on the effects of the environment during pre- and postnatal development on the establishment of particular *set* points of reproductive hormones during adulthood and on the possible mechanisms for how these are acquired. By set points we mean average levels of hormones that appear to be specific to populations when they are compared (see Figure 7-1), although this does not rule out the possibility that variation in set points may also vary across individuals within populations.

In the second part of the chapter, results are presented from a cross-sectional, migration study of Bangladeshi women living in London, UK, designed to empirically test the hypothesis of a developmental component to adult reproductive function. The effects of different formative environments on growth, maturation, and adult reproductive hormone levels are discussed within the framework of evolutionary theory. In the final part of the chapter, the health consequences resulting from the incongruity between conditions in which the human reproductive system evolved and those faced by many contemporary populations are explored, with special reference to breast cancer risk.

VARIATION IN OVARIAN FUNCTION: AGE, ACUTE AND CHRONIC ENERGETIC CONDITIONS

Ovarian function is frequently measured in hormonal profiles of two reproductive steroids—progesterone and estradiol—across an entire menstrual cycle. These hormones, among their other functions, are responsible for oocyte maturation and ovulation and the preparation of the uterine lining (the endometrium) for potential implantation and pregnancy. They can be measured in blood or saliva, while their metabolites (called pregnanediol-3-glucuronide [PDG] and estrone-3-glucuronide [E3G], respectively) can be measured in urine (O'Connor et al., 2003).

Small-scale, community-based studies using bioassay techniques adapted to field conditions and undertaken, for the most part, by biological anthropologists have explored the sources of variation in ovarian function (Table 7-1). Such studies have been undertaken both in traditional populations with subsistence economies, including horticulturalists in the Democratic Republic of Congo (DRC, formerly Zaire) (Bailey et al., 1992; Bentley, Harrigan, & Ellison, 1998; Ellison, Peacock, & Lager, 1986, 1989), agro-pastoralists in Nepal (Panter-Brick, Ellison, Lipson, & Sukalich, 1996; Panter-Brick, Lotstein, & Ellison, 1993), rural farmers in Poland (Jasienska & Ellison, 1998, 2004) and Bolivia (Bentley et al., 2000; Vitzthum et al., 2002), as well as in urban populations living in established market economies in the United States (Lager & Ellison, 1990) and the United Kingdom (Vitzthum et al., 2002). For subsistence-level populations, variation in energy intake, energy expenditure, and energy flux are related to seasonal fluctuations in food availability and/or workloads inherent to their ecology. For urbanized and industrialized populations, energetic dynamics are most commonly related to voluntary dieting and recreational exercise rather than to variables associated with daily subsistence (Ellison, Panter-Brick et al., 1993).

Data from these field studies show that, during periods of energetic stress, ovarian function is temporarily but reversibly suppressed (Ellison, 1990). The observed reductions in hormonal levels may be interpreted in fundamentally different ways. From a clinical standpoint, lower levels of reproductive hormones during energetic stress are

TABLE 7-1 Sources of Variation in Human Ovarian Function

Source of variation	Study design	Main results	Conclusion	Reference
1) Random variation	Comparison of salivary progesterone profiles from consecutive menstrual cycles. Subjects: Boston women of reproductive age within normal ranges of weight for height.	Women tend to have individually characteristic progesterone profiles; the variance between women is approximately three times as great as the variance within women.	Luteal function appears to be fairly integrated within individuals and fairly consistent over time in the absence of other influences.	P. T. Ellison, 1995
2) Variation associated with age	1. Comparison of salivary progesterone and estradiol profiles of Boston women of different age groups (18–48 years old), of stable weight, within normal ranges of weights for height and not engaged in regular strenuous exercise.	Significant differences in progesterone and estradiol profiles between age groups.	Ovarian function as a whole follows a parabolic trajectory with age with increasing function lasting until the early to mid-twenties and declining function evident as early as the mid-thirties.	S. F. Lipson & Ellison, 1992, 1994; O'Rourke & Ellison, 1993
	2. Comparison of progesterone salivary profiles between different age groups of women in quite disparate populations, widely divergent in geography, culture, genetic background and basic subsistence economy (namely Boston women, Lese subsistence farmers from the Ituri forest of Zaire, and Tamang agro-pastoralists from the highlands of Nepal).	Significant differences by age group in all three populations, and significant differences in average levels at every age between populations, with no interaction effect which indicates that the age patterns in the three populations are essentially parallel.	The parabolic pattern of age variation in ovarian function seems to be a common feature of human biology. The consistency of the age patterns suggests that it is due to underlying processes of maturation and aging common to all populations and not to the acute effects of ecological variables that happen to be proportionately distributed by age in all populations.	P. T. Ellison, 1994; P. T. Ellison, Lipson, et al., 1993

3) Variation associated with energetics (changes in energy balance or energy flux)			
Related to changes in energy intake:			
a) Associated with voluntary dieting	Well-nourished Boston and German women of reproductive age.	Moderate weight loss (1–2 kg/month) is associated with lower luteal progesterone and estradiol profiles. Magnitude of weight loss is significantly correlated with the relative degree of steroid suppression in the month following that in which the weight loss occurred. This indicates there is a lag time for the full effect of this energetic stress to be manifested.	Lager & Ellison, 1990; Pirke, Schweiger, Lemmel, Krieg, & Berger, 1985; Schweiger et al., 1987
		Ovarian function is sensitive to energy balance (measured as BMI or body weight change).	
Related to changes in energy expenditure:			
a) Associated with self-imposed aerobic exercise	Young Boston and German women participate in vigorous exercise with increased caloric intake to maintain energy balance.	Lower progesterone and estradiol levels observed among recreational joggers of stable weight, compared with inactive controls of comparable weight and BMI.	Bledsoe, O'Rourke, & Ellison, 1990; Broocks et al., 1990; Bullen et al., 1985; P. T. Ellison & Lager, 1986; P. T. Ellison, Lipson, & Sukalich, 1996; Shangold, Freeman, Thyssen, & Gatz, 1979
		Energy expenditure has negative effect on ovarian steroids independent of energy balance	

continued

TABLE 7-1 *continued*

Source of variation	Study design	Main results	Conclusion	Reference
b) Associated with ecological factors related to subsistence ecology	Well-nourished rural Polish farm women subject to seasonal variation in workload but with stable body weight.	Lower progesterone levels found during the physically demanding season of agricultural work correlated with the amount of energy expenditure but not with energy balance or energy intake.	Energy expenditure has a negative effect on ovarian steroids independent of energy balance.	Jasienska & Ellison, 1998
c) Associated with variation in habitual physical activity	Rural and urban Polish women of reproductive age.	A negative relationship between habitual physical activity (low, moderate, high) and salivary levels of estradiol.	Even moderate energy expenditure associated with lower ovarian function.	Jasienska, Ziomkiewicz, Ellison, Lipson, & Thune, 2006
Related to changes in energy balance due to changes in both energy intake and energy expenditure				
a) Associated with ecological factors related to subsistence ecology	Marginally nourished Lese horticulturalists of the Ituri forest of Democratic Republic of Congo and Tamang agropastoralist	Sustained weight loss over a season associated with lower progesterone levels between and within women in both populations.	Reduced luteal function in periods of negative energy balance. Inconsistent results for estradiol.	Bailey et al., 1992; Bentley, Harrigan, & Ellison, 1990; P. T. Ellison et al., 1986, , 1989; Panter-Brick

	women in the Nepalese highlands subject to negative energy balance due to seasonal food shortage and increased workloads.	In the Lese, sustained populationwide weight loss is associated with lower estradiol, a steady decrease in ovulation frequency and ultimately with a decline in conceptions. No comparable effect of seasonal negative energy balance on estradiol levels among Tamang women.		et al., 1996; Panter-Brick et al., 1993
4) Variation associated with nutritional ecology	Western women	Vegetarian and high-fiber diets, associated with low levels of estradiol compared to omnivorous, low-fiber diets. Conversely, high fats have been associated with elevated gonadal steroid levels.	Dietary composition appears to affect reproductive steroid metabolism.	Armstrong et al., 1981; Barr, Janelle, & Prior, 1994; Goldin et al., 1982, 1986; Persky et al., 1992

considered to be an indication of dysfunction and potential pathology (Castelo-Branco, Reina, Montivero, Colodron, & Vanrell, 2006; Warren & Goodman, 2003). In contrast, an evolutionary perspective would interpret the sensitivity of ovarian function to energetic cues as adaptive and as a mechanism to calibrate and optimize energetic investment in reproduction (Ellison, 2001; Jasienska, 2003).

For human females, reproduction is an expensive enterprise involving long gestations of a large-brained infant, prolonged breastfeeding, and a period of slow postnatal growth of offspring requiring intensive parental care. One would therefore expect human reproductive function to be modulated by mechanisms that can gauge (with some degree of precision) whether investment in a pregnancy at any particular time is likely to compromise the mother's health or survival. Given the taxing costs of reproduction for the human female (Butte, Wong, & Hopkinson, 2001; Dewey, 1997; Durnin, 1991), and the instability and unpredictability of the environment in which modern humans evolved (Lahr & Foley, 1988), a flexible strategy could balance competing reproductive and physiological investments. It would thus be expected to be under positive natural selection and ultimately to yield higher reproductive success (the capacity to pass one's genes to succeeding generations).

In addition to the acute and reversible changes in ovarian function associated with energetics, there is another universal and predictable source of variation in ovarian function, namely age (Lipson & Ellison, 1992; O'Rourke & Ellison, 1993). Throughout a woman's life course, average reproductive steroid hormone levels trace a parabolic trajectory, which parallels that of fertility. This particular trajectory is not linked to energetic factors, but rather to the normal aging processes of the ovary and its declining capacity to produce steroids as the number of follicles decline. The effect of age on hormone levels is observed in all populations regardless of their ecologies (Figure 7-2). The age-related decline in female fecundity and fertility that accompanies lower steroid levels, and the phenomenon of menopause in women, may relate to the increased physiological risks of childbearing for older women (Baird et al., 2005; Ellison, 1995; Swanton & Child, 2005). However, baseline levels of steroid hormones around which age-related variation occurs differ significantly among populations, reinforcing the notion of set points. Populations living in harsh ecological settings have lower age-related, average levels of steroid hormones than populations living in energetically favorable conditions (Ellison, 1996) (Figure 7-2).

Acute, short-term energy challenges that result in changes in hormonal levels also occur relative to specific population-linked, baseline levels (Ellison, 1996). For example, salivary progesterone levels in farming women in DRC, Nepal, and Poland are relatively lower during the energetically expensive harvesting season than during the postharvest period when workloads are less arduous and energy balance is positive (Bentley et al., 1998; Ellison, Panter-Brick et al., 1993; Jasienska & Ellison, 2004; Panter-Brick et al., 1993). But salivary progesterone levels during bounty times in these women are still significantly lower than those of urban women living in Boston, Chicago, or Cambridge (United Kingdom), as illustrated in Figure 7-1.

Although the existence of this significant variation in baseline hormonal levels among different populations has been consistently documented both in anthropological (Ellison, 1996; Ellison, Lipson, et al., 1993) and epidemiological studies (Danutra et al., 1989; Falk et al., 2002; Kamath et al., 1999; Key, Chen, Wang, Pike, & Boreham, 1990; Pinheiro,

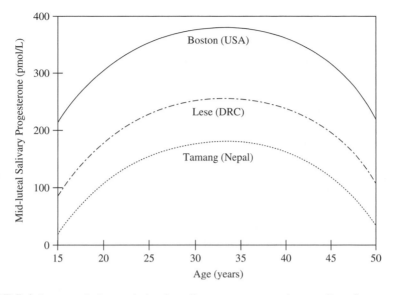

FIGURE 7–2 Interpopulation variation in salivary progesterone by age. Best-fit second-order polynomial regressions of mid-luteal progesterone levels on age for three populations: middle-class Boston women ($n = 136$ cycles), Lese horticulturalists from Democratic Republic of Congo ($n = 144$) and Tamang agropastoralists from Nepal ($n = 45$). (Adapted with permission from Ellison, P. T. (1993). *Ann NY Acad Sci* 709:287–298).

Holmes, Pollak, Barbieri, & Hankinson, 2005), the causes of this variation and its functional significance remain poorly understood. In the epidemiological and clinical literature, differences in steroid hormone levels between ethnically diverse populations have commonly been attributed to factors associated with lifestyle, in particular to differences in dietary composition and caloric sufficiency (Armstrong et al., 1981; Goldin et al., 1986). In contrast, reproductive ecologists suggest that hormonal variation is evidence of *phenotypic plasticity* in response to specific environmental conditions experienced during development and a reflection of diverse, adaptive life history strategies to optimize reproductive fitness (Ellison, 1996; Worthman, 1999).

Fitness is enhanced by adjusting life history traits (such as growth, developmental trajectories, optimal body size, longevity, and determinants of fecundity and reproduction) to the environment in which an individual lives. Life history theory thus posits that resource allocation must be divided into vital functions of growth, maintenance (including immunological defense and somatic repair), and reproduction (Stearns, 1992). Since resources are finite, the demands of one of these three functions over another generate trade-offs, which can be evident in the short or the long term. Decisions on how much, when, and where to invest resources during different stages of the life cycle are dictated by two major variables: the availability of energy/resources, and the selection forces imposed by the environment.

In humans, the compromise between having a relatively large and complex brain and the capacity to walk bipedally has driven the evolution of several of our life history traits: altriciality, longevity, and a relatively slow and prolonged period of postnatal development

(Bogin, 1994). For human females, the postnatal period prior to puberty is critical for the establishment of developmental patterns (such as age at maturation, height, and body condition) that determine future fertility and reproductive success (Ellison, 1981a, 1982). This prepubertal period can also function as a bioassay of the overall level of energy above maintenance costs likely to be available for future reproduction (Cole, 2000). Mechanisms that allow the setting of developmental trajectories to optimize lifelong trade-offs that result in the least wasteful reproductive strategy (i.e., successful gestations) are expected to be advantageous and maintained by natural selection.

The relationship between indicators of environmental quality and tempo of growth and maturation (Cooper, Kuh, Egger, Wadsworth, & Barker, 1996) and their impact on ovarian function (MacMahon et al., 1982) have been documented widely. There is evidence that postnatal conditions of energy abundance conducive to early reproductive maturation (early menarche) are associated with a pattern of high adult levels of ovarian steroid secretion (Apter, 1996; Apter, Reinila, & Vikho, 1989; Apter & Vikho, 1985; Vihko & Apter, 1984). Conversely, situations of high energy flux and/or negative balance lead to late maturation (Frisch, 1987; Malina, Spirduso, Tate, & Baylor, 1978; Warren, 1980) and result in low set points of ovarian hormones (Gardner, 1983; Gardner & Valadian, 1983; Venturoli et al., 1987). It can be argued that given the scenarios of energy insecurity and unpredictability in which modern humans evolved, what appears to be chronically suppressed ovarian function observed in contemporary traditional populations is actually more normal for our species than the enhanced ovarian function and higher hormone levels exhibited by Western populations. The latter living as they generally do in conditions of energy surplus are, in fact, unusual in evolutionary terms (although clinicians regard Western hormone levels as "the norm") and may be implicated in the current patterns of hormone-related disorders such as reproductive cancers (Ellison, 1999).

A number of scholars, beginning with Roger Short in 1976 (Eaton et al., 1994; Ellison, 1999; Greaves, 2000; Strassman, 1999), have already pointed out the association of modern contemporary lifestyles of women and higher risks for breast cancer compared to historical and ancestral populations. These earlier studies, however, focused on several behavioral components common to women in industrialized societies such as delayed childbearing, high rates of contraception, low fertility, and short periods of breast feeding, that together act to increase women's lifetime *exposure* to levels of reproductive steroids.

High levels of ovarian steroid hormones are commonly identified as an important factor in the development and prognosis of breast cancer (Bernstein & Ross, 1993; Key & Pike, 1988; Pike, Spicer, Dahmoush, & Press, 1993). At the cellular level, both estradiol and progesterone act as potent mitogens (inducing cell division) in normal and cancerous breast tissue (Pike et al., 1993). Epidemiological data show that the highest incidence of reproductive cancers is generally found among privileged populations that grow faster, mature earlier, and have higher average caloric intakes and lower average energy expenditures (Bernstein, 2002; Bernstein, Teal, Joslyn, & Wilson, 2003; Clavel-Chapelon, 2002; Henderson & Bernstein, 1991), all factors associated with high levels of gonadal function. Similarly, the rapid transition to high cancer incidence seen in many migrant populations that move from settings of lower cancer incidence is, in the same way, related to the accelerated secular trend in such groups—likely reflecting improved conditions (Shimizu et al., 1991; Thomas & Karagas, 1987; Trichopolous, Yen, Brown, Cole, & MacMahon, 1984; Ziegler et al., 1993).

POTENTIAL MECHANISMS OF VARIATION
IN OVARIAN FUNCTION

The proposed mechanisms through which developmental trajectories may be established and/or modified by contrasting environmental conditions are not fully understood. However, the metabolic axis has been proposed as a likely candidate to function as an integrator of both the acute and chronic energetic cues from the environment and as a coordinator of the allocation of the available energy into growth, maintenance, and reproduction processes (Lipson, 2001). In principle, the quality of the environment during the prepubertal formative years in terms of health, physical activity, and nutrition could determine the basic parameters of a metabolic blueprint that would govern the trajectory of development. This in turn would influence the tempo of maturation and, consequently, baseline levels of adult ovarian function. Data on population differences in some of these metabolic hormones give support to this hypothesis (see Chapter 8).

There is considerable evidence indicating that metabolic hormones, particularly insulin, insulin-like growth factors (IGFs), and leptin, are indeed implicated in determining the timing of the onset of pubertal development, the tempo of the adolescent growth spurt, and the concurrent increase in adrenal steroid levels (Apter, 1997; Chehab, Mounzih, Lu, & Lim, 1997; Foster & Nagatani, 1999; Hindmarsh, Matthews, Di Silvio, Kurtz, & Brook, 1988; Ong, Ahmed, & Dunger, 1999; Smith et al., 1989; Wilson, 1998). In addition to the indirect impact of the metabolic hormones on reproductive function through their association with maturation tempo, the metabolic hormones are also implicated in the regulation of adult ovarian function directly via their actions on the hypothalamic–pituitary–ovarian (HPO) axis (Duleba, Spaczynski, & Olive, 1998; Karlsson et al., 1997; Lipson, 2001; McGee, Sawetawan, Bird, Rainey, & Carr, 1996; Poretsky, Cataldo, Rosenwaks, & Guidice, 1999; Poretsky, Grigorescu, Seibel, Moses, & Flier, 1985; Samoto et al., 1993; Willis, Mason, Gilling-Smith, & Franks, 1996).

PRENATAL EFFECTS ON REPRODUCTIVE FUNCTION

Epidemiological studies in humans (dos Santos Silva et al., 2002; Murphy, Smith, Giles, & Clifton, 2006) and experimental work on other mammals (Fowden, Giussani, & Forhead, 2005) has demonstrated that the adjustment of developmental trajectories according to the prevailing environment is not restricted to the postnatal period but, in fact, can begin before birth. The mammalian fetus uses cues from the uterine environment to monitor the conditions in which it is likely to be born and adjusts metabolic and physiological set points and developmental trajectories accordingly (Barker, 1998; Gluckman, Cutfield, Hofman, & Hanson, 2005; see also Chapter 18). For example, there is evidence that prenatal undernutrition can alter postnatal growth trajectories, with prenatally malnourished offspring growing more slowly, maturing later, and attaining a smaller adult size (Coe & Shirtcliff, 2004; Engelbregt et al., 2004; see also Chapter 17). With respect to the effects of prenatal conditions on *reproductive* function, comparatively little work has been undertaken. The majority of data come from experimental studies on farm animals (Manikkam et al., 2004; Steckler, Wang, Bartol, Roy, & Padmanabhan, 2005), laboratory animals (Guzman et al., 2006; Leonhardt et al., 2003; Zambrano et al., 2005), and captive primates (Abbout, Barnett, Bruns, & Dumesic, 2005). These studies show that female mammals exposed to excess androgen in utero or during early postnatal life are typically smaller in size and show altered reproductive behavior, ovulatory dysfunction, and decreased ovarian reserve.

In humans, most of the understanding of early life influences on reproductive function comes from: (1) the study of the effects of fetal growth restriction on the development of polycystic ovarian syndrome (PCOS) taking individuals born small for gestational age (SGA) as a model (the assumption being that these individuals were malnourished in utero—but see Basso, Wilcox, & Weinberg, 2006; de Bruin et al., 1998; Ibanez et al., 2002; van Weissenbruch, Engelbregt, Veening, & Delemarre-van de Waal, 2005); (2) environmental toxicology data on the effects of pollutants on reproductive function and fertility (Toppari, 2002); (3) epidemiological analyses linking birth weight and/or ponderal index (birth weight/height^3 $\times$ 100) (both used as proxies for early life conditions—but see Basso et al., 2006) with reproductive variables (menarche, menopause, steroid levels) (Adair, 2001; Cresswell et al., 1997; Jasienska, Ziomkiewicz, Lipson, Thune, & Ellison, 2006); and (4) historical data on the effects of birth seasonality on adult fertility (Lummaa & Temblay, 2003). Because of obvious ethical concerns, experimental data on humans are practically nonexistent, as are data from prospective, longitudinal studies, presumably due to the logistical and funding difficulties entailed in such types of research.

Although reproductive development and performance are clearly influenced by prenatal factors, the crucial windows in development and the physiological mechanisms through which environmental influences are transmitted to target organs are, in many cases, complex and poorly understood. There is a large body of literature implicating a role for prenatal programming in the development and functioning of the HPO axis (Rhind, Rae, & Brooks, 2001). For example, the action of gonadotropins—follicle-stimulated hormone (FSH), luteinizing hormone (LH), and gonadotropin-releasing hormone (GnRH)—on reproductive development can be disrupted by maternal food restriction, maternal low body weight (anorexia nervosa), obesity, smoking, and alcohol intake (Davies & Norman, 2002). Other studies have shown that, at earlier stages of fetal development, the normal ontogeny of gonadal development and function can be disrupted by undernutrition or the influence of endocrine-disrupting compounds (Gulledge, Burow, & McLachlan, 2001; Toppari, 2002). Specifically, in female fetuses, the onset of meiosis during oogenesis in the ovary is delayed (Rhind et al., 2001). These data on prenatal programming raise the possibility that several reproductive disorders are influenced by intrauterine factors that alter patterns of gonadotropin release, possibly through the programming of the fetal neuroendocrine axis (Barker, Winter, Osmond, Phillips, & Sultan, 1995). The observation of a positive relationship between ponderal index (an indicator of nutritional status) recorded for women at birth and levels of estradiol measured during their menstrual cycles as adults supports this hypothesis (Jasienska, Ziomkiewicz, Lipson et al., 2006). Results such as these demonstrate that conditions during fetal life influence adult production of reproductive hormones and may contribute to interindividual variation in reproductive function.

As a model to understand the effects of prenatal conditions on the development of the reproductive system, the study of adult reproductive function in SGA individuals is complicated by the fact that individuals who experience a degree of prenatal growth restraint also present a suite of metabolic conditions such as hyperinsulinemia, dyslipidemia, and central adiposity (around the waist) (Ibanez, Ong, Dunger, & de Zegher, 2006). Nevertheless, fetal growth retardation is associated with impaired ovarian development in girls such as lower follicle numbers (de Bruin et al., 1998), lower ovarian steroid production (Ibanez, Potau, & de Zegher, 2000), smaller uterii and ovaries (Ibanez, Potau, Enriquez, & de Zegher, 2000), and reduced rates of ovulation during adolescence (Ibanez et al., 2002). These conditions could indicate female subfertility in adulthood, and a hyposensitive ovarian response to FSH.

Further evidence for the influence of uterine conditions on the establishment of growth and maturation trajectories comes from epidemiological studies implicating birth characteristics (i.e., birth weight, ponderal index, size for gestational age) as factors partially determining age at menarche and even age at menopause. For instance, Adair (2001) has shown that although birth weight was not significantly related to age at menarche, girls who were relatively long and thin at birth attained menarche earlier than girls who were short and thin. Data also show that rapid postnatal growth enhances the effects of size at birth and is related independently to earlier pubertal maturation. That is, the effect of thinness at birth is most pronounced among girls with greater-than-average growth increments in the first 6 months of life (Adair, 2001). Similarly, growth retardation in late gestation, leading to shortness at birth and low weight gain in infancy, may be associated with a reduced number of primordial follicles in the ovary leading in turn to an earlier menopause (Cresswell et al., 1997).

Analyses of data from historical populations (i.e., late nineteenth and early twentieth century) also suggest that early life conditions may play an important role in shaping female reproductive performance across generations. These studies of past groups have found associations between month of birth (related to climatic conditions and presumably food availability) and female reproductive traits, such as early menarche or menstrual disorders (Jongbloet, Kersemaekers, Zielhuis, & Verbeek, 1994), fecundability (Nonaka, Desjardins, Legare, Charbonneau, & Miura, 1990; Smits et al., 1997), menopause, and fertility (Lummaa & Temblay, 2003). For example, women with significantly reduced birth weights who had been exposed to acute, severe famine in utero during the Dutch famine of 1944–1945[1] did not themselves suffer from lower fecundity in adulthood (Lumey, Stein, & Ravelli, 1995), but were more likely to give birth to low-birth-weight (LBW) offspring who had a high frequency of stillbirths and early infant mortality (Lumey & Stein, 1997). Another more recent report, however, indicated the presence of modest but longstanding effects of childhood famine exposure on reproductive function in women. Severe famine exposure during childhood significantly decreased chances of first and second childbirth at any given time after marriage or first childbirth. Similarly, the risk of a medical reason for having no or fewer children than wanted was increased in the severely exposed, as was the risk of a surgical menopause (Elias, van Noord, Peeters, den Tonkelaar, & Grobbee, 2005).

Most of the evidence for the relationship between early life conditions and human reproductive function and performance referred to so far comes from studies of individuals specifically selected either for their birth characteristics (SGA and LBW), exposure to disrupting chemicals, or extraordinary acute conditions (war famine), but for the most part individuals belonged to relatively affluent populations. Conducting studies among these affluent populations limits the opportunities and the degree to which one can assess the kind of variation that would be expected among populations living in more chronically stressed ecologies closer to those in which humans presumably evolved. It is antici-pated that long-term effects of early life conditions on later life history traits would be more easily detected in populations living in harsh conditions and experiencing an energy-limited environment. However, studies in these kinds of environments are few at present and generally short term when they take place. Longitudinal studies are complex, pose numerous methodological and statistical challenges, and are often financially unfeasible.

An alternative strategy to explore the effect of variation in environmental conditions on human plasticity is the use of migrant studies (Lasker, 1995; Lasker & Mascie-Taylor, 1988). One of the main strengths of a migrant study design is that it permits the discrim-ination between genetic adaptation and developmental adaptability. Migrant studies can also prove considerably less expensive and easier to implement than long-term projects. They have been used previously to assess the effect of variation in environmental condi-tions during development on the tempo of maturation (Proos, Hofvander, & Tuvemo, 1991a, b), age at menarche (Leidy, 1998), and adrenal steroids during puberty (Zemel, Worthman, & Jenkins, 1993). The hypothesis for a developmental component impli-cated in the interpopulation variation in baseline levels of ovarian function, although sup-ported by strong theoretical and circumstantial evidence, has been waiting for empirical corroboration.

We have used a cross-sectional migrant design as a natural experiment to evaluate how environmental conditions during growth and development affect adult levels of ovarian hormones and to assess whether there are any critical windows during development when changes in such conditions may have more significant effects (Núñez–de la Mora, 2007a, b). We compared salivary hormonal profiles of healthy women of reproductive age and similar genetic background who, by moving from a country with poor living standards (Bangladesh) to one of significantly higher standards (United Kingdom) have been exposed to contrasting environmental conditions during different phases of their life cycle. The changes in nutrition, lifestyle, and reproductive variables experienced by migrants were assessed through detailed questionnaires and anthropometry.

The study groups were Bangladeshi women who: (1) migrated to the United Kingdom as adults ($n = 56$); (2) migrated to the United Kingdom as children ($n = 42$); (3) second-generation women born in the United Kingdom ($n = 33$); (4) a reference group of women living in Sylhet, NE Bangladesh ($n = 52$); and (5) a reference group of white British women living in London ($n = 50$). Except for the occasional short visit to their home country, all first-generation Bangladeshi migrants had lived continuously in the United Kingdom.

The Bangladeshi migrants in this study originate from relatively affluent, land-owning classes in Sylhet who live in solid dwellings with access to either piped or well water, experience no evident food insecurity, and have low levels of energy expenditure (Gardner, 1995). Nowadays, financial security for this class of Sylheti residents is pro-vided by jobs primarily in the civil service, business sector, or higher education. Many Sylhetis are also supported by remittances received from family members in the United Kingdom or elsewhere. However, despite the seemingly adequate socioeconomic condi-tions, Sylheti inhabitants suffer from chronic exposure to parasites due to prevailing unsanitary conditions. Towns and villages lack appropriate sewage and waste-disposal systems, have limited water-treatment capacity, and are subjected to seasonal floods, resulting in an environment where infection and disease are rife and potable water is scarce (Muttalib et al., 1975; NIPORT, 2001; Northrop-Clewes, Rousham, Mascie-Taylor, & Lunn, 2001). This insalubrious situation is exacerbated by the limited availability and poor quality of health care. Thus, despite the fact that Bangladeshis in the United Kingdom have socioeconomic indicators that reflect their socially disadvantaged position relative to the general population in the United Kingdom (Eade, Vamplew, & Peach, 1996), the overall quality of the British environment and the wide access to health services and a clean water supply are radical departures from conditions in Sylhet. If nothing else, migrants to the United Kingdom are free from chronic exposure to infections. This would be expected to translate into enhanced growth and maturation for migrants (Cole, 2000).

Estimates available from cross-sectional studies show that this latter projection is indeed the case. For example, the growth of infants and children of South Asian background living in the United Kingdom is comparable to 1990 growth standards for white U.K. children (Kelly, Shaw, Thomas, Pynsent, & Baker, 1997). Similarly, data confirm a secular trend towards increased height in succeeding generations, especially in females (Shams & Williams, 1997). With respect to infant and child health, a study in East London where the concentration of Bangladeshi migrants is highest revealed that post-neonatal mortality rates for infants born to Bengali mothers between 1987 and 1990 was 6.9/1000 live births (Hilder, 1994), 10 times lower than Bangladeshi national rates (56/1000 births) (UNICEF, 2006). In an on-going project studying reproductive aging among older Bangladeshi women (aged 35–59), we recently (March 2007) collected data (unpublished) from questionnaires in which we specifically asked women if they have ever or in the past six months, suffered from intestinal parasites ("worms"). From 137 women who answered this question, 91% responded that they had "ever" experienced intestinal parasites, while of 154 women who responded, 14% said they had suffered from intestinal parasites within the past six months. Pinworm, roundworm and hookworm were the most common helminths identified as the source of the problem. Ninety-four percent of women also took anti-helminth medication to treat the problem. These data support the argument that women in the present study are indeed likely to have experienced contrasting environmental conditions during development, depending on their country of birth and the place where they grew up.

We tested the hypothesis that poor environmental conditions experienced during infancy and childhood would result in adult women having lower average baseline levels of ovarian steroid hormones (progesterone and estradiol) than those living in more affluent conditions(Núñez-de la Mora et al. 2007a, b).. We also examined whether a positive change in environmental conditions that impacts developmental tempo is reflected in enhanced reproductive hormonal function—that is, whether migrants who move to an affluent environment while growth and development is ongoing will have higher ovarian steroid levels than nonmigrant Sylheti residents (referred to here as sedentes). Finally, we tested whether alterations in conditions after maturation modify the hormonal set points established during early life.

Our results show that individuals living in more affluent environmental conditions (i.e., second-generation British Bangladeshis and white Londoners) have enhanced growth trajectories with earlier maturation higher levels of salivary progesterone and higher rates of ovulation compared to women living in poorer conditions (i.e., Bangladeshi

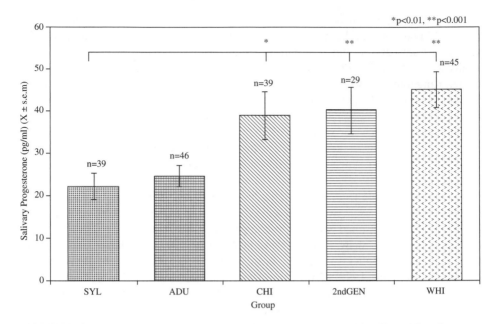

FIGURE 7-3 Average luteal progesterone levels by migrant group. Unadjusted luteal progesterone levels (pg/ml) for one menstrual cycle by migrant group before adjusting for age, age at menarche, and anthropometric variables. Average luteal progesterone values, controlling for anthropometric and reproductive variables, were significantly higher in the child migrant, second-generation, and white groups compared to levels for sedentes. Multiple linear regression model $F_{9,178} = 5.05$; $p < 0.001$; s.e.m. = 0.32: Adj. $R_2 = 0.16$. SYL $<$ CHI $p < 0.01$; 2ndGEN, WHI $p < 0.001$. Child migrants reached menarche at an earlier age ($\bar{x} = 12.2 \pm 0.2$ years) than either Sylheti sedentes ($\bar{x} = 13.2 \pm 0.2$ years), adult migrants ($\bar{x} = 13.0 \pm 0.2$ years), or white women ($\bar{x} = 13.1 \pm 0.2$ years) but at similar ages as second-generation women ($\bar{x} = 12.3 \pm 0.3$ years), who had an earlier menarche than women in Sylhet ($F_{4,210} = 5.3$, $p = 0.001$). Abreviations: Sylheti women resident in Bangladesh (SYL), adult migrants (ADU), child migrants (CHI), second-generation British Bangladeshis (2ndGEN), British white women (WHI).

sedentes), who have delayed maturation and low adult progesterone levels (Figure 7-3). However, the impact of environmental change is contingent on the timing of such improvements. Individuals who migrated to a more affluent environment during infancy or childhood (i.e., first-generation "child" migrants) have significantly higher progesterone levels and attain menarche earlier than individuals who developed in poor conditions (i.e., adult migrants and Bangladeshi sedentes). Moreover, increases in average adult progesterone levels are less pronounced when the environmental change is experienced around the time of adrenarche and are almost nonexistent in the later peri-menarcheal period. The magnitude of the effect of age of exposure to improved conditions can be gauged by the following comparisons: progesterone indices of women who migrated to the United Kingdom as infants are similar to those of United Kingdom–born women, whereas levels of those arriving close to adolescence are indistinguishable from those who migrated as adults and those of Sylhet sedentes (Figure 7-4).

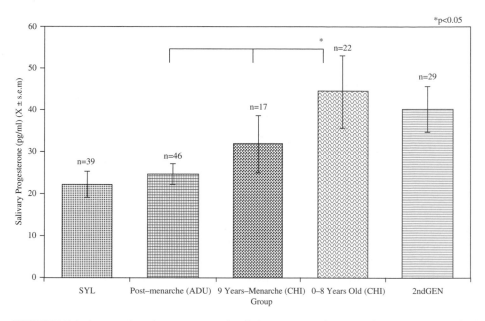

FIGURE 7-4 Average luteal progesterone levels by category of age at migration to the United Kingdom. Unadjusted luteal progesterone levels (pg/ml) for one menstrual cycle. Women who migrated during infancy and early childhood (0–8 years) had significantly higher average luteal progesterone ($F_{2,81} = 3.14$, $p = 0.04$), after controlling for age, anthropometric and reproductive variables than those who migrated at a later stage (including later child migrants from 9 years to menarche [peri-menarche] and adult migrants [postmenarche]). Women who migrated to the United Kingdom during the childhood phase showed significantly earlier age at menarche ($\bar{x} = 11.9 \pm 0.3$ years) than later first-generation arrivals ($\bar{x} = 12.4 \pm 0.2$ years and $\bar{x} = 13.0 \pm 0.5$ years for peri-menarche and postmenarche, respectively) ($F_{3,89} = 3.98$, $p = 0.01$).

Finally, improved environmental conditions experienced during adulthood (post-menarche) do not impact significantly on baseline progesterone levels among first-generation adult migrants. Furthermore, the fact that adult migrants and Sylhet sedentes do not differ significantly in baseline progesterone levels despite their contrasting current environments, physical activity patterns, and body composition indices may be taken as evidence of the "robustness" of the physiological adaptations established during early life that determine set points for ovarian function (Figure 7-3).

First-generation Bangladeshi migrant women who migrated to the United Kingdom as children demonstrate a plastic response to improved preadolescent conditions in their growth, maturation, and ovarian function. This argues against the existence of solely prenatal (uterine) effects on adult progesterone levels, which might limit options if the environment subsequently changes. It can be argued that in a long-lived species like humans a more optimal strategy is to spend a longer period of *postnatal* life monitoring the quality of the environment and adjusting reproductive trajectories accordingly. This more long-term strategy would also offer the opportunity to coordinate the development of the reproductive system with other related systems, such as the skeletal one, which also exhibits a high degree of plasticity and responsiveness to acute changes in the environment (Tanner, 1992).

It remains unclear how growth and maturation rates (and by implication ovarian function) are related, established, and modified during susceptible periods. However, it is evident from the coordination of the final phases of physical growth with reproductive maturation that both processes interact. Ellison (1981, 1982) has suggested that this interaction has a critical adaptive value in ensuring that pelvic skeletal maturation appropriately coincides with other aspects of reproductive maturation to ensure a safe delivery following a potential early conception.

Numerous migrant and refugee studies provide examples of plasticity in developmental tempo. For instance, improvements in conditions that are often the cause of growth faltering during childhood (such as poor nutrition, chronic infection, and psychosocial stress) lead to catch-up growth and growth outcomes equivalent to those of affluent populations (Goel, Thomson, Sweet, & Halliday, 1981; Mjones, 1987; Proos et al., 1991a; Schumacher, Pawsoni, & Kretchener, 1987; Yip, Scanlon, & Towbridge, 1992, 1993). Nutritional intervention and prospective and retrospective studies give further examples of how the tempo of growth and maturation can be affected by nutritional conditions during childhood (Berkey, Gardner, Frazier, & Colditz, 2000).

The importance of the timing of changes in the quality of the environment and its impact on developmental trajectories is illustrated in a longitudinal study of adopted Indian girls in Sweden. In this study, the age at which girls arrived in Sweden determined their subsequent patterns of growth and maturation. Girls adopted close to adolescence showed accelerated growth, hastened maturation, and, consequently, smaller than expected final stature compared to girls adopted in early childhood, who showed equally early maturation but exhibited taller statures. In both cases, adopted girls showed much younger menarcheal ages than their Swedish peers (2–3 years), reflecting their accelerated tempo of maturation upon improvement in environmental conditions (Proos et al., 1991a, b). Unfortunately, our study lacks longitudinal data with which to analyze those components of the growth and maturation trajectories (e.g., height velocity, age at peak velocity, onset of puberty, etc.), which were modified among Bangladeshi women after migration to the United Kingdom.

We also lack data on intergroup variation in metabolic hormones to support the hypothesis suggested earlier that the metabolic axis is the pathway through which indicators of environmental quality translate into a blueprint that governs energy allocation and the trajectory of development. However, the increased susceptibility to type 2 diabetes among Bangladeshi immigrants in the United Kingdom supports the idea of a metabolic blueprint set at low energy parameter that, in conditions of affluence, has turned maladaptive (Erens, Primatesta, & Prior, 2001; Holt, 2004; Mather & Keen, 1985; McKeigue, 1996; McKeigue et al., 1988; Pollard, Unwin, Fischbacher, & Chamley, 2006).

Variation in chronic energy availability can be related to nutritional, energetic, and/or epidemiological factors. Most research in the field of reproductive ecology conducted so far has focused mainly on the first two factors (see Ellison, Panter-Brick et al., 1993; Jasienska, 2001, for reviews), presumably because they have been the most obvious features to study and partly because they are relatively easy to measure, either directly or through proxies, such as changes in body weight and composition, energy expenditure indices, etc. However, ample evidence points to immune factors as inexorably linked to chronic energy availability. For instance, it is widely recognized that chronic illness has a negative impact on growth and maturation (Campbell, Elia, & Lunn, 2003; Moore et al., 2001; Panter-Brick, Lunn, Goto, & Wright, 2004; Solomons, Mazariegos, Brown, & Klasing, 1997; Tanner, 1992). Frequent or chronic diseases provoke persistent stimulation of the body's inflammatory and immune systems with the concomitant lymphocyte proliferation and rise in antibody production. These processes are energetically expensive and may result in restricted growth despite adequate food availability (Stephensen, 1999).

Direct reliable measurements of the energetic costs of continuous and high immune activity and its long-term repercussion on reproductive effort are very difficult to obtain (Long & Nanthakumar, 2004; McDade & Worthman, 1999). However, the prediction derived from lifetime resource allocation and life history theory (Charnov, 2001; Gadgil & Bossert, 1970) is that the experience of recurrent or chronic illness during childhood should be negatively associated with adult rates of reproduction. In mathematical modeling of life history, a reduction in prereproductive mortality results in an acceleration of reproductive maturation and presumably higher reproductive output (Cole, 1954; Gadgil & Bossert, 1970; Schaffer, 1974).

Empirical epidemiological data confirm the prediction that investment in maintenance costs diverts resources away from reproduction; data show that the secular trend in human maturation finds its closest correlate in the declining mortality rates of the demographic transition (underscored by a dramatic shift in patterns of morbidity). By reducing the maintenance costs of immune function, energy for growth and reproduction is freed and maturation is accelerated (Ellison, 1981; Eveleth & Tanner, 1990). Historical analyses provide further indirect evidence for the long-term effects of immune costs on growth. A study in four northern European countries revealed an association between increased adult height and reduced old-age mortality related to a lifetime reduction of infection and inflammation (Crimmins & Finch, 2006).

As outlined above, the adverse energetic conditions experienced by some of the Bangladeshi groups in our study are not related to undernutrition and/or heavy physical workloads as reported in previous research (Ellison, Panter-Brick, et al., 1993) but rather to the costly immunological challenges imposed by the insalubrious environment in Sylhet where many women grew up (Constantine et al., 1988; Muttalib et al., 1975; Northrop-Clewes et al., 2001). Thus, we suggest that the *lower* levels of ovarian function and late maturation among the groups who developed in such challenging immune conditions reflect the trade-offs between maintenance and reproduction predicted by life history theory.

CONCLUSION

But what are the implications from our work for evolutionary medicine and reproductive health? Our findings presented here of a *developmental* effect on adult ovarian function add a new dimension to the study of the etiology and epidemiology of women's reproductive health in later life. Thus, developmental risk factors—younger age at menarche, older age at menopause, increased height, and enhanced ovarian function— are evidently associated with improved health and positive energetic conditions that themselves translate into higher adult lifetime levels of ovarian steroids. The negative health risks attributed to these factors (Okasha, McCarron, Gunnell, & Smith, 2003) are, under normal circumstances, unlikely to be reversed and can be regarded as "built-in" risks for reproductive cancers for women born in affluent environmental conditions. Therefore, it is of crucial importance that specific behaviors (e.g., exercise programs) and/or hormonal interventions, such as those suggested by Short (1976) and others (Eaton et al., 1994), are undertaken to reduce breast cancer risk in the populations that as a result of their developmental characteristics (rapid growth and maturation) are already at comparatively high risk.

In conclusion, in this chapter we have proposed a model for human ovarian function in which chronic energetic conditions *during the postnatal period* establish an overall program of energy allocation into growth, maintenance, and reproduction via the regulation of metabolic hormones such as insulin and/or IGFs (Lipson, 2001; Poretsky et al., 1999). One of the consequences of this program is the establishment of set points for ovarian function around which short-term adjustments are made according to acute fluctuations in energy availability during adult life. From an evolutionary perspective, such fine-tuned regulation should lead to the optimization of reproductive effort and, ultimately, fitness (Ellison, 1996; Lipson, 2001).

The downside of this phenotypic flexibility for modern human females living in affluent conditions is the increased health risk for reproductive cancers in later life that accompanies exposure to higher steroid hormone levels. The value, however, of an evolutionary perspective on reproductive function is that specific behavioral recommendations could be made to reduce the risks of acquiring high ovarian steroid levels. Obviously, we do not want to compromise the nutritional well-being of developing children or their immune status either by restricting food intake or increasing their exposure to pathogens. Nor do we know the potential risks of administering exogenous hormones that might delay menarche but have other long-term side effects. However, schools (and parents) in industrialized countries could promote high levels of exercise for children (at least up until the age of 8 years old and ideally through adolescence) as a healthy, low-risk, and cost-effective means of lowering steroid levels and reducing cancer risks in the next generation of adult women. Framing such health promotion within the context of how far removed we are now (in affluent, industrialized countries) from the kinds of environments in which our human ancestors lived (and expended their energies) for many thousands of years (as has been done by many earlier scholars, e.g., Eaton et al., 1994) is perhaps a fundamental part now of the evolutionary medicine paradigm. But the next step surely, if evolutionary medicine is to move beyond theory, is to try and implement these recommendations in specific settings.

CHAPTER 8

Impaired Reproductive Function in Women in Western and "Westernizing" Populations
An Evolutionary Approach

Tessa M. Pollard and Nigel Unwin

What happens when women live in evolutionarily novel Western environments that promote conditions of obesity, insulin resistance, and hyperinsulinemia? In this chapter Pollard and Unwin describe the significance of high levels of insulin, induced both by high-calorie Western diets and reduced energy output, for women's reproductive function. Hyperinsulinemia promotes high levels of free androgens, mainly by reducing levels of sex hormone-binding globulin. In turn, high levels of free androgens negatively affect reproductive function. Women in "Westernizing" populations undergoing socioeconomic transition often experience particularly high levels of insulin, and there is some evidence to suggest that, as a consequence, they are also likely to face particularly severe impairment of reproductive function. Pollard and Unwin explore this issue in relation to British Pakistani women. They emphasize the importance of studying sex hormone-binding globulin levels in studies of reproductive function. This chapter explores issues that are important for our understanding of reproductive function and are new to evolutionary medicine.

INTRODUCTION

Compared with those living in less affluent countries, women living in Western societies generally experience higher levels of the ovarian hormones progesterone and estradiol (Bentley, Harrigan, & Ellison, 1998; Ellison et al., 1993; Key, Chen, Wang, Pike, & Boreham, 1990; Vitzthum, Spielvogel, & Thornburg, 2004; see also Chapter 7), and ovarian hormone levels in Western women are considered to represent the extreme of the global distribution of ovarian function (Ellison et al., 1993). Within evolutionary medicine and biological anthropology groundbreaking work has highlighted links between these high estrogen and progesterone levels and high rates of breast cancer in the West (Ellison 1999; Jasienska, Thune, & Ellison, 2000). Ellison (2001, p. 213) suggests that such population variation in ovarian function is related to chronic energy availability. Thus high levels of estradiol and progesterone in Western women are the result of environments in which calorifically dense foods are readily available in combination with minimal required energetic expenditure.

For the same reasons, women living in the affluent West are at high risk of pathological changes in the metabolic system, and we show here that these changes are likely to have adverse consequences for reproductive function. In particular, in women of reproductive age there are important interactions between insulin levels and ovarian function. In this chapter we describe the significance of high levels of insulin and consider how, why, and to what degree chronically high levels of insulin can lead to significant problems with reproductive function. We further explore and highlight escalations of these problems among women from populations in socioeconomic transition.

INSULIN RESISTANCE AND INSULIN LEVELS IN AFFLUENT WESTERN POPULATIONS

Insulin resistance is the main underlying pathology of type 2 diabetes and an important risk factor for cardiovascular disease (Reaven, 1988). The main role of insulin is to regulate levels of glucose in the body. Insulin is secreted by the pancreas when blood glucose levels rise as a result of the consumption of carbohydrates. It prompts the uptake, storage, and use of glucose by almost all tissues of the body and suppresses the production of glucose by the liver. It is also an important regulator of lipid metabolism. In people with insulin resistance, skeletal muscle and liver do not respond in the normal way to insulin. As a result the body secretes more insulin, leading to higher insulin levels or hyperinsulinemia, and this may regulate glucose levels successfully for a time. Elevated blood glucose and finally type 2 diabetes result when the pancreas is no longer able to produce sufficient insulin to overcome insulin resistance and maintain normal glucose levels (Greenspan & Gardner, 2004)

Insulin resistance and hyperinsulinemia are strongly associated with excess body weight and physical inactivity (Ryan, 2003), and particularly with abdominal obesity, which is caused by excessive visceral fat (Despres, 2006). In addition, certain types of diet increase the risk of insulin resistance, particularly diets low in fiber and with a high glycemic index (foods that cause a particularly large increase in blood glucose levels) (McKeown et al., 2004). Most refined starchy foods, including bread and starchy root vegetables, have a high glycemic index, whereas nonstarchy vegetables, fruit, and legumes tend to have a low glycemic index (Ludwig, 2002). Levels of obesity are high and levels of physical activity are low in Western societies (Catanese, Koetting O'Byrne & Poston, 2001; Flegal, Carroll, Kuczmarski & Johnson, 1998; Katzmarzyk, 2002), while refined grain products with a high glycemic load now supply 20% of the energy in the typical U.S. diet and high glycemic load sugars supply 16% of energy (Cordain, Eades, & Eades, 2003). For all these reasons, levels of insulin resistance in Western populations are high.

Diet and physical activity levels during most of human evolutionary history were very different, as deduced from studies of modern-day hunter-gatherers, who have very low levels of obesity and high levels of physical activity and usually eat a high proportion of nonstarchy fruit, vegetables, and legumes (Eaton, Eaton, & Konner, 1999; Jenike, 2001). Unfortunately, we have little direct information on insulin resistance or hyperinsulinemia in people living as hunter-gatherers. However, suggestive data were collected by O'Dea (1984), who accompanied a group of overweight diabetic Australian Aborigines while they reverted to a traditional hunter-gatherer lifestyle for 7 weeks. She found that during this period the participants experienced significant weight loss, a striking improvement in levels of insulin resistance, and a reduction in fasting insulin levels.

Thus, persistently high insulin levels are an evolutionarily new phenomenon, and they are an important cause of ill health in affluent Western societies. In addition to type 2 diabetes and cardiovascular disease, increasing numbers of other diseases have been linked to hyperinsulinemia via a number of physiological pathways, including breast, colon, and prostate cancer, myopia, and acne (Cordain et al., 2003).

INTERACTIONS BETWEEN INSULIN LEVELS AND OVARIAN FUNCTION IN AFFLUENT WESTERN POPULATIONS

Lipson (2001) has suggested that metabolic hormones, principally insulin, and the closely related insulin-like growth factor (IGF)-1, as well as leptin, signal energetic conditions to the reproductive system. The ovaries are influenced by an insulin-related regulatory system (Poretsky, Cataldo, Rosenwaks, & Giudice, 1999), and metabolic hormones may also have effects at the hypothalamic level. Several studies have shown that levels of metabolic hormones indicating an energy deficit were associated with disrupted or reduced ovarian function (Lipson, 2001). Lipson (2001) also suggests that, conversely, high levels of insulin and IGF-1 probably stimulate high levels of ovarian steroid concentrations, although this has not been consistently demonstrated in vivo (Poretsky et al., 1999). Early menarche, as seen in Western populations, may be associated with increased insulin concentrations in overweight girls (Lipson, 2001). Thus metabolic hormones appear to provide a mechanism that links energetic availability and ovarian function (Ellison, 2001, see also Chapter 7).

So what happens when women live in evolutionarily novel Western environments that promote conditions of obesity, insulin resistance, and hyperinsulinemia? Obesity is known to be positively associated with risks of oligomenorrhea (infrequent menstruation), amenorrhea (absence of menstruation), and chronic anovulation, and it is thought that hyperinsulinemia is the main cause of these effects (Pasquali, Pelusi, Genghini, Cacciari, & Gambineri, 2003). The main effects of abnormally high levels of insulin do not appear to be on ovarian secretion of progesterone and estrogens (although level of these hormones may be high). Rather, the most important effects are on the ovarian secretion of androgens and the production by the liver of sex hormone-binding globulin (SHBG) (Livingston & Collison, 2002). SHBG is the main binding protein for testosterone and estradiol, and the level of SHBG is an important determinant of levels of free and biologically active testosterone and estradiol in both men and women. Because testosterone has a relatively high affinity to SHBG, any reduction in SHBG increases the bioavailability of circulating testosterone, in particular, and also increases the ratio of free testosterone to free estradiol. Thus hyperinsulinemia promotes high levels of androgens, referred to as hyperandrogenism, in women (Figure 8-1) (Livingston & Collison, 2002; Poretsky et al., 1999). Hyperandrogenism in turn contributes to insulin resistance, leading to a damaging cycle of interaction whereby androgen and insulin levels cycle upwards (Livingston & Collison, 2002). This is illustrated by a recent meta-analysis, which showed that testosterone levels are higher in women with type 2 diabetes than in nondiabetic women. Additionally, in prospective studies, women with lower SHBG levels had a higher risk of developing type 2 diabetes (Ding, Song, Malik, & Liu, 2006).

Androgens have adverse effects on the growth of follicles in the ovary during the early stages of the menstrual cycle (Balen, 1999). It is not surprising then that low SHBG and high free androgens are associated with reduced fecundity in women (van der Spuy & Dyer, 2004). For example, van Hooff et al. (2004) showed that testosterone level at age 15 was positively associated with persistence of oligomenorrhoea at age 18 in girls. Apter and Vihko (1990) showed that women with relatively high serum androgen concentrations conceived at a lower rate than other women.

Low SHBG and high free androgens are also associated with polycystic ovary syndrome (PCOS), one of the "hyperinsulinemic diseases of civilization" identified by Cordain et al. (2003). PCOS is a syndrome of ovarian dysfunction characterized by biochemical and clinical signs of hyperandrogenism, menstrual irregularity, and polycystic ovary morphology (enlarged ovaries with multiple cysts). In PCOS multiple dysfunctional small cysts develop in the ovary, instead of one dominant follicle as in a normal menstrual cycle, and ovulation does not generally occur. PCOS is strongly associated with insulin resistance. It is the most common endocrine cause of infertility in women in the West (Balen, 1999) and is reported to occur in 5–10% of women of reproductive age in affluent populations (Dunaif, 1997). More women (perhaps 20% of Western women (Dunaif, 1997)) have polycystic ovaries but not the full symptomology of PCOS. Dunaif also notes that up to 75% of women with secondary amenorrhoea meet the diagnostic criteria for PCOS. Women with PCOS who become pregnant have an increased risk of miscarriage, preeclampsia, and gestational diabetes (Patel & Nestler, 2006).

Perhaps because PCOS is clearly a pathological aberration of ovarian function, it has been studied mainly by clinicians working in the field of infertility and has largely

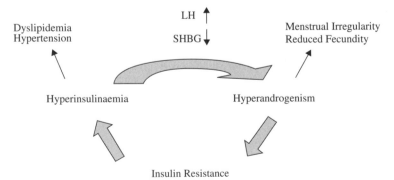

FIGURE 8-1 A simplified representation of the damaging cycle linking insulin and androgen levels in premenopausal women.

escaped the attention of human biologists with an interest in evolutionary theory. Meanwhile, despite the known links with insulin resistance, clinicians have not considered that rates of PCOS may be unusually high in Western populations. It seems clear, however, that we should think of PCOS as one of a number of pathological conditions associated with the novel human experience of living in affluent Western environments. We should also consider it, like type 2 diabetes, as the tip of an iceberg. In this case the invisible part of the iceberg consists of large numbers of women with tendencies towards high androgen levels, irregular menstrual cycles, and low levels of fecundity.

INTERACTIONS BETWEEN INSULIN LEVELS AND WOMEN'S REPRODUCTIVE FUNCTION IN POPULATIONS IN TRANSITION

Insulin Levels in Populations in Transition

We use the term populations in transition to refer to populations that are experiencing changes that are moving them towards the Western lifestyle. The term "nutrition transition" is often used to describe this process in relation to diet (Popkin, 2001). Other terms are also applied to these populations, such as "Westernizing" or "modernizing." We apply the term "populations in transition" particularly to populations living in urban areas of developing countries, but it is also relevant to migrants from developing to Western countries and to indigenous people living in countries colonized by Europeans. Millions of people worldwide fall into these categories.

Very high levels of type 2 diabetes are seen in some populations in transition. The best known examples are groups of indigenous people living in the United States, Canada, and Australia, who have rates of type 2 diabetes that are higher than even the high levels seen in the general populations in those countries (O'Dea, Hopper, Patel, Traianedes, & Kubisch, 1993; Száthmary, 1994; Weiss, Ferrell, & Hanis, 1984). This difference is reflected in high levels of fasting insulin and in the large insulin response to glucose in Australian Aborigines and Native Americans (Guest, O'Dea, Hopper, & Larkins, 1993; O'Dea et al., 1993; Ritenbaugh et al., 2003). In general, these groups of indigenous people followed their traditional subsistence ways of life before the arrival of Europeans, which often had an enormous impact on their social and economic systems, although there was considerable variation in these processes across populations and continents (Kunitz, 1994). In most cases diets are now very poor (high in fats and sugar and lacking in fruit and vegetables) and levels of physical activity are low in these populations (Szathmáry, 1994, Young, Reading, Elias, & O'Neil, 2000). Several groups of Pacific Islanders, most notably the people of Nauru, have also recently adopted Western lifestyles and developed high rates of obesity and type 2 diabetes (Zimmet, Taft, Guinea, Guthrie, & Thoma, 1977). Finally, migrants from some of the poorest parts of the world to the affluent West have been shown to have very high levels of insulin resistance and type 2 diabetes. The best known example is probably that of South Asian populations living in the West, particularly those living in the United Kingdom (e.g., Misra & Vikram, 2004). However, there are other examples, such as the high rates of diabetes suggested by a high relative risk of death from diabetes in Turkish, Moroccan, Surinamese, and Antillean/Aruban migrant groups in the Netherlands (Stirbu, Kunst, Bos, & Jackenback,

2006). Evidence from poor countries, such as India and Tanzania, suggests that the prevalence of type 2 diabetes and associated cardiovascular disease risk factors tends to be much higher in urban compared to rural areas (Aspray et al., 2000; Singh et al., 1997; Vorster, Venter, Wissin & Margetts, 2005).

Competing hypotheses have been posited for the high rates of insulin resistance, hyperinsulinemia, and type 2 diabetes in these populations. Some researchers have focused on putative genetic differences (the "thrifty genotype" hypothesis) (Diamond, 2003; Zimmet et al., 1977), while others have focused on the possibility that slow growth in early life, especially in utero, may increase predisposition to insulin resistance if risk factors for diabetes, such as lack of physical activity, are encountered in later life (the "thrifty phenotype" hypothesis) (Bateson et al., 2004; Drake & Walker, 2004; see also Chapter 18). The thrifty phenotype hypothesis may seem to imply that future generations born into a Western environment will have dramatically improved insulin sensitivity, but intergenerational effects (see Chapter 18) may mean that this will not be the case and that it will take several generations before these populations show levels of insulin sensitivity similar to those in established Western populations.

Whether the increased risk of insulin resistance and elevated insulin levels in Westernizing populations is caused by a genetic predisposition, by a mismatch between early and later environment, or by a combination of both, they have implications for reproductive function in Westernizing populations. These implications are outlined below.

Reproductive Function in Populations in Transition

We should expect high rates of insulin resistance in populations in transition to have adverse consequences for aspects of ovarian and wider reproductive function, as outlined above for Western women. If rates of insulin resistance are very high, then we expect the consequences for ovarian function will be correspondingly greater.

Unfortunately, information on reproductive function in populations in transition is far more sparse than information on insulin resistance, hyperinsulinemia, and rates of type 2 diabetes. However, some relevant work has been done with Pima (Native American) women. In a study of 695 nonpregnant Pima women aged 18–44 years, Roumain et al. (1998) found a history of menstrual irregularity (defined as an interval of 3 months or more between menstrual periods after the age of 18) in 21% of women. This compares with a rate of menstrual irregularity, defined in the same way, of 4% in a Swedish population-based study (Petterson, Fries, & Nillius, 1973; Solomon, 1999). Weiss et al. (1994) set out to test whether Pima women with higher insulin levels had elevated androgens and menstrual irregularities compared to women with lower insulin levels. They found that a high proportion (50%) of women in their "high-insulin" group reported menstrual irregularities. Total testosterone levels did not differ between high- and low-insulin groups of women, however. Given that high insulin levels are known to suppress production of SHBG, the authors speculated that those in the high-insulin group were likely to have low SHBG and therefore higher free testosterone levels. Thus, while no difference in total testosterone was observed between the low- and high-insulin groups, it is still possible that the high-insulin group had more free, biologically active, androgens.

We conducted a study of insulin levels and androgen levels in a group of British Pakistani women, an example of a population in transition. Half of the British Pakistani women were immigrants from Pakistan, while the other half were daughters of immigrant women; our primary aim was to compare these two groups (Pollard, Unwin, Fischbacher, & Chamley, 2006). We present these data here as a relevant case study, comparing the British Pakistani women as a whole with a group of European women.

Insulin Levels, SHBG, and Testosterone Levels in British Pakistani Women: A Case Study

Compared to levels in the general population, there is a high level of coronary heart disease and type 2 diabetes in people of South Asian origin living in the United Kingdom, including British Pakistanis (McKeigue, Shah, & Marmot, 1991). We examined reproductive function and cardiovascular and type 2 diabetes risk factors in premenopausal British Pakistani women, with a main focus on intergenerational change. We were also interested in interactions between risk factors for cardiovascular disease and type 2 diabetes and reproductive function.

The participants were 85 women aged between 20 and 40, of whom 60 were British Pakistani (30 women born in Pakistan, 30 born in the United Kingdom) and 25 were women of European origin born in the United Kingdom (Table 8-1). The women were recruited mostly using snowballing techniques, whereby participants guide the researcher to others who may be eligible to participate in the study (Robson, 1993). Women who reported absent or irregular menses or diabetes were excluded because we wanted to sample estradiol on a specific day of the menstrual cycle (data not reported here). Thus the sample is not representative of the general population of premenopausal British Pakistani women and can only provide information on variation in androgen levels in regularly menstruating women. Of the women born in Pakistan, 4 migrated as young children (<8 years) and 26 migrated aged 15 or over. The majority of migrants had been

TABLE 8-1 Characteristics of Study Group[a]

	British Pakistani	European	p-value[b]
n	60	25	
Age (years)	30.1 ± 5.5	34.6 ± 4.2	<0.001
Height (m)	1.58 ± 0.06	1.63 ± 0.05	0.001
BMI	25.3 ± 4.8	27.3 ± 6.2	0.11
Birthplace			
Pakistan	30	0	
UK	30	25	
Highest educational level			0.45
None	1	0	
Primary	2	0	
Secondary	20	9	
Higher	30	14	
Occupation			0.002
Looking after home	22	4	
Employed	19	18	
Other	11	1	

[a] *Means and standard deviation are given for continuous variables. Sample sizes are given where there are missing data.*
[b] *p-values were calculated using ANOVA for age and chi-squared test for education and occupation.*

born and had grown up in northwest Pakistan, either in the Mirpur district of Azad Kashmir or in the Punjab. These are mainly poor rural areas, although many families who send migrants have benefited from remittances from other family members already in the United Kingdom (Shaw, 2000).

The methods for the study, other than for the assessment of cardiovascular risk factors, are described in Pollard et al. (2006). Briefly, women were visited in their own homes during the morning and following an overnight fast on day 9, 10, or 11 of the menstrual cycle. We assessed body composition using anthropometry, including skinfold measurements, and also levels of serum SHBG and testosterone, allowing us to calculate the free androgen index (as 100 x testosterone (nmol/l) / SHBG (nmol/l)). Fasting levels of glucose and insulin were assessed from serum. Insulin resistance was estimated from fasting glucose and insulin using the homeostasis modeling assessment (HOMA) method (Haffner, Miettinen, & Stern, 1997).

After adjusting for age and BMI using analysis of covariance, the British Pakistani women had significantly higher levels of insulin resistance, as assessed by HOMA-IR, than the European women ($p = 0.03$), although the difference in insulin levels was not

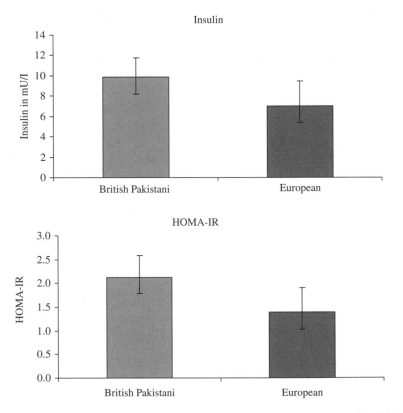

FIGURE 8-2 Geometric means for insulin level and insulin resistance (as assessed by HOMA-IR) adjusted for age and body mass index in British Pakistani women ($N = 57$) and white European women ($N = 24$). Error bars show 95% confidence intervals.

significant ($p = 0.07$) (Figure 8-2). After adjusting for age and BMI, there were also significant differences for SHBG ($p = 0.03$) (British Pakistani women had lower levels than white European women) and for free androgen index ($p = 0.02$) (British Pakistani women had higher levels), but not for total testosterone ($p = 0.39$) (Figure 8-3). There

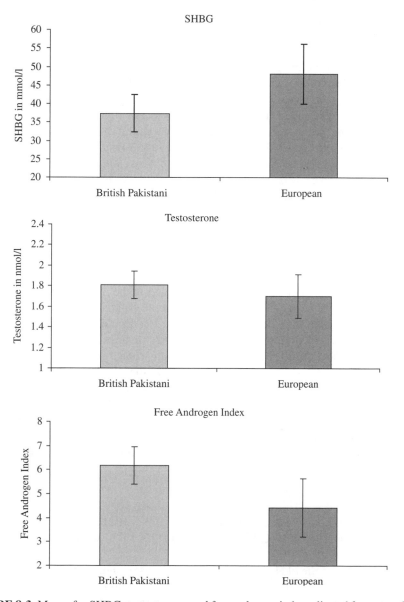

FIGURE 8-3 Means for SHBG, testosterone, and free androgen index adjusted for age and body mass index in British Pakistani ($N = 60$) and white European ($N = 25$) women. Error bars show 95% confidence intervals.

TABLE 8-2 Pearson Correlation Coefficients for Correlations Between Insulin and Insulin Resistance Levels and SHBG, Testosterone, and Free Androgen Index in 85 Premenopausal Women

	SHBG	Testosterone	Free androgen index
Insulin	−0.49***	−0.06	0.41***
HOMA-IR	−0.51***	−0.03	0.45***

$***p < 0.001$

were significant correlations between the insulin and insulin-resistance measures and the androgen-related measures in the expected directions (Table 8-2).

Thus there is evidence in this small group that regularly menstruating British Pakistani women had higher levels of insulin resistance, lower levels of SHBG, and higher levels of free androgens than regularly menstruating British women of European origin for a given age and level of BMI. Higher levels of insulin and insulin resistance were also associated with lower SHBG and a higher free androgen index. These are not surprising results given what we know about high levels of insulin resistance in the South Asian origin population in the United Kingdom and the known relationships between insulin resistance, insulin levels, and levels of SHBG and free androgens outlined above. Two previous studies of people of South Asian origin in the United Kingdom reported lower SHBG levels in South Asian than in European women (Reddy & Sanders, 1992; Reed et al., 1993), and Reed et al. also found higher free testosterone levels in South Asian women. Thus there has been some previous indication of greater androgenicity in women of South Asian origin living in the United Kingdom. There is also some evidence to suggest that PCOS may be more common in South Asian women in the United Kingdom than among European women. Rodin, Bano, Bland, Taylor, & Nussey (1998) described a prevalence of polycystic ovaries on ultrasound, which is more common than PCOS, of 52% in South Asian women in London, which can be compared to rates of around 20% in European populations (Polson, Adams, Wadsworth, & Franks, 1988). Together all these results suggest that there may be a high level of fertility problems in British South Asian women. However, there has been no study of PCOS prevalence rates in the British South Asian population, and we are not aware of any research on levels of infertility in British South Asian women. Such studies are clearly warranted, particularly as fertility is very important to many women of South Asian origin (Pollard et al., 2006).

METHODOLOGICAL IMPLICATIONS FOR STUDIES OF REPRODUCTIVE FUNCTION IN WOMEN

An understanding of the likely existence of high levels of androgenicity and associated problems in affluent Western populations and in populations in transition has important methodological implications for studies of ovarian function in these populations. First, such studies typically rely on the assessment of women experiencing regular menstrual cycles, excluding women with irregular or absent cycles (as we did in our study of British Pakistani women). This is usually done because of the need to assess estradiol and progesterone over a menstrual cycle or at particular points in the menstrual cycle. Such exclusions impose biases on our assessment of ovarian function and reproductive health.

Another methodological message to emerge is the importance of SHBG as a determinant of free hormone levels. In Western and Westernizing women SHBG levels are likely to be low on average because of high levels of obesity and insulin resistance. Low levels of SHBG increase free testosterone and estradiol levels (with the greatest effect on free androgens). Studies of salivary estradiol measure only free estradiol levels and cannot determine the relative influences of ovarian secretion of total estradiol and SHBG levels on free estradiol levels. The importance of SHBG levels is illustrated in work on the effects of the high levels of consumption of phytoestrogens in women in Asia, which appears to provide protection against breast cancer. Although phytoestrogens do not appear to affect ovarian production of estrogen to any great extent, it is thought that they stimulate hepatic production of SHBG, leading to a reduction in free estradiol levels (Adlercreutz, 2002). SHBG levels rise during the luteal phase of the menstrual cycle, but a single serum sample timed in relation to the menstrual cycle has been shown to provide a good characterization of interindividual differences in premenopausal SHBG levels (Ahmad, Pollard, & Unwin, 2002; Plymate et al., 1985).

SHBG levels are also important determinants of levels of salivary testosterone in men. Campbell, Leslie, and Campbell (2006) assessed total testosterone, SHBG, and free testosterone and concluded that population variation in the rates of age-related decline in free testosterone reflect the impact of energetic status on SHBG levels as much as differential decline in testosterone production with age.

In the future, researchers should aim so far as possible (it may not be possible in difficult field situations) to assess salivary free estradiol and testosterone levels in combination with serum levels of total estradiol and testosterone and SHBG. This will provide a much more complete picture of reproductive function, including information on how much observed variation in free estradiol or testosterone levels is due to variation in the gonadal secretion of these hormones and how much is due to variation in SHBG levels.

CONCLUSION

High and increasing levels of obesity, insulin resistance, and insulin in Western and Westernizing populations have potentially harmful effects on ovarian and reproductive function in women. In particular, hyperinsulinemia is associated with hyperandrogenism, irregular menstrual cycles, reduced fecundity, and PCOS. Thus it is appropriate to consider hyperandrogenism, irregular menstrual cycles, PCOS, and associated low levels of fecundity in women as problems created by the evolutionarily novel Western environment, and as conditions that are likely to be experienced at particularly high levels in populations in transition. These are conditions that can profoundly affect quality of life for women. It is also worth noting that hyperinsulinemia may increase reproductive cancer risk (Solomon, 1999). We suggest that the influence of insulin resistance and high insulin levels on reproductive function and reproductive health in Western populations and populations in transition has not yet received the recognition it deserves within evolutionary medicine.

ACKNOWLEDGMENTS

We would like to thank Colin Fischbacher and Jazz Chamley for their collaboration in our work with British Pakistani women. We would also like to thank Gillian Bentley for her helpful comments on a draft of the chapter.

CHAPTER 9

Should Women Menstruate?
An Evolutionary Perspective on
Menstrual-Suppressing Oral Contraceptives

Lynnette Leidy Sievert

Approximately 80% of women in the United States choose to take oral contraceptives at some point in their lives. Many do so in order to eliminate the inconveniences associated with menstrual cycling, as well as for contraception. And while it may appear that such high usage reflects a general ease with hormone alteration, as Sievert indicates, many questions about potential side effects remain unresolved. Indeed, any discussion of whether or not ovulation and menstruation should be artificially or chemically suppressed, including questions pertaining to when and for how long, necessarily cuts across cultural and religious domains, as well as scientific ones. In fact, Sievert points out that menstrual-suppressing oral contraceptives (MSOCs) are often prescribed and/or advertised (even advocated) through various internet websites. Her intent in this chapter, especially for women already using contraceptives, is to provide an array of evolutionary hypotheses about why menstruation may have evolved in the first place, using them as a basis for exploring both empirical and theoretical ideas that might help all women to become more fully informed about reproductive cycling. An important part of this chapter is determining if menstrual-suppressing contraceptive pills actually mimic what has already been described in this volume as the potentially safer hormonal milieu experienced by ancestral hominin women who had a low frequency of menstrual cycles due to repeated pregnancies and periods of lactation (see Chapters 2, 3, 7, and 8). Sievert concludes that in no way are the effects of MSOCs analogous to that experienced in the evolutionary or historic past and that they cannot be used to mimic the beneficial effects of "Stone Age life histories." Her chapter should help initiate and refocus the direction of any discussion of this topic in new ways.

INTRODUCTION

Women who are sexually active and want to prevent pregnancy must choose from among a confusing array of contraceptive options, including pills, patches, injections, vaginal rings, intrauterine devices, barrier methods, and sterilization. Approximately 80% of women in the United States choose to take oral contraception at some point in their lives (Dawson, 1990). Selecting an oral contraceptive narrows the range of birth control options; however, there are more than 50 types of birth control pills on the market. The newest types of pills are menstrual-suppressing oral contraceptives (MSOCs).

Conventional oral contraceptives are generally prescribed in cycles of 21 active pills followed by 7 placebo pills. Women who take conventional oral contraceptives menstruate once per month. In contrast, women who take, for example, Seasonale®, one type of MSOC, take a pill with active hormones for 84 consecutive days (12 weeks) followed by placebo (inactive) pills for 7 days. Women who take Seasonale menstruate once every 3 months—only four times per year.[1]

If women rely on newspaper articles and TV programs for their information about MSOCs, they are aware that some women's health advocates oppose the use of MSOCs because they consider menstruation to be "natural."[2] Many of the debates about the use of MSOCs are consistent with the perspective of evolutionary medicine. On the one hand, some argue that there is a beneficial (adaptive) aspect to menstruation that ought to be considered before menstruation is stopped (Rako, 2003; SMRC, 2003). Others contrast the low frequency of menstrual cycles among ancestral women with the high frequency of menstrual cycles among contemporary women in industrialized nations today. They argue that hundreds of menstrual cycles may actually be pathological in the sense of representing "a *mismatch* between our bodies and novel aspects of the environment; novel, that is, since the development of agriculture, and especially since the industrial revolution" (Nesse and Williams, 1999, p 21, emphasis in original). Novel aspects of the environment include a sedentary lifestyle and greater food security, resulting in more ovulatory menstrual cycles, coupled with access to effective methods of birth control. Both of these points of view—menstruation as adaptation and repeated menstruation as evidence of a mismatch between our genes and our new environment—will be detailed in this chapter.

In addition to the biological aspects of menstrual suppression, the marketing of MSOCs has also capitalized on the assumption that, at least in the United States, menstruation negatively affects women's lives. In response to this negative portrayal of menstruation, the Society for Menstrual Cycle Research issued a position statement recommending that "continuous oral contraceptive use should not be prescribed to all menstruating women out of a rejection of a normal, healthy menstrual cycle" (SMCR, 2003). What is a normal, healthy menstrual cycle? If women are taking an oral contraceptive, does it matter if menstruation is hormonally suppressed?

In the ensuing discussion, a description of the menstrual cycle is followed by various arguments that have been put forth for why, from an evolutionary perspective, women menstruate. This is followed by a discussion of how oral contraceptives work. Following are some thoughts about attitudes toward menstruation, and how those attitudes may create the context for the acceptance or rejection of MSOCs. Finally, the pros and cons of taking MSOCs are examined. This chapter does not examine whether, from an evolutionary perspective, it is a good idea to use oral contraceptives as a method of birth control, although such an argument has been made (see Strassman, 1999). Instead, this chapter considers whether, from an evolutionary perspective, women who are already using oral contraceptives should suppress their menstruation.

THE NORMAL MENSTRUAL CYCLE

The menstrual cycle is a complex process that will not be discussed fully here. Rather, this discussion focuses on the hormones most relevant to the topic of oral contraceptives and menstruation—estrogen and progesterone. The 28-day[3] menstrual cycle results from changing hormone levels. The primary hormones involved in the menstrual cycle are gonadotropin-releasing hormone (GnRH), produced by the hypothalamus; follicle-stimulating hormone (FSH), and luteinizing hormone (LH), produced by the anterior pituitary; and estrogen and progesterone, produced by the ovary (see Figure 9-1). Hormones produced in the ovary are secreted by granulosa and theca cells that make up follicles. Follicles are the cellular envelopes that surround and nourish developing eggs (Peters and McNatty, 1980).

Hormones function in feedback loops, so that GnRH stimulates the pituitary to produce FSH and LH. FSH and LH stimulate developing follicles in the ovary to produce estrogen and progesterone. Estrogen and progesterone loop back to the pituitary and hypothalamus to regulate GnRH, FSH, and LH production (Guraya, 1985; Wood, 1994).

The menstrual cycle is generally divided into two phases. The first is the follicular phase. During this first phase, FSH stimulates ovarian follicular development. As follicles

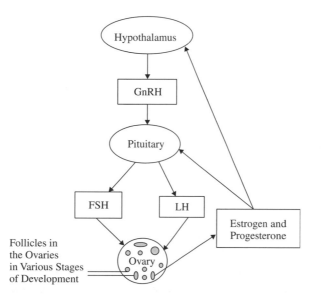

FIGURE 9-1 The hypothalamus–pituitary–ovarian axis. GnRH, gonadotropin-releasing hormone; FSH, follicle-stimulating hormone; LH, luteinizing hormone.

grow, they produce increasing amounts of estrogen. Estrogen levels rise slowly at first, then rapidly reach a peak 24–36 hours before ovulation (Schnatz, 1985), as shown in Figure 9-2. The peak in estrogen production corresponds with a surge in LH, after which estrogen levels fall. LH stimulates the production of progesterone by the ovary.

Rising estrogen levels during the follicular phase of the menstrual cycle stimulate cells in the endometrium (the layer of tissue that lines the uterus) to divide and proliferate, along with a micronetwork of vascular support (Jabbour, Kelly, Fraser, & Critchley, 2006). The proliferation of endometrial tissue peaks on days 8–10 of the menstrual cycle, when estrogen levels are also peaking in the circulation (Bergeron, Ferenczy, & Shyamala, 1988).

The second phase of the menstrual cycle occurs after ovulation and is called the luteal phase. After the release of an egg, the ovarian follicle that nourished the egg changes into the corpus luteum, which functions as a gland. Stimulated by small amounts of LH from the pituitary, the corpus luteum secretes large amounts of progesterone and smaller amounts of estrogen. Progesterone levels peak approximately 8 days after the LH surge (Speroff, Glass, & Kase, 1999), followed by degeneration of the corpus luteum. Estrogen and progesterone levels then fall.

During the luteal phase of the menstrual cycle, the endometrium enters its secretory phase in preparation for the implantation of a blastocyst.[4] The proliferation of cells in the endometrium ends 3 days after ovulation (Speroff et al., 1999). Falling levels of estrogen and progesterone bring about a shrinking of the endometrium, spasms of the spiral arteries, diminished blood flow to the endometrial cells causing ischemia (lack of blood and

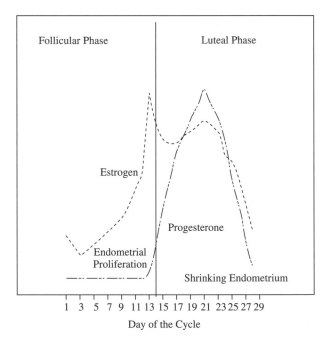

FIGURE 9-2 Fluctuations of estrogen and progesterone across the menstrual cycle. Hormone levels are shown as percent maximum secretion—the highest point of each hormone is the point of 100% maximum secretion. (Adapted from Schnatz, 1985, p. 7.)

oxygen[5] that results in cell death), and a relaxation of the spiral arterioles, resulting in bleeding. Invasion of the endometrium by leukocytes contributes of tissue break down. As tissues break down, intercellular blood enters the uterus (Jabbour et al., 2006; Speroff et al., 1999). The average amount of menstrual blood loss varies from 25 to 35 ml (Fraser and Inceboz, 2000).

In addition to bringing about menstruation, changes in estrogen levels across the menstrual cycle also cause cellular changes in breast tissue. Monthly incremental growth in breast tissue occurs because of cell division, and cells that divide frequently are more likely to develop malignancies. Tissues that grow in response to estrogen (i.e., uterine, mammary, and ovarian tissue) are at increased vulnerability for some forms of cancer (Henderson, Ross, & Pike, 1993; Maynard Smith et al., 1999).

In the evolutionary and historical past it is likely that women started to menstruate at a later age compared to contemporary women in industrialized nations (Bogin, 1999). Ancestral women had their first child at an earlier age, gave birth to more children, and breastfed those children more intensely and for a longer period of time compared to contemporary women living in industrialized societies (Eaton et al., 1994; Short, 1976). Some have argued that the reproductive profile of the Dogon of Mali, millet farmers of the Sahel, is similar to the reproductive profile of our evolutionary ancestors (Strassman, 1999). The Dogon are a noncontracepting population with a total fertility rate of 8.6 live births per woman and a low prevalence of sexually transmitted disease. During a 2-year study (Strassman, 1997), women aged 15–19 years experienced a mean number of 11 menstrual periods, women aged 20–34 had just 4 menstrual periods, and women 35 years and older had 13 menstrual periods. From these data, Strassmann (1997, 1999) estimated that Dogon women experience a median number of 94 menses over the entire lifespan. This is far below the 400–450 menses experienced by women who use contraception in many contemporary societies.

Among contemporary women, risk factors for breast cancer include life history traits that result in more menstrual cycles, such as an early age at menarche, no children or a late age at first birth, and a late age at menopause (Bulbrook, 1991). Because ancestral women had fewer menstrual cycles, they had a lower risk of breast cancer. Some investigators argue that hormonal manipulation of the menstrual cycle through "interventional endocrinology" like oral contraceptives (Eaton and Eaton III, 1999a) may mimic the beneficial effects of "Stone Age life histories" (Nesse and Williams, 1994, p. 181) or "an ancestral hormonal milieu" (Maynard Smith et al., 1999). We will return to this idea after asking why women menstruate at all.

MENSTRUATION FROM AN EVOLUTIONARY PERSPECTIVE

Menstruation is physiologically costly because of the loss of blood, tissue, and iron stores.[6] Menstruation is also costly in terms of reproduction because there is only a brief fertile period during a menstrual cycle when insemination may result in conception. The length of the entire menstrual cycle, including the days spent menstruating, limits the rate of conception and, ultimately, the pace of childbearing (Wood, 1994, p. 115). On the other hand, Strassman (1996, 1999) argues that menstruation is energetically *less* costly than maintaining the endometrium in a ready state between ovulations.

There are several explanations for the evolution of human menstruation: (1) menstruation is the evolutionary byproduct of the menstrual cycle (Finn, 1996; Strassman, 1996); (2) menstruation may be a way of ridding the female reproductive tract of pathogens that are associated with sperm (Profet, 1993); (3) menstruation rids the female reproductive tract of defective embryos (Clarke, 1994); and (4) menstruation is a signal of potential fecundability (Worthman et al., 1992).

HYPOTHESES

Hypothesis 1: Evolutionary Byproduct

Strassman has argued that maintaining the lining of the uterus is so expensive that it is energetically less expensive to regrow the endometrium every 28 days. In other words, menstruation itself is not adaptive, but a byproduct of endometrial preparation for pregnancy (Gosden et al., 1999), and the functional significance of endometrial regression (menstruation) is metabolic economy (Strassman, 1996). If a woman is using a contraceptive to avoid pregnancy, then "the waxing and waning of endometrial cycles is unnecessary" (Strassman, 1999, p. 200). From this point of view, the use of MSOCs is neither beneficial nor deleterious. If menstruation itself is not adaptive, and if pregnancy is being prevented, then it doesn't matter whether a woman menstruates every month or every 3 months.

Finn (1996) also views menstruation as secondary to the reproductive cycle. The implantation of a blastocyst into the wall of the uterus can only occur during a small window, days 21–22, of the menstrual cycle (Speroff et al., 1999). Cells of the blastocyst specialize, or differentiate, into those that will form the embryo itself and peripheral cells (the trophoblast) that invade the mother's tissues at implantation. In humans, the trophoblast actively invades the endometrium, between the epithelial cells. Elevated levels of progesterone protect the blastocyst from maternal inflammatory responses (Finn, 1996). To protect itself from the invading trophoblast, the maternal endometrium transforms into a dense cellular matrix called the decidua, which inhibits the movement of invasive cells (Finn, 1996; Kliman, 2000). These changes that protect the mother from the invasive trophoblast eventually make the uterus unsuitable for implantation. Menstruation returns a nonreceptive decidualized endometrium to a receptive nondecidualized endometrium (Kliman, 2000, p. 1760).

Finn (1996) argues that the evolution of the uterus and the embryo were interlinked. The endometrium reacts to the highly invasive implantation of the early embryo by undergoing decidualization changes in anticipation of pregnancy. When pregnancy does not occur, there is a breakdown of the endometrium. Finn (1996) does not envision a physiological role for menstruation separate from its role in implantation. If menstruation evolved as a byproduct of the mother's defensive response to the anticipated implantation of an early embryo, then the suppression of menstruation by MSOCs among women who are using birth control so as not to get pregnant is neutral—neither beneficial nor deleterious.

Hypothesis 2: Pathogen Removal

Among those who have argued that menstruation is not a by product of the ovulatory cycle, but an end in itself, Margie Profet is most well known. Profet (1993) argued that menstruation evolved as a defense against pathogens transported from the lower reproductive tract to the uterus by traveling sperm. She stated that evidence for adaptive design (for menstruation) is demonstrated by the specialized spiral-shaped uterine arteries that constrict, dilate, and induce menstruation. She argued that menstrual blood lacks many of the normal clotting factors found in venous blood, so that the shedding of the uterine lining can act as a mechanical defense against pathogens. In addition, she argued that menstrual blood delivers leukocytes (white blood cells) to the endometrial tissue to immunologically destroy pathogens.

If menstruation evolved to clean the reproductive tract of pathogens, then the use of MSOCs would result in a higher rate of uterine infections (Gosden et al., 1999; Profet, 1993) and would be considered deleterious. However, arguments for the selection of menstruation as a defense against pathogens have not been substantiated (Coutinho and Segal, 1999). Pathogen load in the reproductive tract is not diminished following menstruation (Strassman, 1996).

However, Profet makes a separate point that is also relevant to the topic of menstrual suppression. Many species of microorganisms can cause endometritis (inflammation and/or irritation of the endometrium), which is associated with heavy or irregular menstrual bleeding. If unusual bleeding is a diagnostic sign of infection, then the use of MSOCs may mask the signs of an infection that could lead to pelvic inflammatory disease and infertility.

Hypothesis 3: Defective Embryos

Clarke (1994) suggested that menstruation may have evolved as an efficient means to eliminate defective embryos. He bases this suggestion on the narrowness of the fertile period (about 6 days), which is determined by the fertile life span of the sperm and the egg—the amount of time either can survive in the female reproductive tract and still be capable of fertilization (Wood, 1994). Noting that this length of time provides an opportunity for fertilization to occur between an aged egg or an aged sperm, and that a high proportion of human conceptions are aborted because of chromosomal abnormalities, Clarke (1994) has argued that menstruation evolved as a device for removing defective embryos before, or at the time of, implantation. In other words, the maternal uterus is the "selection arena" in which defective gametes, zygotes, or early embryos can be eliminated before parents have invested a great deal in the offspring (Stearns and Ebert, 2001). According to this view, the menstrual cycle is designed "not only to maximize the probability of conception in any one cycle, but also to clear the way as quickly as possible for another opportunity should conception not take place" (Wood, 1994, p. 142).

If women are trying to avoid pregnancy through the use of oral contraceptives, then, following Clarke's argument, menstruation is unnecessary because there is no need to clear abnormal gametes or embryos from the uterus. From this point of view the use of MSOCs is neutral. If a woman is not at risk of pregnancy, then it doesn't matter if she menstruates.

Hypothesis 4: Advertising Fertility

Finally, menstruation may have evolved as an end in itself because it serves as a signal of fertility. For example, in many natural fertility populations, including traditional hunting-gathering societies, many women are not menstruating because they are pregnant or lactating (Wood, 1994). It is not unusual, in those circumstances, to have a long inter-val between births of 3 or more years. If men are waiting for an indication of fertility from their partners, then menstruation could serve as an unambiguous sign. Just one menstrual cycle could alert males that a female is fertile. On the other hand, many women experi-ence menstrual cycles when they have a low probability of becoming pregnant, for example, at the beginning and end of their reproductive years (Haig, 1999). Haig won-ders whether this is simply the warming-up and running-down of the female reproductive system, or whether nonfertile cycles have been retained by natural selection because of how menstruation is interpreted by other individuals.[7]

If MSOCs are prescribed to young women who are not yet sexually active for the sole purpose of reducing their menstrual cycles to four times per year (or even less often), then menstruation will not serve as a signal of fertility. But how is menstruation perceived among contemporary women and their partners? Some echo the idea that menstruation provides information: "A healthy, regular menstruation signals that the body is well nour-ished, that we are not overly stressed or under threat, and that we are potentially fertile" (O'Grady, 2005). In this case, the use of MSOCs will interfere with a woman's ability to signal fertility. We will return to this topic after exploring how oral contraceptives work.

HOW ORAL CONTRACEPTIVES WORK

Oral contraceptives that combine estrogen and progestin into one daily pill are thought to inhibit the production of FSH and LH through an effect on hypothalamic GnRH produc-tion and through a direct effect on the pituitary. The estrogenic component suppresses FSH, and thus inhibits follicular development. The progestin primarily targets LH secre-tion, and thus prevents ovulation (Speroff et al., 1999). The constant amount of synthetic steroids provided by the daily pills replaces the normal cyclic production of ovarian estrogen and progesterone. Sometimes the mid-cycle surge of LH is not completely inhibited, in which case oral contraceptives also prevent conception by thickening the cervical mucus, altering the transport of the egg through the fallopian tubes, and chang-ing the endometrium (Sloane, 2002; Speroff et al., 1999; Watkins, 1998).

The estrogen in combination pill oral contraceptives provides stability to the endometrium, preventing irregular bleeding (Speroff et al., 1999). The monthly bleeding that occurs while taking oral contraceptives is fabricated by synthetic estrogen and progestin stimulation of the endometrium during the 21-day pill sequence, followed by withdrawal of the hormones during the 7 days of placebo (Sloane, 2002). Bleeding that women experience while on the pill is generally lighter compared with the bleeding experienced by women who are not using hormonal contraceptives.

When the first oral contraceptive, Enovid, was marketed in the 1960s,[8] the 28-day course of pills was portrayed as imitating the body's "natural processes." Dr. John Rock, one of the developers of Enovid, described the action of the hormones in the contra-ceptive "as simply an extension of the body's normal functioning" (Watkins, 1998, p. 46). Similarly, Seasonale, a type of MSOC, is being portrayed as imitating the more "natural" state of amenorrhea.

Oral contraceptives are associated with a substantial reduction in the risk of ovarian and endometrial cancers, but not breast cancer (Henderson et al., 1993). Stearns and

Ebert (2001, p. 426) suggest that if menstrual suppression results in a decreased frequency of reproductive cancers, "then this will become one of the few cases in which a concrete benefit has resulted from the idea that our bodies are not adapted to our current lifestyle." However, the development of a new contraceptive that would decrease the risk of breast cancer is still in the future (Henderson et al., 1993). The present generation of MSOCs contains the same synthetic estrogen and progestogens as conventional oral contraceptives; therefore using the MSOCs that are currently available provides no additional advantage in terms of the risk of breast cancer.

Superficially, the menstrual suppression offered by MSOCs seems to be similar to the menstrual suppression experience by our ancestors during pregnancy and lactation, but nothing could be further from the truth. When a woman is pregnant, her estradiol and estrone excretion rises to a level about 100 times greater than her nonpregnant levels (see Figure 9-3). In contrast, when a woman is not menstruating because of lactational amenorrhea, her estrogen levels are extremely low because her ovarian follicles are not developing (see Wood, 1994, p. 380). Figure 9-4 shows the difference in maximum levels of secretion between the estrogen and progesterone levels of a normal menstrual cycle and the levels of estrogen and progesterone of a woman taking an oral contraceptive.

Although oral contraceptives were designed to provide monthly withdrawal bleeding, physicians have often prescribed consecutive packages of 21-day active pills for women who want to postpone menstrual periods for special occasions such as a wedding, holiday, or vacation (Glasier et al., 2003; NWHN, 2003; Sloane, 2002).[9] Similarly, women have been prescribed consecutive packages of 21-day active pills in the treatment

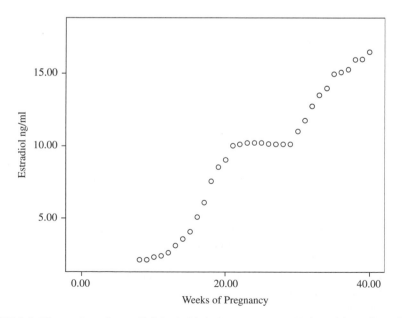

FIGURE 9-3 Fluctuation of estradiol (ng/mL) during pregnancy. (Adapted from Speroff et al. 1999, p. 282.)

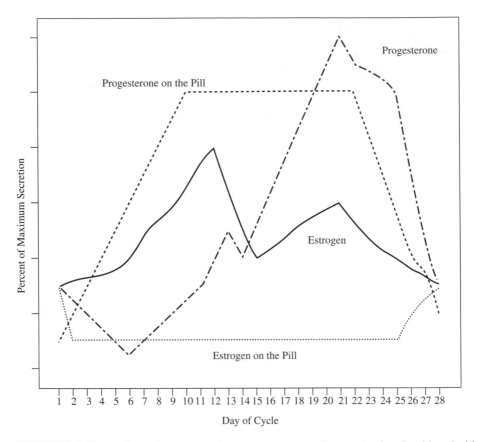

FIGURE 9-4 Fluctuations of estrogen and progesterone across the menstrual cycle with and without use of the contraceptive pill.

of anemia and endometriosis (Coutinho and Segal, 1999; Speroff et al., 1999). Some physicians advocate the avoidance of menstrual periods altogether (Gardner and Miller, 2005). On her web site, Leslie Miller, M.D., instructs women to consult with their health care providers because taking pills to skip periods is not approved by the U.S. Food and Drug Administration (FDA). She then tells women that they will have to take 17 packages of a low-dose, monophasic birth control pill to avoid menstruation for 1 year. She cautions women that they need to be prepared for irregular bleeding for the first 3–6 months as their bodies adjust to the menstrual suppression (www.noperiod. com). Elsimar Coutinho, co-author of *Is Menstruation Obsolete?*, spoke for many when he wrote "Recurrent menstruation... is a needless loss of blood" (Coutinho and Segal, 1999, p. 159).

   In terms of the biological evolution of menstruation, taking MSOCs does not appear to interfere with adaptive aspects of menstruation among women who are already taking oral contraceptives. Culturally, however, the response to the promise of fewer menstrual cycles is harder to summarize.

ATTITUDES TOWARD MENSTRUATION

The widespread existence of menstrual taboos across cultures reflects a shared perception that menstrual blood is "anomalous to a general symbolic, or cultural, order" (Buckley and Gottlieb, 1988). For example, compared to other types of bleeding, menstrual blood is relatively regular, predictable, and uncontrollable. However, despite the widely shared perception of menstrual blood as anomalous, there exists no universal cross-cultural rule of conduct associated with menstruating women. The experience and meaning of menstruation shows a great deal of cross-cultural variation (Snowden and Christian, 1983).

Buckley and Gottlieb (1988, p. 20) posit that "diversity in the symbolic coding of menstruation suggests its arbitrariness and cultural relativity, rather than motivation by any single physical phenomenon." In other words, the physical phenomenon of menstrual blood does not provoke a universal response that results in common meaning, like pollution. Instead of assuming that an anomaly like menstrual blood is always perceived as negative (e.g., polluting), Buckley and Gottlieb suggest that anomalies are perceived as *powerful*. Powerful can have either positive or negative connotations, and this better explains the mixed reaction of women in response to questions about menstrual cycles, menstrual blood, and the idea of menstrual suppression.

For example, Table 9-1 illustrates responses that were recorded on an internet site, the Museum of Menstruation, in answer to the question "Would you stop menstruating if you could?" (http://www.mum.org/stopmen.htm). The answers, while not representative of all menstruating women, give a sense of the broad range of reactions evoked by the topic.

Published survey results also show a range of opinions about menstruation, but also strong support for the idea of menstrual suppression. A study carried out in the northeastern United States surveyed 221 highly educated, mostly white women aged 21–30 years. In response to the lead "Having my period makes me . . . ," women most commonly agreed or strongly agreed with the following three statements: Having my period makes me "know I'm not pregnant" (80%), "believe it's a nuisance" (69%), "avoid sex while bleeding" (56%). Women were interested in menstrual suppression to reduce menstrual pain (63%) and days of bleeding (72%). Fifty-six percent of women agreed or strongly agreed with the statement that they were interested in menstrual suppression, 40% would be "thrilled not to have a period," and 60% said that they "would do it if it did not hurt me" (Andrist, Hoyt, Weinstein, & McGibbon, 2004).

In a telephone survey carried out in The Netherlands, a representative sample of 1301 women was drawn from four age groups. Among menstruating women aged 15–19 and 25–34 years, about one third said they would prefer amenorrhea if they could change their current menstrual bleeding (36% and 32%, respectively). Among women aged 45–49 and 52–57 years, over half would prefer amenorrhea (54% and 64%, respectively). When asked their preferred frequency of menstrual bleeding, women aged 15–19 years most frequently chose once every 3 months (35%), and 26% said never. Among women aged 25–34 years, 24% chose once every 3 months, and 31% said never. Among women aged 45–49 years, 10% said once every 3 months, and 51% said never. When asked their preferred frequency of menstrual bleeding if manipulated by oral

TABLE 9-1 Answers to the Question "Would You Stop Menstruating If You Could?"

Characteristics volunteered by respondents	Answers recorded during May and June 2006
13-year-old, Ohio	"I think in some way I feel like it [menstruation] is a bond with all women, one of my few assurances that I'm normal"
16-year-old, no location	"Despite everyone always going on about how natural it [menstruation] is, I HATE IT!!!"
29-year-old, no location	"I have no clue what's going on with you.... If there's a pill out there that will stop me from having periods, I will take it without looking back"
43-year-old, no location	"This [menstruation] doesn't make me feel like a woman. It makes me feel dirty"
No age, Vancouver, Canada	"To suppress menstruation is to suppress being a woman. When we learn to embrace menstruation as a powerful psychic aspect of who we are, we as humanity will finally start to evolve into stellar beings"
No age, no location	"I would stop in a heartbeat if I could. I have been a teenager bleeding, a young woman bleeding, and a mother bleeding, and now I'm tired of bleeding. My womanhood has been proven!!"
No age, no location	"Our bodies were made to bleed every month for a reason.... It is dangerous and shallow to change years of evolution for the sake of 'convenience'"
No age, Melbourne, Australia, emphasis in original	"Why change something that has been around for as long as millions of years, as long as the history of mankind? Menstruation is purely natural and in my opinion, it is NOT good to interfere with a natural process in your body. It HORRIFIES me how some women just casually say yes to putting hormones and other foreign things into their body to stop this natural process"

Source: http://www.mum.org/stopmen.htm

contraceptives, women aged 15–19 years chose once every 3 months more frequently than once a month (38% vs. 26%), and 22% chose never (den Tonkelaar and Oddens, 1999, p. 361).

Similar findings were reported by Glasier et al. (2003) in Hong Kong ($n = 200$), Shanghai ($n = 200$), Cape Town, South Africa ($n = 201$), and Edinburgh, Scotland ($n = 200$). Women drawn from health care centers were asked "Do you like having periods?" As Table 9-2 shows, the majority of women in Scotland, Hong Kong, and Shanghai said no. In Cape Town 65% of the white women said no, but only 25% of the black women said no. Periods were disliked primarily because of their inconvenience. Given the choice, between 12 and 39% of the women would choose to menstruate every 3 months. Would women consider a method of contraception that stopped their periods? More than half of respondents said yes in Scotland and South Africa. Almost half said yes in Shanghai. In Hong Kong, 37% said yes (32% were undecided).

TABLE 9-2 Cross-Cultural Attitudes Towards Contraception and Amenorrhea

	Hong Kong	Shanghai	Cape Town, South Africa		Edinburgh, Scotland	Sagamu, Nigeria
			White	Black		
"Do you like having periods?" Yes	50%	33%	35%	75%	26%	81%
"How often would you like to have a period?"						
Monthly	42%	43%	30%	49%	33%	71%
Every 3 months	39%	30%	26%	27%	20%	12%
Never	6%	15%	29%	9%	37%	14%
"Would you consider a method of contraception that stopped your periods?" Yes	37%	48%	64%	52%	65%	73%

Source: Glasier et al., 2003.

This same study also included a clinic in Sagamu, Nigeria ($n = 200$). In Sagamu, 81% of women surveyed said that they liked having periods, and 71% said that they would choose to have monthly periods. They viewed periods as a way to "get rid of bad blood." But when these same women were asked, "Provided your periods and your fertility returned to normal immediately after you stopped using it, would you consider a method of contraception which stopped your periods?" a majority of the women (73%) said yes (Glasier et al., 2003). Although attitudes toward menstruation are important for understanding who is more likely to accept menstrual suppression (Johnston-Robledo, Ball, Lauta, & Zekoll, 2003), it is not so easy to assume that attitudes toward menstruation will always predict the use of MSOCs.

Women who switch to MSOCs are strongly motivated to avoid having their monthly menstrual periods, as evidenced by the number of women who quit taking Seasonale, one type of MSOC, because of breakthrough bleeding. In a one-year study that compared Seasonale with a conventional oral contraceptive (Nordette), only 59% (271/456) of the women taking the MSOCs completed the study. Eight percent of the participants quit due to unacceptable bleeding (compared to 2% of the women taking the conventional oral contraceptive) (Anderson and Hait, 2003). In the 2-year follow up, 42% of women discontinued the study; 12 women (6%) reported bleeding and/or spotting as the reason for discontinuation (Anderson, Gibbons, & Portman, 2006).

A WHO study of menstruation published in the early 1980s found that, at that time, most women did not want to give up monthly menstruation or use a method of contraception that would induce amenorrhea (Snowden and Christian, 1983). This differs markedly from the findings of more recent studies (e.g., Glasier et al., 2003 see Table 9-2). Twenty years have passed between the publication of the WHO study and the approval of the first MSOCs by the U.S. FDA. It appears that medical and social factors, including a strong presence of women physicians who vocally support menstrual suppression, have contributed to the cultural selection for the acceptance of MSOCs among women who are already using oral contraception.

PROS AND CONS OF MENSTRUAL-SUPPRESSING ORAL CONTRACEPTIVES

The review above did not produce a compelling reason, in terms of evolutionary theory, to avoid MSOCs among women who are already taking oral contraceptives. Advantages to using MSOCs include (1) effective protection from pregnancy (Anderson and Hait, 2003),[10] (2) reduced cramping, bloating, and other discomforts (migraines, mood changes) associated with periods, (3) the convenience of fewer periods (NWHN, 2003), and (4) a possible reduction in the risk of anemia among women with very heavy bleeding (Coutinho and Segal, 1999). Oral contraceptives have been shown to reduce the risks of uterine and ovarian cancer (Henderson et al., 1993; Strassman, 1999), a protection that will probably be the same with MSOCs. Some argue that MSOCs may be a better method of contraception for adolescents because there are fewer breaks from the hormonally active pills, and therefore young women will be less likely to forget to take their pills at the right time (Kartoz, 2004; Omar, Kives, & Allen, 2005). The safety and efficacy of MSOCs among adolescents is not known, however, because the initial studies of Seasonale, the first MSOC, did not include women younger than 18 (Anderson and Hait, 2003; Anderson et al., 2006).

The side effects of MSOCs are the same as for other combination pill oral contraceptives: increased risk of blood clots, heart attack, and stroke (USFDA, 2003). In addition, MSOCs, like all other oral contraceptives, do not protect against HIV infection or other sexually transmitted diseases (USFDA, 2003). Concerns specific to Seasonale include the unknown effect of 9 weeks of extra hormones each year. The study of the "long-term safety" of Seasonale, to date, followed women from a 1-year phase 3 trial through a 2-year study extension and found few concerns.[11] Long-term studies of breast tissue, bone health, fertility after discontinuation, and other effects of the hormonal changes have not been carried out.[12]

Women taking MSOCs have more unplanned bleeding and spotting between expected menstrual periods compared to women taking conventional oral contraceptives (USFDA, 2003). In the study of Seasonale, women experienced an average of 37.6 (s.d. 38.8) days of breakthrough bleeding and/or spotting during the first year of use (Anderson and Hait, 2003). The median number of bleeding and/or spotting days in the study extension was 8 during the first cycle and 4 during the eighth cycle (Anderson et al., 2006). Women also experienced increased weight, mood swings, and acne (Anderson and Hait, 2003).

The risk of pregnancy while using MSOCs is very low; however, women may not know that they are pregnant for a longer period of time. The monthly period is a signal that women are not pregnant (NWHN, 2003). If a woman is not expecting a period for 2 or 3 months, she may ignore physiological changes associated with pregnancy or attribute those changes to some other cause. This is a serious drawback to a MSOC such as Seasonale because during the first 8 weeks of pregnancy the embryo is particularly sensitive to the teratogenic effects of certain chemicals and pathogens (Moore, 1988). Also, the quantity and quality of menstrual blood may indicate infections (Profet, 1993). Acute infections may be missed if menstruation is suppressed to four times per year.

Finally, women's health advocates are concerned that if menstrual suppression is presented as the preferred contraceptive option, then menstruation will be stigmatized. "This is particularly a concern with respect to young teens who are just beginning to learn about menstruation and are forming a new understanding about the way their bodies function" (NWHN, 2003).

CONCLUSIONS

The purpose of this chapter was to consider whether or not an evolutionary perspective could be applied when making a decision about whether or not to use MSOCs. At a moment when MSOCs are in the news and widely advertised, this is a relevant question, particularly to young women. First, we considered whether or not menstruation serves a beneficial (adaptive) function that could be used to argue against MSOCs. We concluded that, if menstruation evolved as a byproduct of the menstrual cycle to save energy (Strassman, 1996), to rid the uterus of defective gametes or early embryos (Clarke, 1994), or as a byproduct of the inflammatory response of the uterus in anticipation of an invasive trophoblast (Finn, 1996), then menstrual suppression is neither a beneficial nor a deleterious behavior for women who are already using contraception. If menstruation is a sign of health and potential fecundability, then the answer is complicated by the effect of cultural attitudes about menstruation, and no universal recommendation with regard to MSOCs can be made.

Second, this chapter considered whether taking MSOCs results in a mimicking of the hypothesized hormonal milieu experienced by ancestral women who had a low frequency of menstrual cycles due to repeated pregnancies and periods of lactation. We concluded that, instead of imitating the hormonal pattern experienced by our ancestors, the hormonal milieu induced by a MSOC such as Seasonale is in no way analogous to that experienced in the evolutionary or historic past. The lack of cycles due to pregnancy is associated with very high levels of estrogen, and the lack of cycles due to breast-feeding is associated with very low levels of estrogen. MSOC cannot be used to mimic the beneficial effects of "Stone Age life histories" (Nesse and Williams, 1994, p. 181).

ACKNOWLEDGMENTS

I am indebted to the editors of this volume for their helpful comments and to Catherine DeLorey, Christine Hitchcock, Elizabeth Kissling, Geneva Kachman, Kathleen O'Grady, and other members of the Society for Menstrual Cycle Research, who continue to debate the pros and cons of menstrual suppression. I have paid attention to their arguments; however, the conclusions of this chapter are my own, and do not reflect the position of the SMCR.

CHAPTER 10

An Evolutionary Perspective on Premenstrual Syndrome

Implications for Investigating Infectious Causes of Chronic Disease

Caroline Doyle, Holly A. Swain Ewald, and Paul W. Ewald

Interestingly, many of the side effects associated with taking oral contraceptives described in the previous chapter by Leidy Sievert are the same symptoms that are among the hundred-plus included within the premenstrual syndrome, a phenomenon sometimes described by physicians as a "diagnosis by exclusion." Popular culture often dismisses premenstrual syndrome (PMS) as an annoyance that occurs prior to menstruation, rather than viewing it as a medical condition with clearly definable etiological agents, genes, germs, or noninfectious environmental factors. But in this chapter PMS gains much respect, at least as having a predictable but varied set of conditions, and, most importantly, reasons are given for why PMS occurs, illustrating how and why an evolutionary way of thinking can help uncover aspects of disease processes that otherwise might remain hidden. Doyle and colleagues provide a perspective that rounds out and complements the work of Robillard et al. on preeclampsia/eclampsia, Leidy Sievert on menopause, and Pollard and Unwin on high ovarian functioning. The "body of evidence" presented by Doyle et al. suggests that the concept of PMS may be "an artifact of the inadequate knowledge about true categories of disease and effects of immune suppression on their expression." The authors argue that PMS is not by itself an adaptation, but is instead "a heterogeneous collection of adaptations or byproducts of adaptations." Doyle et al. hypothesize that the diverse manifestations of PMS are often byproducts of adaptations that permit fertilization and embryonic development, all of which ultimately can be tied to changes in cell-mediated immunity suppressed during the premenstrual period to enhance implantation, should fertilization occur. This is an important chapter because it shows clearly that natural selection can, while favoring a set of physiological characteristics that is creating a favorable environment for implantation, produce side effects that are sometimes costly for the individual.

INTRODUCTION

Natural selection molds organisms through differences in survival and reproduction. Much of evolutionary medicine has therefore focused on reproduction, particularly health implications of pregnancy and fertility of women. Menopause, for example, poses an evolutionary puzzle because it appears to be a programmed switching off of reproduction (Leidy, 1999). One hypothesis attributes this shut-down to the shorter life span of women during our evolutionary history, and hence to the absence of selection for the maintenance of fertility beyond the fifth decade of life (Leidy, 1999). An alternative hypothesis proposes that natural selection has molded female fertility well into the postmenopausal years, and that menopause is an adaptation that shifts investments toward offspring and other related individuals that have already been born (Leidy, 1999). The benefits of this shift in investment may arise directly from aid to these genetically related individuals and indirectly as a result of increasing longevity, for example, by reducing the probability of death or damage from pregnancy in older ages.

An evolutionary perspective on another aspect of reproduction, childbirth, has compared practices in societies at different phases of the technological advancement (Trevathan, 1999). Modern medical practices differ from those practices that likely have been common throughout evolution of *Homo sapiens*, and may therefore generate unforeseen negative effects on mothers or offspring.

Research within evolutionary medicine has also assessed the possibility that reproductive characteristics may have evolved to protect against vulnerabilities to disease that are inherent to the reproductive process. Profet (1993), for example, hypothesized that menstruation may function to expel infectious agents that would otherwise be able to invade the female reproductive tract, much as the dropping of leaves by deciduous trees may be an adaptation to rid the tree of pathogens that have infected the leaves. This hypothesis has generated criticism and development of alternative hypotheses (Finn, 1996; Strassman, 1996, 1999), which collectively provide the conceptual basis for the additional tests that may resolve the issue.

Health issues related to pregnancy have also been a focus of evolutionary medicine. Complications of pregnancy such as preeclampsia have been hypothesized to result from parent/offspring conflict (Haig, 1993; see Chapter 11). A hypothesis to explain the evolution of pregnancy sickness posits that the sensations of nausea may create an aversion to foods that are chemically dangerous to the developing fetus (Profet, 1992). Reduced intake of such foods could therefore reduce the chances that the fetus will develop abnormally and thus increase the evolutionary fitness of the mother. Flaxman and Sherman (2000) broadened this hypothesis to encompass microbial contaminants of food that may be particularly dangerous during pregnancy.

These examples illustrate the diverse issues related to the reproductive biology of female humans that have now been addressed from an evolutionary perspective. An analysis of premenstrual syndrome (PMS), however, has been lacking in the literature of evolutionary medicine. This absence may reflect the fact that manifestations of PMS are much more heterogeneous than states such as pregnancy sickness, menstruation, menopause, or preeclampsia and do not therefore lend themselves readily to straightforward adaptationist hypotheses. PMS is defined as the collection of manifestations that arise or are exacerbated during the luteal phase of the menstrual cycle (the interval between the release of the ovum and the onset of menstruation) and ameliorate after the onset of menses (Anim-Nyame, 2000; Deuster et al., 1999; L. M. Dickerson et al., 2003). Early definitions of PMS restricted the timing of symptoms to the week before menses, but modern definitions broaden this interval to the entire 2 weeks of the luteal phase (Anim-Nyame, 2000; Frank, 1931; Greene and Dalton, 1953).

More than 100 symptoms have been included within PMS (Hamilton et al., 1984). "Physiological" symptoms of PMS include headache, abdominal and back pain, breast fullness and discomfort, weight gain, abdominal distention, fatigue, and nausea. "Psychological" symptoms include depression, difficulty in concentration, nervousness, irritability, restlessness, and emotional tension (Janiger et al., 1972). Symptoms may vary in intensity and duration from cycle to cycle and from person to person (Dalton, 1994).

This heterogeneity of PMS symptoms provides a clue to its evolutionary basis, because it defies simple adaptive explanations. It raises the possibility that PMS is not itself an adaptation but is instead a sundry collection of adaptations or byproducts of adaptations. In this chapter we investigate the hypothesis that PMS symptoms are often byproducts of adaptations that permit fertilization and embryonic development. Specifically, immune suppression permits this early development but brings with it vulnerability to infection, which in turn leads to symptoms that are grouped together under the label PMS.

An appropriate starting point for this analysis is the recognition that PMS is a diagnosis of exclusion (L. M. Dickerson et al., 2003). If symptoms that occur premenstrually are ascribed to a well-defined illness, they are not included under the PMS umbrella. PMS is therefore characterized by manifestations of unknown etiology (Deuster et al., 1999; Hamilton et al., 1984). It is a collection of manifestations united by their timing rather than by an understanding of etiologies. In reality, PMS may be a catch-all category that includes exacerbated symptoms of chronic diseases that have not yet been well characterized. This chapter addresses this possibility and its implications both for identifying infectious causes of chronic diseases and developing interventions to control them. We begin by summarizing what is known about the general causes of PMS.

HERITABILITY AND ENVIRONMENTAL INFLUENCES

A balanced approach to investigating the causes of chronic illnesses requires that each of the three major categories of causation—infectious, genetic, and noninfectious environmental—be evaluated both logically and empirically (Cochran et al., 2000; Ewald and Cochran, 2000; see Chapter 19). Evidence from twin studies is consistent with some genetic predisposition to PMS (Condon, 1993). Pearson correlation coefficients for concordance of symptoms range from 0.39 to 0.55 for monozygotic twins and from 0.13 to 0.33 for dizygotic twins (Condon, 1993; Kendler et al., 1992; Treloar et al., 2002). These correlations provide a sense of the maximal possible genetic influence rather than a demonstration of genetic influence, because prenatal environments of monozygotic twins may be more similar than those of dizygotic twins (e.g., exposure to pathogens due to sharing of embryonic sacs; see Ledgerwood et al., 2003). Nontwin sibling pairs have not been directly compared with twins, but available information suggests weaker associations among the nontwin siblings than among dizygotic twins, implicating nongenetic influences (Glick et al., 1993). Overall, these familial studies suggest that genetic influences may be present, but that variation in PMS symptoms arises largely from environmental influences.

Suggested noninfectious environmental influences include exposures to tobacco smoke, alcohol, medications, and caffeine (Dawood et al., 1985; Rodin, 1992). Cultural influences have also been proposed, particularly stress, the unconscious mimicking of a mother by her daughter, gender roles, marital status, and education level (Dawood et al., 1985; Rodin, 1992). PMS has been reported throughout the world (Janiger et al., 1972); any environmental explanation of PMS therefore must include exposure to environmental factors that would correspond to the presence of PMS in diverse cultures. Such an exposure has not yet been identified (Deuster et al., 1999; L. M. Dickerson et al., 2003).

Infectious causation has been largely overlooked in studies of PMS. Persistent infections in particular seem feasible because immune function varies across the menstrual cycle. This possibility will be the major focus of the rest of this chapter. We first consider changes in immunological vulnerability to infection during the menstrual cycle.

IMMUNOSUPPRESSION DURING THE LUTEAL PHASE

During the luteal phase of the menstrual cycle, cell-mediated immunity is suppressed and humoral (antibody based) immunity is enhanced. This shift is probably an evolutionary adaptation to reduce the chances that the immune system will destroy the developing embryo (Faas et al., 2000; Grossman, 1985; Scarpellini et al., 1993). The shift appears to be due largely to elevated progesterone during the luteal phase (Clemens et al., 1979; Grossman, 1985; Polan et al., 1988; Valentino et al., 1993). Progesterone suppresses cell-mediated immunity, which reduces the chances of destruction of human cells and promotes humoral immunity (Cerhan et al., 2002; Clemens et al., 1979; Goldsby et al., 2003; Piccinni et al., 1995; Trzonkowski et al., 2001; Wang et al., 1993; White et al., 1997).

Reductions in cell-mediated immunity are associated with less effective control of fungi, viruses, and intracellular bacteria (Boncristiano et al., 2003; Jotwani and Cutler, 2004; Kalo-Klein and Witkin, 1991; Ottenhoff et al., 2003; Qiu et al., 2004; Stobo et al., 1976). Infections by such pathogens may therefore be exacerbated during the luteal phase.

Estrogen also contributes to a shift from cell-mediated to humoral immunity (Salem, 2004; Xiao et al., 2004). Because estrogen rises a day or so before the release of the ovum, estrogen-induced immune suppression would begin just prior to the luteal phase. The vulnerability that arises from this immune suppression may be partially offset by restriction of the nutrient tryptophan through estrogen-induced production of indolamine 2,3-dioxygenase (IDO) (Hrboticky, 1989; Xiao et al., 2004). Restriction of tryptophan is known to suppress viruses, bacteria, fungi, and protozoa (Adams et al., 2004; Bodaghi et al., 1999; Bozza et al., 2005; Grohmann et al., 2003).

The suppression of cell-mediated immunity during the luteal phase raises the possibility that PMS symptoms could result from persistent infections that are less well controlled during the luteal phase. One would expect this exacerbation to be particularly apparent during the late luteal phase for three reasons. First, as the luteal phase proceeds, the cumulative number of days of immunosuppression increases. Second, the response of infectious agents to immunosuppression will inevitably involve a lag. Third, pathogens that are controlled by estrogen-induced tryptophan restriction may fail to rebound until the last few days of the luteal phase, when estrogen declines just prior to the decline in progesterone.

Tryptophan restriction occurs in response to infections in general, apparently as a nonspecific immunological defense (Mellor and Munn, 2004; Taylor and Feng, 1991). Exacerbation of infection during the luteal phase may therefore be compounded by indirect effects, such as depression due to infection-induced tryptophan restriction (Wichers and Maes, 2004; Wirleitner et al., 2003), because tryptophan is the precursor to the neurotransmitter serotonin, which is implicated in depression (Salter et al., 1995; Wirleitner et al., 2003). When pathogens are not well controlled by tryptophan restriction during the luteal phase, women might experience exacerbation of symptoms throughout the luteal phase.

The exacerbating effect of luteal immunosuppression on infection may continue beyond the luteal phase because the restoration of immune competence after the luteal phase will not immediately control infection. The exacerbation of symptoms might even begin just after the luteal phase (i.e., just after the onset of menstruation) if the exacerbations are triggered by cell-mediated responses to the elevated presence of the pathogen rather than to the pathogen directly. If, for example, cell-mediated immunity causes autoimmune damage, enhanced autoimmunity would be expected just after the luteal phase when the cell-mediated immunity is restored. Similarly, if damage is due to inflammation, exacerbation of manifestations would be expected at or just after the onset of menstruation, because inflammatory responses are suppressed during the luteal phase (Clemens et al., 1979; Critchley et al., 2001, 2003; Finn, 1996; Watnick and Russo, 1968). In contrast, if the humoral branch of the immune system causes pathology, the exacerbation of infection could occur during the luteal phase, because the humoral arm is not suppressed during the luteal phase.

In sum, these considerations suggest that cyclic immunological changes could cause exacerbations of infection during the luteal and early menstrual phases. The timing of these exacerbations would depend on the extent to which the immunosuppression during the luteal phase relaxes control of infection, the branches of the immune system that contribute to illness, and the effectiveness of tryptophan restriction in compensating for suppressed cellular immunity during the luteal phase.

EVIDENCE OF PREMENSTRUAL EXACERBATION OF INFECTION

If the suppression of cellular immunity during the luteal phase is clinically relevant, infectious diseases that are controlled by cellular immunity should show exacerbations during the luteal phase. Evidence bearing on this expectation is summarized below.

Bacterial Infections

Some bacterial infections are known to be exacerbated premenstrually (Trzonkowski et al., 2001). Premenstrual increases in positivity for *Chlamydia trachomatis*, for example, range from a doubling to a factor of eight (Horner et al., 1998, Moller et al., 1999; Rosenthal and Landefeld, 1990).

Premenstrual exacerbation has been reported for peptic ulcers (Clark, 1953), which are caused by *Helicobacter pylori*, and bacterial infections of the oral cavity. Gingivitis, which is caused largely by *Porphyromonas gingivalis* (Lovegrove, 2004; Muller and Heinecke, 2004), increases in incidence and severity at puberty in young women (Oh et al., 2002), and some women suffer from "menstruation gingivitis," which is characterized by its premenstrual recurrence (McCann and Bonci, 2001). Some women also experience a premenstrual increase in ulcers of the oral mucosa (Green and Dalton, 1953; McCann and Bonci, 2001), which have been attributed to infections with bacteria such as *Helicobacter pylori* (Fritscher et al., 2004). Glossitis, an inflammation of the tongue, is also exacerbated premenstrually and has been attributed to infections with *Helicobacter pylori, Prevotella melaninogenica, Fusobacterium nucleatum*, and *Peptostreptococcus micros* (Brook, 2002; Gall-Troselj et al., 2001).

In a 10-year study of nearly 43,000 German women, scarlet fever (caused by *Streptococcus pyogenes*) and pneumonia presented more frequently within 3 days of menstruation (Andreas, 1961).

In acne, caused by *Propionibacterium acnes*, an increase in pustule density occurs during the premenstrual period. Accordingly, administration of progesterone has been found to trigger acne (Burton et al., 1973; Tamer et al., 2003).

C. trachomatis, P. gingivalis, H. pylori, P. melaninogenica, F. nucleatum, and *S. pyogenes*, and possibly *P. acnes*, can infect intracellularly (Boncristiano et al., 2003; Delcourt-Debruyne et al., 2000; Dominiak et al., 2003; M. J. Duncan et al., 1993; Hacker and Hesseman, 2002; Han et al., 2000; Lamont et al., 1995; Marouni and Sela, 2004; Peterson and Krogfelt, 2003; Sandros et al., 1993). Accordingly, the infections they cause may become exacerbated during the luteal phase as a result of the shift from cell-mediated to humoral immunity. *Chlamydia* and *H. pylori* are known to be controlled by cell-mediated immunity (Boncristiano et al., 2003; Qiu et al., 2004, Rottenberg et al., 2000). *P. acnes* stimulates cell-mediated immunity; the exacerbation of acne by progesterone therefore suggests that the cell-mediated response is helping to control *P. acnes* (Burkhart et al., 1999; MacDonald et al., 2002).

Viral Infections

Viral infections are also exacerbated during the premenstrual period (Trzonkowski et al., 2001). The number of lesions on the skin (Mysliwska et al., 2000; Tamer et al., 2003) and the oral mucosa (Sciubba, 2003) caused by human herpes simplex virus type 1 (HHSV-1) increases premenstrually. Cervical shedding of cytomegalovirus is significantly increased in the luteal phase until a few days after the beginning of menses (Mostad et al., 2000). Human immunodeficiency virus (HIV) RNA in genital secretions and virions in endocervical fluid peak during the week preceding menses (Reichelderfer et al., 2000). Attacks of pancreatitis, which are associated with hepatitis viruses A, B, C, and E and coxsackievirus (Alvares-da-Silva et al., 2000; Garty et al., 1995; Makharia et al., 2003; Yanagawa et al., 2004; Yuen et al., 2001), usually occur premenstrually (Southam and Gonzaga, 1965). Pancreatitis is exacerbated by HIV, which may cause damage directly or indirectly by suppressing the immunological control of other pathogens (Tyner and Turrett, 2004). In the large study of German women mentioned above, the incidences of "endemic hepatitis" (caused by hepatitis A virus), influenza, and polio were elevated within 4 days before the onset of menstruation (Andreas, 1961).

Fungal Infections

Proliferation of the yeast fungus *Candida albicans* increases just before menstruation (Kalo-Klein and Witkin, 1989). *Candida* can penetrate mucosal cells and proliferate intracellularly (Garcia-Tamayo et al., 1982), and cell-mediated immunity can control proliferation of *C. albicans* through the secretion of interferon-γ, which inhibits germination (Kalo-Klein and Witkin, 1989, 1991; Rogers and Balish, 1980, Romani, 2004). Accordingly, deficiencies in cell-mediated immunity increase the susceptibility to *Candida* infections, whereas deficiencies in the humoral response do not (Rogers and Balish, 1980; Stobo et al., 1976; Witkin et al., 1983). The increased proliferation of *C. albicans* during the premenstrual period may therefore result from the suppression of cellular immunity. Other variables such as glycogen concentration, antibiotic usage, and humidity may exacerbate *Candida* infections, but these variables cannot explain recurrent premenstrual *Candida* vaginitis (Monif, 1985; Rogers and Balish, 1980; Sobel, 1985). IDO-induced tryptophan restriction inhibits *C. albicans* (Bozza et al., 2005); the tendency for *C. albicans* to rise just before the onset of menstruation may therefore be a consequence of the reduced restriction of tryptophan at the end of the luteal phase just before the return of cell-mediated immunity.

Summary of Exacerbations of Infectious Diseases

The preceding examples show that known bacterial, viral, and fungal infections can be exacerbated premenstrually. The pathogens that cause these infections are either known to be controlled by cell-mediated immunity or are generally presumed to be controlled by cell-mediated immunity (as is the case for viruses). Their exacerbation during the luteal phase therefore accords with the idea that luteal-phase suppression of cell-mediated immunity can cause clinically detectable exacerbation of infection.

CHRONIC ILLNESSES OF UNCERTAIN CAUSE

Substantial evidence indicates that many important chronic diseases of uncertain cause are caused by infectious agents (Cochran et al., 2000). If so, the byproduct hypothesis of PMS formulated above predicts that the manifestations of these diseases will often be exacerbated perimenstrually, particularly when their etiological agents are controlled by cell-mediated immunity. This prediction is evaluated in this section by assessing whether chronic diseases that are suspected of being caused by such pathogens are exacerbated perimenstrually. Evaluation of this prediction is important because such exacerbations would often be classified as PMS if they had not previously been assigned to a different disease. Perimenstrual exacerbation of such diseases would suggest that PMS is part of a broader phenomenon that includes not only perimenstrual cycling of known infectious diseases, but of diseases for which infectious causes are suspected as well.

Neurological and Psychiatric Diseases

Manifestations of Parkinson's disease/parkinsonism complex intensify prior to or during menstruation (5 days before to 2 days after menstruation) (Quinn and Marsden, 1986).

Several pathogens are candidate causes of parkinsonism. Influenza A infection early in childhood is associated with the subsequent development of parkinsonism (Takahashi and Yamada, 2001), but unless influenza virus can persist after initial infection, perimenstrual exacerbation of influenza virus would not be a viable explanation for the perimenstrual exacerbation of parkinsonism disease. HIV may exacerbate parkinsonism associated with HIV dementia by causing psychomotor slowing, apathy, and motor disorders (Koutsilieri et al., 2002). As is the case with other AIDS manifestations, this effect may be due to reduced immunological control of persistent infections. Encephalitis lethargica, which is generally categorized as a parkinsonism, has been linked to streptococcal infection (Dale et al., 2004), which is often persistent (Medina et al., 2003; Valentin-Weigard, 2004).

Perimenstrual exacerbations of epilepsy have been recognized since 1885 (Magos and Studd, 1985). This association is so conspicuous that the term "catamenial epilepsy" has been coined to refer to it (Case and Reid, 2001; S. Duncan et al., 1993; Magos and Studd, 1985). Various viral and bacterial pathogens have been associated with seizures. DNA of herpesviruses (HHSV-1, cytomegalovirus, Epstein-Barr virus [EBV], and human herpesvirus-6) has been detected in the temporal lobes at higher prevalences in epileptics than in controls (Donati et al., 2003; Eeg-Olofsson et al., 2004; Lanari et al., 2003). Epilepsy can be induced in mice following inoculation with HHSV-1 (Wu et al., 2003). An elevated seroprevalence of *H. pylori* has also been found among epileptics (Okuda et al., 2004).

Premenstrual exacerbations occur in obsessive-compulsive disorder (OCD) and related conditions (Dillon and Brooks, 1992; Keuthen et al., 1997; Schwabe and Konkol, 1992; Williams and Koran, 1997), for which S*treptococcus pyogenes* is a candidate cause (Church et al., 2003; Leonard and Swedo, 2001; Swedo, 1994; Swedo et al., 1998).

Premenstrual exacerbations of bipolar disorder involve increased occurrences of hyperactivity, irritability, and "periodic psychosis" (Hendrick et al., 1996; Leibenluft, 1996). Borna disease virus (BDV) has been associated with bipolar disorder (Bode et al., 1997, 2001; Taieb et al., 2001).

For over a century, studies of schizophrenics have reported perimenstrual increases in symptom intensity (Bergeman et al., 2002; Hallonquist et al., 1993; Hendrick et al., 1996; Paffenbarger, 1964), particularly increases in the onset or intensity of auditory hallucinations, paranoia, anxiety, depression, hyperactivity, and irritability (Choi et al., 2001; Glick and Stewart, 1980). Hospital admissions for schizophrenia also occur at an elevated rate perimenstrually (Bergemann et al., 2002; Targum et al., 1991).

Many studies in different populations have linked *Toxoplasma gondii* to schizophrenia (Ledgerwood et al., 2003; Torrey and Yolken, 2003; Yolken et al., 2001). In utero *T. gondii* infections in particular are implicated as an insult that is manifested many years later as schizophrenia (Brown et al., 2005; Buka et al., 2000, 2001). Prenatal exposure to influenza has been associated with increased risk of adult-onset schizophrenia in the exposed fetuses (Brown et al., 2004). Maternal infections of HHSV-2 during pregnancy have similarly been implicated with the subsequent development of schizophrenia in the offspring (Buka et al., 2001). HHSV-1 infections have been associated with cognitive deficits in schizophrenics (F. B. Dickerson et al., 2003). Borna disease virus (BDV) has also been associated with schizophrenia (Hatalski et al., 1997; Taieb et al., 2001; Terayama et al., 2003).

"New-onset psychosis" occurs in about 4% of patients with HIV-spectrum illness (DeRonchi et al., 2000; Sewell, 1996). Had it not been associated with HIV from the outset, this ailment probably would have been grouped within schizophrenia. Its existence provides evidence of infectious causation of an illness indistinguishable from schizophrenia, although the mechanism by which HIV induces psychosis remains uncertain.

Gastrointestinal Diseases

Appendicitis is generally presumed to be caused by infection (Gurleyik and Gurleyik, 2003; Pugh, 2000). Its incidence more than doubles during the luteal phase (Arnbjornsson, 1982, 1984). Anecdotal reports and small studies have implicated *Pseudomonas aeruginosa*, *Mycobacteria*, fungi, or multicellular parasites (Lin and Lee, 2003; Bronner, 2004), but the roles of candidate pathogens remain uncertain.

In patients suffering from Crohn's disease, diarrhea and nausea are exacerbated premenstrually; exacerbation of diarrhea continues into the menses (Kane et al., 1998). Infectious causation of Crohn's disease is implicated by familial clustering (Grimes, 2003) and efficacy of antibiotics (Singh et al., 2004). *Mycobacterium avium* subspecies *paratuberculosis* is a candidate pathogen (Greenstein, 2003; Grimes, 2003; Naser et al., 2004).

Appendectomies have been associated with an increased risk of Crohn's disease with complex age dependence (Andersson et al., 2003; Kurina et al., 2002). These associations are consistent with the hypothesis that the appendix is a source of an infectious cause of Crohn's disease that tends not to infect or colonize the appendix prior to age 10.

Irritable bowel syndrome is also exacerbated perimenstrually (Case and Reid, 1998; Houghton et al., 2002; Kane et al., 1998). *Campylobacter, Shigella*, and *Salmonella* have been associated with sudden onset of irritable bowel syndrome (Neal et al., 1997; Spiller, 2003). Each of these pathogens can infect intracellularly (Bloom and Boedeker, 1996; Hacker and Heesemann, 2002) and therefore may be subject to cell-mediated immune control. Such control of *Salmonella* and *Shigella* has been demonstrated or strongly implicated (Ottenhoff et al., 2003; Simor et al., 1989). Treatment of sudden-onset irritable bowel syndrome with neomycin, which is effective against *Campylobacter, Shigella*, and *Salmonella* (Ahmed et al., 2000; Wray and Gnanou, 2000), was associated with an improvement in symptoms relative to placebo-treated patients (Pimentel et al., 2003)

Studies in the United Kingdom and United States categorize 17% and 6% of all cases of irritable bowel syndrome as postinfectious on the basis of sudden acute onset (Longstreth et al., 2000; Spiller, 2003). In a study of 318 gastroenteritis patients in the United Kingdom, the relative risk of postinfectious irritable bowel syndrome after *Salmonella* gastroenteritis was 11.9 (Rodriguez and Ruigomez, 1999).

Osteoporosis

A history of PMS is associated with a nearly twofold increase in risk of osteoporosis in postmenopausal women (Lee and Kanis, 1994). Women with PMS show reductions in bone mineral density in vertebrae and the femoral neck that are accelerated by about a decade (Thys-Jacobs et al., 1995).

Infection with human T-cell lymphotrophic virus type 1 (HTLV-1) and HIV have been linked to osteoporosis (Schachter et al., 2003). These pathogens could cause only a tiny portion of the osteoporosis in Europe and North America, because they are rare relative to osteoporosis, and because osteoporosis was common long before HIV was present in these regions. These associations, however, raise the possibility that other infectious agents could be causally involved by analogously disrupting maintenance of bone density. In the case of HIV, osteoporosis could be enhanced by reduced immunological control of etiological agents.

Osteoporosis is more common and more severe among people with periodontal disease (Garcia et al., 2000; Mohammad et al., 1994). Several pathogens are implicated as agents of periodontal disease, the best studied being *Porphyromonas gingivalis*. Periodontitis, osteoporosis, and *P. gingivalis* infections share many of the same risk factors, such as age, smoking, and concomitant diseases, and each is associated with bone loss (Garcia et al., 2000; Mohammad et al., 1994). These associations raise the possibility that periodontitis and osteoporosis may be two different aspects of the same underlying process, with infectious agents upsetting the balance between bone deposition and bone resorption. If so, the infectious causes of periodontitis, such as *P. gingivalis*, may also be causing osteoporosis.

Diabetes

Premenstrual exacerbations of type 1 and type 2 diabetes involve deteriorations in glycemic control, diabetic ketoacidosis, insulin reactions, and hypoglycemic episodes (Case and Reid, 2001). Nondiabetic women sometimes experience increased glucose intolerance at the time of menstruation (Magos and Studd, 1985).

Type 1 diabetes is associated with enteroviruses (Fohlman and Friman, 1993; Salminen et al., 2004). Although these pathogens are often assumed to be triggers of autoimmune damage that generates type 1 diabetes, they can cause persistent infections (Fohlman and Friman, 1993). If so, the premenstrual exacerbations of type 1 diabetes may result from exacerbations of infections by these agents.

A portion of type 2 diabetes is associated with and probably caused by hepatitis C virus (Khalili et al., 2004; Lecube et al., 2004; Mehta et al., 2000; Shintani et al., 2004). Although hepatitis C infections are not sufficiently common to be responsible for most type 2 diabetes, their association with type 2 diabetes illustrates how persistent infectious agents may be responsible for this illness of uncertain cause.

Migraine Headaches

Migraines, with and without auras, are more likely to occur during the premenstruum than at other times of the menstrual cycle (Case and Reid, 2001; Dzoljic et al., 2002; MacGregor et al., 1990, Magos and Studd, 1985). This association is sufficiently strong to have led to the term "menstrual migraine," which is defined as an attack of migraine, usually without aura that occurs regularly within 2 days of menses (Case and Reid, 2001).

Individuals with aura-associated migraine were infected with the particularly virulent Cag A variant of *H. pylori* twice as often as were those who either did not have migraines or experienced migraines without aura (Gasbarrini et al., 2000). In two different studies, short-term antibiotic treatment ameliorated both types of migraines in most *H. pylori*–infected migraine patients (Gasbarrini et al., 1998, Tunca et al., 2004). Amelioration persisted throughout a 6-month follow-up period (Gasbarrini et al., 1998).

Meniere's Disease

Approximately 5% of women with Meniere's disease reported a premenstrual increase in vertigo, low-frequency hearing loss, and tinnitus, but no patients reported premenstrual amelioration of symptoms (Andrews et al., 1992; Morse and House, 2001).

Meniere's disease arises as a sequella to viral inflammation, infectious otitis media, meningitis, and syphilis (Paparella, 1984; Paparella and Djalilian, 2002; Pulec, 1977). Elevated antibody titers to rubella, mumps, and herpesviruses (HHSV-1, varicella-zoster, and cytomegalovirus) have been reported in Meniere's patients relative to controls; an elevated cell-mediated immune reactivity (assayed by monocyte responsiveness) was found for rubeola, mumps, and herpesviruses (Williams et al., 1987). Cytomegalovirus induces Meniere's-like disease in an animal model (Fukuda et al., 1988).

Fibromyalgia and Chronic Fatigue Syndrome

In a study of 44 Scandinavian fibromyalgia patients, 61% experienced premenstrual increases in generalized pain, fatigue, depression, muscle weakness, muscle tenderness, stiffness, and functional disability (Ostensen et al., 1997).

Various pathogens have been associated with fibromyalgia. Infectious mononucleosis, which is caused by EBV, has been linked to the onset and development of fibromyalgia, with tender points and pain persisting for 6 months in about one quarter of the patients with mononucleosis (Rea et al., 1999). Fibromyalgia has also been linked to *Mycoplasma*, hepatitis C virus, and enteroviruses (Buskila et al., 1997; Nasralla et al., 1999).

Chronic fatigue syndrome patients report more premenstrual symptoms than controls, and less PMS prior to the onset of their chronic fatigue (Harlow et al., 1998). Various *Mycoplasma* species have been detected in patients with chronic fatigue syndrome (Buskila, 2000; Nasralla et al., 1999).

Multiple Sclerosis

Multiple sclerosis is often ameliorated during the bulk of the luteal phase but then exacerbated during the few days before and after the onset of menses. The exacerbations involve worsening of spasticity, weakness, limb paresis, coordination, pain, ocular symptoms, and sphincter disturbances (Sandyk, 1995; Smith and Studd, 1992; Zorgdrager and De Keyser, 1997).

C. pneumoniae, EBV, and human herpesvirus 6 have been implicated as causes of multiple sclerosis (Bulijevac et al., 2003; Fainardi et al., 2004; Haahr et al., 2004; Pender, 2003; Sumaya et al., 1985; Swanborg, 2003). The high prevalence of EBV infection contrasts with the low prevalence of multiple sclerosis, which is generally around 0.1% (Dahl et al., 2004; Ragonese et al., 2004). This discrepancy emphasizes the importance of other contributing factors. *C. pneumoniae* has been associated with multiple sclerosis (Munger et al., 2003; Sriram et al., 1998) and may induce the disease through immunological cross-reactivity with myelin basic protein (Lenz et al., 2001; see Chapter 19). The exacerbation of multiple sclerosis symptoms at the onset of menses is therefore consistent with reduced suppression of *C. pneumoniae* during the luteal phase followed by increased autoimmune pathology at the end of the luteal phase, when reactivated cellular immunity may respond to the elevated chlamydial antigen and myelin basic proteins.

Rheumatoid Arthritis

Rheumatoid arthritis (RA) tends to be ameliorated during most of the luteal phase relative to the preovulatory phase (Latman, 1983). In a study of seven RA patients, maximal finger joint size tended to occur during the very late luteal or early menstrual phases; maximal grip strength never occurred during these time intervals (Rudge et al., 1983).

Viral infections with EBV, cytomegalovirus, hepatitis B and C viruses, and HTLV-1 have been associated with the development of RA (Balandraud et al., 2004; Mehraein et al., 2004; Sawada and Takei, 2005; Tanasescu et al., 1999; Yakova et al., 2005). Antibiotic treatment ameliorated RA symptoms in *H. pylori*–infected patients relative to uninfected RA patients; a significant amelioration persisted during 2 years of follow-up (Zentilin et al., 2002). Streptococcal cell walls have been used experimentally in rats and guinea pigs to produce a remitting and exacerbating arthritis, which is used as an RA model (Al-Mobireek et al., 2000; Kimpel et al., 2003).

Joint pathology involves cell-mediated immune activity (Firestein, 2003), and, like multiple sclerosis, RA is considered a cell-mediated autoimmune disease (Verhoef et al., 1998; Whitacre et al., 1999). As with multiple sclerosis, the perimenstrual exacerbation of RA symptoms can be explained by reduced control of a causal pathogen during the luteal phase followed by increased autoimmune pathology when cellular immunity returns.

Lupus

When systemic lupus erythematosus (SLE) or cutaneous lupus varies with the menstrual cycle, exacerbations tend to occur during the luteal phase (Steinberg and Steinberg, 1985; Yell and Burge, 1993).

SLE patients show elevated positivity for EBV (Moon et al., 2004) and *T. gondii* (Seta et al., 2002). The effectiveness of treatment of SLE with antimalarial medications, such as hydroxychloroquine (HCG) and plaquenil (Wang et al., 1999), is consistent with a causal role for *T. gondii*, because *Toxoplasma* and *Plasmodium* are both apicomlexan protozoa. Perhaps antimalarial compounds ameliorate SLE because they are suppressing *Toxoplasma*.

The premenstrual exacerbation of SLE throughout the luteal phase contrasts with the exacerbation of multiple sclerosis and RA only at the end of the luteal phase. This difference accords with differences in the mechanisms of pathogenesis. RA and multiple sclerosis are cell-mediated autoimmune disorders (Verhoef et al., 1998; Whitacre et al., 1999), whereas SLE is characterized by pathological antibody complexes (Whitacre et al., 1999). Accordingly, exacerbations of SLE occur throughout the luteal phase when humoral immunity and antibody formation are enhanced.

Cardiovascular Disease

Acute coronary events, acute myocardial infarctions, and angina tend to occur within the first week after the onset of menses (Hamelin et al., 2003; Mukamal et al., 2002).

Cardiovascular disease has been linked to infection with cytomegalovirus and oral bacteria such as *P. gingivalis* and *C. pneumoniae*. The link to *C. pneumoniae* has been particularly well documented (Arcari et al., 2005; Belland et al., 2004; Gaydos et al., 1996; Gupta and Camm, 1997; Haraszthy et al., 2000; Kuo et al., 1993; Nerheim et al., 2004; Shor et al., 1992; Maass et al., 1998).

C. pneumoniae apparently damages blood vessels in part by triggering inflammatory responses (Belland et al., 2004; Von Hertzen, 2002), which are suppressed during the luteal phase (Clemens et al., 1979, Critchley et al., 2001, 2003; Watnick and Russo, 1968). The increased incidence of coronary events during the first week after the lutueal phase is therefore consistent with cyclic exacerbation of infection by *C. pneumoniae* and other pathogens during the luteal phase, followed by an inflammatory response to the exacerbated infection just after the return of a fully active inflammatory response.

Asthma

Asthma tends to be exacerbated perimenstrually in about one third of asthmatics (Agarwal and Shah, 1997; Chandler et al., 1997; Shibasaki et al., 1992; Tan, 2001). Asthma has been associated with rhinovirus, parainfluenza virus, respiratory syncytial virus, *Mycoplasma pneumoniae, Hemophilus influenzae,* and *Chlamydia pneumoniae* (Cook et al., 1998; Fayon et al., 1999; Freymuth et al., 1999; Kraft, 2000; Normann et al., 1998; Saikku et al., 1998; Tuffaha et al., 2000). The three bacteria can cause persistent intracellular infections that rebound during suppression of cell-mediated immunity (Ahren et al., 2001; Kroegel and Mock, 2001; Saikku et al., 1998; St. Geme, 2002; Van Schilfgaarde, 1999; Yavlovich et al., 2004). They are therefore candidates for causing asthma that cycles persistently with the menstrual cycle.

ANTI-INFECTIVES

If PMS results from exacerbation of persistent infections, suppression of infectious agents with anti-infective compounds should ameliorate the symptoms. Hypothesizing that premenstrual syndrome may result from a sexually transmitted bacterium, Toth et al. (1988) evaluated whether treatment with doxycycline would ameliorate PMS. They followed 30 patients for 1 month prior to treatments. Half of the patients then received either doxycycline or placebo. After 1 month of treatment, the doxycycline group showed a significant reduction in PMS symptoms; the placebo group did not. The placebo group was then started on antibiotics and experienced a significant reduction in PMS symptoms. All subjects continued to show amelioration of PMS symptoms 6 months after cessation of antibiotic treatment (Toth et al., 1988).

Three years after cessation of antibiotic treatment, 7 out of 20 were symptom-free or virtually symptom-free. At that time 5 of the 13 with PMS recurrence were given intravenous clindamycin and gentamycin and became symptom-free.

ENDOCRINOLOGICAL HYPOTHESES

The hypothesized associations between the menstrual cycle, exacerbation of infections, and exacerbations of illnesses are endocrinological in the sense that the immunological suppression of cell-mediated immunity results from the immunosuppressive effects of estrogen and progesterone. Cyclic expression of symptoms in concert with the menstrual cycle, however, has sometimes been explained by hypothesizing direct effects of reproductive hormones.

The perimenstrual exacerbation of schizophrenia, for example, has been explained by the "estrogen protection hypothesis," which proposes that low perimenstrual estrogen levels increase vulnerability (Seeman, 1996). This hypothesis, however, raises the question, "What is estrogen protecting against?" The estrogen-protection hypothesis is therefore incomplete because it does not include a mechanism of primary causation. In contrast, the exacerbation-of-infection hypothesis proposes that endocrinological changes increase vulnerability to the primary infectious causes of schizophrenia. Estrogen supplementation in postmenopausal women has been associated with amelioration of negative symptoms (e.g., withdrawal and cognitive deficits) of schizophrenia but not positive symptoms (e.g., paranoia and hallucination) (Lindamer et al., 2001). This finding offers some support for the estrogen-protection hypothesis for negative symptoms but suggests that we must look elsewhere to understand the positive symptoms. The support for the estrogen-protection hypothesis, however, still requires an explanation for why the brain would have evolved to generate negative symptoms of schizophrenia. The protective effects of estrogen must protect against negative effects of some other cause, such as an infectious agent or some noninfectious environmental damage, because genetic instructions for a brain that suffered from negative symptoms would tend to be weeded out by natural selection (Ledgerwood et al., 2003).

The documented premenstrual exacerbation of schizophrenia, however, pertains to positive symptoms (Hendrick et al., 1996). The estrogen-supplementation experiment therefore fails to support the estrogen-protection hypothesis as an explanation of the documented perimenstrual exacerbations of schizophrenia.

Direct hormonal effects have been invoked to explain exacerbations of other diseases such as inflammatory bowel disease, irritable bowel syndrome, and asthma (Case and Reid, 1998; Leslie and Dubey, 1994; Tan, 2001). Such interpretations need to be carefully tested before being accepted, because the evolutionary disadvantage of such effects would likely cause them to be weeded out over time.

In one case evidence suggests that a pathogen might respond directly to hormonal changes. *Candida albicans* possesses receptors for estrogen and progesterone, which have been shown to be stimulators of its germination (Powell et al., 1983; Sobel, 1985). It may also be responsive to interferon-γ, a cytokine that is influenced by reproductive hormones and promotes cell-mediated immunity (Kalo-Klein and Witkin, 1990).

ASSOCIATIONS WITH HORMONAL CONTRACEPTIVES AND PREGNANCY

General Effects of Hormonal Contraceptives

Hormonal contraceptives contain estrogen and progesterone in varying doses and proportions. If the changes in illness during the menstrual cycle result from changes in these hormones, oral contraceptives should alter diseases in ways that are analogous to the changes that occur during the menstrual cycle. Because hormonal contraceptives are administered, such alterations implicate hormones as causes of the analogous premenstrual symptoms. At first glance, the expectation of such negative effects of hormonal contraceptives seems at odds with the knowledge that many women use hormonal contraception with little if any side effects; however, approximately one half to two thirds of women who start oral contraceptives discontinue using them within the first year (Berenson et al., 1997; Trussell and Kost, 1987). Side effects are the primary reason for discontinuing oral contraceptive usage (Berenson et al., 1997; Rosenberg and Waugh, 1998).

Many of the side effects of oral contraceptives are similar to symptoms of PMS, suggesting that oral contraceptives may exacerbate the same underlying processes that are exacerbated in PMS. A direct-effect endocrinological hypothesis might explain this similarity by invoking similar direct effects of estrogen or progesterone on human physiology and behavior. If these effects result instead from indirect endocrinological effects on underlying infectious processes, we should see effects of oral contraceptives on infectious diseases that mirror the perimenstrual exacerbations of infectious diseases.

General Effects of Pregnancy

High levels of estrogen and progesterone and a concomitant shift from cellular immunity to humoral immunity persist throughout pregnancy (Al-Shammri et al., 2004). Progesterone falls to luteal phase levels within a day after childbirth and to preovulatory levels after several days; estrogen falls to preovulatory levels by the third day (Greenspan and Gardner, 2004, p. 651). Immunocompetence returns within 3 weeks (Elenkov et al., 2001). Tryptophan restriction occurs throughout pregnancy (Shröcksnadel, 1996); it ends within a few days after birth, except among women with postpartum depression, perhaps indicating a connection between postpartum depression and infection (Maes et al., 2002).

Because the duration of pregnancy is far longer than the duration of the luteal phase, the timing of exacerbations and ameliorations of infections and illnesses during pregnancy may provide insight into the mechanisms by which immune suppression alters manifestations during the menstrual cycle. If, for example, manifestations of an illness are exacerbated at the end of the luteal phase and after the end of pregnancy, the exacerbation at the end of the luteal phase cannot be attributable simply to a lag between the onset of relaxed cell-mediated control of causal pathogen and the growth of that pathogen to damaging levels. More generally, if declines in progesterone and estrogen are responsible for perimenstrual changes in manifestations of illness by causing changes in autoimmunity or through relaxation of tryptophan restriction, analogous changes are expected after birth.

Effects of Hormonal Contraceptives and Pregnancy on Infections

Sexually transmitted pathogens such as *Chlamydia trachomatis, Candida albicans*, herpes simplex virus, human papillomavirus, and HIV tend to have a higher prevalence and incidence among oral contraceptive users (Avonts et al., 1989; Cottingham and Hunter, 1992; Mostad et al., 2000; Oriel, 1972; Powell et al., 1983; Reed, 1992; Sobel, 1985; Spinillo et al., 1995). Although such associations are consistent with increased vulnerability to these infections during the luteal phase, the associations could also be explained by increased exposure to the pathogens among women who use oral contraception relative to those using barrier methods or no contraception. Some studies, however, have accounted for this confounding variable, and still implicate an exacerbating effect of oral contraceptives. Rates of infection with *C. trachomatis* and *N. gonorrheae* were, for example, 70% greater among women on oral contraceptives than among women with tubal ligation or IUDs, even though the frequency of coitus and numbers of sexual partners were not different (Louv et al., 1989). Among HIV-1 infected women, HIV DNA in cervical swabs increased significantly above precontraception levels by the second month after initiation of hormonal contraception (Wang et al., 2004). Similarly, use of oral contraceptives is associated with progression of human papillomavirus infection to carcinogenesis (Ylitalo et al., 1999).

Hormonal contraception and pregnancy can also exacerbate persistent infections that are not sexually transmitted. Oral contraceptives, for example, can exacerbate persistent varicella infections (Krueger et al., 1977) and infections of the oral cavity. Oral contraception contributes to gingivitis (McCann and Bonci, 2001) and has been associated with a 16-fold increase in numbers of *Prevotella* in the gingival microflora relative to women who were not pregnant and not using oral contraceptives; pregnancy was associated with a 55-fold increase (Jensen, 1981). Pregnant women were two to three times more likely to develop infections (osteitis) following tooth extractions (Sweet and Butler, 1977).

Hormonal Contraception, Pregnancy, and Illnesses of Unknown Cause

Illnesses of unknown cause may also be exacerbated by oral contraceptives. Multiple sclerosis, for example, is ameliorated during pregnancy and then becomes exacerbated during the post partum period for up to 3 months (Poser et al., 1979). This amelioration during pregnancy is consistent with the amelioration of multiple sclerosis until the very end of the luteal phase. The amelioration of multiple sclerosis throughout pregnancy indicates that its amelioration during the luteal phase is not attributable simply to delayed effects of the growth of a causal pathogen in response to suppression of cell-mediated immunity. Reduced autoimmunity during the period of hormone-induced immunosuppression could ameliorate multiple sclerosis, which then becomes exacerbated upon the return of a partially effective cellular immune response when the levels of suppressive hormones decline just prior to the menses and just after parturition. Alternatively, the patterns could be explained by causal pathogens that are fairly well controlled by estrogen-induced tryptophan restriction, which diminishes as estrogen declines just prior to menstruation and after parturition.

RA is ameliorated among oral contraceptive users and during pregnancy (Nelson and Steinberg, 1987; Zorgdrager and DeKeyser, 1997). As with multiple sclerosis, this amelioration is consistent with the amelioration of RA until the end of the luteal phase.

Lupus is exacerbated among oral contraceptive users and pregnant women (Krueger et al., 1977; Nelson and Steinberg, 1987; Yell and Burge, 1993). This exacerbation is consistent with the pathology induced by antibody complex formation and is consistent with the exacerbation during the luteal phase.

Psychiatric illnesses often appear to be affected by hormonal changes associated with pregnancy and contraceptive use. With regard to psychoses, the frequencies of admissions, first episodes, and relapses are elevated during the first month after parturition, although the trends specifically for schizophrenia are unclear (Grigoriadis and Seeman, 2002; Paffenbarger, 1964; Pugh et al., 1963). Whether oral contraceptives affect schizophrenia is still uncertain (Felthous and Robinson, 1981). Oral contraceptives are reported to have a mood-stabilizing effect on bipolar disorder (Rasgon et al., 2003). Case reports suggest that implanted contraceptives (Norplant) may contribute to obsessive-compulsive disorder and depression (Wagner, 1996).

Other neurological disorders also vary with use of hormonal contraception. A one-third increase in risk of Meniere's disease was found among women who reported past use of oral contraceptives, and vertigo has been exacerbated by oral contraceptive use (Siegler, 1977; Vessey and Painter, 2001). The evidence on epilepsy is inconsistent. Some evidence associates exacerbations with oral contraceptive use (Sinnathuray, 1988). Other studies have found no increase in the onset or frequency of seizures (Case and Reid, 2001; Vessey et al., 2002). Fibromyalgia is exacerbated in about one third of fibromyalgia patients using oral contraceptives (Ostensen et al., 1997).

Oral contraceptives may improve, worsen (Fajardo, 1981; Grimes, 1999), or cause no change (Couturier et al., 2003; Dzoljic et al., 2002) in migraine symptoms (Ensom, 2000; MacGregor et al., 1990). The frequency of hemorrhagic and nonhemorrhagic stroke is elevated among oral contraceptive users with a history of migraines but not among oral contraceptive users without such a history (Chang et al., 1999; Schwartz et al., 1998; Tzourio et al., 1995).

A tripling in cardiovascular events (i.e., venous thromboembolism, stroke, and myocardial infarction) has been reported in women using pills with higher doses of estrogen and a sevenfold increase in those using newer progestins (Burkman, 2001). The associations of infectious agents with atherosclerosis raise the possibility that oral contraceptives may be increasing the risk of cardiovascular events by affecting infection. The timing of the cardiovascular events may help distinguish such an indirect effect from a direct effect of reproductive hormones. If the hormones themselves were directly causing the pathology, one would not expect the cardiovascular events to occur during the first week of each cycle when women are taking pills that do not contain the hormones. Occurrence of the negative effects during this period, however, would be consistent with infectious causation, because the inflammatory pathology would be expected to flare up during this period of renewed immunocompetence.

Diseases of the gastrointestinal tract have also been evaluated with respect to use of hormonal contraception. In a study of 149 patients with irritable bowel syndrome (Heitkemper et al., 2003), univariate analyses suggested a reduction of abdominal pain, uterine cramps, cognitive, anxiety, and depression symptoms, but none of these reductions were statistically significant when the results were corrected for multiple comparisons. Manifestations of inflammatory bowel disease were ameliorated when the menstrual cycle was eliminated by blocking gonadotropin-releasing hormone (Case and Reid,

1998). When these women were then treated with estrogen and progestin, symptoms often recurred during the progestin phase. The effects of oral contraceptive hormones on irritable bowel syndrome is therefore still unresolved, but the tendency for irritable bowl syndrome to be exacerbated at the end of the menstrual cycle is consistent with an ameliorative effect of estrogen and an exacerbating effect of progesterone. The persistence of exacerbated manifestations into the menstrual phase is consistent with a lag between the immunosuppression of progesterone and a clearing of exacerbated infections a few days after the return of immunocompetence (though not with a direct effect of progesterone).

Patients with Crohn's disease were more likely to be oral contraceptive users than matched controls who did not have Crohn's disease (Corrao et al., 1998). The association between oral contraceptive and Crohn's disease is therefore consistent with the premenstrual exacerbation of Crohn's disease.

Several case reports note an increase in pancreatitis among users of oral contraceptives, with amelioration following discontinuation of hormonal contraception (Liu, 1982; Mehrotra et al., 1981; Parker, 1983). These effects are consistent with the premenstrual exacerbation of pancreatitis.

Contraceptives containing estrogen are protective against osteoporosis (Rickenlund et al., 2004). Formulations containing only progesterone, however, are significantly associated with bone density loss (Cromer, 2003; Scholes et al., 2002). Estrogen appears to have direct positive effects on bone deposition that offset the negative effects of progesterone. The association between PMS and osteoporosis is therefore consistent with negative effect of progesterone on osteoporosis.

The effects of oral contraceptive on asthma are unclear. Some studies report an exacerbation (Derimanov and Oppenheimer, 1998, Forbes et al., 1999). Others report improvement (Haggarty et al., 2003; Tan, 2001) or show no change (Forbes et al., 1999; Lange et al., 2001).

Overall Consistency Between Effects of Hormonal Contraceptives, Pregnancy, and Perimenstrual Manifestations

The effects of oral contraceptives are generally consistent with the fluctuations in illness that occur during menstrual cycles. The general consistency of the evidence lends credence to the hypothesis that hormonal changes are causally involved in the symptoms that recur during the menstrual cycle and that these changes often involve exacerbations of infections. The literature on hormonal contraception, however, provides relatively little evidence to assess hormonal effects on manifestations of persistent infection. The existing body of evidence thus emphasizes the need to investigate effects of hormonal contraceptives on infection rather than simply concluding that hormonal contraceptives are tolerated or not tolerated by different individuals.

AN INTEGRATIVE PERSPECTIVE ON PMS

PMS is often attributed to quirky hormonal effects or psychosomatic illness, in contrast with "true" illnesses that have clearly definable etiological agents (Rodin, 1992). Our cycling defense paradigm, however, provides a more integrated perspective on PMS.

Immunological processes that are known to suppress or exacerbate infectious diseases vary in concert with the menstrual cycle. Persistent infections are exacerbated in accordance with these immunological changes, as are a great variety of diseases for which infectious causes are implicated. For these diseases the accepted or suspected pathogens generally cause damage by mechanisms that accord with the changes in immunological activity that occur over the menstrual cycle. Specifically, the pathogens tend to be controlled by cell-mediated immunity, which is suppressed during the premenstrual period. The pathological mechanisms may involve damage from components of the immune system that are exacerbated premenstrually, as is the case for the antibody complex formation associated with lupus. Or the pathology may involve inflammatory responses that resume during the few days after the onset of menstruation in response to pathogens that have been under less stringent immunological control during the luteal phase, as appears to be the case with myocardial infarction.

We believe that it is unparsimonious to suspect that such a large number of disparate illnesses would be exacerbated by direct effects of estrogen and progesterone for two general reasons. The first reason is mechanistic. Immunological effects of estrogen and progesterone have been well documented. These reproductive hormones suppress cellular immunity and enhance humoral immunity and should therefore exacerbate infections that would otherwise be controlled by cellular immunity, ameliorate autoimmune damage from cellular immunity, or enhance autoimmune damage from humoral immunity. The spectrum of associations documented in the literature accords with these expectations.

The second reason pertains to the restriction of these hormonal effects to diseases of known or suspected infectious causes. We have found no evidence implicating hormonal effects on genetic diseases or diseases caused by noninfectious environmental factors unless the pathology of these diseases is known to or suspected to involve infection (e.g., as is the case with cystic fibrosis).

This argument does not exclude the possibility that reproductive hormones may sometimes have cyclic effects on symptoms that are not attributable to exacerbation of infection. Enlargement of breasts during the luteal phase, for example, is reasonably interpreted as a normal part of the preparation of breast tissue for pregnancy and nursing. But when manifestations such as incapacitating pain interfere with the ability of an individual to function, one must ask how such a handicap would withstand the culling effects of natural selection. This argument is particularly applicable when such manifestations are present only in a portion of the population, because the absence in some individuals indicates that the manifestation is not a necessary consequence of the hormonal fluctuations.

The consistency between effects of hormonal contraception and menstrual changes in hormone levels provides a check on these ideas. This consistency implicates the change in hormones as a cause rather than simply a correlate of cyclic symptomatic changes.

The consistency between menstrual changes and changes associated with pregnancy provides a different kind of insight. By comparing effects of immunological alterations over a 9-month period to those over a 2-week period, the mechanism of immunological effects on infection can be clarified; for example, the amelioration of multiple sclerosis until the end of the luteal phase cannot be attributed simply to a lag in the growth of a causative microorganism in response to suppressed cell-mediated immunity because multiple sclerosis is also ameliorated throughout pregnancy.

This integration of perimenstrual exacerbation of suspected and known infectious diseases provides a framework for integrating PMS with the broader study of chronic disease. Because PMS is a diagnosis of exclusion, we can expect that the causes of PMS will be a grab-bag mix of different illness-producing processes. The pervasive perimenstrual exacerbations of distinct categories of illnesses and the linkage of these illnesses with infection suggests that PMS may be a collection of symptoms caused by a heterogeneous mix of infections; moreover, this body of evidence suggests that the concept of PMS may be an artifact of the inadequate knowledge about true categories of disease and effects of immune suppression on their expression. If a person has been diagnosed with bipolar disorder, for example, an exacerbation of depression would be considered an exacerbation of bipolar disorder. If a person has not been diagnosed as bipolar, premenstrual depression would be considered a manifestation of PMS. Depression is one of the most common symptoms of PMS. A variety of infections could contribute to depression by augmenting estrogen induced tryptophan restriction (via IDO). This IDO-mediated reduction in tryptophan makes it unavailable for the synthesis of the neurotransmitter serotonin. Lowered levels of serotonin have been strongly implicated in depression (Kandel et al., 2000).

This cycling defense model of PMS not only offers a cohesive picture of perimenstrual alterations of wellness, but also provides a basis for future work by emphasizing the need to assess whether the individual manifestations of PMS are associated with exacerbations of infectious processes. If so, treatment of the infections with anti-infectives could be an effective way of controlling PMS symptoms and the cellular pathology that accompanies them.

This integrated perspective also suggests new approaches for determining the causes of chronic diseases. According to the cyclic defense paradigm, perimenstrual exacerbation of a chronic disease implicates infectious causation. Comparisons of assays for suspected agents during the immunosuppressed phase of the cycle with the immunocompetent phase within the same patient will reduce the statistical noise and interpretive ambiguity that arise when comparisons are made among patients. Associations with causal pathogens may therefore become more apparent, and effects of experimental treatment of the suspected pathogens may be easier to detect. Focusing on perimenstrual exacerbations of chronic diseases may therefore facilitate resolutions of any causal role for suspected pathogens as well as treatment of the disease through inhibition of the causal pathogens.

ACKNOWLEDGMENTS

For valuable input we thank C. Corbitt, L. A. Dugatkin, R. A. Goldsby, R. Lewine, A. Toth, W. R. Trevathan, and E. O. Smith.

CHAPTER 11

Possible Role of Eclampsia/ Preeclampsia in Evolution of Human Reproduction

Pierre-Yves Robillard, Gustaaf Dekker, Gérard Chaouat,
Jean Chaline, and Thomas C. Hulsey

Preeclampsia is the consequence of a defective implantation of the placenta that occurs during a critical developmental moment, the second phase of trophoblastic invasion when the human placenta penetrates even more deeply into the uterine wall, presumably due to the increased energy demands of the human fetus. This defect associated with the process of secondary implantation, as Robillard and his colleagues describe, is one of the major causes of intrauterine growth retardation. In an attempt to overcome this failure of implantation, pregnant women exhibit increased blood pressure (gestational hypertension), and the health of both the mother and infant is threatened throughout the rest of the pregnancy. In extreme forms, and when undetected, preeclampsia can lead to maternal seizures and epileptic convulsions (referred to as eclampsia), accounting for about 70,000 deaths of women worldwide. Robillard et al. point out that this type of hypertensive disorder of pregnancy (HDP) is mostly associated with first pregnancies and, more specifically, with women who have not sexually cohabited with their male partners for more than 4 or 5 months. Changing sex partners relatively frequently is another risk factor for preeclampsia. It seems that the longer the father has exchanged body fluids with the mother, therein exposing her to his antigens, the less likely this disease finds expression. Researchers conclude, therefore, that preeclampsia should no longer be considered "a condition of first pregnancy" but more accurately "a condition of first pregnancy *for a couple*" and, thus, a "couples disease." Robillard and colleagues propose that selection favored the loss of estrus (sexual periodicity) among evolving hominins specifically to facilitate more frequent intercourse with the same partner and, hence, longer exposure to male sperm antigens in the female reproductive tract. From an immunological and biochemical perspective, this behavior reduces the chances of the female's immune system rejecting the sperm as if they were foreign invaders, and thus reducing the chances of eclampsia/preeclampsia. In this way, Robillard integrates changes in male–female sociosexual relationships in the hominin lineage with increasing brain size, cranial formation in utero, and loss of estrus, which altogether proposes a new explanation of a significant contemporary health challenge.

HYPERTENSIVE DISORDERS OF PREGNANCY: 10% OF HUMAN PREGNANCIES

Collectively, the different manifestations of hypertensive disorders of pregnancy (HDP) represent the main reproductive burden of human reproduction. Notably, this phenomenon does not occur in other mammals, including primates (Walker, 2000). HDP occur in approximately 10% of human births (approximately 14 million per year of the 136 million births worldwide [WHO, 1999b, 2000]).

Besides the abnormally elevated blood pressure in women with HDP, other major complications can occur, including eclampsia (maternal seizures or epileptic convulsions that could lead to cerebral injury), which represents, without medical intervention, 0.5–1% of human births (approximately 700,000 per year according to the estimates of the World Health Organization [WHO, 1999b, 2000]). More than 95% of cases occur in developing countries, and they often result in the death of the mother as well as the infant. Additionally, in 3% of human pregnancies, HDP will be complicated by generalized endothelial cell disease ("severe preeclampsia") that induces damage to the kidneys (proteinuria due to a glomeruloendotheliosis) or the liver (the HELLP syndrome— hemolysis, elevated liver enzymes, and low platelet count). Severe preeclampsia, without modern medical interventions, results, in one fourth to one third of cases, in cerebral vasculopathy and induces epileptic seizures of eclampsia. Finally, in 7% of pregnancies, women will present with "simple hypertension," which is reversible after birth. HDP is the number one cause of maternal deaths in developed countries and number three in developing areas (after bleeding and sepsis), representing approximately 70,000 maternal deaths per year worldwide out of 530,000 cases (WHO, 1999b, 2000).

The common thread linking all of the complications associated with HDP is that their only known definitive cure is delivery of the fetus and placenta by whatever means possible, including induced labor and cesarean section. As such, preeclampsia is the most common cause of medically induced prematurity. The long-term survival of these newborns depends on access to resources and knowledge of modern neonatology (Brown, 1997).

Preeclampsia is harmful to both the mother and the fetus. Because of poor maternal–fetal vascular exchange, it is the primary cause of intrauterine growth retardation (IUGR), resulting in increased numbers of babies delivered "small for gestational age," or SGA. Throughout the history of humankind, SGA newborns have paid the highest price of infant mortality (Levene, 1985).

In epidemiological terms, HDP are one of the plagues of human reproduction. There are no naturally occurring animal models of HDP and only a few isolated reports from primates including Patas monkeys (Palmer et al., 1979) and lowland gorillas (Baird, 1981). These are reports on single cases of epilepsy during delivery and seem to be infrequent when compared to the number of human births associated with HDP. In rare cases, mammals may present epileptic seizures at delivery because of, for example, hemorrhage or hypoglycemia, but these are not the same as HDP.

Eclampsia (maternal convulsions) has been described in humans from different cultures as early as 4200 years ago (Lindheimer et al., 1999). Eclampsia was probably interpreted as a curse since epilepsy was associated in all past human cultures with possession by evil spirits. It is interesting to speculate that our ancestors may have been able to make the connection between preeclampsia and eclampsia, having observed that young women with edema (abnormal accumulation of liquid in the tissues, one of the signs of renal dysfunction) at the end of pregnancy were likely to develop eclampsia at delivery and/or produced tiny newborns.

WHY THIS REVERSIBLE HYPERTENSION DURING PREGNANCY?

Preeclampsia is the consequence of a defect in the second phase of trophoblastic invasion (Pijnenborg, 1996; Zhou, 1997). This secondary invasion as a normal part of the development of the fetus in humans is unique among mammals. The first trophoblastic invasion occurs at the time of implantation, a few days after fertilization, as in all mammals. In humans, a second invasion occurs 3 months later, after an apparent biological pause, penetrating deep (as much as one third) into the uterine wall. During preeclampsia, this second delayed implantation is incomplete (see Figure 11-1). As a result, vascular exchanges between the mother and the fetus are severely compromised for the remainder of the pregnancy. This secondary implantation failure is the major cause of human IUGR. In an effort to overcome this failure, pregnant women exhibit a

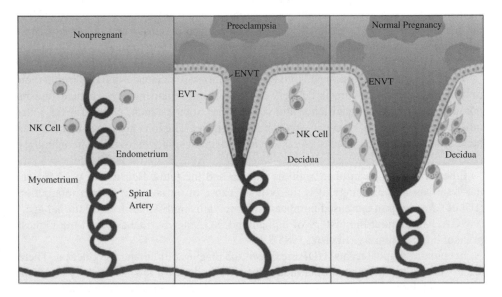

FIGURE 11-1 Endometrium in nonpregnant, preeclampsia, and normal pregnancy.

hypertensive response as a compensatory mechanism to try to provide as much nutrition to the fetus as possible.

The increased fetal nutritional needs at the end of the first trimester result in part from the increasing energy demands of the relatively large developing fetal brain, and this increased energy demand may be implicated in the need for the secondary deep trophoblastic invasion. The success of this second, deeper, penetration at 3 months of pregnancy may require a significant immunogenetic compromise in terms of paternal–maternal tissue tolerance when compared to other mammals characterized by a single trophoblastic invasion.

PREECLAMPSIA, DISEASE OF FIRST PREGNANCIES ALSO A "COUPLE DISEASE"

Complications associated with hypertension in preeclampsia and eclampsia are the result of a global endothelial disease in maternal organisms (Roberts et al., 1989). The complications are particularly likely among women with predisposition to vascular diseases (diabetes, obesity, thrombophilia). In young women (less than 25 years), however, before genetic predispositions for these diseases have been expressed, it has long been observed that HDP most commonly occurs in first pregnancies. It has been well known for three centuries that eclampsia and preeclampsia were "the disease of primigravidae" with rare recurrence in subsequent ones (Chesley, 2000). It has also been recognized for a considerable time that any kind of previous pregnancy (complete to term, spontaneous miscarriage or elective abortion) was protective against preeclampsia in successive pregnancies (MacGillivray, 1983; Seidman et al., 1989). Preeclampsia (and eclampsia) were also found to be essentially absent in primigravid women who conceived after a period of long sexual cohabitation (Marti & Herrman, 1977).

Preeclampsia and eclampsia have been also described in multigravid women with a short period of sexual cohabitation, such as multigravid women who have changed partners. In both multigravidae and primigravidae, HDP occur in approximately 40% of couples with less than 4 months of cohabitation before conception, 25% of those with 5–8 months, 15% of those with 9–12 months, and 5% of those of more than 12 months (and the same father in multigravidae) (Robillard et al., 1994, 1996). These data suggest that HDP/preeclampsia are not just conditions of mothers, but a "couple's disease" (Dekker, 1998; Dekker & Robillard, 2005; Robillard et al., 1994). Considering that HDP/ preeclampsia is a disease of first pregnancy and that multiparous women with a new partner have the same risk as primiparous women, it can be concluded that it is the first pregnancy with a specific partner that is of concern. This recognition is very important, because preeclampsia is no longer viewed as a condition of first pregnancy (primiparas), but more a condition of "first pregnancy for a couple," suggesting a paternal–maternal interaction in its etiology.

Any disease that is more likely to occur in new couples conceiving very shortly after the onset of their sexual relations suggests that it is very disadvantageous for a human female to become pregnant on her first ovarian cycles with a new partner. A relatively long period of sexual cohabitation before conception (at least 6 months) is required to lessen the incidence of HDP/preeclampsia (Robillard et al., 1994). A series of nonconceptive cycles may offer an opportunity for the maternal development of habituation to or a tolerance of paternal antigens. This is accomplished by sperm exposure, which is essentially an antigen challenge in the presence of immunosuppressive factors and tolerance promoting cytokines such as transforming growth factor beta (TGFß) and granulocyte-macrophage colony-stimulating factor (GM-CSF) (Roberson et al., 2003). This leads to immune responsiveness and later tolerance to paternal antigens, allowing the deep secondary implantation of the human trophoblast (Dekker & Robillard, 2005). The development of maternal tolerance towards paternal specific tissues reduces the risk of preeclampsia in subsequent pregnancies with the same partner. In summary, to reduce the risk of preeclampsia/eclampsia, conception in the human female should occur after an extended period of sexual cohabitation, regardless of parity of the female, if it is a first pregnancy for that couple. Interestingly, oral sex (specifically swallowing sperm) is suspected to be protective (Koelman, 2000), whereas using condoms as a regular method of contraception is a risk factor for preeclampsia (Dekker, 1998, 2005).

WHY A VERY DEEP TROPHOBLASTIC IMPLANTATION IN HUMAN PREGNANCY? EVOLUTIONARY CONSIDERATIONS

The very deep trophoblastic implantation in humans suggests that the human fetus exhibits increased nutritional needs as compared with other mammals. The source of these increased energetic demands is the human brain. The fetal human brain requires 60% of total maternal nutritional supplies in utero, compared with the 20% demand on maternal energy in utero in the majority of the 4300 other species of mammals (Cunnane et al., 1993; Martin, 1996).

CRANIO-FACIAL CONTRACTION IN PRIMATES

Since the end of the nineteenth century (Deniker, 1886) and throughout the twentieth (Anthony, 1952; Biegert, 1936, 1957; Delattre, 1952, 1958; Delattre & Fenart, 1954, 1956, 1960; Schultz, 1926, 1936, 1955, 1960), it has been noticed that one of the major evolutionary trends in primate and hominid evolution is an increase in cranial capacity simultaneously accompanied by cranio-facial contractions. The evolutionary changes in the base of the cranium were characterized by varying degrees of occipital flexion and prognathism, depending on locomotory patterns (bipedalism). Gudin (1952) pioneered a global architectural analysis in the sagittal plane, showing that flexure at the base of the skull corresponds to the face riding over the frontal bone. This morphogenetic pattern is found in many living apes and also in the evolutionary phenomenon of hominization. The three-dimensional organization of basicranio-facial architecture is controlled by the processes of flexure at the base of the skull, and this affects the morphogenesis of the two stages of the face, the maxilla and the mandible (Deshayes, 1986, 1988, 1991; Deshayes & Dambricourt Malassé, 1990; Dambricourt Malassé & Deshayes, 1992). This phenomenon, reviewed by Dambricourt-Malassé (1987, 1988, 1993, 2006), is found in all primates and in mammals generally. Cranio-facial contraction is minimal in prosimians, more substantial in monkeys (cercopithecids), even more so in great apes *(Pongo, Gorilla, Pan)* and australopithecines *(Australopithecus)*, and maximal in humans. In all these species, qualitatively, the nature of the process is identical during embryogenesis, but, quantitatively, it is the embryonic amplitude of cranio-facial contraction that differs among the various present-day primates.

SHAPE CHANGES IN THE CRANIUM AND INCREASE IN CRANIAL CAPACITY

In recent papers (Chaline, 2003; Chaline et al., 1998; Millet, 1997; Penin, 1997), differences in the shape of the cranium in some species of great apes, australopithecines, fossil hominids, and modern humans have been quantified by geometric morphometry (David & Laurin, 1992; Felsenstein, 1990; Rohlf & Bookstein, 1990; Sneath, 1967). For eclampsia implications it is interesting to link increased cranial capacity in the *Homo* lineage with ontogeny. The cranio-facial contraction process starts very early in ontogeny, and during this period, neurons duplicate at the rate of 5000 neurons/second. But this process lasts 2 weeks after fertilization in chimpanzees, for example, while it continues for 8 weeks in humans. The extension of this period in humans thus brings about hypertrophy (fourfold) of the brain, and it is interesting to note that the end of this phase corresponds also with the second trophoblastic invasion. Cranial capacity ranges from 282 to 454 cm^3 in chimpanzees, from 350 to 752 cm^3 in gorillas, from 400 to 550 cm^3 in australopithecines, from 510 to 1600 cm^3 in archaic *Homo*, and from 1100 to more than 2000 cm^3 in *H. sapiens*.

According to this view of cranial capacity increase, it is clear that the very deep trophoblastic implantation occurring in humans as a two-phase process may be explained in terms of increased fetal nutritional needs compared with those in mammals with smaller cranial capacities. Thus, the appearance of preeclampsia in humans seems to be linked to the development of a large brain in *Homo*. The most archaic species of the human lineage (*habilis, ergaster, rudolfensis, erectus, heidelbergensis, neanderthalensis*) exhibit less cranio-facial contraction and smaller cranial capacity than *H. sapiens*. The large increase in cranial capacity observed in *H. sapiens* suggests that preeclampsia could be a byproduct of natural selection for that trait.

These considerations suggest a new hypothesis for the disappearance of *H. neanderthalensis* some 30,000 years ago (Chaline, 2003; Robillard, Chaline, et al., 2003). Within the archaic *Homo* bauplan, characterized by reduced cranio-facial contraction compared with *H. sapiens*, *H. neanderthalensis* exhibits the largest increase in cranial capacity of the group, reaching 1600 cm^3, a value that falls within the range of variability of *H. sapiens*. We may ask whether this large cranial capacity was compatible with fetal nutritional possibilities at such a primitive stage of cranio-facial contraction and ontogeny. A hypothetical but possible single-phase process of trophoblastic implantation may have been inadequate for this large increase in cranial capacity, occurring in an archaic structure, and this phenomenon may help to explain, at least partially, the disappearance of Neandertals. The two-phase process of very deep trophoblastic implantation in *H. sapiens* may have been an evolutionary solution, a new character, an innovation, or apomorphy allowing the extended fetal nutrition required by the large increase in cranial capacity.

POSSIBLE BIOLOGICAL CLUES FOR "EXTRAVAGANT" HUMAN SEXUALITY, LOW FERTILITY OF HUMAN FEMALES, AND "LOSS OF ESTRUS" IN HUMANS

Among mammals, the human species presents an apparent "extravagant" sexuality: most human copulations occur at the wrong time to result in fertilization. Copulation takes place throughout the cycle rather than in a period of estrus, and ovulation is concealed from male partner(s) and often even from females themselves (Diamond, 1992; 2000). Further, although extramarital sexuality is ubiquitous in human societies, the human female does not employ the reproductive strategy of her mammalian counterparts, placing the sperm of different males in competition at the time of ovulation. Marriage is an institution in almost all human societies, leading to a longer average fidelity in reproductive couples than in many other mammalian species (Diamond, 1992, 2000; Kaplan et al., 2000). At the same time, the human female displays a rather low rate of fecundity (25% per cycle at the age of maximum fecundity). It has been calculated that in order to conceive a human couple needs, on average (albeit there are numerous individual exceptions), about 100 acts of intercourse. Demographers calculate a mean time until conception in couples without contraception of 7–8 months after the beginning of sexual relations (Léridon, 1993). This is unusual compared with the situation of other mammals, whose sexual relationships during estrus are very fertile. Incidentally, it can be added that once having conceived, the human female has a somewhat high rate of spontaneous miscarriage (15%). At first glance, these facts could suggest that the human female is at some reproductive disadvantage compared to her nonhuman mammalian counterparts (Léridon, 1993). On the contrary, extensive exposure to the sperm of a particular male many times before conception (in fact, the life expectancy of sperm being 3 or 4 days in the female genital tract, even with intercourse twice a week, she is constantly exposed all the year long—a very rare situation among mammals) and many pregnancies with this same partner may be a biological adaptation to the risk of preeclampsia/eclampsia.

As noted, human females exhibit an unusually low fecundity rate when compared to other mammalian females. This seeming paradox is coupled with a risk of HDP as high as 40–45% in new couples with less than 4 months of cohabitation before conception. Low fecundity and risk of HDP with first pregnancy seems like an unusual reproductive strategy. Human females are exposed to a roughly 33% risk of HDP in first pregnancies in societies without modern contraception (Robillard, 1999, 2002). If, on the other hand, we experienced a fecundity rate of 75–90%, 50% of the first pregnancies (with roughly a 20% incidence of severe preeclampsia, and 5% of eclampsia) would experience HDP. Rather than being an advantage, becoming pregnant quickly after onset of sexual relations with a partner becomes a disadvantage with respect to preeclampsia risk. Thus, a fecundity rate of 25% seems to be the best compromise between preeclampsia in first pregnancies without threatening fertility for additional pregnancies (multiparity).

Loss of estrus in the human female remains partially unexplained (Pawlowski, 1999). Because of the apparent advantage of a low fecundability rate in humans due to the reduced risk of HDP, the protective effect of "sexual exposure" with a specific partner (lost with the absence of constant sexual cohabitation in primigravidae [Robillard, 1996]) favored human females who were sexually attractive and receptive across their entire cycle. The protective effect of keeping the antigens of a specific male partner for successive births in women (lost in polyandry) induced a minimal rate of long fidelity in couples, probably not possible in estrus reproduction. The secondary and very deep specific trophoblastic implantation is coupled with the type of placentation, in which there is intimate exchange between maternal and fetal tissues (known as hemochorial placentation; see Figure 11-1). As a consequence, the successful pregnancy requires major maternal immunogenetic compromises in the face of foreign paternal antigens (Robillard et al., 2003a, b).

The cumulative net result arising from these various considerations would support the conclusion that the evolutionary strategy that occurred in humans seems to have been biased towards paternal tissue recognition through long sexual cohabitation in stable couples. Human reproductive characteristics that may also be related include loss of estrus, very low fertility rate, concealed ovulation, non-ovulatory sexuality, permanence of female sexual receptiveness and attractivity, absence of sperm competition in human females at the time of conception, and relatively large testicle size in human males (see Robillard et al., 2003a, b).

ETHNOLOGY: BIOLOGICAL, SOCIAL, AND CULTURAL ADAPTATIONS TO PREECLAMPSIA RISK

Infant as well as maternal mortality as a result of preeclampsia was a powerful selective force on the reproductive process of humans. The costs of preeclampsia are mitigated by exposure to the sperm of a particular male partner before a first pregnancy, providing females the opportunity to develop immunotolerance to foreign cells. This is coupled with a very low fertility rate and significant incidence of spontaneous miscarriage. In addition, there are cultural factors that serve to reduce mortality from HDP. For example, the majority of human cultures encourage marriages of long fidelity in reproductive couples (Diamond, 1992, 2000), and the vast majority of human groups prohibit polyandry (Deliège, 1996c). Further, the risk may have been an important contributing factor to the prohibition of incest in all human cultures (Robillard, Dekker, & Hulsey, 2002).

PREECLAMPSIA AS CONTRIBUTING FACTOR IN PROHIBITIONS OF INCEST AND SYSTEMATIC POLYANDRY

Except for some historical exceptions in royal families (ancient Egypt and Iran, Africa [Deliège, 1996a]), incest has been largely avoided in all human societies. Some anthropological literature states that incest avoidance is neither obligatory, nor properly human, nor a biological necessity, nor a social necessity. Arguments are that, except for genetic disorders, incest (i.e., parents/children, brothers/sisters) may have been a problem in only 1% of births. Even further, some scholars argue that appearance of homozygous deleterious genes by major incest would be advantageous as a means of getting rid of deleterious genes in the next generation (Langaney & Nadot, 1995).

In our view, avoidance of incest as a means to reduce preeclampsia risk may actually have a biological basis more significant than avoidance of the 1% risk of genetic disorders

(Robillard, Dekker, & Hulsey, 2002). Published reports suggest that fertility and pregnancy success is greater when parents are not genetically similar. It would appear that, biologically, females were favored to recognize the father's antigen as foreign (Grob, 1998). Couples with too similar tissue compatibilities often experienced repeated spontaneous abortions (RSAb), and the deleterious role of consanguinity has been extensively reported (Claman, 1993; Hussain, 1998; Surendeer, 1998; Zlotogora, 1997). Furthermore, after two, three, or four miscarriages during the first trimester, consanguineous couples—having finally achieved a "successful" pregnancy—experienced a significant increase of preeclampsia (Seidman, 1989; Thom, 1992). Contemporarily, this RSAb problem (i.e., at least three recurrent spontaneous abortions) occurs in very few couples (0.34%) by the random pairing of histocompatible partners in nonconsanguine populations (Claman, 1993). It would be expected to be much higher in societies where major incest was an accepted method of reproduction.

Concerning preeclampsia, recent data suggest that there is a highly significant increase of the female-to-male human leukocyte antigen (HLA) compatibility in couples experiencing preeclampsia (de Luca Brunori , 2000), but there are only a few epidemiological reports on preeclampsia risks among societies experiencing a high rate of reproduction between consanguines (cousins). Brocklehurst and Ross in 1960 (cited in MacGillivray, 1983) reported in Labrador 10 women with eclampsia in first pregnancy within an isolated group of British descent with considerable intermarriage across generations. Among them, five members of one generation from one family married five members of one generation from the same family. Of these five marriages, one remained sterile, and in the other four the women developed eclampsia. Three eclamptic women were married with cousins in the same family. There were eight cases of eclampsia over the three generations and three cases of eclampsia with the second pregnancy as well. The authors concluded that there was an inherited factor for eclampsia transmitted through the female line. Conversely, Stevenson et al., in 1976 (cited in MacGillivray, 1983), described a case-control approach to a population in Ankara where consanguineous marriages were frequent. Consanguinity was less frequent in women with preeclampsia (they did not present their results of women by primigravidity and other parities and consanguinity).

It is of note that among 565 cultures described (Deliège, 1996b), only two polyandric cultures have been reported: the Toda in southern India and the Nyinba people in Nepal (Deliège, 1996c). Interestingly, in these two groups, polyandrous unions occurred obligatorily, with brothers of the same family (adelphic polyandry) marrying the same wife. Conversely, inside the small high caste of Nayars in Kerala, South India, reproductive unions occurred with apparently total free polyandry. In addition to explanations of low polyandry as a means of ensuring male parental care or patriarchal control of women's fertility, an absolutely free systematic polyandry might have been noticed to contribute to higher preeclampsia/eclampsia risk and thus lower fertility.

ETHNOLOGICAL ASPECTS

Because of the importance of eclampsia in humans, ethnographers should be able to collect information on different human interpretations concerning convulsions and pregnancy.

The association between delivery and seizures should be recorded in one way or another in human memories (e.g., in myths, tales, songs). Cultural development of morals of these stories should be very instructive with regard to their interpretations of convulsions in childbirth. Particularly, it would be interesting to investigate whether this "curse" is directed toward the mother only or toward the couple. If the latter is the case, it may be that past cultures had noticed facts that modern medicine has taken a long time to rediscover.

CONCLUSION

HDP, and especially preeclampsia, are frequent in both the developing and developed world. In developed areas, hypertension is often associated with kidney or liver injury, and hospitalization is usually recommended. In case of threatening signs of eclampsia (maternal convulsions), the only treatment is to perform an emergency cesarean section and deliver the fetus and the placenta. This is a frequent concern of obstetricians and neonatologists and has implications for epidemiologists, biologists, immunologists, demographers, anthropologists, palaeoanthropologists, ethnologists, geneticists, zoologists, and others. Many of these disciplines have not been traditionally included in discussions of HDP.

The authors of this chapter are not aware of any ethnographic report of eclampsia or its associated convulsions and high mortality, notwithstanding that this is a common human reproductive complication factor with both biological and cultural implications. We encourage ethnographers to engage women, sorcerers, shamans, and other healers with the simple question: "What is the meaning of a young woman dying with convulsions giving birth?" Responses should give some clues of the extent to which this problem is known across cultures.

Further research to describe the biological pathways explaining the global reversible endothelial inflammation that is encountered in women presenting preeclampsia/eclampsia (Roberts et al., 1989) and the mechanisms of the paternal–maternal immunological conflicts leading to the poor implantation of certain human trophoblasts (Chaouat et al., 2005, Dekker & Robillard, 2005) is required. At the beginning of this twenty-first century, there are some hopes that these biological clues can be finally fully understood within one or two decades.

For zoologists, anthropologists, and others working in comparative reproduction, knowledge of hypertensive disorders of pregnancy may give clues to understanding certain features of human reproduction, including the two-wave implantation of the human trophoblast, the very low fertility rate of human females, loss of estrus, concealed ovulation, "continuous" sexuality, absence of sperm competition in human females at the time of ovulation, relatively large testicle size in human males, prohibition of incest, and low frequency of systematic polyandry in human cultures (Robillard et al., 2002, 2003a, b). If it is true that the "two-wave" process of implantation of the trophoblast is unique to humans, palaeoanthropologists may hypothesize that the appearance of preeclampsia during hominization may have arisen at a point in human evolution that brain mass of *Homo* fetuses increased to a critical point. Perhaps HDP can even help to explain the disappearance of the Neanderthals (Chaline, 2003).

CHAPTER 12

Breastfeeding and Mother–Infant Sleep Proximity

Implications for Infant Care

Helen Ball and Kristin Klingaman

Research into mother–infant cosleeping with breastfeeding represents a relatively new area for behavioral and physiological investigation inspired by evolutionary thinking. This topic within the evolutionary medicine rubric might well be the furthest along in terms of how much of the data produced by laboratory and in-home field studies is regularly incorporated into medical discourse and public policy, as this chapter by Ball and Klingaman describes. Diverse theoretical and empirical data are used to better understand the ongoing debate in Western industrialized countries concerning where babies should sleep and how and where nighttime infant feedings should occur. According to the dominant Western medical paradigm, infants belong in their own space for sleeping, and only if awake should the mother bring a baby to bed to breastfeed— and then neither can fall asleep until they are back in their proper arrangements. A sleeping mother constitutes a direct threat to the safety of her infant, this view claims. Ball and Klingaman point out, however, that it is only among economically deprived cultural subgroups (where breastfeeding is rare) and where bed sharing is practiced in a dangerous manner that infant deaths are statistically overrepresented. In addition, the authors describe how and why more optimal breastfeeding depends on close sensory mother–infant contact during both the night and day. And, as their review reveals, many mother–infant bed-sharing studies suggest that the mother's body regulates the infant's physiology in many beneficial ways. In turn, the infant's increased breastfeeding frequency, stimulated by maternal proximity, induces positive changes in the mother's uterus while sustaining, if not improving, her milk supply. The ease of breastfeeding with bed sharing also tends to increase the duration that mothers breastfeed. To sleep or not to sleep with baby, then, represents a quintessential anthropological practice that is articulated by Ball and Klingaman's evidence-based and evolutionary-based discussion.

INTRODUCTION

Few topics elicit more passion or prescription, from professionals and the public alike, than infant care. Issues surrounding feeding and sleeping are particularly controversial, having dominated public discourse on infant care for the past century. An anthropological perspective on this discourse highlights the competing ideologies of infancy in the public domain, components of which include popular notions of infant fragility and resilience, the cultural value attached to infant independence, public conceptions of infant development, and the prevailing sense of parental competence. Caregivers seeking guidance on infant care may place their trust in professionals and "experts" or friends and relatives, but they often do not realize that the advice they receive may vary according to the ideological objectives of the person or organization by which it is advocated. Parents seeking guidance on infant feeding and sleeping practices will find that health messages surrounding these issues change frequently as they occupy contested ground between breastfeeding promotion and sudden infant death syndrome (SIDS; also known as crib or cot death) risk-reduction strategies (i.e., "breastfeed through the night" vs. "do not sleep with your infant"). Each position inhabits an ideologically different locale (Rowe, 2003) and inhibits the realization of the other. The intertwined relationship of breastfeeding and mother–infant sleep proximity offers a compelling arena for the application of evolutionary perspectives. In this chapter, therefore, we focus an evolutionary lens upon the mother–infant feeding and sleeping relationship. We consider the recent historical changes in infant care ideology in Western societies that have shaped current ideas regarding infant sleep, explore the implications of infant care trends that have resulted in the decoupling of breastfeeding and sleep behavior, and apply this information to understanding why public health strategies concerning infant feeding and sleeping currently appear to be in a state of impasse.

"Evolutionary pediatrics" is an emerging subfield of evolutionary medicine that examines the link between infant caregiving practices and health issues that affect the entire life history of the individual. Its theoretical framework draws upon cross-species, cross-cultural, historical, and paleoanthropological evidence to inform critical examination of Western postindustrial and biomedical models of infant care. This relatively new aspect of applied anthropology has arguably achieved greater change in medical practice and public consciousness than any other branch of evolutionary medicine to date, as it is increasingly accepted by clinicians and parents alike that many contemporary infant care practices, often driven by medical and/or cultural ideology, are detrimental to infant health, development, and sometimes survival. By providing a counterpoint to the prevailing perspectives on infant care and development, researchers in anthropology and evolutionary medicine have revealed how culturally influenced ideas regarding the way parent–child relationships "should" be structured and the ways in which infants "ought" to behave may clash with the evolved needs and propensities of infants and caregivers (e.g., Hrdy, 1999; McKenna, 2000; McKenna & McDade, 2005; Small, 1998; Trevathan & McKenna, 1994). A mother's urge to cuddle her baby when he cries, for instance, conflicts with the cultural notion (reinforced by peer or intergenerational pressure) that one may "spoil" infants by cuddling. Regardless of their widespread acceptance as "traditional" methods of infant care in Euro-American societies, many practices such as formula feeding, infant schedules, and delayed responses to crying are recently acquired when placed in the broader context of the history of our species (Hardyment, 1983). The three brief examples below provide illustration:

1. The feeding of babies with artificial formula derived from cow's milk became popular throughout the twentieth century for reasons of perceived convenience, status, and modernity (Fildes, 1985), yet formula use introduces babies to allergens and pathogens, denies them the antibodies found in their mother's milk, forces their immature gut to digest the fat-dense milk designed for the infants of ruminant animals, and increases their risk of long-term adverse health outcomes such as hypertension, diabetes, and cancer (e.g., Cunningham, 1995).

2. The popularity of regimented infant schedules is a peculiar example of infant-care practice in Western clock-bound cultures. Scheduled infants who fed, slept, and played by the clock were introduced to British, American and New Zealand mothers by popular parenting expert Frederick Truby King in the early twentieth century, who were provided with sample schedules to follow in his "Mothercraft" manuals (Hardyment, 1983). Parents were advised to keep their infants on strict schedules for both timing and quantities of feeding and sleeping, an approach still in evidence, in modified form, in the routines and "parent-directed feeding" approach to infant care advocated in popular baby manuals today (Ezzo & Bucknam, 1998).

3. The encouragement of infants to "self-soothe" by caregivers resisting the urge to respond to crying and other signals is also unique to Western societies (e.g., Barr & Elias, 1988), where the notions that babies should not be dependent upon caregivers to calm them have influenced infant care practices. The origins of these views can be traced to American behavioral psychologist John B. Watson, who in the 1930s instructed parents on the fostering of self-reliance in their offspring, espousing the view that no child can receive too little affection (Hardyment, 1983). The method of infant "sleep training" known as "controlled crying," advocated in the United States by Richard Ferber (1985) and the United Kingdom by Gina Ford (1999)—whereby parents progressively delay responding to their infants' cries, and then respond only in a limited and prescribed manner—are popular modern descendants of Watson's authoritarian approach to infant care.

These twentieth-century parenting practices have become embedded in the cultural landscape of Western infant care (Valentin, 2005), yet formula feeding, infant scheduling, and controlled crying have all been associated with adverse infant outcomes such as gastrointestinal infection, dehydration, and failure to thrive (Aney, 1998; Howie, Forsyth, Ogston, Clark, & Florey, 1990), and all conflict with the evolutionary predisposition of human infants to be cared for by responsive, emotionally and physically available mothers who provide breast milk according to infant need.

Evolutionarily inappropriate care behaviors are not confined to the realm of parental care; medical care practices in the immediate pre- and postpartum period are also associated with detrimental outcomes for infants. Well-known examples include exposure to opiate analgesics during labor, which make the baby drowsy and unable to root and suckle (e.g., Righard & Alade, 1990); lack of immediate mother–infant skin contact at birth, which has similar consequences in preventing the expression of infant crawling and suckling behaviors in the immediate post-birth period (e.g., Anderson, Moore, Hepworth, & Bergman, 2003); separation of infants from their mothers on the postnatal ward, which hinders effective bonding and breastfeeding initiation (e.g., Waldenstrom and Swenson, 1991); supplementary feeds of water or formula, which reduce the infant's desire to nurse and also have the potential to introduce pathogens to his undeveloped immune system (Royal College of Midwives, 2002); aggressive treatment of moderate cases of neonatal jaundice (e.g., Brett & Niermeyer, 1999) and hypoglycemia (e.g., Hawdon, Ward-Platt, & Aynsley-Green, 1994) involving separation of mother and infant; and/or artificial formula feeding to treat "symptoms" that are normal corollaries of breastfeeding in the period between birth and the onset of full milk production.

INFANT FEEDING AND SLEEPING: THE MISMATCH BETWEEN INFANT CARE FASHIONS, EXPECTATIONS OF INFANT DEVELOPMENT, AND INFANT BIOLOGY

Rapid and dramatic changes took place in infant care practices in many industrializing nations between the mid-nineteenth and twentieth centuries (Hardyment, 1983; Hulbert, 2003). Principal among these were alterations in infant feeding methods and sleeping arrangements. The increasing popularity of "scientifically developed" infant formula, combined with sufficient wealth to permit the majority of families to live in houses with separate bedrooms for parents and children, led to the separation of mothers and infants for both feeding and sleep. One consequence of these cultural changes in infant care was their impact on parental expectations of infant sleep behavior. In the mid-twentieth century, when sleep researchers Moore and Ucko (1957) began documenting the developmental pattern of infant sleep, tables enumerating an infant's month-by-month sleep requirements were hugely popular (Hardyment, 1983; and see, e.g., Good Housekeeping Baby Book, 1956). The results of Moore and Ucko's studies quickly became regarded as normative milestones against which the development of all infants could be assessed. Seventy percent of the 160 babies they studied ceased waking in the night by the age of 3 months—and soon it became the advice of pediatricians and the goal of parents that infants should "settle" (begin sleeping through the night, defined as midnight to 5 a.m.) by 3 months of age (e.g., Better Homes & Gardens Baby Book, 1965). Although Moore and Ucko recognized that feeding type (breast milk or formula) had an impact upon infant sleep behavior, the establishment of prolonged and early sleep habits were their principal priority: "Unsatisfactory feeding is generally the first thing to be looked for in a wakeful baby.... Where breastfeeding proved unsatisfactory, weaning to a bottle or complementary feeds sometimes had an immediate beneficial effect on sleep; in other cases, strengthening the formula or introducing solids settled the child" (p. 338). As decades passed the pursuit of early and unbroken sleep in young infants became a parental priority, and expectations regarding the normal pattern of infant sleep development in both the United Kingdom and United States were culturally codified in pediatric and parenting manuals; the second sentence of the American Academy of Pediatrics' *Guide to Your Child's Sleep* states, "In early infancy, the first task is to help your baby learn to sleep longer at night..." (1999, p. 1). Hundreds of books (not to mention magazine articles and Internet sites) now extol a myriad of techniques for achieving a somnolent baby. What has been overlooked, however, is that the infants upon whom the common yardstick for infant sleep development was based slept in rather different circumstances than infants today: whereas young infants are now predominantly breastfed and sleep in their parents' rooms, in the 1950s most infants received formula milk and were placed to sleep in a separate room from their parents.

Over the last several decades, breastfeeding promotion efforts have succeeded in increasing the proportion of infants breastfed; currently 76% of mothers in the United Kingdom (Bolling, 2006), and 71.4% of mothers in the United States (Li, Darling, Maurice, Barker, & Grummer-Strawn, 2005) provide their babies with breast milk compared with a low of almost 20% in 1956 (www.lalecheleague.org), and breastfed infants exhibit very different sleep/wake development patterns from those of formula-fed infants. It is now apparent that Moore and Ucko's infant population was predominantly composed of formula-fed infants and that they recorded artificially premature settling (consolidation of nighttime sleep) of their subjects, in part due to the soporific effects of cow's milk, and in part due to the separation of infants at night from their mothers, who consequently underestimated their infants' night waking (Anders, 1979). However, the notion of these developmental milestones for infant sleep became cemented in parenting folklore as targets to be attained and subsequently gave rise to conflict between parental expectations that infants should sleep through the night at as early an age as possible (thus conforming to the culturally expected "norms" based upon formula-fed infants) and the biological requirement for breastfed infants to wake and feed frequently throughout the day and night (Carey, 1975; Quillin & Glen, 2004; Wright, McLeod, & Cooper., 1983; Zuckerman, Stevenson, & Bailey, 1987). This conflict has emerged as one of the barriers to breastfeeding in societies where parents of newborn infants value (and strive to obtain) prolonged and unbroken nighttime sleep (Ball, 2003; Greenslade, 1995; Marchand & Morrow, 1994; Pinilla & Birch, 1993).

The differences in sleep patterns between breastfed and formula-fed infants arise largely as a consequence of the human infant's inability to easily digest cow's milk (Raphael, 1976), which causes formula-fed infants (excepting those with a cow's milk allergy [Kahn et al., 1987]) to sleep more deeply and for longer periods at an earlier age than breastfed infants (Butte, Jensen, Moon, Glaze, & Frost, 1992). Infant sleep bouts gradually consolidate into a diurnal rhythm over the course of the first year of life, but breastfed infants— particularly those who are exclusively breastfed for at least 6 months in accordance with current health guidelines (DOH, 2001; WHO, 2001)—do not experience consolidation of nighttime sleep as early as their formula-fed counterparts (Elias, Nicolson, Bora, & Johnston, 1986). Additionally, infants fed artificial formula exhibit significantly different sleep patterns compared with breastfed infants in terms of shorter sleep latency (time taken to fall asleep), longer duration of rapid eye movement (REM; active) sleep, and a larger percentage of REM, while breastfed infants experience significantly more sleep interruptions during the night, are fed more frequently, and consequently have significantly more night feedings (Butte et al., 1992). The "...development of a long unbroken night's sleep by the early age of 4 months is surprising when considered from an evolutionary viewpoint, because human infants, like other primates, are physiologically adapted for frequent suckling and close physical contact with their mothers" (Elias et al.,1986, p. 322). Unrealistic ideals for infant sleep are now, however, engrained in parenting expectations and continue to undermine the confidence of new parents regarding their infants' normal development.

BREASTFEEDING MOTHERS AND BED SHARING

Greenslade comments that "many new mothers are quite unprepared to accept the frequency of breastfeeding which can be seen as often as two hourly because of the easily digestible nature of breast milk, especially when a bottle of formula may keep the infant quiet for four to five hours" (1995, p. 24). This conclusion was echoed by mothers interviewed in the northeast of England, who found the sleep disruption caused by frequent nighttime breastfeeding to be too much to cope with and switched their baby to formula within a few weeks of birth (Ball, 2003). Experienced breastfeeding mothers and lactation professionals acknowledge that minimizing the disruption of nighttime breastfeeding is important in sustaining the breastfeeding relationship over a period of many months. One nocturnal caregiving strategy that accomplishes this is for mother and infant to sleep together, allowing the baby easy access to maternal breasts, as well as requiring minimal sleep disturbance for the mother when the infant needs to nurse. Many U.K. mothers therefore begin the night with their infants in a cot by their bed, bringing the baby into bed at the time of the first nighttime feed, where the infant may subsequently remain to feed and sleep for the remainder of the night (Ball, 2002). We have termed this strategy (which represents the majority of breastfeeding–driven bed sharing) "combination bed-sharing" (Ball, Hooker, & Kelly, 1999), as the infant sleeps in a combination of places over the course of a single night. The existence of an infant care strategy combining breastfeeding and bed sharing is supported by studies of Western mothers in many countries (e.g., Ball, 2002, 2003; Blair and Ball, 2004; Clements et al., 1997; Elias et al., 1986; Ford et al., 1994; McCoy et al., 2004; Mitchell & Scragg, 1994; Rigda, McMillen, & Buckley, 2000). In examining the nighttime caregiving practices of 253 families during the first 4 months of their infants' lives, we found a significant association between breastfeeding and bed sharing: 65% of infants who had "ever breastfed" slept in their parents' bed (at least occasionally), while 33% of formula-fed infants did so (Ball, 2002, 2003), and for infants who were breastfed for a month or more, the association with bed sharing was even greater, with 72% of these infants being bed sharers. Likewise, Rigda et al. (2000), McCoy et al. (2004), Quillin and Glen (2004), and Baddock (2006) report similar significant associations. This indicates that the majority of bed sharing currently carried out in Western societies is done in the context of breastfeeding and that the proportion of infants who bed share will continue to increase as breastfeeding increases across these populations. These points are particularly important given the position recently taken by several national pediatric bodies (e.g., American Academy of Pediatrics) and SIDS organizations to advise parents against bed sharing (see below).

MOTHER–INFANT SLEEP CONTACT AFFECTS LACTATION

The composition of breast milk provides an explanation for the link between bed sharing and breastfeeding. The analysis of human milk composition has identified us as a low-solute, frequent suckling species (Jelliffe & Jelliffe, 1978), meaning that our rather thin and watery milk has a relatively low fat and high sugar content in comparison to that of other animals (Ben Shaul, 1962). Like other primate species with similar milk composition, human infants digest their mother's milk quickly and therefore suckle frequently—and mothers require the stimulation of frequent suckling to trigger milk production. Humans are therefore physiologically adapted for close mother–infant contact day and night— necessary both for the infant's optimal development in receiving the nutritional and immunological benefits of breast milk on a consistent basis (Stuart-Macadam, 1995) and for the maintenance of the mother's milk supply (Woolridge, 1995). Furthermore, as breastfeeding also releases the hormone oxytocin into the mother's blood and milk, it induces sleep in both mother and infant (Dettwyler, 1995; Hrdy, 1999). These interacting factors reinforce the position that sleep contact is an adaptive and common part of mother–infant nocturnal feeding behavior, and therefore that bed-sharing promotes breastfeeding (McKenna, Mosko, & Richard, 1997).

As mechanisms were sought to address the low rates of breastfeeding in postindustrial nations towards the end of the twentieth century, health practitioners began to accept that mother–infant separation undermines the initiation and establishment of breast-feeding (Esmail, Lambert, Jones, & Mitchell, 1995). Evidence concerning the impact of mother–infant separation on breastfeeding drives the current emphasis on practices such as skin-to-skin contact following delivery (Anderson, 2003; DeChateau & Wiberg, 1977; Goldstein Ferber & Makhoul, 2004) and rooming-in on the postnatal ward (DiGirolamo, Grummer-Strawn, & Fein, 2001; Perez-Escamilla, Pollitt, Lonerdal, & Dewey, 1994; UNICEF UK BFI, 2000; WHO, 1999). But despite the importance attached to close mother–infant contact by breastfeeding specialists, clinical research has only examined limited ways in which the brief period of postdelivery skin-to-skin contact currently practiced in delivery suites might be reinforced on the postnatal ward. This provided an ideal situation in which an intervention based on evolutionary medicine could be tested. In most maternity facilities, following 30 minutes of skin-to-skin contact postdelivery, the provision for mother–infant contact involves rooming-in with the infant at the mother's bedside. This is conducted either during the day with the infant removed to a communal nursery at night or (more recently) 24-hour rooming-in with mothers per-forming all aspects of their infants' care (Young, 2005). Research examining the effects of rooming-in has concentrated primarily on sleep and breastfeeding initiation, with studies demonstrating that separation of infants to neonatal nurseries resulted in less fre-quent breastfeeding (Yamauchi & Yamanouchi, 1990) and greater likelihood of breast-feeding failure (Buxton, Gielen, Brown, Paigee, & Chwalow, 1991). However, contrary to the popular belief that mothers sleep better in the immediate postpartum period if their babies are cared for by others, clinical studies have found that nighttime mother–infant separation did not result in an increase in either the quantity or quality of maternal sleep or in maternal alertness the following day (Waldenstrom & Swenson, 1991; Keefe, 1988). Studies have also shown that infants who spend their nights in nurseries sleep sig-nificantly less and cry more than those in their mothers' rooms (Keefe, 1987). Round-the-clock rooming-in is now standard practice in WHO/UNICEF Baby-Friendly accredited hospitals worldwide and in nations with progressive maternity care such as Sweden (Svensonn, Matthiesen, & Widstrom, 2005), but the practice suffers resistance from hos-pital staff and mothers on wards where infant nurseries still exist, and/or infant and maternal care is provided by different nursing teams (e.g., Gokcay, Unzel, Kayaturk, & Neyzi, 1997; Rice, 2000; Svensonn et al., 2005).

Although it is assumed that rooming-in provides mothers and babies with the chance to feed frequently (and rooming-in is clearly more favorable than nursery care), an evolutionary perspective provoked us to question whether a plastic bassinette at the mother's bedside provided sufficient opportunity for the close physical contact needed to reinforce the benefits afforded by delivery room skin-to-skin contact. We hypothesized that if prolonged and unhindered contact was beneficial in promoting the unfolding physiological and behavioral relationship between mother and infant, then facilitating contact for longer periods should lead to more frequent breastfeeding on the postnatal ward, which in turn may improve long-term breastfeeding duration. Our team therefore designed a study to examine the effects of infant sleep location on the postnatal ward of a tertiary-level hospital in Newcastle-upon-Tyne, United Kingdom. Details of the trial design, methods, and clinical results are reported in Ball, Ward-Platt, Heslop, Leech, and Brown (2006), and here we summarize the findings relevant to evolutionary medicine. Sixty-one newly delivered infants (experiencing only vaginal deliveries with no opiate analgesia) and their mothers (with a prenatal intention to breastfeed but little or no prior breastfeeding experience) were randomized to one of three arrangements for the duration of their stay on the postnatal ward: (1) infant in the standard bassinette [cot] at mother's bedside; (2) infant in side-car crib attached to mother's bed; (3) infant in mother's bed with rail attached to bedside—known as the cot, crib, and bed conditions, respectively. Mothers and infants were video-taped throughout their first two postnatal nights using a camera with a night vision lens to film in the dark, and after hospital discharge the participants were followed up by telephone interview at 2, 4, 8, and 16 postnatal weeks. Data from overnight videos were coded and quantified. Those infants randomly allocated to the bed or crib condition exhibited significantly more frequent attempted and successful feeds than those infants randomly allocated to the cot (see Figure 12-1) with no significant differences found in feeding frequency measures between the bed and crib conditions (Ball et al., 2006).

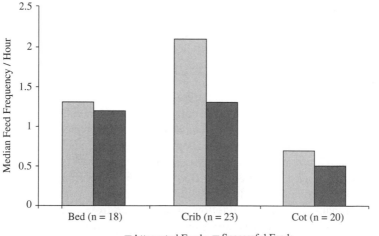

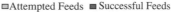

FIGURE 12-1 Median frequency per hour of attempted and successful breastfeeds for mothers and infants by randomly allocated sleep condition. For attempted feeds the difference between bed and cot and crib and cot were significant ($p = 0.012$; $p = 0.008$). For successful feeds the differences between bed and cot and crib and cot were also significant ($p = 0.003$; $p = 0.013$). There were no significant differences between the bed and crib conditions. All comparisons tested using Mann–Whitney U test.

Although superficially similar, as all conditions keep the baby within sight and reach of the mother, in practice the use of the stand-alone bassinette (cot) impedes breastfeeding by introducing a barrier between mother and infant (cot wall), which prevents unhindered contact; inhibits the infant's ability to root and initiate suckling; obscures the infant's cues from the mother; and by its height prevents mothers from retrieving their infants without either assistance or the need for getting out of bed (which following episiotomy or certain types of labor analgesia can be very difficult), thereby substantially hampering the ease and speed of maternal response. Prompt response to infant feeding signals and frequent suckling in the early neonatal period are essential elements in ensuring that mothers establish successful milk production—a process controlled by the hormone prolactin. Each time the infant stimulates the mother's nipple via suckling or touch, prolactin secretion increases rapidly (Johnston & Amico, 1986; Uvnas-Moberg, Windstrom, Werner, Matthiesen, & Winberg, 1990), and during the early postpartum period the amount of prolactin released is directly related to the intensity of nipple stimulation (Neville, Morton, & Umemura, 2001). The mother produces more prolactin each time her baby attempts to feed, so frequent attempts are key. Facilitating close maternal–infant proximity during the nights following birth is doubly important since breastfeeding at night triggers greater prolactin release than daytime feeding (Tennekoon, Karunanayake, & Seneviratne, 1994; Woolridge, 1995). A mother's initial copious milk production (technically known as lactogenesis II, and commonly referred to as the milk "coming in") is modulated by the amount of prolactin she secretes. Research has shown that both the timing of the first breastfeeding and the frequency of breastfeeding on the second postpartum day are positively correlated with milk volume on day 5, suggesting that frequent stimulation of prolactin secretion in the period between birth and lactogenesis II increases subsequent milk production (Neville, 2001). Infrequent suckling, on the other hand, is associated with delayed lactogenesis II (Chapman & Perez-Escamilla, 1999; Sözmen, 1992). The link between frequent early suckling and the timing and volume of copious milk production via the stimulation and operation of the hormone prolactin explains the potential physiological benefit of our infant sleep location intervention. Unhindered mother–infant access facilitates frequent nipple stimulation, frequent suckling, and particularly frequent attempted and successful feeds at night, thereby promoting the earlier onset of lactation and more prolific milk supply.

In addition to being critical for breastfeeding initiation, high initial prolactin levels are also important for successful *long-term* lactation. The maintenance of lactation (known as galactopoeisis) is dependent upon the adequate development of prolactin receptors in the breast tissue (Riordan & Auerbach, 1993), which results from frequent feeding in the early postpartum period (Marasco & Barger, 1999). According to Lawrence and Lawrence (1999) prolactin receptors are laid down in the first 3 months postpartum and are crucial in maintaining lactation following the switch from endocrine control (regulated by the brain) to autocrine control (regulated by local tissue). This means that frequent early feeding attempts will not only lead to effective establishment of milk production, but will enhance its continued maintenance. A common reason given by women in the United States and United Kingdom for quitting breastfeeding is a perceived or real insufficiency in breast milk production (e.g., Hamlyn, Booker, Oleinikova, & Wands, 2002), suggesting that inadequate quantities of prolactin receptors may have been developed in the initial phases of breastfeeding. As this may be a consequence of infrequent feeding bouts, particularly at night, we hypothesized that those infants sleeping in close proximity to their mothers on the postnatal ward in the trial described above (bed or crib condition) would have better long-term breastfeeding outcomes than infants randomly allocated to the stand-alone bassinette (cot) condition as a consequence of their more frequent early feeding pattern. To test this hypothesis, telephone interviews at 2, 4, 8, and 16 postnatal weeks ascertained breastfeeding status following hospital discharge. Figure 12-2 illustrates that although all mothers initiated breastfeeding on the postnatal ward, the proportion of infants from the cot group who were exclusively breastfed at home declined rapidly compared to those in the bed and crib groups. The association between unhindered versus hindered access and cessation of exclusive breastfeeding by 8 weeks was significant ($\chi^2 = 5.1$, df = 1, $p = 0.024$). The same pattern is clear for the decline in any breastfeeding: 43% of infants experiencing the cot condition were still receiving breast milk at 16 weeks compared with 73% of the crib group and 79% of the bed group (Figure 12-3), and also significant ($\chi^2 = 4.2$, df = 1, $p = 0.041$). Although this study was not powered to measure the impact of mother–infant sleep proximity on long-term breastfeeding outcomes, these indicative data suggest that such a trial is warranted.

An evolutionary perspective on early infant life views the mother and infant as a mutually dependent unit, behaviorally and physiologically intertwined via breastfeeding. The removal of neonates from their mothers' bodies for sleep has more serious consequences for successful lactation, and therefore long-term infant and maternal health, than is commonly acknowledged. In the year 2000, 23% of U.K. mothers who initiated breastfeeding in hospital were no longer breastfeeding 2 weeks later, with only 21% of mothers who began breastfeeding still doing so after 6 months (Hamlyn et al., 2002). The introduction of bedding arrangements facilitating unhindered access between mothers and infants on postnatal wards has the potential to increase these proportions dramatically

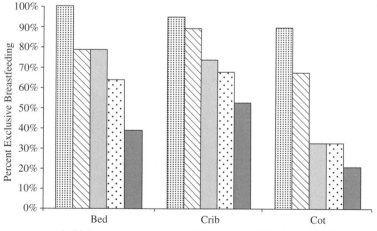

FIGURE 12-2 Percentage of exclusive breastfeeding at birth, 2, 4, 8, and 16 weeks among infants sleeping in one of three randomly allocated sleep locations (mother's bed, side-car crib and stand-alone cot) on the postnatal ward.

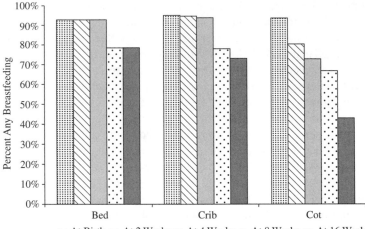

FIGURE 12-3 Percentage of any breastfeeding at birth, 2, 4, 8, and 16 weeks among infants sleeping in one of three randomly allocated sleep locations (mother's bed, side-car crib, and stand-alone cot) on the postnatal ward.

and to educate parents how to work with rather than against the evolved mother–infant relationship.

For most of our history and prehistory, successful mother–infant interaction in the immediate postnatal period was a critical component in infant survival. Natural selection has produced human neonates equipped with a suite of innate characteristics (nonlearned behaviors present from birth such as crying and rooting) that serve to stimulate and elicit maternal care and thereby enhance their own survival chances. A powerful mixture of neurochemicals and hormones primes mothers to respond both behaviorally and physiologically to their infants' cues and signals (Hrdy, 1999). Under the appropriate environmental conditions (e.g., unhindered physical contact in a safe environment with a lack of interruptions), the coevolved system of interaction, feedback, and exchange between a newborn infant and his or her mother unfolds spontaneously according to a predictable sequence (Trevathan, 1987). In suboptimal conditions (e.g., early separation, maternal distraction, lack of safety, maternal anxiety or pain) the process can be so severely disrupted that maternal and infant health, and even infant survival, is compromised (Ball & Panter-Brick, 2000). Only in the last 100 years has the development of medical technologies made it possible for large numbers of neonates to survive the immediate postnatal period without a mother. This is a significant achievement of medical science; but one that carries a price. So successful was medical technology in maintaining infant survival when mothers died or were unavoidably absent that about half a century ago, on the maternity wards of hospitals in industrialized societies, maternal presence in the earliest period of her infant's life began to be considered superfluous (Nusche, 2002). Mothers were confronted with an increasingly passive role in a birth process, which resulted in the removal of their infants to the care of medical experts. Fifty years later, despite all we have learned about the importance of physical contact between mothers and infants, some authorities are now advising mothers that not only is proximity to her body unnecessary for her infant's survival, it is explicitly designated as dangerous on the grounds of SIDS risk and fears concerning overlaying.

IS MOTHER–INFANT SLEEP CONTACT SAFE?

Coroners, pathologists, and epidemiologists are increasingly vociferous regarding the potential dangers to infants of sleeping with their mothers or parents (e.g., BMJ UK Health News, 2002; Byard, 1994; Weale, 2003) and acknowledge little or no value in breastfeeding-related mother–infant sleep contact. Coroners, pathologists, and the U.S. consumer product safety commission have used series of uncontrolled case reports of infant deaths as a basis for arguing that bed sharing results in accidental infant deaths (Drago and Dannenberg, 1999; Kemp et al., 2000; Nakamura, Wind, & Danello, 1999; Scheers, Rutherford, & Kemp, 2003), which have been robustly challenged (e.g., see McKenna & Gartner, 2000; O'Hara, 2000). Epidemiologists, on the other hand, favor odds ratios and relative risks—calculating the probabilistic likelihood of death for infants from SIDS or accidental death under a variety of sleep circumstances, based on the characteristics of infant who died in comparison with matched live control infants in large population-based studies. The assumptions of these studies are much harder to unpick and challenge, and in populations with exceedingly low rates of postneonatal mortality such as the United States and United Kingdom, risk factors for sudden death in infancy assume major concern. Prone infant sleep, parental smoking, poverty, and young maternal age are all well-known factors that increase the risk of unexpected infant death (Fleming, 1994). However, estimates of the relative risk of SIDS in the context of bed sharing vary widely. Although McKenna (1986) hypothesized a reduced risk of SIDS in the context of bed sharing based on an evolutionary perspective, epidemiological studies have so far found no protective effect. Assessments of the impact of bed sharing on SIDS range from no increased risk to the infants of nonsmoking parents to a 12-fold increase for infants sharing a sofa for sleep with a parent who smokes (Blair et al., 1999). Different studies use varied criteria to define what constitutes bed sharing (e.g., Hauck et al., 2003; Carpenter, 2004; McGarvey, McDonnell, Hamilton, O'Regan, & Matthews, 2006) and have produced a confusing array of statistics (see Cote, 2006). Furthermore, such epidemiological case-control studies consistently lack inclusion of infant feeding data in calculating the odds ratios or relative risks associated with bed sharing. Until more appropriate data are collected it is difficult to assess whether breastfeeding–related sleep contact between mothers and infants constitutes a risk to infant safety. However, it is unlikely that any potential risk would be of great magnitude (see Leduc & Camfield, 2006) given that breastfed infants have shown a reduced SIDS risk compared to formula-fed infants in several studies (e.g., Hauck et al., 2003; Hoffman, Damus, Hillman, & Krongrad, 1988). The negative picture of bed sharing that is painted by many epidemiological studies contrasts sharply with the evolutionary anthropological perspective on the importance of close contact and undermines the mother–infant breastfeeding relationship—all of which sets public health programs to prevent SIDS and those to promote breastfeeding at odds.

An anthropological perspective on infant sleep biology and parent–infant sleep behavior, including the evolutionary underpinnings and developmental benefits of mother–infant bed sharing, have been described in numerous publications (McKenna & Mosko,

2001; McKenna, Mosko, Dungy, & McAninch, 1990; McKenna, Thoman, et al., 1993; Mosko, Richard, McKenna, Drummond, & Mukai, 1997). They explain how mother–infant dyads that routinely bed share and breastfeed sleep in close proximity with a high degree of mutual orientation (facing one another) and arousal overlap (waking at the same time). When bed sharing, mothers placed infants in the supine position for sleep, and infants breastfed significantly more frequently and cried less than on nights when they slept apart from their mothers (Richard, Mosko, McKenna, & Drummond, 1996). However, because of the confines of the narrow hospital bed in which mothers and infants slept for these studies, it was unclear whether the orientation, proximity, arousal, and breastfeeding characteristics reported were artifacts of sleeping in cramped conditions or an intrinsic feature of normal bed sharing for breastfeeding mothers and infants. In recent years the results of McKenna and Mosko's studies have been replicated in at least three different settings, and breastfeeding mother–infant dyads have been observed displaying consistent bed-sharing behavior, regardless of whether they slept in a narrow hospital bed, a full-size bed in a sleep lab, or at home in beds ranging from twin to king-sized (Baddock, 2006; Ball, 2006; Young, 2002). Mothers sleep in a lateral position, facing their baby, and curled up around it. Infants, positioned level with their mother's breasts, sleep in the space created between the mother's arm (positioned above her infant's head) and her knees (drawn up under her infant's feet) (Baddock, 2006; Ball, 2006; Richard et al., 1996) (see Figure 12-4). The cumulative results of these studies provide a robust

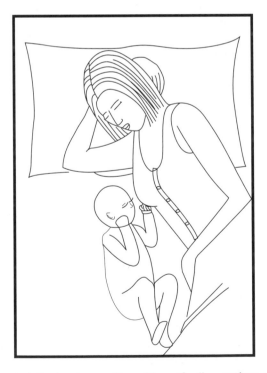

FIGURE 12-4 Characteristic sleeping position of breastfeeding mothers and infants when bed sharing.

understanding of breastfeeding–related bed-sharing behavior and suggest that the characteristic maternal sleep position observed in these studies represents an instinctive behavior on the part of a breastfeeding mother to protect her infant during sleep (Ball, 2006)—a view reinforced by the fact that all primiparous mothers in our team's hospital trials have spontaneously adopted this position without instruction on the first night with their new babies. Although we imagine this behavior to have evolved in a very different sleep context than one adorned with Western beds and bedding, the principle of infant protection is no less effective. When mothers curl up around their infants for sleep, they construct a space in which their infant can sleep constrained by their own body, protected from potentially dangerous environmental factors— be they predators, cold weather, or the suffocation hazards of quilts and pillows. In the current Western context, therefore, bed-sharing breastfeeding infants sleep flat on their mother's mattress, away from pillows, in a lateral or supine position. Despite the fears of coroners and pathologists (e.g., Byard, 1998; Risdon, 2003) that infants may be overlain, when a breastfeeding mother sleeps curled up around her infant in this way she cannot roll forward onto it, and neither can any other co-bed sharers lie on the infant without lying on the mother also.

Bed-sharing infants of breastfeeding mothers appear, then, to avoid the presumed hazards of sleeping in adult beds (e.g., suffocation, overlaying, wedging, entrapment, [Nakamura et al., 1999]) due to the presence and behavior of their mothers. Interestingly, however, notable differences have been observed in bed-sharing behavior between breastfeeding and formula-feeding mothers and infants (Ball, 2006). In a small study comparing 20 families (10 breast- and 10 formula-fed) videoed sleeping in their home environment, the formula-fed infants were generally placed high in the bed, with infants' faces level with parents' faces, and either positioned between, or on top of, the parental pillows. In contrast the breastfed infants were always positioned flat on the mattress, below pillow height and level with the mother's chest. Formula-feeding mothers spent significantly less time facing their infant and in mutual face-to-face orientation than did breastfeeding mother–infant pairs, and they did not adopt the "protective" sleep position with the same degree of consistency. Breastfeeding mothers and infants experienced a significantly greater frequency of arousals from sleep, and significantly more of these were synchronous (mother and baby waking together) for breastfeeding than formula-feeding mothers and infants (see Table 12-1).

The patterning of these differences is consistent with our understanding of the physiological mechanisms mediating maternal and infant behavior, in that breastfeeding mothers experience a hormonal feedback cycle, which promotes close contact with, heightened responsiveness towards, and bonding with infants in a way that is missing for mothers who do not breastfeed (Hrdy, 1999; Small, 1998). The implications of these data—that breastfeeding bed-sharing mothers and infants sleep together in qualitatively and significantly quantitatively different ways than do formula-feeding mothers and infants—indicate that epidemiological studies of bed sharing that have not considered feeding type as a variable for matching cases and controls may have drawn inappropriate results in assessing risk factors associated with bed sharing. One role of evolutionary pediatrics here is to persuade, encourage, and assist epidemiologists to re-examine these issues in ways that take into account the variations in infant care behaviors that are associated with different types of caregiving and which therefore are likely to affect their outcomes.

TABLE 12-1 Comparison of Bed-Sharing Characteristics for Breast-Fed and Formula-Fed Infants.

	Formula-fed	Breast-fed	Significance (Mann-Whitney U-test)
Hours of bed-sharing data (median)	7.6 hours	8.0 hours	ns
Orientation to mother			
Mother facing infant	59%	73%	$p = 0.05$
Infant facing mother	46%	65%	ns
Face-to-face orientation	32%	47%	$p = 0.02$
Orientation to father			
Father facing infant	46%	26%	ns
Infant facing father	20%	9%	ns
Face-to-face orientation	8%	0%	ns
Infant sleep position			
Infant supine	83%	40%	$p = 0.02$
Infant lateral	6%	54%	$p = 0.02$
Infant prone	0%	0%	ns
Parent–infant proximity			
Touching mother	60%	75%	ns
Touching father	20%	6%	ns
Parent–infant sleeping position			
Mother curled up round infant	25%	49%	ns
Father curled up round infant	0%	0%	ns
Height of infant in bed relative to mother			
Infant face level with mother's face or chin	71%	0%	$p = 0.01$
Infant face level with mother's chest	29%	100%	$p = 0.02$
Infant face below mother's chest height	0%	0%	ns
Direction of infant in bed			
Vertical position (perpendicular to headboard)	94%	86%	ns
Rotated between 30–60° to either side	5%	13%	ns
Feeding			
Median feed frequency/night	1.0 bouts	2.5 bouts	$p = 0.009$
Total feeding time	9 min	31 min	$p = 0.007$
Awakening frequency (medians)			
Number maternal arousals per night	2 (range = 0–4)	4 (range = 3–5)	$p = 0.001$
Number of infant arousals per night	2 (range = 0–3)	3 (range = 2–5)	$p = 0.006$
Number of mutual arousals per night	1 (range = 0–2)	3 (range = 1–4)	$p = 0.003$

Source: Modified from Ball, 2006.

EVOLUTIONARY PERSPECTIVES AND INFANT CARE

Anthropological works in the popular and academic domains such as Leidloff's *Continuum Concept* and Eaton, Shostak, and Konner's *Paleolithic Prescription* first applied an evolutionary perspective to infant development and infant care in exploring the mismatch between current parental caregiving practices and infants' evolved expectations. Over the last decade and a half, these themes have become the focus for researchers such as

McKenna and Mosko (2001), Trevathan (1987), and Dettwyler (1995), who have further applied evolutionary reasoning to issues of infancy. Studies of mother–infant sleep proximity, feed frequency, and breastfeeding duration build upon these foundations to demonstrate how the intricate, coevolved relationship between maternal physiology, breastfeeding success, and thereby long-term health outcomes for both infants and mothers are disrupted or reinforced by variation in infant sleep location.

Evolutionary medicine provides a lens through which we can observe the iatrogenic (unintentionally medically induced) effects of changes in infant care—such as the effects on breastfeeding of sequestering newborn infants in neonatal nurseries for the purpose of infection control, or the banning of breastfed infants from mothers' beds due to SIDS odds ratios—providing a perspective that helps to both challenge current practice and identify ways of ameliorating the discordance between culturally sanctioned practice and the evolved needs of infants, such as via the provision of side-car cribs on hospital postnatal wards. An evolutionary pediatric approach to infant feeding and sleep finds that bed sharing makes breastfeeding less "hard work" through enhanced accessibility, reduced sleep disturbance, and more frequent nighttime suckling, which stimulates prolactin release and continued milk production. As increasing numbers of mothers breastfeed their infants, the proportion of infants who bed share will increase, leading to greater conflict between breastfeeding promotion and SIDS-reduction advice and greater confusion for parents. Blanket recommendations against parent–infant bed sharing work antithetically to breastfeeding promotion and undermine programs such as the WHO/UNICEF Baby-Friendly Initiative. Huge successes have been made in the improvement of breastfeeding rates in postindustrial nations over the last decade as mothers have been encouraged to physically reconnect with their infants, so it is tragically ironic to read reports that around the world, and particularly in countries with traditionally high rates of breastfeeding, such as Taiwan and Sweden (e.g., Alm, Lagercrantz, & Wennergren, 2006; Huang & Cheng, 2006), physicians and national institutions are following the lead of the American Academy of Pediatrics in advising mothers to strictly keep their infants out of their beds for fear of SIDS and accidental deaths. By challenging the uncritical acceptance of public health recommendations and biomedical care interventions that disrupt the evolved physical relationship between mothers and infants, evolutionary medicine has begun to influence the recommendations of clinicians, epidemiologists, and policy makers regarding infant care and must continue to encourage a much longer-term view than is currently taken in the realm of infant public health.

CHAPTER 13

Why Words Can Hurt Us

Social Relationships, Stress, and Health

Mark V. Flinn

Many students and other readers of this volume are familiar with coming down with a nasty cold or some other flu-like virus or bacterial infection around the time of final exams and having to spend a good portion of their holidays in bed recovering. The mechanisms by which increased susceptibility to pathogens and illness follow particularly stressful social periods, activities, and disappointments are precisely what Flinn explores in his long-running research among children in a rural community on the island nation of Dominica. He emphasizes that not only can sticks and stones "break *(our)* bones," as in the famous folk saying, but additionally, the unkind words that act as substitutes for sticks and stones can still make children sick. Flinn explores the underlying physiological changes that are associated with social processes and interactions and how they affect or are affected by the human immune system. For example, children he studied in Dominica are more than twice as likely to become ill during the week following a stressful event than children who have not recently experienced any significant stressors. In general, he found that elevated levels of cortisol in response to stress seem to be part of a generalized resistance-lowering response. He broadens his research questions to discuss how and why, from an evolutionary perspective, subjective feelings are often necessary and used to negotiate, sustain, appease, and integrate ourselves into our respective groups and subgroups. Flinn shows here why the long period of childhood (and vulnerability to stress) serves a purpose, along with family systems, to mediate a child's responses to stress, illustrating why understanding cortisol production alone is an insufficient measure by itself to provide a true picture of the relationship of stress and illness. Accordingly, stress related to social situations is but one part of a much larger human adaptive system necessary for acquiring survival-related information and for gaining practice in building and refining the "mental algorithms critical for negotiating social coalitions"—abilities key to the success of our species.

Sticks and stones will break my bones, but words will never hurt me.
English proverb

We humans are highly sensitive to our social environments. Our brains have special abilities such as empathy and social foresight, which allow us to understand each others' feelings and communicate in ways that are unique among all living organisms. Our extraordinary social brains, however, come with some significant strings attached. Our emotional states can be strongly influenced by what others say and do. Our hearts can soar, but they also can be broken. Our bodies use internal chemical messengers— hormones and neurotransmitters—to help guide responses to our social worlds. From romantic daydreams to jealous rage, from orgasm to lactation and parent–child bonding, the powerful molecules produced and released by tiny and otherwise seemingly insignif- icant cells and glands help orchestrate our thoughts and actions. Understanding this chemical language is important for many research questions in evolutionary medicine. Here I focus on the question of why social relationships can affect health—why it is that words *can* hurt children, despite the attempts by parents to protect them with rhymes. Stress hormones appear to play important roles in this puzzle.

Human stress hormone systems are highly sensitive to social challenges. For example, levels of the glucocorticoid stress hormone cortisol increase acutely in response to events such as public speaking (Kirschbaum & Hellhammer, 1994), school exams (Lindahl, Theorell, & Lindblad, 2005), domino matches (Wagner, Flinn, & England, 2002), and a wide variety of other social–cognitive demands (Dickerson & Kemeny, 2004). Elevation of stress hormones can have short- and long-term health costs (Ader, 2006; McEwen, 1998b; Sapolsky, 2005), presenting an evolutionary paradox. We do not have good expla- nations for why there are links between the parts of the brain that assess the social envi- ronment and the hormonal systems that control stress hormones such as cortisol and epinephrine (adrenaline). Furthermore, we do not understand why these links are modi- fiable during child development, such that early experiences may permanently alter hor- monal response to social threats.

Evolutionary medicine is based upon the integrative evolutionary paradigm of Nobel laureate Niko Tinbergen (1963), who emphasized the importance of linking proximate physiological explanations (mechanisms; the nuts and bolts of how our bodies work) with ontogeny (development), phylogeny (ancestry), and adaptive function (how it was favored by natural selection). Using this approach to try and understand the paradox of stress response to social threat involves several steps. First, I briefly discuss why humans evolved what appears to be an unusual sensitivity to social and cultural environments. I then explore relations between physiological stress response and the development of social skills.

Hypotheses are evaluated with a review of an 18-year study of child stress in a rural community on the island of Dominica. My limited objective here is to provide a plausi- ble model and some new pieces of the puzzle linking stress response and health out- comes to the neural plasticity that helps us respond to the dynamic human social environment. Resolution of the paradox of why humans evolved psychological and hormonal systems that can result in "words making us sick" may have significant consequences for public health because it could provide new insights into associations among stress response, social disparities, psychopathologies such as autism, and peri-natal programming.

HORMONAL STRESS RESPONSE TO SOCIAL EVENTS: A BRIEF LOOK AT STRESS IN A CHILD'S WORLD

Danny was roaming the Fond Vert area of the village with two of his closest friends on a rainy Saturday morning. They had eaten their fill of mangoes, after pelting a heavily laden tree with stones for nearly an hour, taking turns testing their skill at knocking down breakfast. Now Danny was up the cashew tree in Mr. Pascal's yard, tossing the yellow and red fruits to the smaller children below who had gathered to benefit from this kindness. Suddenly the sharp voice of his stepfather rang out from the nearby footpath. The bird-like chatter and laughter of the children immediately stopped. Danny's hand froze mid-way to its next prize, and his head turned to face the direction of the yell with a mixed expression of surprise and fright. Ordered down from the tree, Danny headed quickly home, head bowed in apparent numb submission (from MVF field notes, July 14, 1994).

During the event described above, Danny's salivary cortisol level rose from 2.2 to 3.8 µg/dl in little more than an hour. That afternoon, his secretory immunoglobulin A levels dropped from 5.70 to 3.83 mg/dl. Three days later he had common cold symptoms: runny nose, headache, and fever (Figure 13-1). His two companions resumed their morning play, exhibiting a normal circadian decline in cortisol, and remained healthy over the next two weeks.

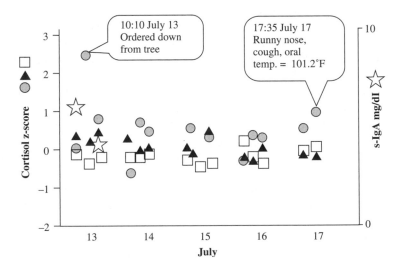

FIGURE 13-1 Morning, mid-morning, and afternoon cortisol levels of Danny (gray circles) and his two friends during summer 1994. Danny's cortisol levels were elevated and his s-IgA levels diminished after being reprimanded by his stepfather on the morning of July 13. Danny exhibits symptoms of an upper respiratory infection with slight fever on the afternoon of July 20. (Adapted from Flinn & England, 1997.)

This anecdotal case example contributes to a common pattern: children in this rural Dominican community are more than twice as likely to become ill during the week following a stressful event than children who have not recently experienced any significant stressors (Flinn & England, 2003). Humans respond to challenges in their social environments by elevating cortisol levels (Dickerson, Gruenewald, & Kemeny, 2004), often with negative consequences for their health (Marmot, 2004). This may be one reason why college students have higher rates of illness associated with final exams. Children lacking social support, including parental warmth and other factors that influence emotional states, seem to be at risk (Belsky, 1997; Davidson, Jackson, & Kalin, 2001; Field, Diego, Hernandez-Reif, Schanberg, & Kuhn, 2003). Why do social interactions, and a child's perceptions of them, affect stress physiology and morbidity? And, more generally, why is the social environment of such paramount importance in a child's world? From the perspective of evolutionary medicine, these "why?" questions ultimately involve understanding the evolutionary design of the psychological development of the human child (e.g., Bjorklund & Bering, 2003).

In Danny's village, located on the east coast of the island of Dominica, where I have lived and studied part-time over the past 18 years, most of a child's mental efforts seem focused on negotiating social relationships with parents, siblings, grandparents, cousins and other kin, friends, teachers, bus drivers, neighbors, shop owners, and so forth. Foraging for mangos and guavas, hunting birds, or even fishing in the sea from rock cliffs are relatively simple mental tasks, complicated by conflicts with property owners and decisions about which companions to forage and share calories with. In this village, children seem more concerned with solving social puzzles than with utilitarian concerns of collecting food. Other populations may have more difficult subsistence practices that require more extensive learning (e.g., Bock, 2005), but negotiating social relationships nonetheless appears universal and cognitively demanding for children in all cultures (Blurton-Jones & Marlowe, 2002; Hewlett & Lamb, 2002, 2005), as it likely was during human evolutionary history (Alexander, 1979; Bowlby, 1969, 1973; Hinde, 1974).

In the following section I review current theories of human life history and the family. I suggest that conspecific social competition was the primary selective pressure shaping the uniquely human combination of physically altricial (helpless) but mentally and linguistically precocial (quick to develop) infancy, extended childhood, and extended adolescence, enabled by extensive bi-parental and kin care. I then turn to the role that the links between psychosocial stimuli and physiological stress response may play in guiding both the acute and long-term neurological plasticity necessary for adapting to the dynamic aspects of human sociality.

EVOLUTION OF THE SOCIAL CHILD

The human child is a most extraordinary organism, possessed of a fantastic mind and yet innocent and helpless—in effect, a larva equipped with an enormous brain. Even relative to other primates, the human infant is unusually altricial and highly dependent upon parents and other relatives for protection, transport, resources (e.g., food), and information (Lamb, Bornstein, & Teti, 2002). The human child has evolved to rely upon extensive investment over a long period of time, often involving multiple care providers in embedded kin networks (Belsky, 2005; Flinn & Leone, 2006; Lamb, 2005; Quinlan & Flinn, 2005). Humans stand out as "the species that takes care of children" (Konner, 1991, p. 427).

The selective pressures responsible for this unique suite of life history characteristics appear central to understanding human evolution (Alexander, 1987, 2005; Bjorklund & Pellegrini, 2002; Flinn & Ward, 2005; Geary, 2005; Kaplan, Hill, Lancaster, & Hurtado, 2000). The delay of reproduction until almost 20 years of age, much longer than that of our closest relatives the chimpanzees and gorillas, prolongs exposure to extrinsic causes of mortality and lengthens generation intervals. What advantages of an extended childhood could have outweighed the heavy costs of reduced fecundity and late reproduction (Stearns, 1992) for our hominin ancestors?

The physical growth of the child, although a little unusual in its timing (Bogin, 1999; Leigh, 2001), does not appear to be especially difficult. The relatively slow rate of overall body growth during childhood, followed by a rapid growth spurt during puberty, may economize parental resources. A small child requires fewer resources than a large one. Hence, delayed physical growth during childhood may have facilitated shortened birth intervals for parents of such children, providing a demographic advantage (Bogin & Marela-Silva, 2003).

Brain growth, however, has a different trend from overall body growth. The baby human has a large brain with high energetic and developmental costs that consume more than half (!) of its total metabolism to build and maintain (Armstrong, 1990; Holliday, 1986; Leonard & Robertson, 1994). Although neurogenesis (nerve cell production) is mostly completed by the third trimester and synaptogenesis (development of connections among the nerve cells) by the third year of life (at a rate of 1.8 million synapses per second!), reproduction is postponed for another 15 years or more. What requires so much additional time to develop? And why burden the growing child, and its caregivers, with such a large brain that requires so much energy for so long? An evolutionary medicine perspective suggests that for natural selection to have favored this unusual life history schedule, there are likely to be some compensatory benefits.

One possibility is that a lengthy childhood is useful for acquiring complex skills: "immatures are enabled to live a protected existence whilst they learn skills necessary for adult life" (Bowlby, 1969, p. 63). But what information is so important and difficult to acquire that many years are needed for its mastery? Most juvenile primates spend considerable effort playing and practicing with their physical environment and developing fighting skills (e.g., Pellegrini & Archer, 2005; Symons, 1978). Compared with other primates, our basic motor skills do not appear significantly more challenging. Children may need time to acquire knowledge for tool use and complex foraging including hunting (Darwin, 1871; Hill & Kaplan, 1999; see also Byrne, 2002a, b). An extraordinarily long developmental apprenticeship is seen as useful for acquiring learned solutions to ecological problems unique to our niche (Bock, 2005; see also Blurton Jones & Marlowe, 2002). Investment in acquiring skills and knowledge via an extended childhood has been suggested to have a fitness payoff from increased adult foraging ability (Kaplan et al., 2000).

An alternative hypothesis for human childhood involves consideration of the brain as a "social tool" (Alexander, 1989; Bjorklund & Rosenberg, 2005; Brothers, 1990; Byrne & Whiten, 1988; Dunbar, 1998; Humphrey, 1976, 1983). This hypothesis suggests that many human cognitive and psychological adaptations function primarily to contend with social relationships, in addition to those necessary for physical ecological demands (e.g., hunting or extractive foraging). It appears that some human cognitive competencies, such as theory of mind, or ToM (this involves abilities such as empathy that help us understand what other people are feeling or thinking about), and language, evolved because of social selection pressures, (Adolphs, 2003; Allman, Hakeem, Erwin, Nimchinsky, & Hof, 2001). Our particularly well-developed mental abilities of general intelligence and executive functions (e.g., Chiappe & MacDonald, 2005; Geary, 2005; Quartz & Sejnowski, 1999) allow us to use mental simulations, "social scenario-building" (Alexander, 1989), and "mental time-travel" (Suddendorf & Corballis, 1997) to construct and rehearse potential responses to changing social conditions. These complex cognitive processes would be more capable of contending with, and producing, novelties of cultural change and individual-specific differences (Bjorklund & Rosenberg, 2005; Tomasello, 1999).

The informational arms race that characterizes human social competition involves substantial novelty (Flinn, 2006b, Flinn & Alexander, 2007) and hence requires unusual phenotypic plasticity. Although knowledge of the basic neuroanatomical structures involved with human social aptitudes has increased dramatically (e.g., Allman, 1999; Damasio, 2003; Gallese, 2005; Moll et al., 2005), the mechanisms that guide their development remain uncertain. Neuroendocrine stress response to stimuli in the social environment may provide important clues.

STRESS RESPONSE MECHANISMS

Physiological responses to environmental stimuli that are cognitively perceived as "stressful" are modulated by a part of the brain termed the limbic system (amygdala and hippocampus). Here we are primarily concerned with what has traditionally been termed the limbic hypothalamic–anterior pituitary–adrenal cortex (HPA) system. The HPA system affects a wide range of physiological functions in concert with other neuroendocrine mechanisms and involves complex feedback regulation. The HPA system regulates a class of hormones that are called glucocorticoids, primarily cortisol, which is normally released from the adrenal glands into the blood stream in seven to fifteen pulses during a 24-hour period (for reviews, see de Kloet, Sibug, Helmerhorst, & Schmidt, 2005; Ellis, Essex, & Boyce, 2005; Weiner, 1992).

Cortisol is a key hormone produced in response to physical and psychosocial stressors. Cortisol modulates a wide range of bodily functions, including (1) energy release, (2) immune activity, (3) mental activity (e.g., alertness, memory, and learning), (4) neural modification, (5) growth, and (6) reproductive function (e.g., inhibition of gonadal steroids, including testosterone). These complex multiple effects of cortisol make it difficult to sort out its adaptive functions. The demands of energy regulation must orchestrate with those of immune function, and so forth. Cortisol regulation allows the body to respond to changing environmental conditions by preparing for, and recovering from, *specific* short-term demands (Mason, 1971; Munck, Guyre, & Holbrook, 1984).

These temporary beneficial effects of glucocorticoid stress response, however, are not without costs. Persistent activation of the HPA system is associated with immune deficiency, cognitive impairment, inhibited growth, delayed sexual maturity, damage to the hippocampus, enhanced sensitivity of amygdala fear circuits, and psychological maladjustment. Stressful life events—such as divorce, death of a family member, change of residence, or loss of a job—are associated with infectious disease and other health problems during adulthood (Cohen, Doyle, Turner, Alper, & Skoner, 2003; Maier, Watkins, & Fleschner, 1994; Marmot & Wilkinson, 1999).

Current psychosocial stress research suggests that cortisol response is stimulated by significant perceived uncertainty (Dickerson & Kemeny, 2004; Kirschbaum & Hellhammer, 1994). From a child's view, important events are going to happen, but she is uncertain how best to respond. Cortisol release is associated with unpredictable, uncontrollable events that require full alert readiness and mental anticipation. Temporary moderate increases in stress hormones (and associated neurotransmitters such as dopamine) may enhance mental activity for short periods in localized areas of the brain and prime memory storage, hence improving cognitive processes for responding to social challenges (Beylin & Shors, 2003; LeDoux, 2000). Mental processes unnecessary for appropriate response may be inhibited, perhaps to reduce external and internal "noise" (Servan-Schreiber et al., 1990).

Chronically stressed children may develop abnormal cortisol response, possibly via changes in binding globulin levels and/or reduced affinity or density of glucocorticoid, corticotropin-releasing hormone (CRH), oxytocin, and vasopressin receptors in the brain (De Kloet, 1991; Fuchs & Flugge, 1995). Early experience—such as maternal licking of rat pups (Meaney et al., 1991; Takahashi, 1992; Weaver et al., 2004), some types of prenatal stress of rhesus macaques (Clarke 1993), insecure maternal–infant attachment among humans (Spangler & Grossmann, 1993), and sexual abuse among humans (De Bellis et al., 1994; Heim et al., 2002)—can permanently alter HPA response.

Early theoretical models of stress response did not attempt to directly explain the apparent evolutionary paradox of sensitivity to the social environment. Current perspectives view stress response as an optimal resource allocation problem (Korte, Koolhaas, Wingfield, & McEwen, 2005). Energy resources are diverted to muscular and immediate immune functions and other short-term (stress emergency) functions at cost to long-term functions of growth, development, and building immunity. Under normal conditions of temporary stress, there would be little effect on health. Indeed, there may be brief enhancement of immune (Dhabbar &McEwen, 2001) and cognitive function. Persistent stress and associated hyper- or hypocortisolemia (unusually high or low cortisol levels), however, is posited to result in pathological immunosuppression, depletion of energy reserves, and damage to parts of the brain (e.g., Santarelli et al., 2003; Sheline, Gado, & Kraemer, 2003). This highlights the problems with a stress response system that evolved to cope with short-term emergencies. The chronic stress produced by modern human social environments may present novel challenges that the system is not designed to handle, potentially resulting in maladaptive pathology (Sapolsky, 1994).

The chronic social stress hypothesis, however, is difficult to reconcile with the long evolutionary histories of complex sociality in primates, perhaps especially in our human ancestors. Why, given all the extensive evolutionary changes in the human brain, would selection not have weeded out this apparent big mistake of linking stress response with social stimuli? Modern human environments have many novelties that can elicit stress response (for example, roller coasters, final exams, and traffic jams), but social challenges in general seem to have a much more ancient evolutionary depth and, as suggested in previous sections, may be a key selective pressure for the large human brain. One possibility is that the energetic, immunological, and mental preparations for potential dangers is an unavoidable costly insurance, akin to expensive febrile (fever) response to pathogens such as the common cold viruses, that are usually benign—the "smoke-detector" principle (Nesse & Young, 2000). The idea is that although physiological stress response to social challenges is costly, and most often wasteful, it may have helped our ancestors cope with rare and unpredictable serious conflicts often enough to be maintained by selection. The benefit/cost ratio could be improved by fine-tuning stress mechanisms in response to environmental conditions during development.

A complementary approach to the mismatch hypotheses suggests that neuroendocrine stress response may guide adaptive neural reorganization, such as enhancing predator detection and avoidance mechanisms (Buwalda, Kole, Veenema, Huininga, De Boer, Korte, & Koolhas, 2005; Dal Zatto, Marti, & Armario, 2003; Le Doux, 2000; Meaney, 2001; Wiedenmayer, 2004). For example, in mice stress response from exposure to cats can have long-term effects on the central amygdala (right side), resulting in increased fear sensitization (Ademec, Blundell, & Burton, 2005; see also Knight, Nguyen, & Bandettini, 2005). The potential evolutionary advantages of this neural phenotypic plasticity are apparent (Rodriguez Manzanares, Isoari, Carrer, & Molina, 2005). Prey benefit from adjusting alertness to match the level of risk from predators in their environments. Social defeat also affects the amygdala and hippocampus, but in different locations than does predator exposure (Bartolomucci et al., 2005), suggesting that stress response helps direct changes in the brain to the appropriate places.

Glucocorticoids, perhaps in combination with other hormones and neurotransmitters, appear to facilitate the neurological processes that underlie some types of learning. The potentiating effects of cortisol on emotional memories and other socially salient information may be of special significance in humans (Fenker, Schott, Richardson-Klavehn, Heinze, & Düzel, 2005; Jackson, Payne, Nadel, & Jacobs, 2006; Lupien et al., 2005; Pitman, 1989).

Adaptive Developmental Changes in Response to Social Environment

> Environmental stimuli (in children mainly psychosocial challenges and demands) exert profound effects in neuronal activity through repeated or long-lasting changes in the release of transmitters and hormones which contribute, as trophic, organizing signals, to the stabilization [NE] or destabilization [Cortisol] of neuronal networks in the developing brain . . . destabilization of previously established synaptic connections and neuronal pathways in cortical and limbic structures is a prerequisite for the acquisition of novel patterns of appraisal and coping and for the reorganization of the neuronal connectivity in the developing brain (Huether 1998, p. 297).

If physiological stress response promotes adaptive modification of neural circuits in the limbic and higher associative centers that function to solve psychosocial problems, then the paradox of psychosocial stress would be partly resolved. Temporary elevations of cortisol in response to social challenges could have advantageous developmental effects useful for coping with the demands of an unpredictable and dynamic social environment. Elevating stress hormones in response to social challenges makes evolutionary sense if it enhances specific acute mental functions and helps guide neural remodeling (e.g., see Bartolomucci, Palanza, Sacerdote, Panerai, Sgoifo, Dantzer, & Parmigiani, 2005; Buwalda, Kole, Veenema, Huininga, De Boer, Korte, & Koolhas, 2005; Francis, Diorio, Plotsky, & Meaney, 2002; Maestripieri, Lindell, Ayala, Gold, & Higley, 2005; Mirescu, Peters, & Gould, 2004; Weaver, Cervoni, Champagne, D'Alessio, Sharma, Seckl, Dymov, Szyf, & Meaney, 2004). In the following sections we will examine the relationships between stress hormone levels, social challenges, and health in the everyday social environments of the children living in Danny's village.

SOCIAL ENVIRONMENT, STRESS RESPONSE, AND HEALTH: THE DOMINICA STUDY

Assessment of relations among psychosocial stressors, hormonal stress response, and health is complex, requiring: (1) longitudinal monitoring of social environment, emotional states, hormone levels, immune measures, and health; (2) control of extraneous effects from physical activity, circadian rhythms, and food consumption; (3) knowledge of individual differences in temperament, experience, and perception; and (4) awareness of specific social and cultural contexts. Multidisciplinary research that integrates human biology, psychology, and ethnography is particularly well suited to these demands. Physiological and medical assessment in concert with ethnography and coresidence with children and their families in anthropological study populations can provide intimate, prospective, longitudinal, naturalistic information that is not feasible to collect in clinical studies. For the past 18 years (1988–present) I have conducted such research with the help of many colleagues and students and the extraordinary cooperation of a wonderful study population.

The Study Village

Bwa Mawego, the village that Danny lives in, is a rural community located on the east coast of Dominica. About 500 residents live in 160 structures/households that are loosely clumped into five "hamlets" or neighborhoods. The population is of mixed African, Carib, and European descent. The community is isolated because it sits at the dead end of a rough road. The community of Bwa Mawego is appropriate for the study of the relationship between a child's social environment and physiological stress response for the following reasons: (1) there is substantial variability among individuals in the factors under study (family environments, social challenges, and stress response), (2) the village and housing are relatively open, hence behavior is easily observable, (3) kin tend to reside locally, (4) the number of economic variables is reduced relative to urban areas, (5) the language and culture are familiar to the investigator, (6) there are useful medical records, and (7) local residents welcome the research and are most helpful. The study involved 282 children and their caregivers residing in 84 households. This is a nearly complete sample (>98%) of all children living in four of the five village hamlets during the period of fieldwork from 1989 until 2006.

Methods and Field Techniques

Our initial objective in 1989 was to assess each child's general stress level as determined by the level of cortisol in their saliva. The idea was to see how this hormone was associated with a child's family environment. We also were fortunate to have saliva samples from different times of day in this initial collection and quickly recognized that very precise control of circadian patterns—in particular sleep schedules and wake-up times—was critical to accurate assessment of HPA stress response (Flinn & England, 1992). More than 30,000 saliva samples later, it seems we have more questions than answers.

In this study, monitoring cortisol levels over long periods of time is used to assess physiological stress response to everyday events, including social challenges. Saliva is collected from children by members of the research team at least twice a day, wherever the children happen to be (usually at their household). The large sample size of cortisol measures for each child (more than 100 samples for most children) in a variety of naturalistic contexts provides a much more extensive and reliable picture of HPA stress response than small sample designs. In the next section I briefly review some of the results from this study that may provide useful insights into relations between health and stress response to psychosocial threats.

Cortisol Response to Naturally Occurring Social Threats

Our analyses of naturally occurring stressors in children's lives in Bwa Mawego indicate that social threats are important stressors, with the emphasis upon the family environment as both a primary source and mediator of stressful stimuli (Flinn & England, 1995, 2003). Temporary, moderate increases in cortisol are associated with common activities such as eating meals, active play (e.g., cricket), and hard work (e.g., carrying loads of wood to bay oil stills) among healthy children. These moderate stressors—"arousers" might be a more appropriate term—usually have rapid attenuation, with cortisol levels diminished to normal within an hour or two (some stressors have characteristic temporal "signatures" of cortisol level and duration).

High-stress events (cortisol increases from 100 to 2000%), however, most commonly involved trauma from family conflict or change (Flinn & England, 2003). Punishment, quarreling, and residence change substantially increased cortisol levels, whereas calm, affectionate contact was associated with diminished (-10 to -50%) cortisol levels. Of all cortisol values that were more than two standard deviations above mean levels (i.e., indicative of substantial stress), 19.2% were temporally associated with traumatic family events (residence change of child or parent/caretaker, punishment, "shame," serious quarreling, and/or fighting) within a 24-hour period. In other words, family problems that we were aware of accounted for about a fifth of all the high cortisol levels, more than any other factor that we examined. In addition, 42.1% of traumatic family events were temporally associated with substantially elevated cortisol (i.e., at least one of the saliva samples collected within 24 hours was >2 SD above mean levels). Hence, family problems appear to reliably elevate cortisol levels.

There was considerable variability among children in cortisol response to family disturbances. Not all individuals had detectable changes in cortisol levels associated with family trauma. Some children had significantly elevated cortisol levels during some episodes of family trauma but not during others. Cortisol response is not a simple or uniform phenomenon. Numerous factors, including preceding events, habituation, specific individual histories, context, and temperament, appear to affect how children respond to particular situations.

Nonetheless, traumatic family events and social emotions such as guilt and shame (Flinn, in press a) were associated with elevated cortisol levels for all ages of children more than any other factor that we examined. These results suggest that family interactions were a critical psychosocial stressor in most children's lives, although the sample collection during periods of relatively intense family interaction (early morning and late afternoon) may have exaggerated this association.

Children residing in households with a stepparent have high cumulative mean cortisol levels relative to their half-siblings in the same household (Flinn, 1999; Flinn & Leone, in press). Children in bi-parental households have moderate cortisol levels (Flinn & England, 1995), with a higher proportion of elevations occurring in the context of positive affect situations such as competitive play, physical work, and excitement regarding novel situations.

Although elevated cortisol levels are associated with traumatic events such as family conflict, long-term stress may result in diminished cortisol response. In some cases, chronically stressed children had blunted response to physical activities that normally evoked cortisol elevation. Comparison of cortisol levels during "nonstressful" periods (no reported or observed crying, punishment, anxiety, residence change, family conflict, or health problem during the 24-hour period before saliva collection) indicates a striking reduction and, in many cases, reversal of the family environment–stress association (Flinn & England, 2003). Chronically stressed children (those in households with high—top quartile—rates of observed and reported stressful events) sometimes had subnormal cortisol levels when they were not in stressful situations. For example, cortisol levels immediately after school (walking home from school) and during noncompetitive play were lower among some chronically stressed children than their peers (see Long, Ungpakorn, & Harrison, 1993). Some chronically stressed children appeared socially "tough" or withdrawn and exhibited little or no arousal to the novelty of the first few days of the saliva-collection procedure. These subnormal profiles may be similar in some respects to those of individuals with posttraumatic stress disorder (e.g., Yehuda, Engel, Brand, Seckl, Marcus, & Berkowitz, 2005).

Although elevated cortisol levels in children are usually associated with negative affect, events that involve excitement and positive affect also stimulate stress response. For example, cortisol levels on the day before Christmas were more than one standard deviation above normal, with some of the children from two-parent households and those having the most positive expectations exhibiting the highest cortisol (Flinn, in press b). Cortisol response appears sensitive to social challenges with different affective states. Other studies further suggest that the cognitive effects of cortisol may vary with affective states, such as perceived social support (Ahnert, Gunnar, Lamb, & Barthel, 2004; Quas, Bauer, & Boyce, 2004).

There are some age and sex differences in cortisol profiles, but it is difficult to assess the extent to which this is a consequence of neurological differences (e.g., Butler, Pan, Epstein, Protopopescu, Tuescher, Goldstein, Cloitre, Yang, Phelps, Gorman, Ledoux, Stern, & Silbersweig, 2005), physical maturation processes, or the different social environments experienced, for example, during adolescence as compared with early childhood (Flinn et al., 1996). For instance, young adult women have a higher incidence of depression and associated abnormal cortisol profiles than children or young men in this community.

The emerging picture of HPA stress response in the naturalistic context from the Dominica study is one of sensitivity to social threats, a finding consistent with clinical and experimental studies. The results further suggest that family environments are an especially important source and mediator of stressful social challenges for children. In the next section data on the longitudinal effects of early traumatic experiences are examined to assess the domain specificity of changes in stress response; that is, does exposure to early trauma result in sensitivity to some types of stressors but not to others?

Ontogeny: The Early Trauma Leads to HPA Dysfunction Hypothesis

Early experiences can have profound and permanent effects on stress response. Exposure to prenatal maternal stress or prolonged separation from mother in rodents and nonhuman primates can result in life-long changes in HPA stress response (Meaney 2001; Suomi, 1997; see also Levine, 2005). Research on the developmental pathways has targeted the homeostatic mechanisms of the HPA system, which appear sensitive to exposure to high levels of glucocorticoids during ontogeny. Glucocorticoid receptors (GRs) in the hippocampus that are part of the negative feedback loop regulating release of CRH and adrenocorticotropic hormone can be damaged by the neurotoxic levels of cortisol associated with traumatic events (Sapolsky, 2005). Very high levels of cortisol can actually kill off the nerve cells that are responsible for turning off further cortisol release. Hence, early trauma is posited to result in permanent HPA dysregulation and hypercortisolemia (abnormally high levels of cortisol), with consequent deleterious effects on the hippocampus, thymus, and other key neural, metabolic, and immune system components (Mirescu, Peters, & Gould, 2004). These damaging effects may have additional consequences resulting from the high density of GRs in the prefrontal cortex in primates (de Kloet, Oitzl, & Joels, 1999; Patel, Lopez, Lyons, Burke, Wallace, & Schatzberg, 2000; Sanchez, Young, Plotsky, & Insel, 2000), where much of the executive function or higher learning processes occur.

The specific mechanisms affecting relations between exposure to trauma early in development and subsequent HPA system function in humans are not as well documented as in animal studies. Nonetheless, a similar causal linkage appears plausible (e.g., Essex et al., 2002; Heim et al., 2000; Lupien et al., 2005; O'Conner, Heron, Golding, Glover, & ALSPAC study team, 2003; Teicher, Andersen, Polcari, Anderson, Navalta, & Kim, 2003).

Children in the Bwa Mawego study who were exposed to the stress of hurricanes and political upheavals during infancy or in utero do not have any apparent differences in cortisol profiles when compared to children who were not exposed to such stressors. Children exposed to the stress of parental divorce, death, or abuse (hereafter "early family trauma" or EFT), however, have higher cortisol and morbidity (Figure 13-2) levels at age 10 than other children. Based on analogy with the nonhuman research discussed previously, two key factors could be involved with these results for EFT children: (1) diminished hippocampal GR receptor functioning, resulting in less effective negative feedback regulation of cortisol levels, and (2) enhanced sensitivity to perceived

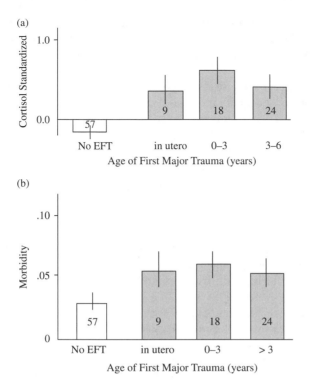

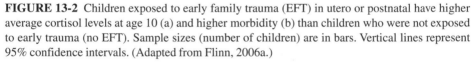

FIGURE 13-2 Children exposed to early family trauma (EFT) in utero or postnatal have higher average cortisol levels at age 10 (a) and higher morbidity (b) than children who were not exposed to early trauma (no EFT). Sample sizes (number of children) are in bars. Vertical lines represent 95% confidence intervals. (Adapted from Flinn, 2006a.)

social threats. Children usually elevate cortisol in response to strenuous physical activity, but rapidly return to normal levels. If EFT has affected the negative feedback loop, then recovery to normal cortisol levels would be slower. Resumption of normal cortisol levels after physical stressors, however, is similar regardless of early experience of family trauma (Figure 13-3). Cortisol profiles following social stressors, however, indicate that EFT children sustain elevated cortisol levels longer than non-EFT children (Figure 13-4).

The enhanced HPA stress response of children in this community that were exposed to EFT appears primarily focused on social challenges, suggesting that the developmental effects of early trauma on stress response may be domain-specific and even context-specific. These results are consistent with studies of the effects of social defeat in rodents and nonhuman primates (e.g., Kaiser & Sachser, 2005; Wiedenmayer, 2004).

Stress and Health Outcomes

A large and convincing research literature confirms commonsense intuition that psychosocial stress affects health (Ader et al., 2006). Retrospective studies indicate that

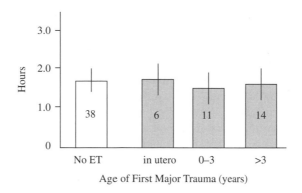

FIGURE 13-3 Children exposed to early family trauma (ET) do not have slower recovery to normal cortisol levels after physical stressors than no-ET children do. Sample sizes (number of children) are in bars. Vertical lines represent 95% confidence intervals. (Adapted from Flinn, 2006a.)

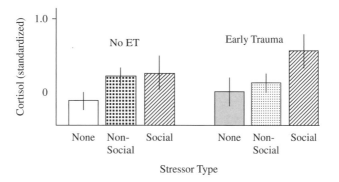

FIGURE 13-4 Children exposed to early family trauma (ET) have higher cortisol levels in response to social stressors, but not nonsocial stressors, than no-ET children. Vertical lines represent 95% confidence intervals. (Adapted from Flinn, 2006a.)

traumatic life events, such as divorce or death of a close relative, are associated with subsequent health problems, such as cancer or cardiovascular disease. Clinical studies indicate that individuals with stressful lives are more susceptible to the common cold (Mason et al., 1979).

Stress response may deplete cellular energy and immune reserves. Although cortisol may provide short-term benefits, the body needs to replenish energy reserves to provide for immunity, growth, and other functions. Hence chronic stress and high average cortisol levels are predicted to be associated with frequency of illness. Chronically stressed children with high cortisol levels tend to be ill more frequently than children in normal stress environments (Flinn & England, 2003). Short-term temporal patterns of cortisol and observed stressful events also are associated with increased risk of illness, as anecdotally illustrated in the previous example of Danny (Figure 13-1), in which illness follows a high stress event. Children in Bwa Mawego have a nearly twofold increased risk of illness for several days following naturally occurring high-stress events such as a family crisis (Figure 13-5).

These prospective data suggest that stress increases vulnerability to infectious disease; however, they do not demonstrate a direct effect of cortisol. Sleep disruption and poor nutrition often accompany social trauma. Stressful events may be associated with increased exposure to pathogens, resulting, for example, from trips to town by family members or residence changes. Stressful events may be more likely when family members are ill. Common infectious diseases are more prevalent during stressful seasonal periods such as Christmas, start of school, and carnival. A more direct causality would be indicated by immunosuppressive effects of stress.

Numerous (hundreds) of specific interactions between stress endocrinology and immune function have been identified (Ader et al., 2006). Indeed, so many different and complex mechanisms appear to be involved in psychoneuroimmunological (PNI) interactions that a general explanation remains elusive. It seems paradoxical that an organism would suppress immune response during periods of stress when exposure and vulnerability to pathogens may be high.

Several nonexclusive, complementary hypotheses appear feasible:

1. Allocation of energy to "emergency" demands may favor diversion from immunity (Sapolsky, 1994).
2. Overactive defensive responses to stress can result in autoimmunity; anti-inflammatory effects of glucocorticoid stress hormones may be protective of some types of tissues (Munck, Guyre, & Holbrook, 1984).
3. The possibility of damage to peripheral tissues generating novel antigens (e.g., collagen in joints) during exposure to stressors, such as disease and strenuous physical or mental activity, may require particular suppression of immune function.

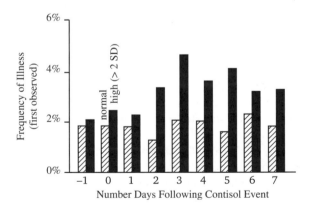

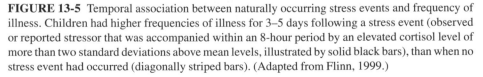

FIGURE 13-5 Temporal association between naturally occurring stress events and frequency of illness. Children had higher frequencies of illness for 3–5 days following a stress event (observed or reported stressor that was accompanied within an 8-hour period by an elevated cortisol level of more than two standard deviations above mean levels, illustrated by solid black bars), than when no stress event had occurred (diagonally striped bars). (Adapted from Flinn, 1999.)

4. The movements of immune cells may be enhanced or focused by localized overrides of the general immuno-suppressive effects of cortisol.

The complexity and dynamics of the immune system make assessment of immune function difficult. We have conducted an exploratory investigation of several components of immune function among children in Bwa Mawego using saliva samples. Preliminary analyses of these data suggest that psychosocial stress may have different effects on the different components of immune function. Apparent differences between immune functioning of chronically stressed and normal children include lower levels of s-IgA and neopterin (Flinn & England, 2003). These measures change in response to stress events and illness. Temporal patterns of immune function appear to differ slightly between normal and chronically stressed children. We do not know if these differences affect morbidity for any specific pathogen, but they are suggestive of possible links among psychosocial stress, immune function, and illness.

SUMMARY AND CONCLUDING REMARKS

Hormonal stress response may be viewed as an adaptive mechanism that allocates energy resources to different bodily functions, including immunity, growth, muscle action, and cognition (McEwen, 1995; Sapolsky, 2005). Understanding stress response is important because of consequences for health and psychological development. The perspective of evolutionary medicine provides new ways of looking at this important problem.

The objective of the long-term bio-cultural study in Bwa Mawego is to monitor children's social and physical environment, behavioral activities, health, and physiological states in a naturalistic setting so as to better understand relationships among family environment, stress responses, and health. Analyses of data indicate that children living in households with intensive, stable caretaking usually had moderate cortisol levels and low frequency of illness. Children living in households with nonintensive, unstable caretaking were more likely to have abnormal (usually high and variable, but sometimes low) cortisol levels. Traumatic family events were associated temporally with elevated cortisol levels. Some children with caretaking and growth problems during infancy had unusual cortisol profiles. These associations indicate that family environment was a significant source of stress and illness risk for children living in Bwa Mawego. The variability of stress response, however, suggests a complex mix of each child's perceptions, neuroendocrinology, temperament, and specific context.

Relationships between family environment and cortisol stress response appear to result from a combination of factors. These include frequency of traumatic events, frequency of positive affectionate interactions, frequency of negative interactions such as irrational punishment, frequency of residence change, security of attachment, development of coping abilities, and availability or intensity of caretaking attention. Probably the most important correlate of household composition that affects childhood stress is maternal care. Mothers in socially secure households (i.e., permanent amiable co-residence with mate and/or other kin) appeared more able and more motivated to provide physical, social, and psychological care for their children. Mothers without mate or kin support were likely to exert effort attracting potential mates and may have viewed dependent children as impediments to this. Hence, co-residence of father may provide not only direct benefits from paternal care, but may also affect maternal care (Belsky et al., 2005). Young mothers without mate support usually relied extensively upon their parents or other kin for help with childcare (Flinn & Leone, in press).

Children born and raised in household environments in which mothers have little or no mate or kin support were at greatest risk for abnormal cortisol profiles and associated health problems. Because socioeconomic conditions influence family environment, they have consequences for child health that extend beyond direct material effects.

Returning to the paradox of why natural selection favored sensitivity of stress response to social stimuli in the human child, several points emerge. Childhood is necessary and useful for acquiring the information and practice to build and refine the mental algorithms critical for negotiating the social coalitions that are key to success in our species. Mastering the social environment presents special challenges for the human child (e.g., Lamb, 2005). Social competence is difficult because the competition—one's peers—is constantly changing and similarly equipped with theory of mind and other cognitive abilities. Results from the Dominica study indicate that family environment is a primary source and mediator of stressful events in a child's world. The sensitivity of stress physiology to the social environment may facilitate adaptive mental responses to this challenging aspect of a child's world.

Coping with social problems, however, can have significant health consequences, ranging from dysregulation of emotional control and increased risk of psychopathology (Gilbert, 2001; Nesse, 1999) to broader health issues associated with social and economic disparities (Marmot & Wilkerson, 1999). The potential for intergenerational cycles that perpetuate social relationships that affect stress (Belsky, 2005; Belsky, Jaffee, Sligo, Woodward, & Silva, 2005; Maestripieri, Lindell, Ayala, Gold, & Higley, 2005) and poor health are especially concerning.

We are still far from identifying the specific mechanisms linking stress response to psychological development and health outcomes. An evolutionary medicine perspective can be useful in these efforts to understand this critical aspect of a child's world by integrating knowledge of physiological causes with the logic of adaptive design by natural selection. It reminds us that medical practice and public health can benefit from consideration of our evolutionary history as extraordinarily social creatures. We evolved to have feelings and thoughts focused on social relationships. Our thoughts and feelings, however, are not without costs; they can affect our health, sometimes in very important and significant ways. Cancer, atherosclerosis, infectious disease, and many other health problems are linked to our social and emotional well-being (Ader et al., 2006). Our stress response systems appear to have an important evolved role in this connection.

CHAPTER 14

Why Are We Vulnerable to Acute Mountain Sickness?

Cynthia M. Beall

Have worldwide fluctuating oxygen levels influenced human evolution? This is a fascinating question that is used as the background to introduce us to Beall's exploration of acute mountain sickness, a human physiological response to decreased oxygen pressures at higher elevations. A variety of data suggest that during the last 2 billion years the earth's oxygen levels have fluctuated between about 10 and 30% as compared to 21% today. It was not low during the geological time periods that frame human evolution, perhaps a good thing. Beall observes that throughout hominin evolution natural selection did not favor oxygen storage in human tissues, which suggests that it might not have been useful to evolve that particular characteristic. Throughout her contribution Beall reviews the physiology and clinical characteristics of acute mountain sickness experiences. She uses an evolutionary line of questioning to determine, among other things, if this potentially life-threatening response to lowering oxygen pressure at increased elevations is a defect or a defense against hypoxia. She explores the more difficult question of whether it is a short-term acclimatization process, much like tanning, or a true adaptation—an evolved response, which enhances both immediate and long-term survival and reproductive success under more diverse environmental conditions. She asks if mountain sickness can be seen as a genetic adaptation or as a simple epiphenomenon, i.e., if it can be better explained by something else, perhaps quite independently, and not just as an evolved protective response. It may well be that what we call mountain sickness is a general reflection of how we respond to stress and how the evolved biochemical system, in relation to the central cardiopulmonary control systems, struggles to make the best out of a very bad immediate situation. The answer to several of these questions is as Beall concludes: we simply do not know.

Next, one comes to Big Headache and Little Headache Mountains.... They make a man so hot that his face turns pale, his head aches, and he begins to vomit...

Too Kin, original translation in Gilbert, 1983, p. 316

259

This passage, written by a Chinese diplomat traveling through the Karakoram Range in western China sometime between 37 and 32 B.C. describes vividly a case of acute mountain sickness (AMS), a "constellation of symptoms in the context of a recent gain in altitude..." (Barry & Pollard, 2003, p. 915). Millions of people travel to high altitude (frequently defined as 2500 m [8250 ft] or higher) for pleasure and business every year. Many experience headache, loss of appetite, nausea, dizziness, or insomnia, typically 6–12 hours after arrival and often after the first night at high altitude (Bartsch & Roach, 2001; Basnyat & Murdoch, 2003). AMS is considered "a benign, self-limiting illness" (Bartsch & Roach, 2001, p. 731) that typically resolves after a few days at high altitude as biological responses engage. A small proportion of people develop life-threatening high-altitude pulmonary edema or high-altitude cerebral edema, but it is not clear whether these are severe forms of AMS or separate diseases. This chapter focuses on AMS, the relatively mild high-altitude illness that affects a large proportion of travelers to high-altitude areas.

The environmental cause of AMS is a relative lack of oxygen (hypoxia) due to the progressive fall in barometric pressure that accompanies high altitude and the consequently fewer molecules of air, including oxygen, per volume of air. For example, at altitudes of 1500 m (5000 ft), 3000 m (9900 ft), and 4500 m (15,000 ft), each liter of air in a breath contains 17%, 32%, and 44%, respectively, fewer oxygen molecules than at sea level. High-altitude or hypobaric (low-pressure) hypoxia is the term for less than the normal sea-level amount of oxygen in the air.

Inhaling fewer oxygen molecules severely disrupts homeostasis because air is the only source of the oxygen that is essential for terrestrial animal life. Animals, including humans, depend on oxygen-using metabolic energy production, also called aerobic or oxidative metabolism, which uses 95% of the oxygen we consume (Babcock, 1999). Oxygen is both vital and dangerous: it reacts rapidly and destructively with other molecules. Thus, organisms do not store oxygen, but instead require an uninterrupted supply.

While the environmental cause of AMS is clear, a number of recent authoritative reviews agree that the pathophysiology—the proximate cause—is unknown, despite decades of research (Barry & Pollard, 2003; Bartsch & Roach, 2001; Basnyat & Murdoch, 2003; Gallagher & Hackett, 2004; Roach & Hackett, 2001; Rodway, Hoffman, & Sanders, 2003). The purpose of this chapter is to take an evolutionary medicine approach to addressing the question: "Why are we vulnerable to acute mountain sickness?" This approach considers both the ultimate evolutionary explanation for the existence of AMS and the proximate explanation for its biological basis.

EPIDEMIOLOGY OF AMS

Because there are no clinical tests or objective measures, diagnosis of AMS relies on self-report of symptoms. Scoring systems based on responses to standardized questionnaires have been developed to allow data collection and reporting that is comparable across studies (Roach, Bartsch, Hackett, Oelz, & Committee, 1993; Sampson, Cymerman, Burse, Maher, & Rock, 1983). According to the widely used Lake Louise scoring system, "A diagnosis of AMS is based on a recent gain in altitude, at least several hours at the new altitude, and the presence of headache and at least one of the following symptoms: gastrointestinal upset (anorexia, nausea, or vomiting), fatigue or weakness, dizziness or lightheadedness and difficulty sleeping" (Roach et al., 1993, pp. 272–273).

The prevalence of AMS increases with altitude (it is rare below 2500 m [8250 ft]). For example, the prevalence of AMS among climbers in the Swiss Alps increased from 9% at 2850 m (9405 ft) to 13% at 3050 m (10,065 ft), 34% at 3650 m (12,045 ft), and 53% at 4559 m (15,045 ft). At the highest altitude, 73% of the climbers reported headache, 35% reported anorexia or nausea, 11% reported vomiting, 13% reported dizziness, and 66% reported insomnia (Maggiorini, Bartsch, & Oelz, 1997). Children seem to have the same incidence of AMS as adults, although there is much less information available on this subject (Pollard et al., 2001). AMS usually resolves in 2–3 days (West, 2004). Descent to lower altitude—removal of hypoxia—relieves the symptoms promptly.

It is not clear why some people fall ill with AMS and others do not. Interestingly, individual characteristics including age, sex, and physical fitness are not important risk factors for AMS, but a past history of AMS, rapid ascent, or physical exertion increases the risk. A slow ascent and recent exposure to high altitude can counterbalance an individual's susceptibility (Bartsch, Bailey, Berger, Knauth, & Baumgartner, 2004; Basnyat & Murdoch, 2003; Schneider, Bernasch, Weymann, Holle, & Bartsch, 2002).

GEOLOGICAL AND EVOLUTIONARY HISTORY OF ADAPTING TO LOW OXYGEN LEVELS

Two billion years of aerobic evolution have resulted in mammalian cells and tissues that are extremely oxygen dependent.

Webster, 2003, p. 2911

The geological history of oxygen in the atmosphere is under continuing investigation, but the broad outlines are understood (Kerr, 2005). Oxygen is generated solely by photosynthesis. It reached detectable low levels about 2.2 billion years ago after roughly 0.5 billion years of photosynthesis by single-celled organisms (Bekker et al., 2004; Des Marais, 2005; Raymond & Segre, 2006). As oxygen accumulated in the water and atmosphere, some organisms adapted to the newly available element with the evolution of oxygen-metabolizing and oxygen-detoxifying pathways and other characteristics that enormously expanded the number of potential niches (Falkowski, 2006; Graham, Dudley, Aguilar, & Gans, 1995).

The first fossils of cells with nuclei and organelles such as mitochondria appeared about 1.9 billion years ago. Mitochondria evolved from oxygen-metabolizing, aerobic bacteria that were incorporated into non–oxygen-metabolizing, anaerobic, single-celled organisms with nuclei; they are the structures in cells where oxygen-using metabolism produces heat and energy (Wallace, 2005). Aerobic metabolism converts dietary energy and oxygen into heat, energy, carbon dioxide, and water and enabled the evolution of complex animal life. The enormous advantage of aerobic over anaerobic metabolism is higher energy production (Webster, 2003). It yields 19 times more metabolic energy per molecule of glucose fuel (Nathan & Singer, 1999).

Selective advantages resulting from higher aerobic energy production include larger body size, the evolution of circulatory systems because simple diffusion does not provide enough exchange of oxygen and carbon dioxide with the atmosphere, and the evolution of features requiring high energy expenditure such as walking or regulating body temperature. Other selective advantages accrue from new metabolic pathways to which oxygen contributes directly or indirectly. Oxygen-using organisms have at least 1000 oxygen-dependent enzymatic reactions (Falkowski, 2006; Raymond & Segre, 2006). Examples include metabolic pathways for synthesizing steroids (including some vitamins and hormones) and antibiotics (including penicillin) (Falkowski et al., 2005). Oxygen concentration in the atmosphere finally reached approximately modern levels around 600 million years ago (Brocks et al., 2005; Kerr, 2005). Levels have risen and fallen substantially many times since then. Fossil evidence for the earliest multicellular animals dates to about 575 million years ago and is quickly followed by the fossils of large animals (Kerr, 2005).

While many new features related to the presence of oxygen evolved over these millions of years, a key aspect of aerobic metabolism itself remained the same. It originated in aquatic organisms under conditions of low partial pressure of oxygen that diffused from the surrounding water into the cells. Mitochondria still operate today at very low oxygen levels even if oxygen is delivered by circulatory systems. They appear to retain an "ancestral" low oxygen environment (Massabuau, 2001, 2003) in the sense that cellular levels of oxygen have remained relatively unchanged throughout 2 billion years of evolution. Consistent with the stability of the cellular environment, "the basic cellular machinery has been established since the early days of evolution" (Massabuau, 2003, p. 857). This suggests that humans' cellular mechanisms for using and sensing oxygen and responding to fluctuations in oxygen level are highly conserved traits, meaning they are shared with many species that have inherited them from an ancient common ancestor.

Why have cellular oxygen levels remained low despite presently high levels of ambient oxygen and the evolution of oxygen-delivery systems? Low levels limit the unavoidable production of a group of highly reactive and destructive forms of oxygen. For example, highly reactive forms of oxygen damage DNA, proteins, fats, and organelle walls and contribute to biological aging changes. Even at the low oxygen levels in the mitochondria, about 5% of the metabolized oxygen generates the highly reactive forms of oxygen (Nathan & Singer, 1999). Antioxidants have evolved that counter this damage by chemically converting the highly reactive forms into less reactive or harmless molecules.

A balance is struck between the benefits of high-yield oxygen metabolism and its dangers: the low oxygen levels are both "primitive" (evolutionarily conserved) and "protective" (against generating too many of the highly reactive forms of oxygen) (Massabuau, 2003). However, a consequence of the low oxygen levels is a precarious homeostasis for cells and the evolution by natural selection of precise, rapid responses in order to survive fluctuations in oxygen supply.

Thus, people ultimately adapt to hypoxia because of descent from lineages that survived hundreds of millions of years at very low levels of oxygen and tens of millions of years of life at low levels of oxygen, as compared with today. Humans continue to use the ancient cellular machinery in features that evolved later in our unique lineage. Furthermore, people encounter transient hypoxia during everyday life, for example, during intrauterine life and sleep. We retain a well-equipped biological toolbox capable of effective response to short- and long-term fluctuations in oxygen levels, including those that occur when traveling to high altitude.

SYSTEMIC RESPONSES TO HYPOXIA AND EXISTING HYPOTHESES ABOUT PROXIMATE CAUSES

Despite many decades of study, the proximate cause of AMS is unknown. Common study designs used to detect the cause or causes include natural experiments with temporary visitors (such as mountain climbers) and true experiments with healthy volunteers at high altitude. Most investigations have focused on systemic aspects of oxygen delivery.

Oxygen moves along what is called a "cascade" of drops in oxygen levels from ambient air to inspired air to alveolar air (alveoli are little pouches at the far ends of lungs) to arterial blood to the blood in the tiniest capillary vessels to the cells and mitochondria and finally to venous blood. Diffusion from higher to lower oxygen levels is the main mechanism for moving oxygen. The rate of oxygen diffusion is proportional to the difference in levels: smaller differences slow the movement. Figure 14–1 illustrates the effect of high-altitude hypoxia on the transport of oxygen. It compares the cascade at sea level (solid, top line) with that at 4540 m (~15,000 ft) (dotted line). The general pattern of steep drop in oxygen level from inspired air to arterial blood is illustrated at both altitudes. However, the high-altitude cascade starts with a lower level of oxygen that results in a smaller total drop. The lower "head of steam" at the top of the high-altitude cascade elicits a number of biological responses in order to deliver adequate oxygen to cells and mitochondria. Regardless of altitude, cells and mitochondria operate at oxygen levels well below that of inspired air. For example, oxygen levels are about 1–3 mmHg in muscle cells and <1 mmHg in mitochondria (Ward, Milledge, & West, 2000).

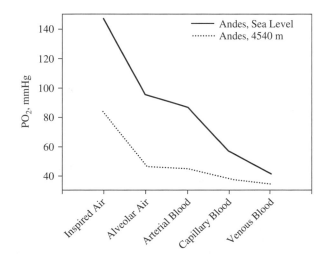

FIGURE 14-1 Oxygen transport cascade at sea level and high altitude of 4540 m (14,982 ft) illustrates the oxygen levels at all points of oxygen delivery. (From Hurtado, 1964.)

Traveling quickly from sea level to high altitude (3800–4500 m), called acute expo-sure, causes an immediate, profound fall in the body's oxygen levels and in the volume of oxygen circulating in the blood (hypoxemia). Figure 14–2 illustrates this fall using two physiological indicators of hypoxic stress: the partial pressure of oxygen in arterial blood (solid line) and the percent of oxygen saturation of hemoglobin (dashed line). People remain hypoxemic during the first days after acute high-altitude exposure when there is a risk of AMS, i.e., the biological responses during the first days at high altitude that prevent AMS or allow its occurrence and recovery take place despite the ongoing hypoxemia.

Although "[t]he physiological effects of the hypoxia of high altitude on the human body are legion" (West, 2004, p. 790), some effects have been investigated particularly for a hypothesized relationship to AMS. For example, it seems common sense to reason that individuals who are relatively more hypoxemic are at greater risk. There is variation about the mean values presented in Figure 14–2, but the degree of hypoxemia does not appear to be an important risk factor for AMS (Bartsch & Roach, 2001).

Turning to one of the key organ systems involved in oxygen transport, the lungs are the interface with ambient air. One of the most important adaptations to hypoxia is an imme-diate increase in breath rate and volume. This hyperventilation can partly offset the fewer oxygen molecules in each breath (Lenfant & Sullivan, 1971; Ward, Milledge, & West, 2000) and improve diffusion into the arterial blood. The increase in ventilation is the result of a reflex called the hypoxic ventilatory response (HVR). Measured as the

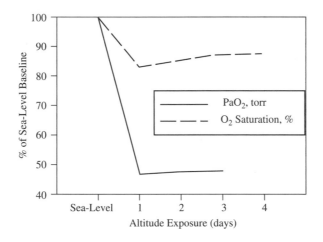

FIGURE 14-2 Physiological indicators of high-altitude stress. The data describe healthy adult lowlanders who were transported to 3800–4500 m [12,540–14,850 ft] or higher in a single day and tested in the following 3–4 days. Because biological characteristics change rapidly, it is important to compare results from people who took about the same amount of time to reach roughly the same high altitude and who provided measurements in the first few days at high altitude when AMS is most likely to occur or be avoided. In order to compare measurements of different physiological systems made in different biological units, sea level baseline is presented as 100% and later measurements on days 1 to 4 at high altitude are expressed as percentages of the sea level baseline. (From Goerre, Wenk, et al., 1995.)

increase in ventilation relative to the decrease in arterial oxygen level, it is an indicator of the effectiveness of the ventilation response. HVR is controlled by oxygen sensors in the carotid body, a tiny, pea-sized tissue in the neck where the carotid artery branches from the aorta to carry blood to the head and neck. At high altitude, the carotid body senses the lower level of oxygen in the arterial blood flowing through it (see Figure 14–1, dashed line) and responds by releasing neurotransmitters into the nerve connecting it to the respiratory center in the brain. Figure 14–3 shows that ventilation (solid line) and HVR (dots) both increase markedly during the first few days at altitude when there is a risk of AMS and when it resolves, if it occurs. The hyperventilation is beneficial, yet there is also a cost. Hyperventilation causes a rise in arterial pH, a trait that is tightly regulated within a very narrow range (Ward et al., 2000). Kidney responses lower the pH toward normal, although this takes a few days and may not be complete during the usual period of risk for AMS.

Considering that ventilation is such a vital response to acute high-altitude hypoxia, a longstanding hypothesis about the proximate cause of AMS proposes that individuals with low HVR have a higher risk of AMS. It reasons that a relatively low ventilation response could lead to lower levels of oxygen in the lung, less oxygen diffusion into the artery and greater hypoxemic stress. Some, although not all, retrospective studies found

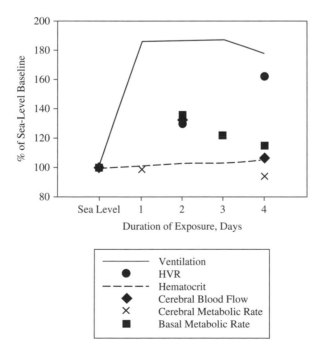

FIGURE 14-3 Physiological changes during the first four days at high altitude. (From Basu, Selvamurthy, et al., 1996; Butterfield, Gates, et al., 1992; Sato, Severinghaus, et al., 1994; Severinghaus, Chiodi, et al., 1966.)

relatively low HVR among people with a history of AMS. However, large prospective tests of this hypothesis found that HVR measured at sea level does not correlate with the development of AMS symptoms (Milledge et al., 1991; Milledge, Thomas, Beeley, & English, 1988).

Another widely studied response to high-altitude hypoxia is an increase in hematocrit, the number of red blood cells per volume of blood (Figure 14–3, dashed line). This increases the oxygen-carrying capacity of blood, although it does not restore sea level capacity because oxygen saturation remains low (Figure 14–2, dashed line). During the time when AMS typically occurs, the increase in hematocrit is caused by a reduction in the volume of the noncellular portion of the blood, plasma, which in effect concentrates the red blood cells (Ward et al., 2000). At sea level, a high hematocrit is a risk factor for headache, the defining symptom of AMS (Aamodt et al., 2004). That relationship has apparently not been evaluated as a risk factor for AMS.

Another homeostatic response thought to be relevant to AMS is an increase in cerebral blood flow, detectable within minutes of exposure to hypoxia. Figure 14–3 illustrates that cerebral blood flow (diamond) remains elevated throughout the first few days at high altitude when there is a risk of AMS. Higher blood flow could also increase pressure in blood vessels, perhaps stimulating pain receptors or increasing vessel permeability (Bartsch et al., 2004; Sanchez del Rio & Moskowitz, 1999). Therefore, another hypothesis about the proximate cause of AMS reasons that the increased blood flow can cause brain swelling and higher intracranial pressure, which in turn cause the headache and other symptoms of AMS (Roach & Hackett, 2001). However, there is only weak evidence in support of that hypothesis (Bartsch et al., 2004). On the contrary, a benefit to increased cerebral blood flow is a higher rate of oxygen and glucose delivery, which allows cerebral metabolic rate to remain stable during the first few days at high altitude (Figure 14–3, crosses) (Severinghaus, Chiodi, Eger, Brandstater, & Hornbein, 1966).

Another recent hypothesis suggests that the increased production of highly chemically reactive forms of oxygen damages the blood-brain barrier—tightly joined cells that line the brain's blood vessels (Bartsch et al., 2004). Damage to the blood-brain barrier lessens its effectiveness, perhaps causing headache and associated symptoms. Normally, the barrier prevents pathogens or other potentially harmful substances from entering the brain (Francis, Van Beek, Canova, Neal, & Gasque, 2003). Oxygen and carbon dioxide diffuse freely across the blood-brain barrier, whereas many substances, including glucose, must cross with the aid of transport proteins. Possibly relevant for the AMS symptom of nausea, the barrier is not as tight in an area of the brain that initiates the vomit reflex in response to chemical cues (Miller & Leslie, 1994). The brain may be particularly vulnerable to molecular damage because it has a high density of mitochondria that generate the chemically reactive forms of oxygen and has a relatively low level of counteracting antioxidants (Bailey, 2003). However, a recent test of this hypothesis suggests that blood-brain barrier damage due to highly reactive forms of oxygen does occur, but is not an important proximate cause of AMS (Bailey et al., 2006).

These rapid responses to acute high-altitude hypoxia—hypoxemia, hyperventilation, increased cerebral blood flow, and blood-brain barrier damage—form the bases of some of the leading current hypotheses about the proximate cause or causes of AMS. None provides an entirely satisfactory explanation for the proximate causes of AMS. An approach from an evolutionary medicine point of view may supply new hypotheses as a result of asking why these physiological responses exist. This approach examines the integration of genes and their products with cellular events and the physiological responses of individuals acutely exposed to high-altitude hypoxia.

CELLULAR RESPONSES TO HYPOXIA: CLUES TO PROXIMATE CAUSES

> HIF1 [hypoxia inducible factor 1] may have originally evolved in simple multicellular animals to regulate cellular energy metabolism... according to O_2 availability. In contrast, elaborate [hematological], cardiac, vascular, and respiratory systems are required to adequately supply O_2 to adult mammals (many of which consist of $>10^{13}$ cells) and HIF1 is required for the establishment and utilization of each of these systems.
>
> Semenza, 2001, p. 1

Animal cells respond to hypoxia with increased levels of a protein called hypoxia inducible factor 1 (HIF1), a transcription factor that induces the transcription and expression of at least 70 and probably many more genes (Semenza, 2004). HIF1 has two subunits: HIF1β and HIF1α. The HIF1β subunit is always produced and remains at a constant level in cells, where it participates in other pathways as well. The HIF1α subunit is produced continuously, but is also degraded continuously when oxygen is at normal levels. Hypoxia in the "physiological range" causes virtually instantaneous stabilization and an exponential increase in level of the HIF1α subunit and thus the HIF1 protein (Iyer et al., 1998; Semenza, 2001). Reoxygenation causes resumption of HIF1α degradation and low HIF1 levels. As a result, "changes in gene expression can occur that are both rapid and graded with respect to duration and severity of the hypoxia stimulus" (Lahiri et al., 2006, p. 268). HIF1 or similar molecules are found in all multicellular animals investigated so far, including insects, fish, birds, and mammals (Webster, 2003). HIF1 is called the "master regulator" of cellular and systemic oxygen homeostasis because it initiates the process of synthesizing molecules that increase oxygen delivery or modify metabolism and allow cells and organisms to survive fluctuations in oxygen levels. The following review describes some links between HIF1 target genes and systemic responses to hypoxia. Each systemic response is regulated by a number of factors; here the focus is on HIF1.

HIF1 AND CELLULAR METABOLISM AND THE FIRST DAYS AT HIGH ALTITUDE

The earliest adaptive benefit of HIF1 in simple multicellular animals was probably to regulate switching between oxygen-consuming aerobic metabolism ("new" in the past 2 billion years) and non–oxygen-consuming anaerobic metabolism (the more ancient form used by organisms before oxygen), depending upon oxygen availability (Semenza,

2001). There is a cost to the switch because anaerobic metabolism is energetically less efficient in the sense of yielding fewer energy molecules per molecule of glucose fuel, but cell survival, normal tissue function, and organism survival are huge benefits.

Mitochondria use the oxygen in the air we breathe and the calories in the food we eat to produce energy in the form of ATP. We do not have reserves of oxygen, and cells die within minutes of oxygen depletion. Many foods are converted into glucose, the usual energy source for human cells, which is carried into cells by transport proteins. Glucose is broken down in the cytoplasm by a process called glycolysis, a series of chemical reactions catalyzed by enzymes that do not require oxygen. This is the ancient anaerobic metabolic pathway for generating energy. The end product of glycolysis is pyruvate, which either can be converted into lactate, which performs other functions, or can enter the mitochondria and the oxygen-using pathway of ATP production. (Amino acids and fatty acids directly enter the oxygen-using pathway in the mitochondria and do not undergo glycolysis.) Thus, pyruvate links the anaerobic and aerobic pathways. HIF1 target genes help flip the switch between the two pathways, depending upon oxygen availability.

The genes for two proteins that move glucose into cells (and across the blood-brain barrier) are HIF1 targets. The genes for all 11 enzymes in the glycolytic pathway are HIF1 targets. The gene for the enzyme that converts pyruvate to lactate is also a HIF1 target gene. Furthermore, under hypoxia, the aerobic mitochondrial pathway is actually blocked by the protein product of a HIF1 target gene (Simon, 2006). The combination of enhancing glucose transport and the non–oxygen-consuming glycolytic pathway and impeding the oxygen-consuming pathway increases glycolysis under hypoxia so that energy production in the low-efficiency, yet non–oxygen-using pathway can supply energy needs in the cell. The glycolytic genes are highly conserved—glycolysis is thought to have been the first energy-generating metabolic pathway to evolve (Semenza, 2002b; Webster, 2003). HIF1-induced proteins enable this metabolic switch from aerobic to anaerobic metabolism, which is an extremely important, ancient cellular adaptive response to lowered oxygen.

The glycolytic switch, discovered in yeast cells, occurs in a variety of human tissues in cell cultures such as heart muscle and white blood cells (Baierlein & Foster, 1968; Okuda, 2006), illustrating again the ancient evolutionary origin of our response to highaltitude hypoxia. There is evidence that a metabolic shift favoring the uptake of glucose and the anaerobic pathway occurs among people in the first days after arrival at high altitude (Braun et al., 1998; Roberts, Butterfield, et al., 1996; Roberts, Reeves, et al., 1996; Young et al., 1991). The details of energy metabolism have apparently not been evaluated as risk factors for AMS.

Mitochondria normally operate at very low oxygen levels, and there is no evidence that levels fall even closer to zero when the organism is under hypoxic stress. What is the benefit of the metabolic switch to lower mitochondrial oxygen consumption? One obvious benefit is less oxygen fuel consumption overall when the supply is limited. Another benefit may derive from having a little oxygen left over to diffuse into distant tissue. Oxygen diffuses out of the capillary and into the cells from higher to lower oxygen levels (Figure 14–1). If oxygen is nearly completely consumed in cells near the capillary, then very little will diffuse to distant tissues. Alternatively, if less oxygen is consumed in cells near the capillary, then some may diffuse to cells further away (Hagen, Taylor, Lam, & Moncada, 2003).

HIF1 AND ANTIOXIDANTS AND AMS

A high cost to downregulating aerobic metabolism in the mitochondria is generating more of the highly reactive forms of oxygen. The increase is puzzling, but seems to occur because the usual dampening reactions are curtailed under hypoxia (Wallace, 2005). The process of evolution by natural selection has tinkered with this and incorporated the highly reactive forms of oxygen into the response to hypoxia. They stabilize the HIF1α subunit and raise HIF1 levels (Hoppeler, Vogt, Weibel, & Fluck, 2003). Thus, highly reactive forms of oxygen may be a two-edged sword capable of causing damage as well as enabling HIF1 regulation and cell survival under low oxygen levels. Many antioxidants (chemicals that limit damage caused by these highly reactive forms of oxygen) have evolved, and some are the products of HIF1 target genes. One is erythropoietin (EPO), an antioxidant that is detectable in the blood stream within a couple of hours of arrival at high altitude. EPO may be particularly important to protect neural function in the brain, a major site of the synthesis of EPO and its receptors (Buemi et al., 2003; Marti, 2004; Milano & Collomp, 2005). EPO concentration in the blood increases dramatically during the first few days at high altitude (Figure 14–4). Another HIF1 target gene catalyzes the synthesis of bilirubin, also a powerful antioxidant (Pachori et al., 2004).

These and other findings suggest that AMS may result from a temporary imbalance between highly reactive forms of oxygen that can cause cellular damage and antioxidants that can limit the damage. During the time when AMS typically occurs, there is evidence of such an imbalance in muscle and nervous system tissue (Bailey, Kleger, Holzgraefe, Ballmer, & Bartsch, 2004; Bailey et al., 2006; Jefferson et al., 2004). Exercise exacerbates the imbalance, consistent with the evidence that exertion increases the risk of AMS. One study found that indicators of this imbalance did not differ in those who remained well as compared with those who suffered from AMS (Bailey et al., 2006). In another study, a group of mountaineers took powerful dietary antioxidants, including vitamin C, during their ascent, and had lower AMS scores than the control group (Bailey & Davies,

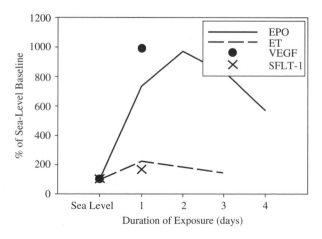

FIGURE 14-4 Circulating protein levels of HIF1 target genes. (From Abbrecht and Littell, 1972; Goerre, Wenk, et al., 1995; Tissot van Patot, Leadbetter, et al., 2005.)

2001). The contributions of highly reactive forms of oxygen and the counteracting antioxidants to the processes of high-altitude acclimatization may be a promising line of investigation into the proximate cause of AMS.

HIF1 AND THE BLOOD AND AMS

HIF1 target genes regulating the supply of red blood cells containing oxygen-carrying hemoglobin include EPO, transferrin, and the transferrin receptor (Semenza, 2002a). EPO, described earlier as an antioxidant, also stimulates the differentiation of red blood cell precursor cells. A marked, rapid increase in EPO at high altitude (Figure 14–4, solid line) results in the formation of new red blood cells containing hemoglobin, a process that takes about a week. New red blood cells require iron for their hemoglobin molecules. Transferrin receptors are necessary for the red blood cell precursors to bind and absorb iron transported by the transferrin protein. The rise in EPO has been suggested as a cause of AMS (Le Guen, 2004), but there appears to be no difference between circulating EPO levels of those who suffer from AMS and others (Mansoor et al., 2005). The delayed timing of the increase in the number of red blood cells suggests that this effect is not relevant to AMS. Instead, natural selection apparently tinkered with the rise in EPO to serve a second function protecting the brain.

HIF1 AND BLOOD FLOW AND AMS

Higher blood flow increases the rate of oxygen delivery and potentially offsets lower arterial oxygen content. Blood flow increases or decreases as a result of vasodilation (increasing the diameter of blood vessels) or vasoconstriction (decreasing the diameter). Acute hypoxia causes vasodilation of most blood vessels, with the important exception of the lung. As a result, blood pressure generally remains the same or falls slightly during the time that AMS is most likely to occur (Ward et al., 2000).

HIF1-regulated proteins or products of the pathways in which they participate cause vasodilation or constriction. One HIF1 target gene codes for nitric oxide synthase 2 (NOS2), an enzyme that catalyzes the synthesis of nitric oxide, a vasodilator. Nitric oxide–caused vasodilation contributes to the increased cerebral blood flow under hypoxia (Van Mil et al., 2002), generally considered beneficial because of the need to meet the unchanging oxygen demands of the brain. However, laboratory studies have shown that experimental doses of nitric oxide can induce headache, the primary symptom of AMS (Ashina, Bendtsen, Jensen, & Olesen, 2000). Similarly, a field experiment boosting nitric oxide synthesis with dietary supplements reported an increase in high-altitude headache (Mansoor et al., 2005). Thus, nitric oxide may contribute both to the beneficial high cerebral blood flow and the costly headache during the first days at high altitude. Nitric oxide may simply increase brain blood flow and stimulate pain receptors, or it may modify the sensation of pain (Benjamin, 1999; Parsons, 2006).

Maintaining cerebral blood flow may be particularly important for humans because of our large brain-to-body size ratios. Our brain uses 20–25% of our energy budget, although it accounts for just 2% of total body weight (Leonard, Robertson, Snodgrass, & Kuzawa, 2003). Brain metabolism is stable and cannot be downregulated (except during sleep). Perhaps meeting the energy demands of our large brains is so important for maintaining normal function that painful consequences are a relatively small cost.

In contrast to vasodilation outside the lungs, hypoxic vasoconstriction occurs in the lungs. Endothelin is a potent vasoconstrictor active in the lung that probably contributes to the hypoxic pulmonary vasoconstriction. Endothelin (ET-1) and its receptor (ETR) are also HIF1 target genes. Circulating ET-1 is elevated by about 200% on the first 2 days at high altitude and remains nearly 50% higher on the third (Figure 14–4, broken line). Levels of the vasodilator nitric oxide are decreased, even though NOS2 is a HIF1 target gene, because the enzymatic activity of NOS is downregulated by hypoxia (Dweik et al., 1998). This illustrates that there are multiple inputs into each response to hypoxia. Hypoxic pulmonary vasoconstriction has been interpreted as beneficial because it may improve oxygen diffusion (Ward et al., 2000).

Blood flow is also influenced by the number of blood vessels, another feature of oxygen delivery influenced by HIF1 target genes including vascular endothelial growth factor (VEGF) and its receptor (sFLT-1) (Semenza, 2004). VEGF contributes to the growth of new blood vessels from existing ones, a process called angiogenesis. Additional blood vessels improve oxygen diffusion and delivery because more tissue will be close to capillaries. While that outcome is beneficial, there may an associated cost. Another term for VEGF is vascular permeability factor because it also increases the flow of materials from the blood to the surrounding tissues, an effect that may increase the risk of AMS. A sample of travelers who remained well at high altitude experienced a 10-fold increase in circulating VEGF and a 50% increase in its receptor (Figure 14–4, circles and crosses, respectively), whereas those who suffered AMS had a comparable increase in VEGF but not its receptor (Tissot van Patot et al., 2005). The inference was that free VEGF may play a role in AMS by causing leaks in the blood-brain barrier.

This description of a few HIF1 target genes gives a glimpse of the array of effects or potential effects on oxygen delivery of any one HIF1 target gene. HIF1 is instrumental in effecting the metabolic switch to increase glycolysis and spare oxygen, in defending against harmful forms of oxygen generated under hypoxia, increasing the production of new red blood cells, increasing cerebral blood flow that maintains brain metabolism, and stimulating the growth of new blood vessels that may improve diffusion. As future studies evaluate the responses of the many HIF1 target genes and their effects and interactions during the first few days at high altitude, a clearer understanding of the integration of genes, organ systems, and organismal responses to hypoxia will emerge. Meanwhile a population with chronically high levels of HIF1 is informative.

HIF1 AND CHUVASH POLYCYTHEMIA

About 6% of the population of Chuvashia in central Russia has an autosomal recessive disorder that mimics the process of acclimatization to high altitude. The mutation causing Chuvash polycythemia impairs the normal ongoing degradation of HIF1α and results in continuously high levels of HIF1 (Ang et al., 2002; Bushuev et al., 2006; Gordeuk & Prchal, 2006; Perrotta et al., 2006; Smith et al., 2006). Because the HIF1 hypoxia-response pathway is continuously engaged, the natural experiment of Chuvash polycythemia removes some of the confounding factors that influence studies of AMS such as an individual's previous history of high-altitude exposure or rate of ascent. People with Chuvash polycythemia report more frequent headache, dizziness, and difficulty breathing upon exertion, symptoms also characteristic of AMS. Study of the pathways from HIF1 to its target genes and to systemic characteristics of Chuvash polycythemia finds parallels with AMS, although it is not an exact model.

People with Chuvash polycythemia have elevated concentrations of the products of HIF1 target genes as compared with normal Chuvash controls. These include genes associated with glucose uptake and glycolysis, red blood cell differentiation, hemoglobin synthesis, and blood flow. Many physiological characteristics of Chuvash polycythemia mimic the systemic response to high-altitude hypoxia, including higher breathing rates and hypoxic ventilatory responses, elevated hemoglobin concentration, indicators of vasoconstriction in the lungs and vasodilation in other blood vessels. People with Chuvash polycythemia respond to mild experimental hypoxia like acutely exposed lowlanders, indicating that HIF1 levels can increase further when appropriate. There is wide variation among Chuvash polycythemia patients in traits such as the level of ventilation or pulmonary artery pressure. Other factors must influence those responses among the Chuvash and, by extension, among visitors at high altitude.

Chuvash polycythemia is a lifelong disorder, in contrast with AMS, which is benign, self-limiting, and situation specific. Although most patients are treated with regular blood letting to reduce blood values to the normal range, survival to age 65 is about one-half that of controls. Individuals with Chuvash polycythemia have high morbidity due to bleeding episodes, blood clots, and brain blood vessel abnormalities. Whether the acute and temporary increase in HIF1 among travelers to high altitude produces similar risks is not known. Chuvash polycythemia is a valuable model of acclimatization to high-altitude hypoxia because it isolates the contribution of the HIF1 pathway to the usual physiological response to high-altitude hypoxia.

Future studies seeking to link the constellation of AMS symptoms to the HIF1 system will need to consider that HIF1 accumulation is influenced by factors in addition to hypoxia, including heat stress and levels of insulin, nitric oxide, vitamin C, and iron. In addition, HIF1 target genes are influenced by other factors, including hormones and nutrients. These findings imply that any given response to hypoxia via HIF1 integrates a number of influences, depending upon the particular individual, the target gene, and the tissue (Bilton & Booker, 2003; Knowles, Raval, Harris, & Ratcliffe, 2003; Lahiri et al., 2006; Maloyan et al., 2005). Furthermore, natural selection depends on genetic variation. Genetic variation in a number of HIF1 target genes has been reported, although there has been little success in linking a variant of any one gene with an indicator of high-altitude illness (Rupert & Koehle, 2006). Integrating the molecular biology of HIF1 with organismal biology is crucial to understanding why we are vulnerable to AMS.

CALORIES AND HYPOXIA AND AMS

> ...mitochondria [are] at the intersection between environmental factors such as calories and cold and the human capacity to energetically cope with the environmental challenges in different regions of the globe.
>
> Wallace, 2005, p. 392

This statement could appropriately add hypoxia to the list with calories and cold; the addition would direct attention to the metabolic requirement for both calories and oxygen. Responses to acute high-altitude hypoxia require metabolic energy precisely when the limiting fuel, oxygen, is in short supply. A striking feature of the first few days at high altitude is the increase in basal metabolic rate (BMR, the amount of energy required for essential functions such as breathing, heart rate, and regulating body temperature) and the associated increase in energy requirements. For instance, one study reported a 17–27% increase over sea-level baseline during the time that there is a risk of AMS (Figure 14–3, squares) (Butterfield et al., 1992).

Humans appear to have an energetically costly set of responses to hypoxia. Responses that are likely to increase energy demand include the increase in ventilation and cerebral blood flow. A response that decreases energy demand occurs in human infants and adult animals from small-bodied species ranging from protozoa to mammals —including the mouse, rat, cat, pig, rabbit, sheep, and pygmy marmoset. They downregulate body temperature upon exposure to acute hypoxia and use less energy to keep warm (Mortola, 2004; Singer, 1999, 2004; Steiner & Branco, 2002; Tattersall, Blank, & Wood, 2002). However, human adults, along with members of other large-bodied animal species, do not use that energy-conserving response.

Body temperature in people at high altitude is not well documented in the literature. Two studies report no change in a sample of people who remained healthy at high altitude, in contrast with a substantial increase of about $1°C$ ($1.8°F$) among those who suffered from AMS (Bailey et al., 2006: Maggiorini et al., 1997). Fever would increase oxygen demand and exacerbate hypoxic stress. If the association is confirmed in future studies, fever and its determinants may offer important clues to identifying the proximate causes of AMS.

Fever is a feature of the sickness response, also called the acute phase reaction, a set of immune system defenses against nonspecific stress or infection (Dalal & Zhukovsky, 2006; Kluger, Kozak, Conn, Leon, & Soszynski, 1996; Mackowiak, 1998; Watkins & Maier, 2000; Wieseler-Frank, Maier, & Watkins, 2005). Cells of the immune system release chemicals that increase the temperature set point to cause fever, an adaptive defense against pathogens. Remarkably, HIF1 target genes include those that produce some of the molecules that cause fever (interleukin [IL]-1, IL-6, and tumor necrosis factor [TNF]α) (Dalal & Zhukovsky, 2006; Schmedtje & Yan-Shan, 1998). The sickness response itself has not been studied during acute exposure to hypoxia. However, one study reported a significant elevation over baseline of one of these fever-causing molecules (IL-6) in the cerebrospinal fluid of those with AMS as compared with healthy controls (Bailey et al., 2004, 2006). Factors raising the body temperature set point could be offset by others lowering it, including some, such as nitric oxide, that are also the products of HIF1 target genes (Steiner & Branco, 2002). Taken together, these findings suggest the possibility that HIF1 target genes exerting different counterbalancing influences on body temperature may influence the risk of AMS.

HIF1 AND HYPOXIA IN EVERYDAY LIFE AND IN COMMON DISEASES

Millions travel to high altitude every year and acclimatize to high-altitude hypoxia, but everyone experiences long-term hypoxia during intrauterine life as well as episodes of transient hypoxia after birth, and perhaps during the course of illness. These are the situations in which the HIF1 response engages routinely and rapidly in response to fluctuations in oxygen level. Natural selection acting during these events has shaped the responses we have today because they recur every generation and in everyone's life.

Hypoxia is essential for normal embryonic development, and HIF1 and its target genes play a role. For example, VEGF is essential to the development of a variety of tissues with tubes, including the placenta, blood vessels, kidneys, and lungs (Bernhardt et al., 2006; Gebb & Jones, 2003). HIF1 may play a role in maintaining vasoconstriction in the fetal lungs. Indeed, one hypothesis reasons that hypoxic pulmonary vasoconstriction evolved to perform this function during hypoxic intrauterine life and actually serves no function postnatally (Ward et al., 2000)

Hypoxia accompanies chronic illnesses affecting over one tenth of the U.S. population, including some 30 million Americans who are ill with chronic obstructive pulmonary disease, asthma, or sleep apnea (Kochanek & Smith, 2004; Lethbridge-Cejku, Schiller, & Bernadel, 2004; National Center for Health Statistics/Centers for Disease Control and Prevention, 2002; Young, Peppard, & Gottlieb, 2002; No authors listed, 1994). Sleep apnea is an example of a group of diseases called sleep-disordered breathing that are associated with a disproportionate amount of sleep time at very low oxygen saturations as a result of transient cessations of breathing. Sleep apnea is associated with elevated EPO and VEGF (Schulz, Hummel, Heinemann, Seeger, & Grimminger, 2002).

Hypoxia is associated with two thirds of the deaths each year in the United States (Semenza, 2000). Cardiovascular disease is a leading cause of death. Narrowing of the blood vessels of the heart decreases blood flow and oxygen delivery and can result in elevated HIF1 and VEGF levels. If these induce branching and remodeling of blood vessels, then the response could restore blood flow and relieve hypoxia, and HIF1 would play a beneficial role in recovery (Paul, Simons, & Mabjeesh, 2004). In contrast, cancer is a leading cause of death in which HIF1 plays a detrimental role. The high growth rate of cancer cells consumes oxygen and can cause hypoxia in tumors. The resulting high HIF1 levels induce high levels of the anaerobic metabolism (glycolysis) enzymes, while higher VEGF levels initiate the development of new blood vessels that deliver oxygen to the tumor cells and allow them to grow. HIF1α levels are elevated in more than 70% of human cancers and are associated with an increased risk of death from many types of cancers (Bel Aiba, Dimova, Gorlach, & Kietzmann, 2006; Hirota & Semenza, 2006). Higher HIF1 levels may promote survival for people ill with heart disease, and yet compromise survival for people ill with many forms of cancer.

ASSEMBLING THE SYSTEMIC AND CELLULAR CLUES

Hypoxia and the cellular and systemic responses are features of human biology at all altitudes and have been throughout human evolutionary history. During travel to high altitude when there is the risk of AMS, hypoxia is unchanging and has an environmental source rather than a source in normal human biology or pathology. The distinctive source, magnitude, and duration of high-altitude hypoxia may contribute to the phenomenon of AMS.

Despite a number of promising hypotheses, there is still no clear understanding of the proximate causes of AMS. Hypotheses based on systemic responses (such as cerebral blood flow) and those based on cellular mechanisms (such as those due to highly reactive forms of oxygen) have been posed and tested, yet not found fully convincing. However, there is enormous potential to develop a new understanding of AMS as scientists learn more about cellular defense systems and their integration into systemic responses.

The overview presented in this chapter identifies some general topics for future research. One is the finding that HIF1 and its target genes overlap or intersect with systems of defense against other stressors, including infection. In addition, there is evidence that recent heat acclimatization enhances the response of laboratory animals to acute hypoxia by inducing the transcription of many HIF1 target genes even when there is no hypoxia (Maloyan et al., 2005). Cross-tolerance is the term for the phenomenon of exposure to one stress improving response to a later one. Perhaps AMS should not be viewed in isolation from other cellular defenses.

Another topic to pursue in order to better understand AMS is that of energy metabolism, both aerobic and anaerobic. Learning the allocations of energy and oxygen resources among the various tissues or responses may identify reasons for the constellation of symptoms. For example, considering why BMR increases while cerebral metabolic rate is stable may offer insight into the reason for some AMS symptoms.

WHY ARE WE VULNERABLE TO AMS?

The ultimate cause of AMS is our inheritance of an ancestral ability to adapt to fluctuations in oxygen availability. Consequently, we can adapt to severely limited supplies of our essential fuel, oxygen, and we can survive in high-altitude environments. The proximate causes of AMS remain unknown. Despite a conviction that "there is certain to be a population at risk [for high-altitude headache and AMS]" (Sanchez del Rio & Moskowitz, 1999, p. 150), it is still not clear what defines that population.

A principle of evolutionary medicine is that there are just a few categories of evolutionary explanations of disease (Nesse & Williams, 1994). One potentially relevant category of evolutionary explanation consists of illnesses that are manifestations of a mismatch between our current environment and the environment in which we evolved. In the case of AMS, modern technology provides the means to expose more people to high-altitude hypoxia more rapidly. Because a fast rate of ascent increases the risk, transportation that delivers people to high-altitude destinations much faster than they could walk contributes to the observed prevalence of AMS. Yet, as the unfortunate Too Kin observed in the opening quote of this chapter, arrival on foot or horseback does not prevent AMS. The current environment probably accounts for some of the prevalence because it facilitates exposure in a manner that increases the risk, but it does not account for the phenomenon of AMS itself.

Another potentially relevant category of evolutionary explanation of illness is defense (Nesse & Williams, 1994). Several features of a defense can be assessed to evaluate whether AMS is a defense, analogous to fever.

1. "A defense is unpleasant, but useful" (Nesse & Williams, 1994, p. 26). AMS is unpleasant, but could it be useful? If headache were a cue that an organism is under stress, it might be useful if it triggers a response that relieves the stress. In the case of

AMS, if headache prompts an individual to descend (descending just a few hundred meters can relieve high-altitude headache), then perhaps it could be interpreted as useful. Similarly, if headache slows physical activity, it may assist in adjustment to high-altitude hypoxia by avoiding the added oxygen consumption.

2. Was AMS shaped by natural selection specifically to fight hypoxia? This is not known presently. Natural selection shaped the HIF1 transcription factor and target genes to counteract hypoxia, but it remains unclear whether they account for the symptoms of AMS.

3. Are the drugs used to treat AMS blocking or interfering with the normal defense? Acetazolamide and dexamethasone are drugs commonly used to prevent and treat AMS. Both interfere with the normal defense in the sense that both act to counter responses that are initiated by HIF1 target genes. The drug acetazolamide enhances ventilation and oxygen levels, speeds the regulation of pH by the kidney, and relieves symptoms of AMS (Gallagher & Hackett, 2004). It acts by inhibiting the activity of a kidney enzyme that is a HIF1 target gene (Ivanov et al., 1998; Wykoff et al., 2000). Dexamethasone is used to relieve the symptoms of AMS, although it does not increase ventilation or oxygen levels. It is an anti-inflammatory drug, typically used to relieve symptoms of immune response to general tissue injury, a response that includes the expression of several HIF1 target genes. Dexamethasone may work by interfering with that defense. Thus, it seems that the drugs are blocking the normal defense, although this has not been studied explicitly.

4. Does the drugs' interference with the response put people at higher risk of subsequent illness? They do not increase physiological hypoxia as measured by oxygen saturation of hemoglobin; indeed acetazolamide does the opposite. One way to answer this question would be to evaluate whether treatment of AMS increases the risk of more dangerous forms of mountain sickness, high-altitude pulmonary edema, and cerebral edema.

5. Does the drug delay an adaptation that would otherwise take place? In the case of acetazolamide, it is thought to accelerate the adaptation.

Currently there is insufficient evidence to assess whether AMS is an example of a defect—"a happenstance result with no particular utility" (Nesse & Williams, 1994, p. 8)—or an example of "a coordinated defense shaped by natural selection and activated when special sensors detect cues that indicate the presence of a specific threat . . ." (Nesse & Williams, 1994, p. 8). There is an elegant integrated defense against high altitude and other forms of hypoxia. Whether AMS is a part of that defense or simply a painful and useless accompaniment remains to be discovered.

CHAPTER 15

Evolution and Modern Behavioral Problems

The Case of Addiction

Daniel H. Lende

Is addiction simply a state of mind, a genetic process, an evolved character-istic of our species, part of an emotional system found in all cultures? Is it strictly speaking a biological issue at all? Is it all biological? Can it ever be adaptive? Is it psychologically maladaptive? Can certain personalities be predicted to be vulnerable to particular types of addiction? Is addiction cul-turally specific? Could our early ancestors have found anything to be addicted to? How do cultural values and ideologies and friendships and fam-ily relationships and expectations create patterns of behavior that increase or decrease the likelihood of addictions? Lende offers a remarkably thorough beginning point that plots out a systematic methodology for answering some of these questions. Similar to Worthman's discussion of sleep, he uses an integrated ecological and developmental model framed by evolutionary thinking to describe a methodology to study addiction that forces us away from peripheralizing the components around which it is constituted in favor of a conceptual perspective that identifies addictive behaviors as being part of an otherwise expectable response at least to certain psychological dilem-mas, circumstances, or contexts. Interestingly, Lende's discussion leads us to understand how addictive sequences often mimic "normalcy" but are instead expressed to a degree that rather than looking "normal," the behavior hovers on one or the other end of a behavior continuum. Certainly, for treating those addicted, and for lessons in how to study and interpret addiction, Lende eliminates easy categorical boundaries. He gives us some tools to appreciate the manner in which the human personality can come to positively interpret and even enjoy the very behavior by which it is victimized. It is an important therapeutic insight.

INTRODUCTION

Using the case study of addiction, this chapter addresses how to build a research-based approach to behavioral psychopathology using evolutionary theory. The chapter charts a middle ground between evolutionary psychology and behavioral ecology, while further developing the evolutionary mismatch approach. Taken together, this synthesis provides for a robust approach to modern behavioral problems that proves complementary to research in psychiatry, neuropsychology, and medical anthropology.

After summarizing the problem of substance abuse, the chapter presents some general assumptions for research, covers central steps to building an evolutionary approach, and finally considers how to translate this approach into method. Throughout, substance abuse will provide the relevant example, but the theoretical map itself is applicable to a broad range of problems such as overeating, compulsive behavior, and gambling. This is a how-to guide for studying these problems, derived from the challenges of actually doing such research on substance use and abuse.

BACKGROUND

Several reviews of how evolution applies to addictive behavior already exist, including a comprehensive chapter on the basic Darwinian approach to substance abuse in the first edition of this volume (Smith 1999). Other general reviews include Lende & Smith (2002), Nesse & Berridge (1997), and Saah (2005). Specific topics have also been analyzed, including the phylogenetic roots of substance abuse (Dudley 2000, 2002; Levey, 2004; Panksepp et al., 2002; Sullivan & Hagen, 2002), life history theory (Hill & Chow, 2002; Lende & Smith, 2002), animal models (Gerald & Higley, 2002; Panksepp et al., 2002), related problems like smoking (Pomerleau, 1997) and gambling (Spinella, 2003), and evolutionary discordance (Pani, 2000). Several articles that have focused on reward and decision making in substance abuse are also considered here (Kelley, 2004; Lende & Smith, 2002; Nesse & Berridge, 1997; Newlin, 2002; Pani, 2000).

Despite this growing body of research, most researchers focus either on animal models or on proposing how adaptive models help us make sense of addictive behavior. In particular, these models offer analyses that show how characteristics of addiction can be consistent with the theory of natural selection. At present, there is a need for a research program that systematically addresses the interconnected issues in addiction. In the remainder of the chapter I will outline the basic steps that were utilized in my research on adolescent drug use and abuse in Colombia (Lende, 2003, 2005). The overall study included a broad anthropological analysis of substance use and abuse, using both epidemiological and ethnographic methods. As such, the evolutionary component of this research was conceived as being complementary to a wider biocultural view of substance abuse (see also Hruschka et al., 2005).

The general anthropological basis of my research required a reworking of core proposals of evolutionary psychology and human behavioral ecology. Both bodies of theory present specific research programs based on derivations of modern evolutionary theory (Cosmides & Tooby, 1997; Daly & Wilson, 1999; Smith, Borgerhoff Mulder & Hill, 2000; Winterhalder & Smith, 2000). The problem for addiction, as for many modern behavioral problems, is that these theoretical approaches are simply not applicable. Behavioral ecology, highly reliant on optimality theory and evolutionary stable strategies,[1] does not provide the necessary insight into the very costly, even pathological problem of substance abuse. With evolutionary psychology, there is no "universal module" for addictive behavior of the sort that evolutionary psychologists generally propose. These modules are generally seen as solving adaptive problems in past environments. Given the phylogenetic novelty of concentrated psychoactive substances, there is no past adaptive problem that substance users directly solve by taking drugs in large quantities. The theoretical problems of both behavioral ecology and evolutionary psychology are related to their particular derivations of evolutionary theory (e.g., optimality and universal modules). As shown here, a return to general evolutionary theory—the processes of natural selection and descent with modification that Darwin originally proposed—proves important for developing an evolution-based approach to modern behavioral problems.

This research also required a more critical application of evolutionary medicine. Evolutionary medicine often uses a discordance model, which focuses on how modern environments change the functioning of adaptations (often in negative ways). However, consuming drugs has not provided a consistent adaptive benefit or cost over evolutionary time, which means that addiction is not an evolutionary problem in itself. Thus, a simple discordance model does not work well. For example, several researchers propose that drugs provide "false" fitness benefits due to their evolutionary novel impact on brain structures (Nesse & Berridge, 1997; Panksepp et al., 2002). These benefits are then assumed to account for the problem of addiction. In this approach, addiction is reduced to the novel effects of drugs alone. This type of analysis misses out on the numerous ways that evolutionary theory can be applied to the *behaviors* involved in addiction. These researchers also overlook the significant sociocultural aspects of substance use and abuse, from difficult family relations to the important role that friends play in drug use (Compton et al., 2005).

Thus, alongside basic evolutionary processes such as natural selection and descent with modification, a sophisticated consideration of the present-day environment is central to understanding modern behavioral problems. In today's world, many sociocultural and environmental processes and contexts that powerfully affect our behavior simply did not exist during evolutionary time. The impact of these environmental factors places a considerable demand on the evolutionary approach to work with other bodies of knowledge, such as sociocultural anthropology. This synthetic approach offers the possibility to produce more robust explanations of modern behavioral problems by attending to the multiple facets inherent in these behavioral problems.

ADDICTION: OUTLINING THE BEHAVIORAL BIOLOGY

A crucial step in developing this evolutionary approach is a clear description of current understandings of addiction. Too often, evolutionary theory confines itself to what initially appears as theoretically relevant, without engaging the actual complexity of the problem under consideration (e.g., the false fitness benefit model discussed earlier). This section aims to rectify this problem by outlining the biological and behavioral aspects of addiction (see Table 15-1).[2]

TABLE 15-1 Behavioral Biology of Addiction

Function	Reward and liking	Seeking and desire	Habitual action	Association learning	Stress	Self control and cognitive biases
Relation to drug use	Positive sensations linked to drug use	Urge to seek out drugs and wanting to use drugs	Routinized searching and using behaviors	Environmental cues get linked to liking and wanting drugs	Heightens sensitivity to drug cues, reduces self-control	Inability to stop seeking or using, focus on benefits of use
Brain areas	Nucleus accumbens, substantia nigra	Mesolimbic dopamine system, ventral tegmental area, orbitofrontal cortex	Dorsal striatum, caudate-putamen	Hippocampus, amygdala	Hypotha-lamus, prefrontal cortex	Prefrontal cortex

a This table summarizes those aspects of behavioral biology discussed throughout the chapter. The "related brain areas" serve as a rough guide, for the actual neurobiology is not so localized and is more interconnected. Certain neuropsychological processes that are relevant to addiction are not included, such as long-term potentiation in memory and management of attention in the prefrontal cortex. Withdrawal, central to some drugs, is also not included, as it can be substance specific (e.g., alcohol) while also creating aversive states similar to stress (Koob & Le Moal, 2005). Topics discussed later can also be linked to the behavioral biology. Ritualized behavior has links with the category "habitual action," and the importance of meaning involves the prefrontal cortex (indeed, Everitt and Robbins [2005] argue that the prefrontal cortex plays a central role in "post hoc commentary" on sensory perceptions linked to drug use).

Two core behavioral patterns define addiction. First, over time the individual transitions from intermittent substance use to compulsive involvement with drugs (Everitt & Robbins, 2005; Koob & Le Moal, 2004). This amplification of one activity (drug use) with neglect of other areas of life (e.g., social responsibilities of family and work) is central to substance abuse. Second, addiction is also defined by "relapse," which means a reversion to the intense engagement with substance use (DeJong, 1994; McLellan et al., 2000). This return to old behavioral patterns can happen months or years after an individual has stopped using drugs, and thus is not always directly related to withdrawal from drugs.

Thus, "intensification" and "reinstatement" are two defining behaviors for substance abuse. It is in this sense that addiction is often defined as a chronic, relapsing disorder (Leshner, 1997; McLellan et al., 2000). Three often-used diagnostic criteria provide a more concrete view of the specific individual problems related to these behaviors (American Psychiatric Association, 2000; Deroche-Gamonet et al., 2004): (1) high motivation for drugs, with everyday activities focused on obtaining and using drugs; (2) difficulties in stopping or limiting drug use, and (3) continued use despite high personal and social costs (e.g., medical and family problems). In general terms, substance abuse is marked by heightened desire for and engagement in drug-related behaviors, compromised ability to control drug use and/or switch to other activities, and altered views of the costs and benefits of drug use.

Multiple brain systems underlie these different aspects of abuse. Although by no means delineated with clarity, mesolimbic dopamine systems play a central role in facilitating wanting and seeking of drugs (Hyman, 2005; Kelley & Berridge, 2002) and the prefrontal cortices mediate aspects of control (Kalivas & Volkow. 2005).[3] The alteration of costs and benefits relate both to drug-specific effects (e.g., opiates on opioid systems) and to neural systems that produce sensations of pleasure or "liking" in the brain (Berridge & Robinson, 2003; Hyman, 2005; Kalivas & Volkow, 2005). A main point of this discussion is that addiction involves multiple brain systems, and it is the interaction of these brain systems with environments and drugs that plays a formative role in developing substance abuse.

Given this behavioral interaction of drugs and individuals, addiction is not a genetic problem per se. The vast majority of people who try drugs do not end up addicted to them (Anthony et al., 1994). Studies indicate that some variation in the vulnerability for drug abuse can be genetic, and genetics should not be overlooked as an important component of substance abuse (Young et al., 2006). However, it is equally clear that environmental circumstances can create these same vulnerabilities (Drake et al., 2002; Piazza & Le Moal, 1996). Thus, both having alcoholic parents (genetics) and growing up with alcoholic parents (environment) contributes to the risk for substance abuse (Newlin et al., 2000). Since genetics and environment play a role in substance abuse, the function of the proximate mechanisms (such as brain systems) offers the means to understand how these different sources of vulnerability interact during an individual's development.

In terms of drugs and their pharmacological impact on the brain, psychoactive drugs have three types of effects (Kelley & Berridge, 2002; Nesse & Berridge, 1997). First, they can provide natural rewards through intrinsic reinforcement within the brain (such as pleasure and/or relief of stress). Second, psychoactive drugs alter the functioning of the brain, for example, generating new connections between neurons or creating tolerance to the effects of certain neurotransmitters. Finally, drugs—given their purity and their availability—provide evolutionarily novel impacts. In the modern world people can ingest highly concentrated drugs and they can do so frequently. During our evolutionary history, this sort of access to drugs simply did not exist. In summary, it is the combination of purity with the mimicking of natural reward and the altering of functioning that can play such havoc with brain systems.

Finally, it is important to mention a central issue related to costs and benefits. Addiction has been linked to psychosocial stress and to the management of negative affect (Cooper et al., 1995; Koob & Le Moal, 2005). Indeed, in many ways, the functional use of drugs provides an important behavioral guide to understanding why individuals decide to use drugs (Boys & Marsden, 2003; Quintero & Davis, 2002). Individuals' reasons for using drugs are crucial and can be linked to both internal states (emotions, feelings, and the like) and social contexts and cultural norms (Boys & Marsden, 2003; Moore, 2004). Thus, desire, control, and costs and benefits should be understood in relation to how individuals view drugs and what drugs can do for them, and not simply as a manifestation of hard-wired brain circuits.

FIVE STEPS FOR EVOLUTIONARY-BASED RESEARCH ON BEHAVIORAL PROBLEMS

The remainder of this chapter presents five steps that, taken together, provide a framework for how to conduct evolution-based research on problematic modern behaviors like substance abuse. The first step presents some basic assumptions for research, summed up as "the human organism point of view." The next three steps are adaptive analysis, phylogenetic comparison, and discordance and malfunction. The final step focuses on methods, particularly how the conjunction of adaptive analysis and an embodied view of behavior offer important insights into how to carry out evolutionary based research. All five steps are summarized in Table 15-2.

TABLE 15-2 Evolutionary Analysis of Modern Behavioral Problems

	Specific steps	Application to addiction
1: Human Organism Point of View	(a) Focus on how people actually behave, with consideration of proximate mechanisms and positive and negative outcomes (b) Take a biocultural view, where evolutionary and cultural explanations work together in explaining behavioral problems	(a) Addiction can be highly costly, where the behavioral biology plays a major role in explaining maladaptive outcomes (b) Drug use both biological (pharmacology) and cultural (subcultures of use)
2: Adaptive Analysis	(a) Critical assessment of biomedical and sociocultural approaches (b) Proximate mechanisms reveal the outcome of natural selection (not a priori modules) (c) Present benefits and costs shape behavior, along with sociocultural factors	(a) Addiction not simply driven by "hard wired pleasure" or cultural learning of expected drug effects (b) Address "reward" as an evolutionary problem related to foraging and reproduction, and shaped by the limitations of past environments (c) Drug-using lifestyle can reinforce drug use, e.g., through sexual behavior often considered as a "risk" factor
3: Phylogenetic Comparison	(a) Proximate mechanisms (e.g., neuropsychological processes) appeared in different phylogenetic periods (b) Use animal models and research, while still maintaining a biocultural view	(a) Addiction involves the interaction of ancient limbic motivational systems and the more recent prefrontal cortex (b) Wheel running provides a model for compulsive use, with the understanding that cage environments significantly shape animals' behaviors
4: Malfunction and Discordance	(a) Malfunction reveals functioning of particular proximate mechanisms that work together to produce behavior (b) Discordance can focus on how modern environments promote malfunction—what specific factors encourage nonadaptive behavior? why are specific people vulnerable?	(a) Mechanisms for "seeking" excessively active due to drug use (b) Sexual and competitive benefits associated with use reinforce drug use, while drug availability and stress promote involvement in drugs due to heightened vulnerability and short-term focus
5: Methods	(a) Focus on specific experiences and behaviors (b) Engage the viewpoint of the individual—what does the behavior accomplish from their perspective? (c) Use an epidemiological approach to examine factors that impact maladaptive behavior, including both evolutionary and cultural hypotheses	(a) Subjective experiences of "wanting" and "seeking" drugs significant predictor of being addicted (b) Shift away from painful subjective states important reason to use (c) Compulsive involvement and endorsement of cultural models differently related to addiction and poly-drug use

Step One: Guiding Assumptions—"The Human Organism Point of View"

For an evolutionary approach to be complementary with other fields of inquiry, two main assumptions are crucial: (1) that human nature is essentially biocultural, for it involves the interaction of culture and human biology, and (2) the individual point of view provides a unique perspective for applying evolutionary theory. Evolutionary theory often proceeds from a theory of inclusive fitness and/or optimality. Neither of these approaches is biocultural at its core. However, human evolution is (Fuentes, 2004; Richerson & Boyd, 2005). Local behavioral traditions such as those demonstrated by chimpanzees likely predate our hominid lineage (Wrangham et al., 1994), tool manufacture and use dates back at least 2 million years (Klein, 1999), and symbolic activity (such as bead making) dates back at least 100,000 years (or approximately 4000 generations) (Vanhaereny et al., 2006).

The corollary of this assumption is that many modern behaviors are not good candidates to be broken into biological parts that can be categorized as phylogenetically ancient and cultural parts that are a recent veneer. In the past, eating was presented as the result of either Paleolithic tastes (Eaton & Konner, 1985) or recent cultural history (Harris, 1986). However, recent analyses highlight the interaction of biology and culture in eating (Goodman et al., 2000; Rozin, 1996). With addiction, biocultural interactions also play a role, such as the previously mentioned "reasons to use." Another biocultural aspect of addiction that deserves further analysis is ritual-like behavior (i.e., repeated stereotypical actions). Substance abusers can display these sorts of behaviors in the precise steps they take while preparing and consuming drugs (Lende, 2003). Ritual-like behaviors have roots in animal behavior (Eilam et al., 2006), and recent cultural analyses of ritual are amenable to behavioral analysis (Bell, 1997). Human ritual has also been analyzed from an evolutionary point of view (Donald, 1991; Boyer & Lienard, in 2006). Thus, the links between the evolution of ritual and the behavior of ritually preparing and using drugs represents one way in which a biocultural approach could be made more explicit in the analysis of addiction.

Inclusive fitness and maximization both take perspectives that limit their view of how organisms develop, negotiate their environments, and engage in successful or unsuccessful behaviors. Maximization, with its emphasis on an ideal solution for all individuals in a population, does not focus sufficiently on the particular mechanisms and processes by which organisms (or individuals) accomplish specific ends, nor does it consider how individuals might vary in these mechanisms. Inclusive fitness, by emphasizing the role of genetics and inheritance, also leaves little room for an understanding of how a specific organism actually goes about living a life (e.g., how it makes choices about what sorts of things to eat). Put differently, between the population-level rationality of optimality and gene-level adaptive modules, the point of view of the human organism—of actual people—is often lost.

The human organism point of view is addressed at different points in this chapter, from the actual biological mechanisms involved in addiction to understanding people's intentions. The thread that ties these areas together is the consistent focus on building an understanding of how organisms (in this case, people) actually function on the ground. Optimality and adaptive modules posit theories for how organisms *should* behave. The organism point of view presents the challenge of building an evolutionary understanding based on how people actually behave. For this chapter that means the focus on people who engage in extremely costly and repetitive consumption of drugs.

Step Two: Adaptive Analysis

With a concern for both adaptive design and behavior, evolutionary theory can provide a critical assessment of some biomedical portrayals of substance abuse as well as improvement of neuropsychological theories of decision making. Beginning with research by Olds (1958) on the self-stimulation of the brain in rats, there is a long history of biomedical research that views substance abuse as the result of the overwhelming pleasure produced when hard-wired brain circuits are stimulated (either by electrical current or by drugs of abuse) (Blum et al., 1996).

This approach has all the makings of an adaptive just-so story (Gould & Lewontin, 1979), a speculative account without necessary analysis (Lende & Smith, 2002). Initially the story might have sounded plausible. However, subsequent research has shown that not all animals respond equally to stimulation and that the quality of the environment (e.g., enriched cages with other things to do besides self-stimulating) plays a central role in rates of stimulation (Wurbel, 2001). Furthermore, the reduction of reward (in the psychological sense of how animals respond to the environment) to pleasure does not make adaptive sense. To use the example of food, nutritional quality shapes food choices as well as pleasurable tastes (Goodman et al., 2000). With drugs, having friends who use drugs can be as important as the drugs themselves in rates of substance use and abuse (Beyers et al., 2004; Lende, 2005).

A growing number of researchers have become interested in understanding how reward works through a sophisticated combination of neurobiological, behavioral, and computational analyses (Redish, 2004; Schultz, 2000; Wise, 2002). This research breaks down reward into separate components (such as wanting/seeking and liking/consuming) (Berridge & Robinson, 2003). It also pays attention to the idea of "natural rewards," or how appropriate responses can lead to enhanced survivorship or reproduction (not simply pleasure) (Kelley & Berridge, 2002). Nevertheless, this research paradigm retains its experimental focus on how animals respond (e.g., whether rats prefer sugar or cocaine), rather than a theoretical focus on how decision making affects fitness.

This problem hampers the application of the reward paradigm to addiction, for it places undue emphasis on drugs as the cause of addiction—drugs as sensitizing neurological systems (producing maladaptive responses like substance abuse) and/or providing exceedingly high reward to individuals whose genetic variability make them susceptible. An evolutionary approach would also look at the design of decision-making systems in relation to the structure of past environments (Lende & Smith, 2002). In the past, foraging and reproduction have consisted of two general phases: finding food or partners and then engaging in eating or sex. The two phases of decision making correspond to the different components of wanting/seeking and liking/consuming that neurological research has outlined (Robinson & Berridge, 2001, 2003). The design perspective can further elaborate the seeking phase. In past environments there was a relative scarcity of food and sexual partners (Lende & Smith, 2002). This limitation indicates that there was no selective reason to build a system that automatically self-regulates (i.e., to prevent eating too much or having too much sex). For humans, this sort of design places much greater emphasis on higher levels of cognitive control, which are generally compromised in substance abusers.

The emphasis on drugs as reinforcers also limits our understanding of evolutionarily important sources of reward in present environments. Drug-related behaviors can lead to adaptive outcomes, such as enjoyable sexual situations and positive outcomes to dominance or competitive interactions. In other words, from an evolutionary point of view, sexual behavior can be a potent reinforcer. In the substance abuse field, however, sex and violence are generally cast as dangerous "risk behaviors." Research rarely examines how environmental and behavioral links between drug use and "sex and violence" might actually encourage further use. In summary, these proximate reinforcers can help explain why people maintain certain lifestyles (a topic developed further later in this chapter), even if from the biomedical point of view these individuals are putting themselves at risk.

In summary, the adaptive analysis proposed here focuses on both adaptive design and behavior with an emphasis on the proximate level. Rather than attempting to come up with a module that matches a proposed adaptive problem, an adaptive analysis considers research on neuropsychological mechanisms as revealing the outcome of evolutionary processes. These outcomes can then be analyzed to understand how adaptations developed in the past and how today's environment shapes the adaptive functioning of neuropsychological systems.

Step Three: Phylogenetic Comparison

A robust evolutionary approach to behavioral problems can also draw on the strengths of phylogenetic and comparative cross-species analysis. This approach leads to greater understanding of substance abuse by drawing on the vast research on animal models of abuse (Berridge, 2003; Cardinal & Everitt, 2004; Deroche-Gamonet et al., 2004; Kelley & Berridge, 2002; Olmstead, 2006). Today it is evident that the dopamine systems involved in substance abuse are among the most ancient that we possess. Dopamine receptors appeared before the split of vertebrates and invertebrates (Cravchik & Goldman, 2000), and there are invertebrate models of dopamine function (Wolf & Heberlein, 2003). Thus, the typical approach of identifying the Pleistocene as the "environment of evolutionary adaptedness" (the time when psychological adaptations were formed) is mistaken because many core brain systems that mediate motivation and emotion emerged far earlier in evolutionary time (see Panksepp & Panksepp, 2000, for a more elaborate version of this argument).

At the same time, as mentioned earlier, the prefrontal cortices have been implicated in substance abuse (Kalivas & Volkow, 2005). These have emerged over the last 1.6 millions years of human evolution (Semendeferi et al., 2001; Streidter, 2006). Thus, addiction involves the interaction of phylogenetically recent and ancient brain systems, which appears common to many behavioral health problems (Bechara et al., 2000; Cardinal et al., 2002; Davidson et al., 2000). This model highlights the necessity for sophisticated phylogenetic thinking about how brain systems interact and what roles they play in modern behavior.

Here it helps to return to the animal research. It is important to emphasize the individual variation that can result from these ancient systems (Cravchik & Goldman, 2000)—while universal, these systems should not be considered "uniform." With respect to addiction, it is clear that there are animal lines that respond more to certain substances than other genetic varieties (e.g., mice that like to drink alcohol) (Crabbe, 2002). At the same time, the comparative view highlights the role of environmental conditions in encouraging the repetitive use of drugs, even in the studies taken as paradigmatic (e.g., cocaine-using rats neglecting food and water until near death) (Badiani & Robinson,

2004; Garner & Mason, 2002; Wurbel, 2001). First, these animals need to be trained to exhibit this behavior, and second, there needs to be a nearly complete lack of other behavioral options (i.e., an unenriched cage, even if food and water are available, is not a behaviorally rich environment, something that most zoos have finally realized). Thus, the animal research points to addiction as a more complex disorder than is commonly appreciated. An evolutionary analysis, therefore, cannot simply rely on proposals about "false fitness benefits" or reward systems gone awry due to drugs.

An interesting animal model exists for a comparative approach to modern abnormal behavior—wheel running by rodents (Rhodes et al., 2003; Sherwin, 1998). This is a behavior not exhibited in the wild (similar to addiction); nonetheless, some animals will spend an extraordinary amount of time and effort doing this. Wheel running can even displace drug consumption as a preferred behavior (Cosgrove et al., 2002)! Sherwin (1998) and I agree— a behavior-based approach is crucial to understanding these sorts of obsessive activities. Each behavior is related both to the activity itself (wheel running or drug taking) and to the surrounding environment (the cage or a drug lifestyle that reinforces use). For humans with their enlarged cortices, there is an added level of complexity due to the meaning drug use can have for people (e.g., "reasons to use"). For example, the shifts in wanting and attention related to changes in dopamine activity have corresponding interpretations by the person (Lende, 2005). In my research, an adolescent girl with a troubled home life spoke of how drugs put her into a "video" that she contrasted with her life at home.

In summary, drawing on an understanding of brain evolution and the use of animal models is central to developing an evolutionary medicine of behavioral disorders. Researchers who do not take this step run the risk of reverting to simplistic and often mistaken proposals about adaptive benefits, rather than building on the wealth of knowledge that already exists on the comparative biology of behavior.

Step Four: Malfunction and Discordance

Evolutionary medicine's concern with malfunction provides the field with a considerable advantage over evolutionary psychology and human behavioral ecology. Both of these approaches generally assume optimal design, but malfunction can reveal adaptive function just as well. As I show below, this approach proves particularly fruitful in illuminating the function of proximate components that are often glossed over in assumptions about optimal modules or behaviors.

Berridge and Robinson (2003) discuss how reward can be parsed into at least three components: learning (including associative conditioning and cognitive processing), affect and emotion (implicit "liking" and conscious pleasure), and motivation (wanting and seeking). For over a decade, Robinson and Berridge (1993, 2001, 2003) have argued that pathological functioning in the brain components mediating wanting and seeking is central to drug abuse. Drugs, given their pharmacological impact on the mesolimbic dopamine systems of the brain (the wanting system), can produce sensitization, a progressive amplification in neuronal responding. This sensitization leads to extremely strong desire and searching for drugs. The process can happen even as the pleasurable rewards provided by drugs decline due to tolerance in the "liking" system. Thus, there is a relative dissociation of wanting and seeking from pleasure, with heightened seeking a core problem in addiction.

Other research supports this view of the mesolimbic dopamine system. Salamone et al. (2003) examined the role of dopamine in responsiveness to conditioned stimuli and the activation of behavior (for example, searching for food at the sound of a bell). Their research indicated that dopamine mediates the amount of effort put into reaching a goal (particularly in vigorous responding by mice and rats, such as climbing barriers to reach food). Similarly, Cannon and Bseikri (2004) showed how the lack of dopamine leads to deficits in goal-directed behavior. Finally, Redgrave et al. (1999) argued that dopamine plays a central role in switching animals' attention to unexpected and behaviorally important environmental stimuli. In summary, overinvolvement in wanting and seeking drugs and heightened sensitivity to conditioned cues that signal environmental availability of drugs (so as to start seeking them) represents a core "malfunction" at the heart of addictive behavior.

Even given the role of drugs in sensitizing the dopamine system, the overall malfunctioning is still environmentally shaped (Crombag & Robinson, 2004). Here is where a sophisticated understanding of modern environments produces a great pay-off in expanding how the discordance concept can be used. Normally, discordance focuses on the mismatch between past and present environments. For example, our evolved taste for salt makes evolutionary sense, for salt was an important but limited nutrient in past environments. Today the abundance of salt can lead to health problems such as hypertension. This mismatch is easy to recognize, and can be further developed by examining why certain people consume more salt than others and what sorts of environmental factors encourage salt consumption. This approach places emphasis on examining *how* modern environments shape the maladaptive responding of evolved traits. Turning to drug use, both the pleasurable effects of drugs and the proximate benefits associated with drug use help establish drug taking as a goal. Sharing drugs with friends, part of establishing social relationships and long-term reciprocities, should also not be overlooked as another way in which drug taking becomes established. These behavioral and environmental factors can favor the move from the initial goal of drug use to compulsive involvement with drugs (Everitt & Robbins, 2005; Hyman, 2005; Wise, 2002).

The discordance view highlights two other ways in which modern environments promote addiction—drug availability and psychosocial stress. Epidemiological research has shown the role that drug availability plays in increased rates of substance use (Compton et al., 2005), although availability on its own does not automatically promote drug use (indeed, an integrated suite of sociocultural factors can mediate against drug use even in environments where drugs are readily available, such as Colombia [Lende, 2003]). With psychosocial stress, behavioral biology has confirmed its importance in heightening vulnerability for drug use, in particular through heightened responsiveness to reward (Koob & Le Moal, 2005; Kreek et al., 2005; Weiss, 2005). Thus, from the discordance point of view, environments that share high availability and high stress are those most likely to promote drug taking and seeking. Inner city environments where drug selling is active can be particularly stressful (Bourgois, 2003). These types of environments often promote intense drug using. Similarly, families in which parents abuse drugs or alcohol present the same mix of availability and high stress for children, and this combination should be considered a major reason why substance abuse runs in families (alongside genetics) (Compton et al., 2005; Kreek et al., 2005).

What is ironic, and ultimately maladaptive, is that these same stressful environments promote risk-taking behavior and a focus on short-term benefits by the participants

(Lende & Smith, 2002). These are precisely the environments in which the pleasures of drugs, the proximate benefits of a drug-using lifestyle, and the importance of friends can help establish initial drug taking. Subsequent use can then be enhanced due to both the aversive costs of stopping (e.g., reduction in pleasure, increase in stress, physiological aspects of withdrawal— see Koob & Le Moal, 2005) as well as the conscious recognition by users that using drugs takes them away from the stresses and difficulties of their every-day lives (Lende, 2005).

Overall, modern environments play a central role in the establishment of drug taking and in the reasons individuals return to drug use. The discordance and malfunction views help amplify the understanding provided by adaptive analysis and phylogenetic compar-ison, producing a more comprehensive approach to substance abuse than any one type of analysis on its own.

Step Five: Methods

In turning the varied considerations of this chapter into a research paradigm, strategic choices need to be made. Given the complexity of substance abuse, a focus on key behav-ioral components represents one fruitful approach that is elaborated upon here, although the modern environment, the role of ritual, and the interaction of genetics and develop-ment represent other research possibilities.

Even after an initial choice of research focus, the step from evolved behavioral biol-ogy to research is not one of simple prediction and testing. Returning to our initial assumptions, it is important to rely on the "human organism point of view." This view-point—emphasizing what matters to the individual—places considerable emphasis on actual experiences and behaviors. In contrast, evolutionary psychology generally relies on judgments by informants (say, of attraction), rather than focusing on how and why individuals actually experience attraction. With abstract judgments, cultural symbolism and biases often shape how individuals respond. The obvious impact of culture opens up the evolutionary psychology approach to easy, repeated, and often vehement critiques (Buller, 2005; McKinnon & Silverman, 2005; Rose & Rose, 2000).

Human behavioral ecology faces a similar problem given its core question: Does the behavior match the theoretical prediction? This approach often does not consider what the behavior accomplishes from the viewpoint of the individual, something that ethnog-raphy can provide. Moreover, its theoretical aim is not always useful for research on health. Human behavioral ecologists rely on abstract "outcomes" that might be theoreti-cally relevant (e.g., optimal foraging) but are not necessarily relevant to what shapes adaptive or maladaptive behavior (e.g., what environmental factors favor healthy eating). In contrast, an epidemiological approach offers the tools to analyze what factors are asso-ciated with unhealthy dietary habits or what risk factors predict substance abuse.

In my previous research, ethnography contributed to understanding participants' experiences of compulsive wanting and seeking (Lende, 2005). Psychometric techniques were used to develop a scale that examined "compulsive involvement" in substance abuse by focusing on these subjective experiences. This measurement proved to be an impor-tant predictor of addiction (Lende, 2005). Indeed, this approach—using ethnography to explore experiences and behaviors and then developing the interconnections between these reports and the behavioral biology of substance abuse—represents an alternative way to do evolutionary analysis.

Similarly, rather than being focused on expected benefits about drugs (a judgment approach), this research looked at actual patterns of behavioral reinforcement of the drug-taking lifestyle. By asking how many times respondents had been involved in agreeable sexual situations and had won competitions or fights due to substance use, this research emphasized the significant differences between addicted and nonaddicted individuals (defined in Lende, 2005). Using a summary variable of evolutionary benefits (the sum of both sexual and competitive benefits), addicted individuals reported 2.76 total benefits versus 0.98 benefits for nonaddicted individuals ($p < 0.001$, two-tailed t-test).

This *experience-and-behavior* approach shares many similarities with an embodied view of human behavior. Embodiment refers to the central role that bodily states and interactions with the environment play in cognition and behavior, rather than abstract reasoning and symbolism (such as the computer model of the brain). Evolutionary psychology, based on an information-processing model, and human behavioral ecology, with its emphasis on assumed rationality, both contrast sharply with recent understandings of how organisms (including people) engage in successful cognition and behavior in specific environments. From understandings of how to build successful robots (and not just computer programs) (Clark, 1996) to the ecological view of psychology (Reed, 1996; Rosch, 1996) to embodied views of perception and neuroscience (Barsalou, 1999; Barsalou et al., 2003; Gibbs, 2006) to categorization and even philosophy (Lakoff & Johnson, 1999), this emerging approach is one that evolutionary theory can engage successfully, provided it remains rooted in the selectionist and phylogenetic analyses that are its main strengths.

Combining ethnography and epidemiology also permits the examination of other competing hypotheses to explain substance use and abuse. For example, compulsive involvement was not a significant predictor of poly-drug use even though it was for addiction (Lende, 2005). However, endorsement of a cultural model emphasizing social distance from the world of drug use was a significant negative predictor for poly-drug use, even though endorsement of this model had no significant statistical relationship with addiction (Lende, 2005).

Similarly, risk factors derived from other research paradigms can actually end up being quite complementary to an evolutionary approach. Previous epidemiological research in Colombia revealed the importance of friends' drug use and of experiencing violence as predictors of marijuana use (Brook et al., 1998). In my research, these two factors were major predictors of addiction alongside compulsive involvement (Lende, 2005). Friends' drug use provided both drug availability and an adaptive benefit (particularly given the importance of social relationships in the high-risk environments associated with using). Experiencing violence captured the extreme stress involved in compulsive use of drugs, which often takes place on the "street" in Colombian cities. This high-risk environment also accentuates short-term benefits such as positive sexual encounters and winning competitive encounters—respondents often reported feeling stronger and "crazier" due to drug use.

Thus, the evolutionary approach can be fully compatible with approaches developed in other fields, while also providing novel interpretations for how and why individuals behave the way they do. From compulsive involvement and adaptive benefits to making sense of how modern environments can push individuals to engage in short-term behaviors, evolutionary medicine—drawing on an approach that begins with the experiences and behaviors of actual individuals—places itself in a position to provide novel understandings of modern behavioral problems like addiction.

CONCLUSION

This chapter highlights three important components in the evolutionary analysis of addiction. First, it is crucial to use adaptive considerations and phylogenetic comparisons when considering the behavioral biology that underlies problematic behavior. Particular processes, like wanting and seeking, can malfunction. This malfunction can be affected by specific adaptive benefits and/or vulnerabilities (from genetics and development to local environments, such as a drug-using family). This focus on malfunction and the factors that shape malfunction can apply to other behavioral problems, such as eating disorders. Obesity is a modern epidemic, and recent research (Berthoud, 2004; Kringelbach, 2004; Wang et al., 2004) is compatible with many of the points developed in this chapter.

It is also useful to consider the interaction between more phylogenetically ancient motivational systems and more recent systems of cognitive and symbolic control. Environments that are stressful and that encourage short-term behavioral strategies can sensitize phylogenetically older systems so they become overly reactive. At the same time, systems of inequality (which control local resources and access to long-term successful behavioral strategies) can reinforce this sort of immediate decision making, even as advertising and global economic development present a wealth of options to satisfy cravings.

Finally, modern lifestyles seem to bundle together evolutionarily relevant factors in ways that worsen compulsive involvement in behaviors. With friends, availability, adaptive benefits, and subjective escape all wrapped up into drug taking, this lifestyle has an immediate appeal and ease, especially in contrast to stressful environments with few available long-term options. This sort of lifestyle can be reinforced by the particular cultural scenes and attitudes that provide ways to further define a drug-using lifestyle. Overall, the parsing of lifestyles and environments in evolutionarily relevant ways (while maintaining a biocultural approach) represents a logical next step for research, given how evolutionary analyses already address the separate components of behavioral decision-making systems. This type of approach will significantly increase the validity and applicability of the discordance hypothesis in evolutionary medicine.

ACKNOWLEDGMENTS

I thank the editors, especially Neal Smith, for their substantial comments, which significantly improved this chapter. Portions of the research discussed here were supported by grants from the National Institute of Drug Abuse and the Fulbright Program.

CHAPTER 16

After Dark

The Evolutionary Ecology
of Human Sleep

Carol M. Worthman

Until relatively recently, studies of the sleep of human adults or infants ignored the human adaptive context and circumstances within which human sleep evolved. Perhaps a consequence of this is that medically trained sleep researchers missed opportunities to understand the kinds of environmental pressures and needs for which both contemporary adult and infant sleep architecture and arousal patterns were originally designed. Worthman's chapter provides a novel and innovative analysis of what various forms of human sleep are good and not good for and what factors best explain conundrums such as the apparent human inability to prevent sleep restriction alongside and in relationship to the ubiquity of insomnia in modern life. The need in the past and present for nighttime vigilance is one of the more important aspects of her discussion. She also examines the dissociation between objective measures of sleep (quantitative data) and what people subjectively report (i.e., how people describe a "good" or "adequate" nights sleep). Further, she notes that sleep researchers worry about Westerners sleeping less when, according to epidemiological studies, death is more likely for someone that sleeps more, rather than less. Similar to other anthropologists who study sleep from an evolutionary point of view and have challenged the Western cultural notion that infants should sleep alone, or that necessarily uninterrupted early consolidated sleep is "good" or safe for babies, Worthman flips around conventional understandings of how and why adult sleep responds to local conditions as it does and what it all means for human health. Her contribution illustrates what evolutionary medicine seems to do quite well, i.e., not mistaking adaptation for pathology in the same way that it forces a more careful distinction between defense and defect. Worthman's broad ecological analysis includes new considerations of the evolutionary origins and contexts of sleep. Her functional explanations expose instances in which cultural ideologies are mistaken for more empirically based, species-wide science. For example, she answers the question of why adults might sleep less than research suggests is ideal. What a surprise it is to learn that one possible answer is that we are not supposed to! Is it possible that there may be better things to do with our time than sleep, activities that more effectively promote our mental and physical health at that particular time? Worthman suggests that this might well be one answer to why Westerners sleep as they do! Perhaps this is good news for students, who never seem to find time to get enough sleep.

INTRODUCTION

Why do we sleep? Remarkably, we still don't know (Rechtschaffen, 1998). What we do know is that sleep is as essential to life as oxygen or food: sleep disruption erodes psychobehavioral performance and alters bodily function, and complete sleep deprivation can lead to death nearly as swiftly as does starvation (Roth, 2004). The gap in knowledge about the essential biological functions of sleep limits the efforts of sleep scientists and clinicians to explain and identify treatments for sleep disorders, advise patients on best sleep practices, and suggest public health guidelines for prevention of sleep problems. In the absence of a complete account of sleep function, a more broadly grounded understanding of the sources and sequelae of sleep problems might help, nevertheless, to address some of these concerns. This possibility will be explored in light of expanding knowledge about the physiology and phenomenology of sleep along with evolutionary and comparative ethnographic analysis.

The stakes for understanding sleep are rising as globalization inadvertently transforms sleep practices around the world. Virtually universal introduction of schooling and new forms of labor over the last 50 years have regimented daily schedules in new ways, while the spread of electricity and media has altered capacity, options, and demands for activity around the clock. Such spectacular technological and sociological transformations have attracted both credit and blame for sleep restriction and sleep-related problems, including accidents, psychiatric disorders, insomnias, obstructive sleep disorders, and chronic physical diseases. The effects on sleep from striking structural and technological sources have tended to eclipse other more subtle ones, including changes in the conditions under which people sleep. Adoption of modern forms of housing, beds and bedding, and climate control alter the ecology of sleep, as does erosion of cosleeping practices with increased secure space, changing notions of childhood and human development, and the rise of the postmodern family. This essay will consider how the newly configured material, social, and psychological contexts of sleep may exert not only direct effects on sleep behaviors and related health problems, but also indirect ones through interactions with lifestyle-defining macrosocietal shifts in technology, labor, and social structure.

Another, larger question colors the struggle to understand linkages between changing sleep habits and health. Sleep habits are highly plastic, shifting to meet the demands of circumstance and motivation in ways that sleep researchers argue can be deeply injurious (Bonnet & Arand, 1995; Dawson & Reid, 1997; Harrison & Horne, 2000; Landrigan et al., 2004). *Why* such plasticity? If sleep is so important, strong countervailing pressures should restrict the human capacity to adjust sleep behaviors in ways that adversely affect health. A broader comparative and evolutionary view suggests some answers to this question, and furthermore suggests why, when, and how disturbed or curtailed sleep becomes problematic. Specifically, the present analysis identifies situations that provoke sleep restriction and discovers the role of stress and stress physiology in the causes and consequences of disrupted sleep. Identification of conditions that act as *triggers* for sleep restriction can guide individuals and caregivers to avoid, detect, and cope with the situations that stimulate sleep restriction. Insights into the bearing that the extensive knowledge about stress ecology and physiology has on understanding the sources and sequelae of sleep behavior may resolve old questions and change scientific, clinical, and popular views of why and how we sleep.

HUMAN SLEEP

For most people, sleep occupies about a third of the day and, as such, represents the most common human behavior. Outwardly, sleepers are quietly disengaged from the world, eyes closed, limbs relaxed, and habitually withdrawn to a designated comfortable location. Yet the apparent behavioral quiescence of sleep belies its characteristic intense, complex, and patterned physiological activity (Table 16-1). A brief review of this complex state provides valuable background to understanding the nature and ecology of sleep and how it may be disrupted (reviewed in Buysse, 2005; Hobson & Pace-Schott, 2002; Rama, Cho, & Kushida, 2006). Virtually all systems and their functions are altered as sleep sequences through distinctive physiological patterns that run in 90- to 100-minute cycles between phases of nonrapid eye movement (NREM) and rapid eye movement (REM). Usually, sleep begins with a progression through the four stages of NREM sleep, moving from a brief period of Stage 1 drowsy sleep (3–8% of sleep), to Stage 2 light sleep (45–55%), to the deep and very deep slow wave (δdelta) sleep comprising Stages 3 and 4 (15–20%). In the coma-like depths of slow wave sleep, several body functions (e.g., respiration and heart rate, thermoregulation) are slowed, muscles relax, and directed thought is sharply diminished. Brain activity alters, and not only in the distinctive overall electroencephalographic (EEG) signatures of each sleep stage: some brain areas active in waking become inactive, while others inactive in waking become active. The contrast between external and internal activity states becomes greatest in REM sleep, during which a very active brain occupies an immobilized body. Thermoregulation and muscle tone are nearly absent, heart rate and respiration become slow and more irregular, and eyes move in characteristic staccato bursts. REM sleep hosts dreaming. The qualitatively distinctive mental activity experienced in this stage features hallucinatory over directed thought, absence of self-reflective awareness, attenuated analytical thought, and lack of voluntary control over dream content.

Sleep Regulation

How does the body "know" when to sleep and to wake? Orienting to the world and maintaining appropriate levels of arousal constitute critical features of effective functioning for any organism. Hence, these features are subject to redundant mechanisms that negotiate meeting immediate demands such as evading a predator or foraging for food

TABLE 16-1 Characteristics of Wake and Sleep States

Behavioral state Functional state	Wake Awake—somnolent	NREM Stages 1–4	REM Tonic—phasic
Physiological			
EEG	Fast, low voltage	Slow, high voltage	Fast, low voltage
Brain activity	+++ (vary by region)	+++ (vary by region)	+++ (vary by region)
Eye movement	Varies with vision	Slow / irregular	Rapid, phasic
Muscle tone	++	+	0
Heart rate, blood pressure, respiration	+++ (variable)	++ (regular)	+ (variable)
Response to hypoxia, hypercarbia	+++	++	+
Thermoregulation	+++	++	0 to +
	Physiological + behavioral	Physiological, sweat/shiver	Physiological
Behavioral			
Eyes	Open, blink	Closed	Closed
Posture	Erect	Recumbent	Recumbent
Body movement	Continuous, voluntary	Episodic, involuntary	Immobile—twitches
Responsiveness	+++	+ /++	0/+
Cognitive			
Mental activity	Vivid, external origin	Absent or dull	Vivid, internal origin
Conscious thought	Logical, progressive	Logical, perseverative	Illogical, distorted
Memory	Acquisition, retrieval	Consolidation (declarative and nondeclarative)	Consolidation (declarative and nondeclarative)
Proportion of sleep period			
Infancy (16–18 h/day)	Gradual consolidation, reduction of sleep quota		50%
Adolescence (9 h/day)		Intense SWS	20–25%
Adulthood (7–8 h/day)	<5%	75–80%	15–25%

Source: Buysse 2005; Hobson & Pace-Schott 2002; Rosenthal 2006; Roth 2004, Walker & Stickgold 2006.

against ongoing homeostatic needs that are met during sleep. Accordingly, regulation of sleep and wake states is the product of two interacting mechanisms, a circadian pacemaker and homeostatic drive. The internal circadian pacemaker manages alertness and operates through the suprachiasmatic nucleus of the hypothalamus: entrained primarily by external environmental light, the nucleus tracks ambient time and synchronizes activity of the body's systems and organs to both clock time and seasons (Pace-Schott & Hobson, 2002; Richardson, 2005). Circadian drive for alert wakefulness—indexed by activity of arousal systems in brain stem, basal forebrain, and hypothalamus—peaks at 8–9 p.m. and thereafter drops precipitously to a minimum during the latter half of the habitual sleep period, or between 3 and 6 a.m., whereafter it rises throughout the day (Wright, Hull, Hughes, Ronda, & Czeisler, 2006).

Reciprocally, homeostatic sleep drive constitutes sleep pressure that accumulates during wakefulness and resolves during sleep (Borbély & Achermann, 2000). Homeostatic regulation of slow wave activity, or slow oscillations in membrane potential of cortical neurons during sleep, manifests in increased slow wave activity after wakefulness and declines to baseline during sleep. Slow wave activity may reflect synaptic changes that generate the cellular "drive" for sleep (Tononi, 2005). Thus, slow wave activity increases during sleep in specific brain regions after learning tasks that target those regions (Huber, Ghilardi, Massimini, & Tononi, 2004). In this homeostatic model of sleep need, the longer the time since the last sleep episode, the greater the drive; conversely, the longer the time elapsed in a sleep bout, the lower the homeostatic drive for sleep. Further, insufficient sleep incurs a "sleep debt" reflected in residual sleep drive manifested in subjective sleepiness and objective latency to fall asleep (Littner et al., 2005) and produced by inhibition of wakefulness-promoting neurons as adenosine levels rise with duration of wakefulness (Basheer, Strecker, Thakkar, & McCarley, 2004). Hunger and food consumption provide a well-studied behavioral parallel: the greater the hunger, the more intense the feeding, and the more that has been eaten, the lower the hunger drive (Lima, Rattenborg, Lesku, & Amlaner, 2005). The physiological bases of homeostatic sleep drive are uncertain, but biomarkers for extent of sleep drive comprise amount and intensity of slow wave activity, or delta EEG activity during NREM sleep, and possibly the amount of EEG theta activity during wakefulness (Buysse, 2005). Sleep loss potentiates a compensatory catch-up response manifested in more and greater intensity of slow wave sleep and longer sleep episode. In sum, current formulations of sleep drive aim to explain patterns of sleepiness, but the physiological bases remain fuzzy: the gap in our understanding of the bases of sleep need leads to reliance on amount and timing of slow wave sleep as markers of sleep drive or deficit.

Interactions of the circadian pacemaker and homeostatic drive direct the sleep–wake cycle through inputs to hypothalamic nuclei regulating wakefulness, particularly the hypocretin/orexin system, to adaptively adjust the amount and timing of sleep (Saper, Cano, & Scammell, 2005). Yet sleep is also immediately reversible. Capacity for reversibility inheres in the neuroarchitecture of sleep and permits acute demands, such as the cry of a hungry infant or the ring of an alarm clock, to counterbalance the ascendant states of arousal regulating systems. Brain activity states that potentiate condition-specific arousal responses (micro-arousals) are systematically distributed throughout sleep and alter the threshold for reaction to external stimuli: the cyclic alternating pattern of such states in NREM sleep is thought to permit sleep reversibility even during the otherwise coma-like periods of deep sleep (reviewed in Halász, Terzano, Parrino, & Bódizs, 2004). Generally, micro-arousals may organize a capacity for filtered monitoring of the external environment during sleep by sensitizing endogenous processes of sleep to internal and external conditions. Density of micro-arousals is increased after a stressful day or in anxious individuals and has been associated with nonrestorative sleep (poor sleep quality) even where sleep efficiency (percent actual sleep during sleep period) is maintained: treatments that reduce micro-arousals in insomniacs improve subjective sleep quality (Halász, Terzano, Parrino, & Bódizs, 2004).

The picture of sleep that emerges, then, is of a behavior state that is highly regulated and structured through endogenous neurological processes, yet is entrained by external cues and acutely reversible by momentary demands. In other words, perhaps more than any other behavior, sleep combines powerful physiological regulation with inbuilt sensitivity to context, both internal and external. Unlike other behaviors, the course and content of sleep lies largely outside voluntary control (Hobson & Pace-Schott, 2002).

EVOLUTIONARY BACKGROUND

Regular or cyclic variation in the environment (diurnal, seasonal, trophic) presents adaptive opportunities and challenges for resident organisms. Accordingly, life forms universally display capacities to vary activity states in synchrony with patterns of light–dark, warm–cold, or feeding opportunities. Although sleep has been studied most extensively in mammals, characteristic sleep-like behavior has been observed in invertebrates such as cockroaches and fruit flies, amphibians and fish such as tree frogs or carp, and reptiles and birds such as lizards or hummingbirds (Lesku, Rattenborg, & Amlaner, 2006; Tobler, 2000). Data on the comparative physiology of sleep and activity states remain patchy but can be generalized to suggest that the hallmarks of sleep-like behavior include characteristic posture, reduced activity, altered arousal thresholds, and homeostatic regulation manifested in rebound or compensatory responses after rest/sleep deprivation. Despite the ubiquity of behavior that meets these criteria, substantial variation in sleep budget, or the amount and distribution of sleep behavior, has been observed both within and between taxa. Species-characteristic sleep quotas, or daily amount of sleep, vary among mammals from 3 hours in horses and 4 hours in elephants to 19 hours in opossum and nearly 20 hours in brown bats (Siegel, 2005 source materials). The underlying architecture and physiology of sleep differ among taxa as well. At one extreme, dolphins and other cetaceans lack REM and are never completely asleep; rather, one hemisphere goes into slow wave "sleep" and the contralateral eye closes while swimming and navigation continue. Other extremes include short wake cycles in small animals, down to 7 minutes in 15.5 g big brown bats, and long ones in large animals, up to 2 hours in 3500 kg Asiatic elephants (Siegel, 2005).

Debated Functions of Sleep

Of the many functions ascribed to sleep, the most prominent concern rest and recuperation, conservation of energy, safety and predator avoidance, and memory consolidation and affective processing (Siegel, 2005). Those who emphasize that sleep is by the brain for the brain underscore a role in brain development and function (Walker & Stickgold, 2006). While there is evidence that some of these functions are necessary, none has been found to be a sufficient role for sleep. For instance, the primacy of rest is undercut by observations that periods of hibernation or torpor, such as in bears or hummingbirds, are followed by profiles of brain activity in sleep indicative of sleep deprivation. A role for energy sparing is limited by the high energetic cost of REM and the observation that "[t]he metabolic savings of sleep over quiet wakefulness has been estimated at approximately 10 to 15 percent; from the standpoint of energy savings, a night of sleep for a 200-pound person is worth a cup of milk" (Rechtschaffen, 1998, p. 364). Absence of sleep in newborn dolphins and killer whales argues against the crucial role of sleep in brain development (Siegel, 2005). Compelling evidence for the role of sleep in brain plasticity and memory consolidation (Hairston et al., 2005; Huber, Ghilardi, Massimini, & Tononi, 2004; Wright, Hull, Hughes, Ronda, & Czeisler, 2006) nevertheless fails to account for the near-absence of postpartum maternal sleep or sleep rebound in cetaceans (Siegel, 2005).

The continued mystery surrounding its function motivates interest in the comparative study of sleep for clues from its evolutionary history. Comparative evolutionary approaches have focused on features thought to be related to the putative functions of sleep. Thus, brain and body size, metabolic rate, diet (carni-, omni-, and herbivore), and neonatal characteristics (birth weight, altriciality) all have been considered as life history traits that influence the need for energy conservation, predator avoidance through inactivity and concealment, buffering or restoration of wear and tear, or demands of development, especially brain development. As such, taxonomic correlations between these life history traits and key parameters of sleep (sleep quota, amount of NREM and of REM sleep, and duration of sleep cycle) have been consulted to identify possible functional constraints that shape the evolution of sleep (Allison & Cicchetti, 1976; Tobler, 2000). Phylogenetic studies have concentrated on the more extensive data available for the well-studied mammalian order and repeatedly have linked taxonomic variation in sleep parameters with size of body and brain, metabolic rate, and neonatal characteristics (Elgar, Pagel, & Harvey, 1988; Zepelin, 2000). A recent definitive multivariate analysis has superceded previous reports by taking the critical step of accounting for evolutionary effects related to body size, or allometry, as well as removing statistical artifacts (Capellini, Barton, McNamara, & Nunn, in press). Capellini and colleagues' results, summarized in Table 16-2, demonstrate the pervasive effects of allometry on sleep parameters and substantially clarify evolutionary relationships. In particular, this clarified view prunes the list of candidate functions for sleep. That brain mass is unrelated to any sleep parameters refutes direct functions of sleep for brain restorative processes. Similarly, absence of association between neonatal brain mass and sleep parameters militates against a direct role for sleep in brain development (Rechtschaffen, 1998). The failure to find constraints on sleep parameters related to metabolic rate argues against hypothesized restorative need for relief of oxidative stress from metabolic turnover (Siegel, 2005) as well as against a straightforward role in energy conservation for sleep (Berger & Phillips, 1995).

Most prominent among Capellini and colleagues' findings that support proposed sleep functions are the multiple relationships of life history characteristics to sleep parameters that suggest effects of predator pressure (Lima, Rattenborg, Lesku, & Amlaner, 2005): short gestation length and low birth weight are related to lower sleep quotas, both

TABLE 16-2 Comparative Evolutionary Analysis of the Correlates of Mammalian Sleep

Phenotypic feature	Sleep quota	NREM	REM	Sleep cycle length
Body mass	—	Negative	—	Positive
Brain mass	—	X	—	X
Basal Metabolism	X	X	—	X
Gestation length	Negative	Negative	Negative	X
Body mass, neonatal	—	Negative	Negative	X
Brain mass, neonatal	—	X	—	X
Total sleep				Negative
NREM quota			Positive	—
REM quota				Negative

—, *Association tested, not significant.*
X, *Association removed by controlling for allometry.*
Blank, Test for association not reported, presumably positive.
Source: Data from Capellini et al., in press.

REM and NREM, which may reflect reduced investment in maintenance. Then, the association of longer sleep cycles with less total and REM sleep supports the proposed trade-off between vigilance and sleep need whereby the reduced vigilance characteristic of REM is more widely spaced and diminished when total sleep is increased. Nevertheless, as Capellini and colleagues emphasize (Capellini, Barton, McNamara, & Nunn, in press), the phenotypic features included in their analysis account for little taxonomic variation in sleep parameters (9–40%): that so much diversity remains unexplained powerfully indicates that other factors are at work and much remains to be explored. For instance, the greater the body mass, the longer the length of sleep cycle. This association mediates all other phenotypic relationships to cycle length; even so, the body mass–cycle length relationship explains only a third of the phylogenetic variance in cycle length. Note also that phylogenetic analyses of this global kind cannot evaluate possible brain region– or function-specific roles such as memory consolidation (Walker & Stickgold, 2006) or cortical plasticity (Hobson & Pace-Schott, 2002) and suggest the need to ally physiological with field research to link experimental with phenotypic, demographic, and ecological information and accelerate progress on understanding the functions of sleep.

Viewed from a comparative evolutionary perspective, the characteristics of human sleep are not distinctive (Siegel, 2005). Given both the brain-based understandings of sleep and that so much else in human behavior and cognition has been considered extraordinary, its unexceptional character in humans is worth remarking. Quotas for total, REM, and NREM sleep, ratio of REM to NREM, and sleep cycle length do not stand out in phylogenetic analyses, although overall and specific regional size and organization of the human brain do (Allison & Cicchetti, 1976; Rilling, 2006).

The strong focus on sleep architecture—structure of the sleep cycle by stage and NREM/REM—by comparative studies for insight into function has tended to overshadow the role of ecological factors in the evolution of sleep behavior and physiology. Sleep is a risky behavior, because it includes periods of blunted awareness, relative physical unresponsiveness, reduced or absent thermoregulation, and a stationary site (Lima, Rattenborg, Lesku, & Amlaner, 2005). Sites, surfaces, and social groupings for sleep all would have direct bearing on important ecological challenges incurred for sleep, including thermal exposure, physical safety and comfort, and vulnerability to predators and parasites (Anderson, 1998). Extensive field studies of primates document that avoidance of predation drives selection of sleeping sites, exemplified by use of tree holes by prosimians and tamarins, cliff faces by Hamadryas baboons, and tree crowns or outer branches by many primates, from smaller monkeys to apes (Anderson, 1998; Kappeler, 1998). Widespread practice of nest building among the great apes even may represent evidence for instrumental tool use and observational learning, or culture (Fruth & Hohmann, 1996).

Sleep in Human Evolution

The record of evolutionary history for human sleep is sketchy (see Nadel et al., 2004). Sleep sites, whether nests in trees or beds on the ground, leave little, if any, trace in the fossil record. Skeletal evidence provides clues to where hominids might have slept: advancing skeletal modifications in the evolution of bipedalism diminished agility in trees and decreased access to and usability of arboreal sleeping sites. Loss of hair that limited infant capacity for clinging would have made tree occupation even more cumbersome and dangerous. Hair loss also increased thermal pressure from heat loss during sleep and required sources of heat or covering in exposed arboreal settings. The ground-dwelling ancestral ape lineages became ground-sleeping in hominids, who have been presumed to have relied on protection from tools, social groupings, then fire, and eventually physical structures to fend off predators during waking and sleeping. Thence, one must turn to the record of occupation sites themselves. Residence in and exchange with social groups is seen as characteristic of the human lineage: an influential theory proposed that emergence of a home base for convergence after foraging and sharing of food, information, and sociality formed a crucial step in social evolution (Isaac, 1981). But sharing and other features of home base are not unique to humans, and unambiguous identification of such home bases in the paleoanthropological record has proven difficult (Sept, 1998). Disputed evidence for hominid association with fire begins in Africa 1.4–1.5 million years ago and is uncontestably accepted as widespread systematic, controlled use at around the onset of the last Ice Age in the later middle Pleistocene (~110,000–130,000 B.P.) in conjunction with appearance of anatomically modern humans (Wrangham, Jones, Laden, Pilbeam, & Conklin-Brittain, 1999). Convergently, characteristic human occupation sites that combine use for living, production, and food sharing also appear during the same period in sub-Saharan Africa. Use of caves and traces of posts for huts around hearths appear by 500,000 B.P. (Nadel et al., 2004).

For much of human evolution, security in sleep depended upon sources other than fire or housing, which undoubtedly have shaped the features of sleep and sleeping behavior. Features of the evolutionary bioecology of human sleep are summarized in Table 16-3. Although limitations in the archeological record may produce conservative estimates of the dates by which humans customarily used fire and lived in physical structures that

TABLE 16-3 Elements of Human Sleep Ecology

Microecology	Evolutionary Bioecology
Proximate physical ecology	Group living
Bedding	Ground dwelling
Presence of fire	Subsistance foraging
Sleeping place or structure	Equatorial
Proximate social ecology	Intense social relations
Sleeping arrangements	Sharing, reciprocity
Separation of sleep—wake states	Food
Biotic macro- and microecology	Labor
Domestic animals	Information
Parasites and nighttime pests	Protection and care
Macropredators (animal, human)	Use of tools and (later) fire
Macroecology	Dual inheritance
Labor demands	
Social activity	
Ritual practices	
Beliefs about sleep and dreaming	
Status (social status, class, gender)	
Life history, lifespan processes	
Ecology, climate	
Demography and settlement patterns	

afforded protection from predators and the elements, these practices nonetheless came late in the evolution of human sleep. Thence, an evolutionary picture of human sleep ecology as "extremely safe" and safer than in any other mammal (Allison & Cicchetti, 1976) would appear overoptimistic.

COMPARATIVE PERSPECTIVES

Surprisingly, anthropology and behavioral ecology have not systematically engaged the-most prevalent of human behaviors. In consequence, the empirical grounds for comparative analysis of sleep behavior are exceedingly thin. Documentation of cross-cultural patterns and variation in sleep, sleep quota, napping, objective and subjective sleep quality, sleep architecture, and life course trajectory has barely begun (see BaHamman, 2003; Liu, Liu, & Wang, 2003; McKenna, 1986, 2000; McKenna & McDade, 2005; McKenna, Mosko, Dungy, & McAnninch, 1991; McKenna et al., 1993; Reimao et al., 2000a, 2000b; Reimao, Souza, Medeiros, & Almirao, 1998; Worthman & Brown, 2007 (see also Chapter 12). The physical and social ecology of sleep is, by contrast, more accessible in ethnographic and historical accounts (Ekirch, 2005; McKenna et al., 1993). Humans inhabit a wide range of physical settings and distinctive cultures associated with strikingly different personal and social landscapes of meaning, thought, and action. The pervasive impact of culture extends to sleep and informs where, when, how, and with whom one will sleep at any age and physical or social condition, along with the meanings and interpretations of sleep and its wider social–emotional frame. With ethnographic information from colleagues having society-specific expertise (Robert Bailey, Fredrik Barth, Magdalena Hurtado, Bruce Knauft, Mel Konner, and John Wood) and using an analytical framework outlined in Table 16-3 (left side), we undertook a preliminary comparative analysis of human sleep ecology (Worthman & Melby, 2002). This analysis revealed areas of commonality and diversity in the proximal conditions or microecology under which people sleep and documented the pervasive effects of social, cultural, and physical ecological factors, or macroecology, on patterns of sleep.

Our comparative analysis yielded unexpected findings, particularly by identifying unusual characteristics of contemporary sleep ecology and practices. Across societies we reviewed, sleep settings were social and solitary sleep rare; bedtimes fluid and napping common; bedding minimal; fire present; conditions dim or dark; and conditions relatively noisy with people, animals, and little or no acoustic and physical barrier to ambient conditions. As such, sleep settings offered rich and dynamic sensory properties, including security and comfort through social setting, fuzzy boundaries in time and space, and little climate control. By contrast, postmodern industrial societies emerged as having relatively impoverished, stable sensory properties including solitary or low-contact sleep conditions, scheduled bed- and waketimes and consolidated sleep, padded bed and profuse bedding, absence of fire, and darkness, silence, and high acoustic as well as physical boundaries to sleep spaces. These much more static sleep conditions typically offer security and comfort through physical setting, rigid boundaries in time and space, and climate control. Although contemporary postmodern industrial Western conditions did stand out as unusual, there were favorable contrasts that included the relative absence of parasites and vectors of disease, fear of predators and ambush, discomfort from harsh temperatures or rough bedding, or disruptions from crowding, noise or activities of others. Other features may make sleep regulation more challenging, including habitual solitary sleep or limited cosleep from infancy onwards; a "lie down and die" model of sleep in restricted intervals with few, brief sleep–wake transitions; and sensory deprivation of physical and social cues in sleep settings. An untested question is whether these unusual habits and settings place high and sustained burdens on sleep–wake regulation systems that contribute to contemporary sleep problems and disorders.

Comparative analysis also reveals common features of sleep behavior among humans. Human nights are filled with activity and significance, and nowhere do people typically sleep from evening to dawn. Across cultures, humans also show a range of arousal states that blur binary sleep–wake distinctions, including capacities for sustained somnolence or resting wakefulness, for adjusting level of vigilance in sleep, and for nonconsolidated sleep patterns including napping and night waking. When and as necessary, humans can and will restrict sleep for extended periods. They also will opportunistically sleep, tolerating long resting bouts they may not need.

The risky conditions under which human sleep evolved likely promoted both complexity of sleep architecture and capacity for vigilance in sleep (Lima, Rattenborg, Lesku, & Amlaner, 2005). We know that a sure way of increasing the proportion of REM is to lengthen the bout (Siegel, 2005), but we do not know how culture-based lifetime differences in sleep patterns and settings influence sleep architecture, or amounts and quality of sleep, or even memory, the capacity for state regulation, and mental health. These compelling questions await future study.

NOT GETTING ENOUGH? SLEEP DIFFICULTIES AND DYSFUNCTIONS

Sleep problems affect an estimated 50–70 million Americans (Strine & Chapman, 2005). Sleep scientists and clinicians habitually point to dramatic statistics documenting national and international escalation in sleep problems and threats to sleep adequacy (U.S. Department of Health and Human Services, 2003). Recent Sleep in America Polls provide vivid evidence for the nature and extent of adult Americans' sleep problems and poor sleep habits (National Sleep Foundation, 2005). In its most recent report, the survey found that barely half of Americans (49%) say that they regularly "had a good night's sleep," and 17% of respondents reported that they felt tired or not up to par on all or most days. Unsurprisingly, respondents also reported a daily average consumption of 2.5 caffeinated beverages. In another national survey, 26% of adults reported experiencing sleep insufficiency on 14 or more of the past 30 days (Strine & Chapman, 2005). Sleep problems constitute a personal and a public concern: they not only affect mental and physical health and well-being, but also represent a major source of traffic and work-related accidents and errors, and lateness or low productivity at work or school.

To the evident frustration of advocates, the public on the whole appears unmoved by sleep matters, and sleep habits remain poor by scientific accounts. Before considering further why sleep problems are so widespread and why they continue to advance in the face of medical advice, a brief review of the nature and extent of sleep disruptions and disorders is in order.

Sleep Difficulty

The most prominent sleep complaint is insomnia, defined as difficulty in entering or sustaining nighttime sleep or poor sleep quality (Brown, 2006). One third of contemporary Americans report having one or more current insomnia symptoms (Ohayon, 2002), and the lifetime prevalence of having the disorder itself is 16.6% (Breslau, Roth, Rosenthal, & Andreski, 1996). Prevalent as it is, insomnia arises from multiple causes and presents informative complexities that were brought to widespread attention by Mendelson's important observation that patients taking benzodiazepine had objectively poor sleep but experienced better subjective sleep quality (Mendelson, 1990). Cognitive processes since have been recognized to play specific major roles in sleep quality and insomnia (Harvey, Tang, & Browning, 2005). Related to Mendelson's observation, insomniacs' common experience of sleep onset as more delayed and quality of sleep as lower than is objectively the case provides further evidence for the significance of sleepers' distorted perception in poor sleep quality. Studies that alter subjective sleep quality by using placebo, manipulating attribution, or modifying unhelpful beliefs about sleep have demonstrated the importance of expectation. Associations of reduced reported sleep quality with selective attention to markers of delayed sleep onset and of poor sleep quality upon waking illustrate the contributory role of attention in insomnia (Harvey, Tang, & Browning, 2005; Tang, Schmidt, & Harvey, 2007).

Psychiatric manuals recognize a wide array of other sleep disorders with organic and psychiatric origins (Buysse, 2005), but only one will be considered here because of its rising prevalence and visibility, namely sleep-related breathing disorders and particularly obstructive sleep apneas. Epidemiological reports in the 1990s drew attention to these conditions by finding a startlingly high prevalence in several countries. Characterized by frequent sleep-related apnea and hypopnea (obstructed/interrupted and shallow breathing, respectively) with daytime sleepiness (Stradling & Davies, 2004), prevalence ranges from 1 to 28%, depending on level of severity (Young, Peppard, & Gottlieb, 2002). Risk factors include gender (men two- to threefold more often than women), overweight and obesity, smoking, and age (Tesali & Van Cauter, 2002). The worldwide trends to increased obesity, smoking, and aging population structure contribute to escalating rates in obstructive sleep apnea. This condition, in turn, contributes to risk for hypertension and other vascular disease, as well as exposure to the consequences of sleepiness and impaired cognition (Young, 2004).

Sleep Loss

By contrast with sleep difficulties, sleep loss is directly linked to psychological, behavioral, and social-structural factors. The sleep quota among Americans has declined over the last 24 years (1982–2005), from 8 to 6.9 hours a day (Kripke, Garfinkel, Wingard, Klauber, & Marler, 2002; National Sleep Foundation, 2005). In a recent poll, modal reported sleep per night was 6.8 hours, contrasting to the recommended 7–9 hours, depending on age and other factors affecting need. Yet of respondents to that poll, only 22% reported getting less sleep than they needed, and 40% said they got more than needed (National Sleep Foundation, 2005).

Youth are a focus of particular concern because they appear especially vulnerable to disordered sleep patterns associated with severe consequences reflected in spiking rates of accidents and suicide or even school failure (Dahl, 2006). Sleep need in adolescence remains high (at around 9 hours), and youth show later onset and offset of sleep along with an increased penchant for resisting sleep in favor of more stimulating pursuits (Carskadon, 2002). Such youth-specific risks to educational, emotional, and physical well-being are thought to have increased because the percentage of young adults who sleep fewer than 7 hours per night has more than doubled during the last 40 years (1960–2001), from 16 to 37% (Spiegel, Tasali, Penev, & Van Cauter, 2004).

Consequences of Sleep Loss and Disruption

Gauging the actual impact of sleep deprivation is challenged by the lack of a direct measure for sleep need or deficit (Littner et al., 2005). The measurement problem relates to ignorance about the "true" function of sleep, for how can sleep sufficiency be assessed or lack of sleep detected when the target outcome is unknown (Young, 2004)? Nevertheless, both intensive research and human experience recognize the effects of acute and chronic sleep deprivation. Impact on cognitive performance includes gaps in attention and responsiveness, rapid decay in performance on tasks, reduced capacity for multitasking, errors in perception and response, increased variability in performance, and impaired executive functioning, working memory, and emotion regulation (Durmer & Dinges, 2005). The greater the sleep deficit and the more disrupted the sleep episodes, the more severe is the impact of sleep disruption and loss.

Sleep deprivation evokes distinctive compensatory neurophysiological profiles in sleep (Tobler, 2000): in particular, sleep latency is dramatically reduced and slow wave sleep activity is increased, especially time in Stage 4 sleep. Lost sleep apparently can be replaced with substantially less recovery sleep than the original deficit. For instance, up to 10 days' sleep deprivation can be recouped within one to three 8-hour nights of sleep (Bonnet, 2000).

Rapid recovery of sleep parameters from sleep restriction and the lack of parity between sleep lost and compensatory sleep might imply that the "costs" of sleep loss need not be fully repaid. Other consequences of sleep restriction contradict this conclusion (Table 16-4). A burst of recent research has demonstrated that physiological effects of chronic sleep debt contribute to risk for and severity of chronic health problems (Spiegel, Leproult, & Van Cauter, 1999). Indeed, merely 6 days of sleep restriction induces endocrine and metabolic changes that may contribute to chronic conditions such as obesity, diabetes, and hypertension (Spiegel et al., 2004; Spiegel, Knutson, Leproult, Tasali, & Van Cauter, 2005). The changes associated with sleep loss include decreased glucose tolerance, increased sympathetic activity, increased cortisol, and decreased thyroid activity. Simply stated, sleep has been discovered to drive energy regulation, and thus, sleep duration moderates body weight and metabolism (Taheri, Lin, Austin, Young, & Mignot, 2004). Sleep restriction results in endocrine changes, including increased ghrelin and decreased leptin, with a consequent increase in appetite (Spiegel, Tasali, Penev, & Van Cauter, 2004). Unsurprisingly, multiple large population studies have found increased BMI or greater future risk for obesity among those who sleep less than 7 hours per day (Cizza, Skaarulis, & Mignot, 2005).

Brain and endocrine activity maintain a bidirectional relationship in sleep (Steiger, 2003), so sleep disruption alters endocrine profiles and vice versa. For instance, ghrelin stimulates not only appetite, but also endocrine activity (growth hormone; cortisol and its

TABLE 16-4 Correlates of Sleep Restriction

	Parameter	Change postrestriction
Acute		
Endocrine	Leptin	—
	Ghrelin	+
	Catecholamines	+
	p.m. cortisol	+
	Cortisol: diurnal variation	—
	TSH: mean	—
	TSH: diurnal amplitude	—
Metabolic	a.m. glucose tolerance	—
	Insulin sensitivity	—
Autonomic	Heart rate variability	+
	Sympathovagal tone (S/ParaS)	+
Cognitive	Hunger, appetite	+
	Perceived stress	0
	Executive function, working memory	—
	Multitasking	—
Behavioral	Response accuracy	—
	Performance consistency	—
Chronic		
	Obesity	+
	Metabolic syndrome	+
	Hypertension	+

Source: Brown, 2006; Durmer & Dinges, 2005; Irwin, 1999; Sekine et al. 2002; Spiegel 1999; Spiegel, Tasali et al., 2004; Spiegel, Leproult et al., 2004; Taheri et al. 2004.

releasing hormone, adrenocorticotrophic hormone) (Schmid et al., 2005). In consequence, increased ghrelin from sleep restriction leads to increased cortisol and growth hormone, which, in turn, influence multiple systems, including metabolism. Reciprocally, changes in ratios of the releasing hormones for growth hormone and cortisol alter sleep propensity (Steiger, 2003).

These lines of inquiry have galvanized public health concerns that link the documented decline in the amount of daily sleep to the concurrent surge in national rates of obesity: during the dramatic rise in obesity rates over the last two decades, the proportion of adults of all ages whose nightly sleep averages 6 hours or less has increased from roughly 20 to 30% (Centers for Disease Control and Prevention, 2005b). Obesity is firmly associated with inactivity (Vioque, Torres, & Quiles, 2000), so why should sleep reduction contribute to overweight?

Mounting laboratory, clinical, and statistical evidence for the health-eroding effects of sleep deprivation must confront a repeated set of epidemiological findings that fail to confirm such evidence at the population level. Two large epidemiological samples (1 and 1.1 million adults, respectively) drawn 20 years apart and questioned prospectively found essentially identical results linking mortality to sleep extension, rather than sleep restriction (Kripke, Garfinkel, Wingard, Klauber, & Marler, 2002; Kripke, Simons, Garfinkel, & Hammond, 1979). Mortality is lowest among men and women who report sleeping 7 hours (6.5–7.4 hours) daily. At more than 7.5 hours of reported daily sleep, mortality steadily increases as amount of sleep increases. Remarkably, the mortality associated with shorter sleep durations of 4.5–6.5 hours was less than that of the near majority who sleep longer than 7.5 hours. Insomnia was not related to mortality.

Quality of life aside, how can one reconcile these findings with the alarm sleep scientists and clinicians express over the recent declines in sleep quota among Americans, given that quotas have fallen from amounts (8 hours on average) associated with greater mortality risk to those (6.8 hours) associated with lowest risk? The analyses treat sleep behavior independent of lifestyle and context; hence, one cannot know *why* individuals slept more or less and whether factors that determine number of hours slept also influence well-being. Sleep behavior may be as much a consequence as a cause in pathways to differential health. Impact of lifestyle, including the eroding effects of poor health and environmental quality that confront disadvantaged populations, will be considered below.

PERPLEXING PARADOXES OF SLEEP AND HEALTH

The course of the discussion so far has encountered several puzzles regarding human sleep behavior and its relationships to well-being and health. These conundrums include:

- Why are humans able to rack up enormous sleep debts if the interest paid on that debt is so high in terms of function, well-being, and health? Why do mechanisms that regulate sleep behavior fail to prevent accumulation of injurious sleep debt?
- Why are objective and subjective sleep quality dissociated?
- Contemporary Western populations are privileged, with perhaps the most uniformly excellent health and living conditions in human history: why are rates of insomnia and other sleep disorders so high?
- Why is sleep restriction related to obesity?
- Why are sleep researchers concerned about declining sleep quotas if the epidemiological evidence links lower quotas to lower mortality risk?
- Given the statistics showing declining sleep quotas, why do nearly three quarters of Americans (72%) say that they get enough or more than enough sleep?

We now turn to consider potential solutions for these puzzles suggested by evolutionary adaptationist analyses, first by identifying a set of common threads that run through these disparate questions, and then by extracting key underlying factors that contribute to sleep problems and thus may merit greater attention in treatment and prevention.

SLEEP AND STRESS

Rapid reversibility distinguishes sleep from states such as coma, unconsciousness, or hibernation. Yet the vital capacity for reversibility carries a sting: sleep can be fragile and difficult to maintain or even to attain. Such difficulties can reach epidemic proportions, as with the high prevalence of insomnia symptoms (Ohayon, 2002) and sleep-related psychiatric disorders (Abad & Guilleminault, 2005). An adaptationist perspective emphasizes the value of stepping back to pose teleological questions of design concerning the purposes of sleep, the impact of conditions and pressures under which it evolved on its organization and regulation, capacities for response to challenge, and sensitivities to competing demands or functions. Such a perspective draws attention to two distinguishing features of sleep: (1) plasticity in sleep behavior and capacity to carry and redress sleep debt and (2) regulation by convergent ecological, cognitive–emotional, and physiological processes (Saper, Cano, & Scammell, 2005).

Sleep Disruption as a Response to Stressors

Many factors can influence the timing, duration, stability, and quality of sleep (see Table 16-5), which contribute to the elasticity of sleep behavior and its capacity to accommodate other life demands. The nature of these factors merits scrutiny and reveals a common feature: the conditions that disrupt sleep represent stressors, or demands on time, energy, or attention. As such, stressors challenge an adaptive response that commands a reallocation of resources. Stressors related to sleep disruption operate in three dimensions: as demands on time and energy, as cognitive demands or burdens, and/or as direct moderators of sleep/wake regulation. Sources of influence can be categorized in these three dimensions by their dominant pathways for affecting sleep (Table 16-5, columns on right). Thus, workload represents vital subsistence activity that directly influences schedule and defines times for sleep. Shift work represents a conspicuous example, including approximately 14.8% of U.S. workers (~14.8 million persons) whose hours fall or extend outside the regular daytime shift (6 a.m. to 6 p.m.) (United States Census Bureau, 2006). On an epic scale, globalizing shifts from agrarian to wage labor are transforming daily schedules and altering sleep patterns worldwide.

In contrast to social conditions, ecological factors such as day length operate largely through physiological pathways, reflecting the deep evolutionary origins of activity–rest regulation for adaptation to environmental conditions. Similarly, endogenous conditions such as age, health, or neuroregulatory capacities directly influence regulation and structure of sleep. Illness and infection, in particular, disrupt sleep patterns by inducing lassitude and sleep via the potent prosomnogenic cytokines (particularly interleukin [IL]-1β and tumor necrosis factor [TNF]-α) produced during inflammatory responses (Krueger, Majde, & Obál, 2003).

Turning to psychological factors, both cognitive and affective processes powerfully influence sleep. Cognitive loads can erode sleep budgets, not only by taking up time but also by maintaining wakefulness for planning, problem solving, or rumination. But by far the most powerful influence on wakefulness is emotional, particularly feelings of insecurity, threat, and fear. Anxiety-laden cognitive activity and the burden from perceived threats are forceful stimulants to arousal that antagonize sleep (Semler & Harvey, 2004). Whatever the objective validity of concerns and fears, cognitive framing translates social and personal experience into signals of reassurance or threat to the organism that inform motivational states and arousal regulation (Saper, Cano, & Scammell, 2005). Social marginalization, uncertainty, and threat or shame are the key elicitors of physiological and affective stress responses (Dickerson & Kemeny, 2004; Sapolsky, 1998). The linkages are adaptive because these emotions signal challenge and the potential need for response (McNamara, 2004).

TABLE 16-5 Sources of Sleep Disruption

Source	Routes of influence on sleep	Time, energy	Cognition– emotion	Physiology
Behavioral				
	Subsistence and domestic demands, workload	X		x
	Monitoring/tending the vulnerable (juveniles, sick; livestock)	X	X	
	Food consumption patterns			X
	Context maintenance (fire, position)	x	X	
	Vigilance, defense	x	X	
	Social life, ritual practices	X	x	
Ecological				
	Temperature			X
	Noise		X	x
	Light			X
	Posture, physical discomfort			X
	Bed: substrate, covering, sharing		X	X
Psychological				
	Insecurity, threat, fear			
	Psychological (distress)		X	
	Physical (malaise, self-monitoring)		X	
	Social (rumination)		X	
	Ecological (monitoring)		X	
	Beliefs about sleeping, dreaming		X	
	Planning, problem solving	X	X	
	Bad dreams, nightmares			X
Endogenous				
	Infection, illness	X		X
	Age (sleep quota, consolidation, NREM/REM cycle, phase shift)	X		X
	Genetic/organic conditions, state regulation, need for sleep			X

Sources: Lima, 2005; Stephan, 2002; U.S. DHHS, 2003.Worthman & Melby, 2002.
X Strong association
x Weak association

Accordingly, subjective and objective sleep experience comprise related but distinct aspects of sleep quality that are governed by divergent influences. Findings from recent studies of American populations illustrate these contrasting dimensions. Influences on objective sleep quality include day length, body mass index, stimulant and medication use, employment, level of sleep debt, prior emotion and learning states, and current health status. Subjective sleep quality is influenced by loneliness, depression, poor perceived health, unemployment and economic difficulties, back pain, and obesity (Jacobs, Cohen, Hammerman-Rozenberg, & Stressman, 2006; Tworoger, Davis, Vitiello, Lentz, & McTiernan, 2005). As the literature on insomnia has discovered, cognitive processes (beliefs, stressful thoughts, expectations, attributions, metacognition, or thinking about thinking) indeed influence objective sleep onset and maintenance, but the influence pales beside their eroding effects on recall and subjective experience of sleep and sleep quality

(Harvey, Tang, & Browning, 2005). Poor subjective sleep quality maintains the signal that conditions are unfavorable or challenging and adjusts psychophysiological and behavioral responses accordingly (Capaldi, Handwerger, Richardson, & Stroud, 2005; Fisher & Rinehart, 1990).

In sum, the multiplicity of factors influencing sleep behavior and regulation promotes adaptation to meet present demands and challenges. Whether they are demands on energy, time, or attention in important life domains, including subsistence and material welfare, social status and integration, physical survival and well-being, and pursuits of meaning and value, such demands signal the need and capacity to reallocate resources toward or away from sleep. In brief, all are stressors or markers of stressful conditions that trigger an adaptive response at the physiological, cognitive, and behavioral levels. This insight provides us with a possible answer to the puzzle about why sleep restriction would be related to obesity. A review of the physiological responses to sleep restriction listed in Table 16-4 confirms a profile of resource redeployment very similar to the classic stress response, with elevated cortisol, increased sympathetic activity, and maintenance of blood sugar levels levied to meet immediate demands. The parallels to stress extend further: the ability to restrict or adjust sleep to meet acute demands is a real advantage in the short run, but this ability carries real costs if invoked too often. Similar to effects of chronic stress and cumulative stress burden (allostatic load), potential consequences include increased risk for the chronic conditions of diabetes, obesity, and cardiovascular disease (McEwen & Seeman, 1999; McEwen & Wingfield, 2003). Sleep debt is never fully repaid in the currency of sleep, but it is paid in the currency of allostatic load.

A Human Propensity for Sleep Debt

The view of sleep regulation as designed to strike an adaptive balance among competing demands and constrained resources furthermore suggests an answer to another set of puzzles concerning why sleep is so vulnerable to restriction and why sleep regulation is not more robust against disruption. The very complexity of running dual systems of sleep regulation, homeostatic drive, and circadian pacemaker both increases regulatory capacity and flexibility and reduces resistance to overdetermination from acute external or internal states. Furthermore, the complex three-stage neurointegration involved in regulating circadian rhythms is thought to permit flexible daily schedules (Saper, Cano, & Scammell, 2005), coordinating sleep–wake states with patterns of food consumption, temperature and light cycles, and physical activity (Stephan, 2002). The powerful influence of affective and cognitive states on arousal levels and sleep patterns finds firm neurological footing in identification of inputs from limbic areas to hypothalamic systems regulating arousal (Saper, Cano, & Scammell, 2005).

Motivational and affective states press the wedge of arousal levels into ongoing sleep–wake systems. Particularly in an intensely social, meaning-driven species, this wedge presents demands that are as critical to survival and well-being as sleep itself. Consequently, the excitements and demands of social life compound the pre-existing capacity to stay awake under pressure from physical and survival demands (e.g., demands of foraging or fear of predators) to enhance the human capacity for context-dependent wakefulness or vigilance and, thus, the risk for incurring sleep debt.

Shades of Sleep and Declensions of Wakefulness

An adaptationist account of sleep's integral role in resource allocation inevitably turns to appraisal of the sharp distinction of sleep from other activity states, which is customarily drawn in sleep science (Allison & Cicchetti, 1976; Zepelin, 2000). In noting mosaic patterns in sleep onset and the difficulties of identifying the moment of transition to sleep, Carskadon and Dement (2000, p. 17) write of the "wavering of vigilance" before the physiological conditions of sleep are established. Recent analyses suggest the need to go much further and survey activity-arousal states as a spectrum of which sleeping forms a part. In a recent behavioral ecological examination of the role of vulnerability to predation in the evolution of sleep behavior and physiology, Lima and colleagues (Lima, Rattenborg, Lesku, & Amlaner, 2005) argue that sleeping animals are not "dead to the world." Rather sleep architecture has evolved to meet both the functional need for a "blacked out" brain and the security need for risk detection. They contend that the complexities of sleep architecture reflect the competing demands of homeostatic drive against predation risk by modulating levels of arousability, environmental monitoring, and intensity of neuroactivity throughout a bout of sleep.

Sleep science itself refers to "states of vigilance" regarding levels of consciousness in wakefulness and the stages of sleep (Massimi et al., 2005). Independent of adaptationist accounts, sleep research has begun to recognize the spectrum of arousal states and investigate how the capacity for arousal is built into sleep. A "dead to the world" cultural view of solid sleep, a clinical emphasis on consolidation as diagnostic of "good sleep," and associations of arousals with sleep disorders have led to the treatment of intrusions of consciousness as sleep problems. As noted in a recent report (Halász, Terzano, Parrino, & Bódizs, 2004, p. 1):

> The nature of arousals in sleep is still a matter of debate. According to the conceptual framework of the American Sleep Disorders Association criteria, arousals are a marker of sleep disruption representing a detrimental and harmful feature for sleep. In contrast, our view indicates arousals as elements weaved [sic] into the texture of sleep taking part in the regulation of the sleep process.

These investigators point to specific EEG configurations as micro-arousals that represent transiently altered thresholds for monitoring incoming stimuli and transitioning out of sleep. Thus, sleep physiology incorporates ongoing monitoring of external conditions and gated attention to incoming stimuli, providing a neurophysiological basis for vigilance and a dynamic capacity for reversibility in sleep.

Security and the Sentinels of Sleep

As previously discussed, much of human history preceded the routine use of fire and solid dwellings to ensure security in sleep. Hence, security for ground-sleeping hominoids and early humans would have relied on both residence in a group and a capacity for vigilance and responsivity in sleep. This scenario supports an expectation that sensitivity to cues that predict and track vulnerability would be adaptively important. Several lines of evidence suggest that this is the case. Consider again the architecture of human sleep. The stages of sleep differ markedly in reversibility and sensitivity to external cues, from Stage 1 sleep, from which the easily awakened sleepers often claim they had not been asleep, to the deep and inattentive stages of slow wave sleep (SWS) and REM. A sleep bout progresses through sleep stages in approximately 90-minute cycles that ensure variability in levels of information processing, vigilance, and reversibility throughout. Moreover, humans spend relatively little total sleep time in profound SWS (Stage 3: 3–8%; Stage 4: 10–15%) and much more in shallower states of SWS (Stage 1: 2–5%; Stage 2: 45–55%) (Roth, 2004). Finally, as reviewed in the preceding paragraph, the microarchitecture of sleep provides ongoing momentary capacity for sampling of salient cues and wakening.

A well-honed capacity for vigilance combines with the attentiveness to cognitive–emotional cues, as discussed earlier, to set the stage for sensitivity of sleep onset and maintenance to cognitive framing and ambient cues to security or vulnerability. Indeed, humans may rely on such cues for falling asleep and staying asleep by depending on sensory stimuli that indicate safety, including the undisturbed presence of others, benign weather conditions, or feelings of contentment. Therefore, an absence of cues that signal safety may increase the risk for poor sleep and insomnia. Comparative analysis (as outlined above and in Table 16-3) and species evolutionary history suggest that human sleep evolved as densely social and sensorily rich. By contrast, we have seen that sleepers in contemporary Western societies sleep in conditions that are sensorily and socially impoverished, and thus provide few immediate cues to safety. Low sensory inputs may potentiate the impact of cognitive framing for sleep, in which the baggage of material, social, or personal insecurity and worry is imported into the system of vigilance and safety monitoring within sleep processes (Semler & Harvey, 2004). Indeed, this picture coincides with clinical profiles of insomnia.

This line of reasoning suggests a model of sleep as dependent on signals of safety or insecurity that regulate levels of vigilance. In the common contexts for sleep identified in the earlier comparative discussion, the gentle crackling of a well-maintained fire, the warmth and breathing of cosleepers, and the quiet munching of animals all give direct cues of social and material security. Similarly, an unreflective sense of social and material security, with the prospect of similar conditions on the morrow, conduces to relaxed vigilance. A cue-dependent view of sleep yields a possible answer to another puzzle, namely, why rates of insomnia and other sleep disorders are so high among Americans and other privileged postindustrial populations whose health and living conditions appear exceptionally good. The cue-dependency model of sleep suggests that the absence of dense sensory cues to security may increase the reliance on and impact of internal cognitive–emotional cues to insecurity or distress. In addition, the salience and burden of uncontrollable threats that are physically remote but cognitively present may be increased by globalized media and community: 80% of Americans watch television within the hour before bed, and 45% say they worry about current events (National Sleep Foundation, 2005). Alternatively, a playing radio or television could provide the sensory stimuli needed for establishing and maintaining sleep, a virtual electronic hearth or community.

Life After Dark: The Value of Wakefulness

The regulation of sleep and wakefulness bears an adaptive imprint in another respect. Recall that the arousal system is built into the circadian pacemaker that generates cycles of wakefulness. Circadian waking drive grows during the day, peaks during evening hours, and drops precipitously in the later evening (Saper, Cano, & Scammell, 2005). Thus, peak wakefulness occurs mid-evening, shortly before homeostatic sleep pressure combines with falling wakefulness to result in sleep onset. It is surprising to learn that peak wakefulness occurs so late in the day. This point is easily overlooked when the focus is on sleep and sleep maintenance, but is important with respect to understanding the adaptive context of arousal regulation. Across the breadth and depth of human societies and history, crucial elements of daily subsistence and community life have transpired during the evening period between sundown and onset of the night's sleep. Food, information, gossip, ideas, and stories are shared, plans are laid, efforts coordinated, disputes aired and conflicts negotiated, relationships cemented, and social, healing, and religious rituals planned and performed. In any society, evening is a time for sharing and social "work" once the day's productive work is done and members of the social group return from the day's activities. The regular use of fire supports extension of activity after dark.

Two aspects of wake–sleep adapt humans for these patterns. First, humans require far less sleep than there are hours of darkness, which opens the evening for sustained activity. Second, wakefulness is greatest in the evening, which keeps people on line and tuned up for sustained engagement. The demands or stimulation of evening activities and contents may converge with the drive to maintain engagement to create momentum for sustained wakefulness at the expense of sleep (Hull, Wright, & Czeisler, 2003). This insight raises another possible reason for chronic sleep restriction or insomnia in contemporary populations. As possibilities for evening engagement escalate (due to lighting, climate control, safety, transport, or media), whether for paid or domestic work, entertainment, social life, or other pursuits, the push to "take back the night" and sustain increased evening wakefulness becomes intensified. This logic offers a solution to another conundrum: perhaps three quarters of Americans say they are getting enough sleep or more despite national trends to the contrary, because they are getting the amount they want given the attractions of rewarding activities.

THE SLEEP RESTRICTION RESPONSE

Convergent lines of evidence point to a sleep restriction response in humans that is highly attuned to signals of insecurity and threat. People do not just lose sleep, they stay awake because they want or need to. Factors heretofore considered disruptive of sleep (Table 16-5) alternatively may be viewed as triggers for sleep restriction. Sleep restriction triggers include time and energy demands (childcare, work), threats to physical survival (illness, fear), and social challenges (real or feared loss, marginalization). Triggers to sleep restriction also include positive pursuits and rewards, including novelty seeking, eating and food sharing, acquisition of information or meaning, social integration, social security, relaxation, and entertainment. Many activities that fill the nights of human societies represent such pleasurably engaging, reinforcing pursuits: they include rituals, dining, gossiping, politicking, singing and dancing, hanging out, and storytelling.

Triggers to sleep restriction therefore address negative as well as positive motivational dimensions, by activating aversive (unease, vigilance) or appetitive (excitement, reward) responses that promote wakefulness states in regulatory systems (Dahl, 2002). Recognition of the power of these triggers for sleep restriction may help to explain the patterns that so concern sleep scientists and clinicians. Attention to the positive and negative triggers to sleep restriction in clinical and research settings should advance the understanding of why people stay up too long or cannot fall asleep, why they restrict sleep or suffer from insomnia. Active consideration of the sleep restriction response and its triggers broadens the understanding of sleep and sleep problems to incorporate the physical, social, and affective contexts for sleep behavior, and provides a framework for prevention and treatment efforts.

SLEEP AND HEALTH INEQUALITIES

Beyond the obvious impact on sleep patterns by objective conditions like workload, temperature, or season, emotional dynamics and social situation have emerged as critical contexts for sleep that signal level of security or threat. Loneliness, fear, and insecurity as well as social marginality and bereavement index the burden of stressors and profoundly erode sleep. Such psychosocial effects not only disturb objective sleep quantity and efficiency, but also diminish subjective sleep quality (Allaert & Urbinelli, 2004; Cacioppo et al., 2002; Jacobs, Cohen, Hammerman-Rozenberg, & Stressman, 2006). As discussed above, sleep disruption induces physiological changes akin to stress responses. Further, poor subjective sleep quality sustains an internal signal of stress and maintains mobilization of resources for coping with stressors. Emotional and social conditions that sustain disruption of sleep by both objective and subjective criteria thereby promote chronic stress responses that potentiate chronic physical diseases and risk to mental health.

Such insights have prompted attention to the role of sleep in relating social disparities to health inequalities (Van Cauter & Spiegel, 1999). Chronic sleep disruption or poor sleep quality from work (Galinsky, Kim, & Bon, 2001), emotional distress, worry (Hall, Bromberger, & Matthews, 1999), and poor living conditions all increase with decreasing socioeconomic status (SES) (Hunt, McEwen, & McKenna, 1985; Moore, Adler, Williams, & Jackson, 2002). Studies in two countries, Japan and the United States, have identified subjective sleep quality rather than quantity as a significant contributor to mental and physical health risk. Among Japanese, reported sleep quality mediated the relationship of employment grade to both mental and physical health among men but not women (Sekine et al., 2005). In the U.S. sample, sleep quality mediated a pathway from income to physical or mental health that was independent of the direct relationships of income to health (Moore, Adler, Williams, & Jackson, 2002). These findings confirm the evolutionary analysis developed here by highlighting the vulnerability of sleep to stressors and its place in adaptive responses that mediate relationships between stressors and health.

CONCLUSION

Rather than being an escape from this world, sleep emerges from this discussion as coextensive with our engagement in it. As with virtually all other systems, sleep and sleep regulation reflect the trade-offs and tensions between the needs of the organism and the demands and opportunities it confronts. The two systems regulating sleep strike a balance between the demands for wakefulness from the circadian system and the demands for slumber from sleep drive. Comparative evolutionary analysis reveals that human sleep quotas, physiology, and architecture are unexceptional. The capacity to respond to threats to survival by restricting sleep or increasing vigilant sleep with reduced sleep quality is well developed in humans as in other organisms. Furthermore, parallels between physiology of sleep restriction and that of stress physiology are prominent in humans as in other species, involving the reallocation of resources to meet acute demands at the expense of other, deferrable needs. Hence, physiological profiles of sleep restriction resemble those of chronic stress and carry similar risks for stress-related chronic disease.

How we sleep may matter as much or more than how *much* we sleep. Human evolutionary history and cross-cultural analysis suggest both how reliant we have been on social contexts for safe sleep and how thoroughly culture defines both the physical and social conditions for sleep. Alongside these is a third set, the critical emotional–cognitive conditions for sleeping. While physical and social factors determine the nature and quality of sleep conditions, emotional–cognitive factors introduce appraisal of these conditions to inform vigilance. Feelings—loneliness, fear, worry—represent appraisals of insecurity and disrupt sleep. The vulnerability of humans to widespread insomnia reflects the power of cognitive appraisal processes in sleep onset and maintenance. That subjective rather than objective criteria furthermore drive the experience of sleep quality sustains the signal of poor or insecure environments that require vigilance and mobilization of resources to meet acute stressors.

The insight that sleep disruption and its related physiology constitute responses to stressors draws attention to the cues that trigger or allay sleep restriction. Cues to security assuage wakefulness and support sleep drive. Triggers of the sleep restriction response turn out to be not only negative, aversive experiences such as insecurity, but also positive, appetitive ones such as excitement and pleasure. Extensive after-dark activities of humans are supported by a sleep need much below the hours of darkness and by the rewards of activities such as eating, socializing, and entertainment. Engagement in these rewarding and important pursuits promotes wakefulness and thus triggers the sleep restriction response just as potently as do negative conditions; either way, resources are allocated away from the functions represented by sleep and toward those represented by immediate demands for waking.

The insights obtained by viewing sleep from an adaptationist perspective sleep also illuminate sleep problems and their health consequences. Appreciation of the links between sleep and stress is key. Grasping the strong evolutionary underpinnings for dependence of sleep on emotional–cognitive states indexing levels of social and material insecurity or threat may yield a thread by which to unravel the role of sleep in health inequality and mental health. Similarly, grounded appreciation for the sleep restriction response could inform treatment and prevention of some sleep problems by reinforcing attention to the triggers of the response and tailoring interventions to resolve or remove those triggers. Warnings about sleep restriction are unlikely to be effective so long as people have "good reasons" for their sleep habits and problems that are firmly founded in the ambient triggers to vigilance or reward that maintain wakefulness.

CHAPTER 17

Evolutionary Medicine and Obesity
Developmental Adaptive Responses
in Human Body Composition

Jack Baker, Magdalena Hurtado, Osbjorn Pearson,
and Troy Jones

Baker and colleagues reinforce a recurrent theme about the significance of "conditioned responses" and individual variability in their work exploring fetal–adult developmental continuities. They test a variety of research models looking for consistencies in associations between fetal growth patterns and both body composition and neurological development beginning in utero and during childhood. They also include adolescence–adulthood continuities. One inference from their work is that often statistical associations are dependent on the type of method used to analyze them. Even so, one important consistent finding is that individuals who experience reduced fetal growth also experience deficits in brain size (assessed by imaging techniques and anthropomorphic measurements including head circumference) and neuron formation. When all populations and circumstances across societies were considered, they found mixed support for the link between reduced fetal growth and later fatness or obesity. They discuss the possibility that it may not be so much that the relationship is not real but that other factors also play important roles in the expression of adult phenotypes. That muscle mass, brain size, and abdominal fatness may at times be affected differentially in relationship to in utero conditions may be best accounted for, they argue, by considering the time at which each individual is measured and the possibility that later "fatness" is increased under some conditions but not others. Rather than asking if reduced fetal growth leads to later obesity, they suggest that perhaps a better strategy, one reminiscent of foraging evolutionary models (i.e., models that examine how food quantity, quality, and collecting/harvesting/preparation patterns are fitted to the local ecologies), is to ask under what conditions reduced size at birth leads to obesity—a solution that no doubt the next wave of researchers will implement.

OBESITY AND CHRONIC DISEASE IN THE MODERN WORLD

Currently, obesity looms as perhaps the greatest long-term health threat for humans in both developed and developing countries (Frisancho, 2003; World Health Organization, 1998). Because of its relationship with a host of chronic diseases, including heart disease, hypertension, and even certain forms of cancer, understanding the determinants of obesity has important implications for both clinical practice and public health strategies (Bjorntorp, 1990, 1997b; Bjorntorp & Eden, 1996). It has been suggested for over 40 years that evolutionary biology might provide important perspectives on the development of obesity (Knowler, Pettitt, Savage, & Bennett, 1981; Neel, 1962; Neel, Weder, & Stevo, 1998; West, Bailey, Coniglione, Smith, Scroggins, & Ellison, 1974). Recent epidemiological findings linking reduced fetal growth to changes in body composition at birth, during childhood, and into adulthood have renewed interest in the evolutionary origins of human obesity and the role of developmental responses in shaping the process (Cameron & Demerath, 2002; Gluckman & Hanson, 2004; Gluckman, Hanson, Moran, & Pinal, 2005; Kuzawa, 2005).

People who experienced reduced fetal growth have an increased risk of becoming obese, but their phenotype is characterized by some interesting features in addition to increased fatness. These individuals also tend to have reduced muscle mass and greater storage of body fat within the abdomen, sometimes called a centralized pattern of fatness or, colloquially, an "apple-shaped" physique (Bjorntorp, 1990, 1997; Bjorntorp & Eden, 1996; Frisancho, 2003). Reduced muscle mass and more abdominal fatness increase risk for diabetes, heart disease, and hypertension above the risk from increased fatness alone (Bjorntorp & Eden, 1996). Many studies have linked each of these aspects of body shape and composition to reduced growth in utero (Barker, Robinson, Osmond, & Barker, 1997; Cameron & Demerath, 2002; Erikkson, Forsen, Tuomilehto, Osmond, & Barker, 2001; Euser, Finken, Kejzer-Veen, Hille, Wit, & Dekker, 2005; Jaddoe & Witteman, 2006; Kahn, Narayan, Williamson, & Valdez, 2000; Kensara, Wootton, Phillipps, Patel, Jackson, & Elia, 2005; Koziel & Jankowska, 2002; Labayen, Moreno, Blay, Blay, Mesana, & Gonzalez-Gross, 2006; Laitenen, Pietilainen, Wadsworth, Sovio, & Jarvelin, 2004). Interestingly, it has been suggested that these changes might have an adaptive basis that help to prepare the growing fetus for the world it will inhabit. If so, the link between slowed growth in utero and altered physiology and body composition later in life should be explicable via developmental models adopted from evolutionary biology (Levins, 1968; Schlichting & Pigliucci, 1999).

This chapter reviews the perspective that evolutionary medicine offers for understanding the relationship between obesity and reduced fetal growth resulting in small size at birth. Two different evolutionary models of chronic disease risk may be proposed to explain obesity later in life among those born small: (1) the predictive adaptive response (PAR) and (2) the brain optimization rule. The conceptual feasibility and empirical predictions of both models are compared, then contrasted with a third, more general model, that physiological "damage" during stunted fetal growth produces all of the observed changes in adults. The predictions of each model are tested using the conclusions from epidemiological research. The chapter closes with a discussion of the implications of these findings for clinical practice and epidemiological research.

EVOLUTIONARY MEDICINE AND EVOLUTIONARY
MODELS OF DEVELOPMENTAL OBESITY

The field of evolutionary medicine contends that while we may live in the Space Age, our bodies and physiology remain firmly planted in our Stone Age past (Strassman & Dunbar, 1999). Human physiology was shaped by natural selection over millions of years throughout the course of mammalian and later human evolution. Because of this, human physiology is best understood as an adaptive system, which was optimized to increase our survival and reproduction in these ancestral environments (Lappe, 1994; Nesse & Williams, 1994). If so, many human diseases may arise from—or be exacerbated by—a mismatch between a physiology prepared to meet evolutionary needs of our ancient ancestors and the very different environment in which we now live that has resulting from unprecedented and rapid cultural change during the last 10,000 years (Boyd Eaton & Eaton 1999; Nesse & Williams, 1994; Strassman & Dunbar, 1999). Advocates of evolutionary medicine suggest that both clinical practice and research on public health could be improved by incorporating these principles (Lappe, 1994). Over the past 15 years, evolutionary perspectives have increasingly been incorporated into clinical and public health research as interest in Darwinian thinking has grown among health care providers and epidemiologists (Stearns, 1999).

Evolutionary thinking is characterized by a careful consideration of how phenotypes are designed to increase biological "fitness," which can be broadly defined as the production of viable offspring (Stearns, 1999; Williams, 1966). While measuring fitness is straightforward, producing viable offspring is a complicated process that involves several steps. The offspring must survive to maturity, choose a mate, gestate and give birth to their own offspring, and finally support those offspring to their own maturity (Stearns, 1992). In mammals, the period of dependency after birth includes both lactation by the mother and an intense period of learning by the offspring before they are able to fend for themselves (Wood, 1994). This general feature of juvenile mammals is even more pronounced among primates whose offspring often do not reach maturity for several years to more than a decade (Kaplan, Hill, Lancaster, & Hurtado, 2000). These lengthened periods of dependency create evolutionary challenges.

Because the energy (usually food) available to an animal is always limited, the animal must make physiological trade-offs between spending its energy on functions including growth, maintenance of its body, locomotion, and reproduction. The relative costs and benefits of dividing resources between these competing functions ultimately determine fitness (Stearns, 1992; Zera & Harshman, 2001). As a species evolves, it must navigate an inherent antagonism between having traits that would increase fitness the most and the disruption that those traits might cause to the existing delicate balance of trade-offs between competing physiological functions. Over time, the process of natural selection tends to produce phenotypes that best balance these trade-offs and produce higher levels of fitness across the range of environments that individuals have experienced over time and space (Levins, 1968). The phenotypes that are most affected are those that directly affect survival and reproduction (Williams, 1966). Some flexibilty in the form of developmental and physiological plasticity exists, however, and it is likely that the ability to have this type of short-term developmental or physiological responses has also been favored by selection. Phenotypic plasticity is shaped by developmental experiences that induce physiological changes that probably act to increase survival, reproduction, and ultimately fitness (Levins, 1968; Bateson et. al., 2004).

Although one might not immediately equate body composition with survival, it is also shaped by physiological trade-offs that may have evolutionary benefits. During fetal growth, trade-offs between tissues such as fat and muscle can have long-term effects on body composition. During gestation, tissues experience simultaneous "critical" periods of development. During these periods, the number of cells and size of tissues such as muscle, brain, or fat may be "programmed" for the entire life course (Barker, 1995, 1997; Cameron & Damerath, 20002; Gluckman & Hanson, 2004; Gluckman et. al., 2005; McCance & Widdowson, 1974). When such "programming" occurs, it is assumed to affect later responses, making the tissues more or less responsive to the environment (Schmalhausen, 1949). When energy is limited, investments in each tissue may be altered to reflect the "preferences" of a physiological design that evolved to maximize fitness (Schlichting & Pigliucci, 1999). Zera and Harshman (2001) referred to these "preferences" as "priority rules" that can be described in models that predict how scarce nutrients during fetal development should be divided among the growing brain, musculo-skeletal system, and fat mass in order to maximize lifetime fitness. The predictions may then be tested with the results of previous research to evaluate their adequacy.

What are the most "adaptive" or fitness-enhancing responses to the environment during growth and development? Adaptive responses differ from other physiological characters because they improve survival or reproduction within specific environments (Curio, 1973; Williams, 1966). They are not simply byproducts of random processes or damage to tissues during development; instead, they link specific experiences (known as "exposures" in epidemiology) to specific physiological characteristics that clearly increase survival and reproduction within specific environments (Gould & Lewontin, 1979; Stearns, 1992). Models that emphasize adaptation through the process of development differ from other models that invoke random processes such as tissue damage during development (in which all cells have equal chances of deleterious effects) as potential explanations (Bateson et. al., 2004). In those born small but later obese, adaptive models of development predict specific relationships between brain, muscle, and fat tissues. They propose that these relationships are adaptive in nature, enhancing fitness through increases in either survival or reproduction. Developmental damage models make no such claims.

PREDICTIVE ADAPTIVE RESPONSE, BRAIN PRESERVATION, OR DEVELOPMENTAL DAMAGE?

Predictive Adaptive Response (PAR) Model: Variation in Body Composition Modulates Energy Expenditure

Gluckman and Hanson (2004) suggested the PAR model as an explanation for chronic disease. In the present context, this model suggests that lowered muscle mass, greater fat mass, and more abdominal obesity tend to co-occur in individuals who have small size at births and function as an energy-saving response to early life signals that (presumably) that the individual will face greater energetic scarcity (or more periods of scarcity) across his or her life span. Well-developed theory borrowed from microeconomics supports this model, suggesting that in times of scarcity, individuals tend to spend or invest less and save more to avert shortfalls (Hirschleifer, 1966; Winterhalder, Lu, & Tucker, 1999). In terms of obesity among those who were born small, several physiological facts are relevant. First, the amount of energy used during activity or while at rest is largely determined by the amount of muscle that an individual has (Arslanian, 1996; Ravussin, 1995). Decreasing muscle mass lowers total energetic requirements. Second, greater fat mass results in greater energetic storage per unit of body mass. One gram of fat stores 9 kcal, while carbohydrates (which may be stored in the liver or muscles) and proteins store only 4 kcal per gram (Groff & Groper, 2000). Last, abdominal fat cells are more sensitive to hormonal signals that cause release of fats into the bloodstream (Bjorntorp, 1990, 1997a, b; Bjorntorp & Eden, 1996; Rebuffe-Scrive, Enk, Crona, Lonnroth, Abrahamsson, & Smith, 1985; Rebuffe-Scrive, Bronnegard, Nillson, Eldh, Gustaffson, & Bjorntorp, 1990; Streeten, 1993). Thus, lowering muscle mass, increasing fat mass, and storing relatively more of the total fat in the abdomen results in (1) reduced total energetic requirements, (2) greater storage against shortfalls, and (3) easier access to these stores during shortfall. A physiology characterized by these changes would be primed to perform well in environments characterized by energetic scarcity (Neel, 1962; Neel et. al., 1998). The PAR model predicts that individuals who experience reduced growth due to energetic shortfalls in utero become physiologically primed for precisely this kind of a "feast or famine" environment.

Brain Optimization Rule: The Evolution of a Trade-Off Between Brains and Brawn

The brain optimization rule model further develops the line of reasoning that physiological trade-offs may underlie some chronic diseases. It postulates that if a scarcity of nutrients occurs in utero, especially during the second trimester when the brain and muscle tissues are both in a critical period, the body will favor the growth of the brain at the expense of muscle (Barker, 1995, 1997; Yajnik, 2000, 2004). According to this model, the priority of brain tissue is accomplished by restricting sugar uptake by muscle. Normally, the hormone insulin signals all cells to take up glucose, fats, and proteins from the blood; however, in individuals who experienced reduced growth in utero, the muscle cells are induced to become resistant to the effects of insulin, thus leaving a greater amount of sugar in the blood stream to fuel brain development (Barker, 1995, 1997; Reaven, 1998; Yajnik, 2000, 2004). Since these effects occur during the critical period of muscle development, they are long term in nature and result in life-long resistance to insulin resistance (a step toward obesity and diabetes) and reduced muscle mass (Cameron and Demerath, 2002). It is important to emphasize that any proposal that a priority rule has evolved to favor brains over brawn is a hypothesis rather than an empirically documented fact. However, the proposition is plausible given the fact that an overriding trend in human evolution has been the reduction of muscle mass and increase of brain mass (Kaplan, Hill, Lancaster, & Hurtado, 2000; Klein, 1999).

The primary prediction of the brain optimization rule model is that a negative relationship between brain mass and muscle mass should be observed among people who had a small size at birth. Similarly, people who are born small, but do not have later deficits in brain mass or function as adults, should also be found to have lowered muscle mass. The model could also explain the observation that people who had small size at births tend to be fatter, perhaps due to insulin resistance induced in their muscles in utero. The body's typical response to the resistance of a tissue to a hormonal signal is to increase production of the signaling hormone (Arslanian, 1996; Groff & Groper, 2000). In the case of insulin, increased production to compensate for resistance would result in more rapid clearance of sugars from the blood, leading to quicker return of hunger after meals. This could lead to overeating and ultimately, greater fatness (Neel, 1962; Neel et. al., 1998). The brain optimization rule makes no particular prediction concerning abdominal fatness.

Developmental Damage: An Explanation Based on Clinical Pathology

Where possible, evolutionary models should always be tested against a null expectation that variation is produced by random processes (i.e., chance) or without any particular adaptive target (Curio, 1973; Stearns, 1992). In the case of relationships between reduced fetal growth and later obesity, a null model is available. The developmental damage model invokes clinical damage of tissues as a plausible, null alternative that could potentially produce all of the phenotypic changes noted people who experience reduced fetal growth and later become obese (Gluckman & Hanson, 2004; Gluckman et. al., 2005; Kuzawa, 2005). The developmental damage model suggests that all tissues should be simultaneously damaged because all of them are subject to the same lack or resources. In such a case we would expect that the growth of the brains, muscles, and fat should all be stunted. Since it is likely that the glands (hypothalamus, pituitary, adrenal glands) that produce the hormones that regulate the storage of fat in the abdomen may be damaged by the same nutritional shortfall, this endocrine damage may also contribute to abdominal obesity (Jaddoe & Witteman, 2006). If true, the developmental damage model could explain increased relative fatness in the abdomen without the need to invoke any adaptive responses across development.

Discriminating Between the Three Models

Each model makes specific predictions about the relationships that should be observed between muscle, brains, and fat in people who experienced slowed fetal growth (Table 17-1). The model of a PAR predicts that these people should have (1) lowered muscle mass, (2) greater fatness, and (3) greater abdominal fatness. It makes no statement about brain development. The brain optimization rule makes two possible predictions. From one perspective, the model might predict a negative relationship between muscle mass and brain mass. A slightly different perspective might argue that brain mass will be no different between those born small and with stunted muscle mass and those born of normal size, but will be diminished in those born small but with normal levels of muscle mass. Though it is not a specific prediction of this model, it also allows for increases in overall fat mass as a side effect of insulin resistance in muscle tissue.

The developmental damage model predicts uniform stunting of all tissues including muscles, the brain, and fat. It allows for greater relative fatness in the abdomen through damage of the endocrine glands that regulate abdominal obesity. Since the models make very specific predictions about the body composition, they may potentially be discriminated

TABLE 17-1 Evolutionary Models of Obesity Among Those Born Small: Model Predictions and Supporting Evidence[a]

Model	Discriminating predictions	Supporting evidence
Developmental damage (DD)	Brains, muscle, and fat tissues all stunted in those born small.	Simultaneous reduction in brain mass or cognitive function, muscle mass, and fat mass.
Brain optimization Rule (BOR)	Discriminated from the DD model because of non-uniform stunting of tissues. Brain preserved but muscle mass stunted in those born small.	No differences in brain growth or cognitive function in those born small, but reduced muscle mass. Allows for increased fatness, but makes no prediction about abdominal fatness.
Predictive adaptive response (PAR)	Discriminated from the DD model by specific pattern of changes: 1) reduced muscle, 2) increased fatness, 3) relatively greater abdominal fatness. Clear support requires rejection of the BOR model, with no relationship between brain and muscle development.	Strongest support with rejection of both DD and BOR models. Consistent findings relating reduced fetal growth lowered muscle mass, increased fatness, and more abdominal fatness.

[a] *Adaptive and neutral evolutionary models may be discriminated based on their predictions. The DD model requires stunting of all tissues. The BOR model is discriminated because brain development is not stunted when muscle mass is sacrificed among those born small. The PAR model is discriminated from the DD and BOR models by a clear and specific pattern of nonuniform stunting of tissues.*

through a survey of the literature reporting associations between reduced fetal growth and later obesity, brain development, and body composition. We collected the results of a large series of studies that have tested for associations between measures of size at birth and later body composition or brain development. Studies suggesting positive or negative relationships or no effect were compiled, used to arrive at a consensus of the studies' findings, and compared to the predictions of each model to determine which model has the most support. This process should reveal if either of the adaptive models better explain the findings than the null model of clinical damage to tissues.

Discriminating between all three models is complicated because some of their predictions overlap. Logically, the null model (developmental damage) should first be eliminated. If the consensus findings suggest that uniform stunting of all tissues occurs, then the developmental damage model would be supported. If not, then the alternative adaptive models should be tested, beginning with the brain optimization rule model. If brain mass is preserved while muscle mass is sacrificed among those born small, then this model would find support. The PAR model does not predict that brain mass should receive priority, but postulates that abdominal fat stores are particularly useful. Both of these predictions allow it to be distinguished from the brain optimization rule model.

EMPIRICAL SUPPORT FOR EACH MODEL

We reviewed available studies that examined associations between reduced fetal growth and both body composition and neurological development in utero and during childhood,

TABLE 17-2 Consensus Empirical Findings of Association Between Small Size Birth and Later Body Composition[a]

Outcome measure	Total studies	Increased in those born small	Decreased in those born small	No relationship	Qualitative consensus conclusion
Fat mass/percentage	12[b]	5	2	5	No clear consensus finding.
Skeletal muscle mass	7[c]	0	7	0	Small size at birth negatively impacts long-term muscle mass.
Abdominal fatness	12[d]	8	0	4	Small size at birth increases abdominal fatness.
Brain development	15[e]	0	13	2	Brain development negatively impacted by small size at birth.

[a] *The literature suggests lowered muscle mass, reduced brain development, and greater abdominal fatness among those born small. It provides only equivocal evidence of effects of reduced fetal growth on overall fatness.*

[b] *Binkin et al., 1998; Euser et al., 2005; Kensara et al., 2005; Laitenen et al., 2004; Larciprete et al., 2005; Lebayen et al., 2006; Padoan et al., 2004; Ravelli et al., 1976, 1999; Sachdev et al., 2005; Stanner et al., 1977.*

[c] *Euser et al., 2005; Hediger et al., 1998; Kahn et. al., 2000; Kensara et. al., 2005; Lebayen et al., 2005; Wells et al., 2005; Sachdev et al., 2005.*

[d] *Barker et al., 1997; Kensara et al., 2005; Koziel and Jankowska, 2002; Lebayen et al., 2006; Laitenen et al., 2004; Law et al., 1992; Malina et al., 1996; Ravelli et al., 1999; Sachdev et al., 2005; Schroeder et al., 1999; Stanner et al., 1977; Valdez et al., 1994.*

[e] *Amin et al., 1997; Georgieff et al., 1985; Gross et al., 1978; Gutbrod et al., 2000; Hack et al., 1984, 1989; Hediger et al., 1998; Kitchen et al., 1980; Monset-Couchard and Bethman, 2000; Pena et al., 1998; Stanley and Speidel, 1985; Vohr and Oh, 1983.*

adolescence, and adulthood (Table 17-2). These studies reported results measuring the effects of reduced fetal growth on later brain development, overall fatness and muscularity, and abdominal fatness. These outcomes were measured using body measurements (head circumference, body mass index, skinfold measures) as well as cellular measures of brain cell development (the reader is referred to Roche, Heymsfield, & Lohman, 1996, for several chapters reviewing these methods of assessment). Twelve studies reviewed examined relationships between reduced size at birth and later overall fatness. Seven studies tested for relationships of reduced fetal growth and later muscle mass. Fifteen studies reviewed the effects of reduced fetal growth on either head circumference or neurological development. Twelve studies tested for associations of small size at birth with later abdominal fatness.

Overall, these studies provide no support for the brain optimization rule, but fail to discriminate convincingly between the developmental damage model and the PAR. It is clear that brain mass is stunted among people who have experienced reduced fetal growth. Thirteen of 15 studies confirmed the fact that those who experienced reduced fetal growth also experienced deficits in brain size and neuron formation. Those born small also displayed reduced muscle mass: seven of seven studies reported this association.

Eight of 12 studies reported greater abdominal fatness in people who were born small. Of the 12 studies testing for relationships between reduced fetal growth and overall fatness, 5 reported greater fatness in those born small. Two studies found the opposite effect; both of these used measurements obtained through imaging technology while growth restriction was occurring in utero. Five studies found no association at all between the obesity later in life and small size at birth, which suggests that reduced fetal growth results in greater overall fatness only under certain conditions.

While the review clearly suggests that the brain optimization rule model may be rejected because simultaneous stunting of brain and muscle occurs, it does not allow one to clearly discriminate between the predictive adaptive response and developmental damage models. Observations of the reduction of both muscle and brain mass tend to support the idea that developmental damage creates the observed relationship between reduced fetal growth and body composition later in life. Two studies that were able to use medical imagery to track the effects of reduced growth in utero found these fetuses to have lower fat mass than average-sized fetuses, providing further support for the hypothesis that reduced growth in utero adversely affects all tissues (Larciprete, Valensise, Di Pierro, Vaspollo, Casalino, Arduini, et al., 2005; Padoan, Rigano, Ferrazzi, Beaty, Battaglia, & Galan, 2004). Studies of body composition in childhood, adolescence, and adulthood provide mixed results for the effects small size at birth on later fatness. At present, it appears that reduced fetal growth leads to greater fatness only under certain conditions—conditions that currently remain somewhat unclear (Cameron & Demerath, 2002).

The balance of the evidence suggests that the developmental damage model adequately explains relationships between reduced fetal growth and later body composition. These conclusions are tentative because the PAR model cannot be ruled out without findings that establish a firmer link between small size at birth to greater fatness later in life. Future studies could attempt to do this by examining relationships between reduced fetal growth and all three tissues in the same individuals, thus overcoming a shortcoming of a literature review that cannot compare differences in each of these tissues simultaneously.

Given the mixed results of the studies that investigated the link between reduced fetal growth and later fatness, it is highly likely that the factors that create this link in certain cases are quite complex. The relationship may be produced by uncontrolled confounding factors, unexamined interactions between factors, or even threshold effects (in which a threshold of growth deficit in utero must be experienced to produce the effect later in life, a threshold that may differ depending on the individual's genotype or that of the mother). The results of Ravelli, Stein, and Susser (1976) strongly suggest that greater fatness occurs in those whose mothers suffered through a famine while pregnant with them, but subsequent studies have found it difficult to replicate these effects, even in animal models (Armitage et. al., 2004). Ravelli, Stein, and Susser's (1976) study measured obesity risk in 19-year-old Dutch Army recruits whose mothers suffered semi-starvation during the World War II. During this time, caloric intakes were severely reduced among pregnant women to as little as one third of the necessary requirement for pregnant and lactating women (2100 kcal per day for 62-kg women [Insel, Turner, & Ross, 2002]). The study found a 50% increase in risk among the recruits, but these conclusions were seriously weakened when a follow-up study on 50-year-old men and women from the same cohort found no effects (Ravelli, Van der Meulen, Osmond, Barker, & Bleker, 1999). As a case in point for the difficulty in replicating such findings, a study conducted on the population of Leningrad, which was exposed to a similar famine during World War II, failed to produce evidence of this relationship (Stanner, Bulmer, Andres, Lantseva, Borodina, Poteen, & Yudkin, 1997). While a handful of studies have suggested increased risk for obesity among those born small (Erikkson, Forsen, Tuomilehto, Osmond, & Barker, 2001), the contradictory evidence from other studies shows that other factors also play important roles in adult phenotypes (see Cameron & Demerath, 2002, for a similar opinion).

Does the failure of either evolutionary model to convincingly explain the data sound the death knell for evolutionary models for obesity? Probably not: more likely, it highlights the usefulness of further evolutionary modeling along a new, innovative line. Conditional strategies for dealing with environmental variation during postnatal growth are widespread in nature (Parker & Maynard-Smith, 1990). In the current study, for example, we applied a coarse-grained assumption that phenotypic changes occurring in utero will hold across the entire life span. In the case of muscle mass, brain mass, and abdominal fatness this assumption seems to hold, but studies of actual fetal growth restriction show that fetal fat mass is also sacrificed (Larciprete et. al., 2005; Padoan et al., 2004). Postnatal studies indicate that fatness is increased under some conditions and not under others and that these effects may vary depending upon the time at which individuals are measured. These observations suggest that conditional models of postnatal development might be viable strategies that make good evolutionary sense. Understanding these strategies could be accomplished within an evolutionary framework that models trade-offs between sets of costs and benefits and their complicated-interactions while relaxing the assumption *that in utero* effects will hold across the life span.

IMPLICATIONS FOR CLINICAL PRACTICE, EPIDEMIOLOGY, AND EVOLUTIONARY MEDICINE

Clinical practitioners face the unique challenge of integrating the results of research studies based on populations with their need to treat individuals who may have greatly differing phenotypes (Lappe, 1994). Links between epidemiological research on infectious diseases and evolutionary theory are direct—it is easy for clinical practitioners to understand that natural selection directly affects host/pathogen dynamics. Understanding chronic diseases in an evolutionary framework is more challenging. While many clinicians have embraced the evolutionary idea of "thrifty" genes (Knowler et. al., 1981; Neel, 1962), the idea that adaptive developmental responses might provide useful insights for treating patients suffering from obesity and related chronic diseases is not so straightforward. A greater understanding of the dynamic physiological responses potentially produced by evolution, as well as the limits imposed by developmental experiences, can only enhance the individual practitioner's clinical intuition. However, the incorporation of evolutionary approaches into medical practice will not alleviate each practitioner's need to interpret a research literature that often contains conflicting results. This issue is no different than other issues within evidence-based medicine. Ultimately, adding an evolutionary "intuition" (Stearns, 1992) to the deep understanding of biochemistry endowed within a medical education can enhance clinical practice within a variety of settings ranging from family practice to endocrinology.

The implications of this study are much brighter for the introduction of evolutionary models into epidemiological research and public health practice. Epidemiology works by testing of alternative hypotheses, progressively eliminating of their predictions in order to narrow the possibilities to find the most consistent relationships between experiences associated with disease and pathological outcomes (Aschengrau & Seage, 2003). The models reviewed here produced specific, testable predictions that may be falsified empirically. As such, they become useful tools for the design of epidemiological research. By generating research based on evolutionary principles, such a process promises to truly integrate evolutionary perspectives into epidemiology.

Along these lines, the findings of this study may be particularly important in shaping future evolutionary epidemiological research. Particularly, the equivocal findings regarding the relationships between reduced fetal growth and later obesity suggest that reframing research on this outcome within a framework based on conditional responses (a well-developed tool within evolutionary biology [see Parker & Maynard Smith, 1990, for a review]) might be useful. Rather than asking whether reduced fetal growth leads to later obesity, perhaps a better strategy is to ask under *what conditions* reduced size at birth leads to later obesity. Forging evolutionary models that incorporate flexible postnatal responses based on exposures in childhood and in utero may provide new and better avenues for understanding relationships between reduced fetal growth and later body composition. These perspectives would certainly be evolutionary in nature, but would incorporate additional dynamics. Moreover, they would once again produce testable hypotheses that could be examined using standard epidemiologic research designs and methods. The result could be a marked improvement in strategies to prevent obesity, which typically have been unsuccessful thus far (Caballero, 2004; Kaur, Hyder, & Poston, 2003).

Testing hypotheses derived from evolutionary models is important for the field of evolutionary medicine as well. Explanations for diseases or adaptations that seem evolutionarily plausible are really hypotheses that need to be tested. Not all phenotypes are produced by the process of adaptation—neutral variation also exists within nature (Gould & Lewontin, 1979). By testing specific, empirical predictions of evolutionary models, we stand to gain insights into whether natural selection or clinical pathology has shaped a phenotype or not. Understanding the targets of selection involved and the potential "design" of physiological responses is enhanced when specific empirical predictions are tested (see Stephens & Krebs, 1986, Chapter 13, and Parker & Maynard Smith, 1990, for useful reviews of the importance of evolutionary modeling and hypothesis testing within evolutionary biology). By putting evolutionary hypotheses to the test, practitioners of evolutionary medicine will sharpen their understanding of the nature of the characters they study while avoiding the pitfalls of evolutionary "storytelling" that occur when the criterion plausibility alone is used to understand biological variation (Gould & Lewontin, 1979).

CHAPTER 18

The Developmental Origins of Adult Health

Intergenerational Inertia in Adaptation
and Disease

Christopher W. Kuzawa

Lower weight babies end up as smaller adults with reduced muscle mass and changes in metabolism, making them more prone to developing diabetes and cardiovascular disease. In this chapter Kuzawa illustrates how a woman's nutritional status at conception can serve as an important cue for the developmental direction of the fetus. Perhaps even more interesting is that the early nutritional stress encountered by a fetus is useful for predicting the likely health status of the same individual much later in life. Kuzawa proposes a possible answer to one of the most important questions confronting initiatives aimed at improving global health: Why is it that "transitioning" populations have elevated cardiovascular disease when they experience much lower average intakes of fat, traditionally have low blood pressure, and experience much less populationwide obesity than is characteristic of industrialized nations?

EVOLUTIONARY MEDICINE AND THE RISE OF CARDIOVASCULAR DISEASES

More people die from heart attacks and stroke than from any other cause (MacKay et al., 2004). This global statistic is unsettling, but it is also rather remarkable considering that cardiovascular diseases (CVDs) were a minor contributor to human suffering and mortality until recent history. There are good reasons to suspect that our ancestors were not afflicted with CVDs during most of human evolution, and that several recent changes have contributed to their emergence as important health problems. The first and most straightforward is that many of us are now living longer than our ancestors likely did and, as a result, are more prone to chronic degenerative diseases that only afflict individuals lucky enough to reach old age (Omran, 1971). The second includes the changes in lifestyle, behavior, and diet that have swept across the globe in recent generations to radically transform the environments that we confront in our daily lives. The classic biomedical model views CVD as the cumulative result of unhealthy lifestyle practices that interact with the specific genetic susceptibilities that we inherited from our parents at conception.

From an evolutionary perspective, the rapid emergence of chronic diseases like CVD has been explained as a result of the fact that cultural practices like diet may change at a pace that is far more rapid than can be accommodated by the gradual process of adaptive evolution operating on gene frequencies (Neel, 1962). With respect to human diet and energy balance, our ancestors subsisted for millions of years as small bands of highly active foragers who rarely had access to concentrated sources of carbohydrates, fats, or salt. As a species, our metabolism and the human body's "expectations" for nutrients were sculpted during this long era of high physical activity and balanced dietary intake, and there has been little opportunity for natural selection to modify our genetic constitution to match the changed realities of contemporary human ecologies. The resultant "mismatch" between our "Paleolithic" genome and our changing way of life is assumed to help explain conditions like obesity, diabetes, and hypertension, and, through these, the now global epidemic of CVD (Eaton & Konner, 1985).

Is a Gene–Environment Model Sufficient to Explain the Current Global CVD Epidemic?

Although this concept of gene–environment mismatch is intuitively appealing, there are reasons to question whether "genes" and "environments" are the only factors influencing the development of conditions like CVD, and thus, whether an amendment to the model might be due. This interpretation is supported by the aforementioned status of CVD as a cause of mortality. The current global CVD epidemic is occurring very rapidly in societies that were scarcely afflicted by it a mere generation or two ago (MacKay et al., 2004). Although it is expectable that disease patterns will shift as life expectancy improves and lifestyles change, there are differences in the disease experiences of these populations compared to the prior experiences of populations that went through a similar but more gradual transition in places like western Europe and the United States. Many currently transitioning populations have an elevated risk for CVD at lower levels of exposure to unhealthy lifestyle or environmental factors (Colin Bell et al., 2002). In the Philippines, for instance, adolescents have high levels of cholesterol in the absence of obesity or high intakes of dietary fat (Kuzawa et al., 2003), while the increase in blood pressure that accompanies weight gain is also more severe, leading to higher risk of hypertension at any given level of body mass index (Colin Bell et al., 2002; Deurenberg-Yap et al., 2002; Lear et al., 2003). A pattern of high CVD susceptibility and CVD risk factor clustering has been documented among such diverse groups as Brazilians (Sawaya et al., 1998), Venezuelans (Molero-Conejo et al., 2003), Native Americans (Benyshek et al., 2001), Australian Aboriginals (Gault et al., 1996), and Indians (Yajnik, 2004), to name only a few.

If CVD is a simple product of a mismatch between our evolved genome and our current lifestyle, how do we make sense of these heterogeneities in the global experience of disease change? One possibility is that these recently transitioning populations have genes that make them respond more adversely to lifestyle change. Although this would be in keeping with the general framework of the gene–environment mismatch model, it seems quite unlikely that populations as unrelated as Indians, Filipinos, and Native Americans should share high frequencies of high-risk genes that are not shared by populations that experienced these transitions several generations prior. Similar patterns of high disease susceptibility in genetically unrelated populations point to the need for an alternate explanation for these differences in CVD risk.

Refining the Model: The Developmental Origins of Health and Disease (DOHaD)

Insights into this problem are coming from a rapidly growing new area of medical research. Starting in the late 1980s, David Barker and his colleagues at Southampton University in Britain published a series of papers showing that the risk of dying from CVD, or of suffering from conditions that precede CVD like hypertension or diabetes, is higher among individuals who were born small (Barker et al., 1989, 1994). Although earlier studies had found evidence for similar relationships between deprivation during childhood and subsequent adult mortality rates (Forsdahl 1977; Kermack et al., 1934), Barker and his colleagues were the first to link these associations to a biological marker—birth weight—that hinted at possible mechanisms to account for them. Building from the assumption that a baby born small had been a poorly nourished fetus, they proposed that these relationships were the byproduct of adjustments made by the fetus in response to a compromised intrauterine nutritional environment. They reasoned that a fetus faced with undernutrition would be forced to adapt to this stress. It would slow its growth rate as a strategy to reduce nutritional requirements, but might also change its metabolism and physiology in such a way that would linger into adulthood to influence the risk of developing chronic disease. These permanent alterations to an organism's metabolism, physiology, or organ structure in response to early environments have been described as developmental "programming" (Lucas 1991), and more recently, "induction" (Bateson, 2001).

The hypothesis that adult risk for CVD could be programmed by prenatal nutrition was initially greeted with skepticism (Kramer & Joseph, 1996; Paneth et al., 1996). Most of the early studies documenting these relationships merely linked death records or adult health characteristics with birth weight data that had been recorded many decades earlier in birth records. This allowed an evaluation of relationships between birth weight and adult health or mortality, but largely ignored other aspects of lifestyle or environment that could influence the development of cardiovascular risk between birth and the onset of adult disease. This left open the possibility that birth weight was merely serving as a marker for other unmeasured factors that are known to influence CVD risk. For instance, small babies are born into lower income households, and perhaps birth weight was merely an indirect measure of social class or socioeconomic status.

There have now been hundreds of human studies documenting similar relationships, many of which incorporate longitudinal data on a wider range of lifestyle and environmental influences that might confound associations with birth size. Small birth size relates to an elevated risk of developing hypertension (reviewed by Adair and Dahly, 2005), insulin resistance and diabetes (Eriksson et al., 2002; Yajnik, 2004), abnormal cholesterol profiles (Kuzawa & Adair, 2003), an abdominal or visceral pattern of fat deposition (Oken & Gillman, 2003), and an elevated risk of suffering CVD and cardiovascular mortality (Leon et al., 1998). Although birth weight is an admittedly crude measure of intrauterine nutrition, animal model studies now number in the hundreds as well and show that restricting the nutritional intake of pregnant rats or sheep has similar adverse effects on blood pressure, insulin resistance, and cholesterol levels of adult offspring (reviewed by Langley-Evans et al., 2003; McMillen & Robinson, 2005; Seckl & Meaney, 2004).

Although programming of fetal biology has received most research attention, developmental responses continue to be important during infancy and childhood. For instance, small size in infancy is also associated with higher CVD risk in adulthood, while breastfed infants have lower rates of hypertension (Lawlor et al., 2005), obesity, and diabetes as adults (Arenz et al., 2004). There is also evidence that prenatal and postnatal exposures interact to influence adult health. Being born small but then experiencing rapid "catch-up" growth after birth, itself suggestive of an improvement in nutrition, predicts the same constellation of adult diseases (Adair & Cole, 2003; Ong, 2006). Small birth size is particularly deleterious among individuals who put on more weight or body fat later in life, which is associated with high CVD risk (Oken & Gillman, 2003). In Cebu City, the Philippines, individuals from higher income households eat more fat, have lower levels of physical activity, and have more body fat (Kuzawa et al., 2003). Although still relatively lean by U.S. standards, higher income adolescents in this population have higher

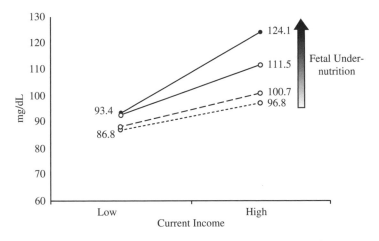

FIGURE 18-1 Low-density lipoprotein cholesterol by current household income among Cebu males, and stratified by different criteria of prenatal undernutrition (after Kuzawa, 2001). The lowest (dotted) line represents the entire male sample, while the second (dashed) line is limited to males with lower than average birth weights (<3 kg). The third and fourth lines use maternal characteristics to further restrict the lower-birth-weight subsample to individuals who likely ended up small as a result of fetal growth restriction. Line 3 (solid line, hollow dots) represents lower-birth-weight individuals born to taller-than-average mothers, while the top line (solid line, solid dots) further restricts this subgroup to the offspring of tall mothers with poor nutritional status, as indicated by triceps skinfold during pregnancy.

levels of low-density lipoprotein (LDL) cholesterol ("bad cholesterol"). What is intriguing is that the effect of living in a higher income household on LDL cholesterol differs among individuals who vary in fetal nutritional sufficiency (Figure 18-1). In these relatively lean adolescent Filipinos, the combination of fetal undernutrition followed by relative affluence after birth is associated with highest cholesterol levels (Kuzawa, 2001).

EVOLUTIONARY APPROACHES TO THE DOHaD LITERATURE

Although seemingly paradoxical, the finding that early life *undernutrition* may heighten the disease impact of *overnutrition* experienced later in the life cycle just might make sense if the fetus is calibrating its nutritional requirements on the basis of its prenatal experiences. Building from this idea, Hales and Barker (1992) proposed that adult risk of diabetes might trace to developmental adaptations made in response to prenatal undernutrition. They cited evidence that the nutritionally stressed fetus is forced to reduce the growth of nonessential organs like muscle or liver, while also inducing changes in insulin metabolism, in part to protect the large and glucose-demanding brain. According to their hypothesis, the resultant "thrifty phenotype" helps the fetus survive a difficult pregnancy, but later predisposes that individual to diabetes and CVD when faced with adequate or abundant postnatal nutrition and weight gain.

More recently, researchers have hypothesized that the adjustments made by the fetus may be designed to do more than merely help it survive gestation, but could also help improve its fit with the postnatal world (Bateson, 2001; Bateson et al., 2004; Gluckman & Hanson, 2005; Kuzawa, 2001, 2005; Wells, 2003). To the extent that prenatal exposures like nutrition or hormone levels are a response by the mother to the external ecology, these resources may act as cues, providing the fetus with opportunities to fine-tune its biology to better match the realities of the world that it will be born into. In one recent formalization of this idea, Gluckman and Hanson (2004a) propose that the adjustments made *in utero* are an example of a *predictive adaptive response* (PAR) "... made during the phase of developmental plasticity to optimize the phenotype for the probable environment of the mature organism" (p. 1735). According to these newer proposals, a rapid pace of environmental change within a single lifetime might lead to a new form of mismatch—not between our environment and our Paleolithic genome, but between *postnatal* environments and a biological imprint established in response to a *prenatal* cue signaling a marginal future nutritional ecology (Gluckman & Hanson, 2005; Wells, 2003). Like the biological equivalent of the linguistic accent that we learn as young children, this imprint could serve us well if we stay in place and the ecology remains stable, but might lead to a form of developmentally based mismatch, heightening risk for CVD, when individuals experience a brisk pace of nutritional or lifestyle change within their lifetimes.

If this model of developmental adaptation is correct, the pace and magnitude of recent change in nutrition or lifestyle may be an important influence on a population's pattern of disease risk, in addition to the more widely acknowledged role of genetic background and lifestyle. This might help explain the heterogeneity of disease risk observed across populations and between ethnic groups within nations. But just how plausible is this idea of developmental prediction? Are there comparable examples from other species, and, if so, what similarities and differences are there between them and the types of responses that we see in humans? And perhaps most importantly, does the human fetus have access to an ecological cue of sufficient reliability to allow it to predict the nutritional ecology that it is likely to confront decades after birth?

In this chapter I review examples of predictive developmental plasticity in other species as a basis for critically evaluating the plausibility that a similar process is at work in humans. As will be discussed, some mammals have evolved elaborate strategies that allow true "forward-looking" prediction based upon intrauterine cues. Humans, in contrast, have few options but to rely upon a form of "backward-looking" prediction based upon a signal reflecting the past nutritional experiences of recent ancestors. This capacity to anchor nutritional expectations to past experiences allows the fetus to calibrate its developmental biology to typical local conditions, but can heighten risk for diseases related to metabolism, such as CVD, when the ecology changes rapidly within a single generation. A developmental approach to CVD reveals that the lingering biological imprint of the past is not limited to our "Paleolithic" genome. Instead, there are multiple potential causes of biological mismatch that trace to different mechanisms of inheritance, each designed to cope with ecological change operating on different temporal scales (Kuzawa et al., 2007).

PREDICTIVE DEVELOPMENTAL PLASTICITY

Predictive Developmental Plasticity: Lessons from Amphibians

Developmental plasticity refers to the ability of a gene or genome to produce a range of different phenotypes[1] in response to the environmental conditions that an individual experiences during development (West-Eberhard, 2003). Because plasticity is a process of altered development, it is generally not reversible and is often sensitive to conditions experienced early in the life cycle. The differences in behavior or biology of identical twins reared apart attest to the power of plasticity (Heller et al., 1993). Many European nations witnessed a decline in menarcheal age from around 17 to 13 years in little more than a century, which is far too rapid to be due to changes in the genetic composition of these populations (Tanner 1962). Instead, this secular trend may be traced to the effects of improvements in hygiene and nutritional status on plasticity in growth rate and maturational timing (Eveleth & Tanner 1990).

Although not all plasticity is beneficial to the organism, the animal kingdom is filled with examples of species that have evolved an adaptive capacity to modify development in response to ecological characteristics that vary across the species' home range or that vary from generation to generation (West-Eberhard, 2003). The western spadefoot toad (*Scaphiopus hammondii*) provides a particularly interesting and relevant example. The spadefoot inhabits dry grasslands in areas like eastern California. Given the aridity of its ecology, the adult spadefoot spends much of the year in damp underground burrows, only to emerge after a heavy downpour to lay its eggs in one of the newly formed pools. Although this is a safe strategy for an amphibian living in an arid ecology, the ponds are temporary and have an unpredictable life, making it impossible to know in advance the amount of time available for the tadpoles to complete their growth. This lack of predictability does not leave the tadpole without recourse, because there are certain cues that are correlated with the pond's rate of drying, which the tadpole senses and uses to calibrate its pace of maturation. The spadefoot has evolved a remarkable capacity to shift the timing of metamorphosis from aquatic tadpole to terrestrial adult to match the life of its pond (Denver, 1999).

Research into the hormonal control of this developmental plasticity led to a finding that is as surprising as it is fascinating (reviewed in Crespi & Denver, 2005). A tadpole that senses that its pond is drying speeds up the timing of the developmental transition into the adult stage by producing a peptide called corticotropin-releasing factor (CRF). In amphibians, as in mammals, CRF (also called CRH) is a key regulatory molecule for the stress hormone system. This same peptide is produced by the fetuses of certain mammalian species, including humans, and it is believed to help initiate parturition early in the event of a difficult pregnancy (Challis et al., 2005). Thus, CRF and the stress hormone axis modulate the timing of key developmental transitions in response to ecological signals in these distantly related species, acting like a larval escape signal in each— in the case of the tadpole initiating early morphogenesis and exit from the pond, and in the human fetus speeding up the transition from intrauterine to extrauterine life (Denver, 1999).

What should we make of this odd parallel between the developmental biology of toads and humans? It is a fundamental principle of evolutionary biology that when a complex structure or trait is found in two species, it was very likely already present in their last common ancestor.[2] Considering the toad and human, our last common ancestor very likely had four legs and reproduced sexually. It was also bilaterally symmetrical, had two eyes, one mouth, and a gastrointestinal tract. Such patterns of "homology" are one basis for inferring that all living species share common ancestors if we go back far enough in evolutionary time. Research on developmental plasticity in the spadefoot helps extend the concept of homology to the hormonal architecture that regulates how bodies develop, including in this case the capacity to adjust the timing of key life history transitions in response to stressful challenges. Mammals evolved from early reptile-like amniotes that split from amphibians more than 300 million years ago (Carroll, 1997). Because the CRF peptide and the stress hormone system are present in humans and toads, this implies that this system has been around for at least that many years, and that some of the basic components that regulate its effects on the developing organism have been conserved since then.

In light of these similarities, it seems likely that the CRF–stress hormone system present in the human fetus is built from a template that was already present in rough outline among ancient amphibians. It likely evolved a capacity to respond to developmental cues that were directly experienced by the embryo in the outside world, not unlike the functioning of the system in the modern spadefoot tadpole. With the eventual evolution of internal fertilization in placental mammals, the embryonic environment shifted inside the mother's body. This allowed the mother to buffer the embryo by maintaining a constant temperature and by mobilizing nutritional stores to offset deficits when dietary intake is scarce. But it also created new channels for the mother to communicate ecological information to the fetus—through stimulation of systems like CRF and the stress hormone axis, but by no means limited to this. As a type of sensory modality, the information conveyed in the various nutrients and hormones crossing the placenta allow the mammalian fetus to monitor and track many features of the future environment into which it will be born and live out its life. And importantly, because this signal is communicated by the mother via the placenta, this opens up opportunities for natural selection to modify the information that the signal encodes and, as will be discussed, to enhance its reliability as a cue.

Research on the developmental origins of health and disease has documented detailed examples of fetal biological systems that are influenced by maternal nutritional or hormonal cues, and it was proposed above that a form of predictive signaling could go some way towards explaining the differences in how populations are experiencing the burden of CVD as nutrition and lifestyle change across the globe. Might these responses to prenatal nutrition also be part of a broader strategy of plasticity allowing the human fetus to shift its adaptive priorities dynamically in anticipation of the outside world? Given that most human research on early life developmental plasticity focuses on outcomes like cholesterol levels or diabetes, it is rarely certain whether these human responses might be part of a developmental strategy that initially evolved to help the organism predict and adapt to postnatal life. These traits may have great significance for human health, but their functional role or adaptive importance is more ambiguous and thus difficult to interpret. Luckily, there are clear examples of other mammals that have evolved adaptive capacities to predict their future ecology in response to prenatal cues, providing a useful starting point for considering the possible function of the responses documented in humans.

Predictive Intergenerational Signaling in Mammals: The Montane Vole

Some of the best examples of intergenerational signaling in mammals come from rodent populations that inhabit highly seasonal environments in places like Siberia and the intermountain west of North America. Here I borrow from the work of my colleague at Northwestern, Terry Horton (Horton, 1984). Starting in the early 1980s, Horton and her colleagues, then at the University of Utah, helped pioneer the study of predictive developmental responses in mammals, working with the Montane vole (*Microtus montanus*) (Negus & Berger, 1987; Negus et al., 1992). This species provides fascinating insights into the strategies of intergenerational signaling that mammals have evolved to help them adapt to dynamic environments.

Given their short life spans of 1 year or less, and the even shorter length of the breeding season, these rodents have one chance to reproduce and are forced to adopt one of several developmental strategies depending on when in the yearly cycle they are born (Negus & Berger, 1987). Individuals born in the spring enjoy a period of increasing day length and food availability. Given this, the best strategy for an animal born in the spring is to grow rapidly and mature at a young age, which allows it to reproduce during the height of the summer breeding season. This is an effective strategy, but the offspring of these matings are then born later in the same year, and thus during a very different stage in the seasonal progression—a period that will soon shift into autumn and a severe and protracted winter. If the offspring attempted to breed this late in the year, their own offspring would be too small to survive the extended winter and would die. For these later-born individuals, it thus makes sense to grow to a body size adequate to survive winter, while delaying reproduction until the following spring.

This extreme plasticity in development is an ingenious strategy. However, what is particularly fascinating about it is that an individual vole has already started to set its developmental trajectory *before birth* (Figure 18-2), before it has had a chance to experience the seasons for itself (Horton, 1984). Work by Horton and others has shown that these developmental responses are in part dependent upon the mother having an intact pineal gland, and that these predictive developmental responses in offspring may be manipulated by injecting her with the hormone melatonin during pregnancy (reviewed in Goldman, 2003). Endogenous production of melatonin by the pineal gland is regulated by the body's biological pacemaker and is acutely suppressed by sunlight, resulting in circadian dynamics in circulating melatonin that mirror cycles of light and dark. The body uses the diurnal changes in melatonin to entrain biological rhythms such as the sleep/wake cycle to the daily cycle of light and dark. It has the same effect in the vole mother, but it also crosses her placenta, providing the vole fetus with this information as well. If after birth the offspring senses increasing day length—as mirrored in the *change* in the circadian dynamics of melatonin relative to what was sensed *in utero*—it infers that it has been born early in the year, while a decrease in day length signals that birth has occurred later in summer or fall. By monitoring changes in melatonin across late gestation and the period of lactation, the offspring is able to sense the current position in the seasonal cycle, allowing it to set its long-term developmental and reproductive strategy in a predictive fashion.

This is not the end of the predictive challenge faced by the young vole, because the spring melt and the onset of new plant growth may shift by 6 weeks or more from year to year, which is a very long time for a species that matures as early as 4–6 weeks of age

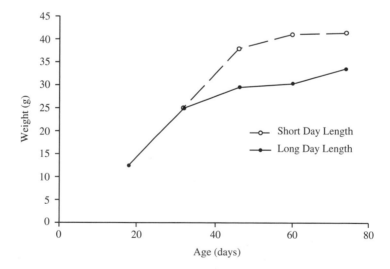

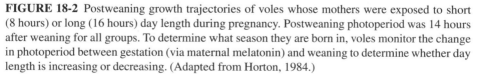

FIGURE 18-2 Postweaning growth trajectories of voles whose mothers were exposed to short (8 hours) or long (16 hours) day length during pregnancy. Postweaning photoperiod was 14 hours after weaning for all groups. To determine what season they are born in, voles monitor the change in photoperiod between gestation (via maternal melatonin) and weaning to determine whether day length is increasing or decreasing. (Adapted from Horton, 1984.)

(Negus et al., 1992). Given that the vole has a single opportunity to reproduce, it must fine-tune the timing of reproductive maturity with greater precision than it could achieve using photoperiod alone as a cue. It manages this with the aid of a second cue conveyed by the mother across the placenta. In addition to the transmission of photoperiod cues, a chemical produced in abundance by grasses during their early spring growth also passes across the placenta, providing the fetus with information about the vole's primary food resource. The presence of this metabolite in the maternal diet during pregnancy has the effect of speeding the pace of postnatal growth and reproductive maturation in offspring (Berger & Negus, 1992; Epstein et al., 1986; Frandson et al., 1993). Thus, the fetus uses information on prenatal and postnatal photoperiod to sense its position in the seasonal cycle, while additional cues from the diet provide finer-grained information on the more variable timing of plant growth during its particular year of birth.

This elaborate system of intergenerational communication has helped this short-lived species, and others with similar life histories, to thrive in challenging environments marked by extreme seasonal shifts in temperature, day length, and food availability, which are compounded by year-to-year variation in the onset of important ecological events. Similar systems of maternal–fetal signaling have been documented in other high-latitude short-lived species, including the Siberian or Djungarian hamster (*Phodopus sungorus*) (Weaver & Reppert, 1986) and the meadow vole (Lee et al., 1989).

THE FUNCTION OF DEVELOPMENTAL RESPONSES TO FETAL NUTRITION IN HUMANS

The ecology and life history of the Montane vole make this species a perfect candidate for the evolution of predictive developmental plasticity based upon maternal–fetal signaling. There are enormous shifts in ecology during the year that are regular and therefore predictable. Because this cycle is both severe and long relative to an individual vole's life expectancy, when one enters it places important constraints on that individual's possible developmental and reproductive strategies. What's more, the mother's body produces a hormone that not only signals current position within the seasonal cycle with high reliability, but also passes across the placenta to a fetus already endowed with receptors capable of sensing it. Her ingestion of certain plant metabolites is tightly correlated with the onset of spring vegetative growth, providing additional information on the availability of plant resources. Given this convergence of conditions, it is almost unthinkable that this species would *not* have evolved a capacity to fine-tune postnatal life history in response to maternal cues.

The response of the human fetus to prenatal nutrition clearly *is* an example of developmental plasticity. Less certain is whether this response is *adaptive*, implying that it evolved by natural selection to help the organism survive or reproduce. Did some of the long-term effects that fetal undernutrition have on human metabolism and physiology evolve to improve the developing organism's fit with the postnatal environment, akin to what we see in the vole and its predictive developmental plasticity? Several conditions must be met for this type of strategy to have evolved. First and most obviously, there must have been ecological variability—an ability to adjust to postnatal ecology is of no use if the ecology does not vary. This assumption seems reasonable. As generalists, humans are not tied to narrow niches, latitudes, or climatic zones, and thus inhabit ecologies that vary in both the quantity and consistency of resource availability. The paleoclimate record shows that climate change compounded this challenge of coping with ecological variability. In contrast to the highly unusual climate stability of the past 10,000 years, the preceding millions of years were marked by chaotic shifts that led to locally rapid ecological change (reviewed by Roy et al., 1996; Potts, 1998). Data from pollen cores, ocean sediments and glacial cores show that there were large and unpredictable climate shifts that occurred on the scale of centuries and even decades. Although natural selection operating on gene frequencies can adjust a population to changing conditions, this process is slow in comparison to these shifts. Thus, our ancestors would have required more rapid modes of biological adaptation to cope with this ecological variability (Potts, 1998).

In light of this challenge, having an ability to predict the present state of the environment might provide the human fetus with certain advantages. The human and animal model literatures show that prenatal nutrition influences postnatal traits like blood pressure, glucose metabolism, and lipid metabolism. Although researchers focus on these outcomes for their obvious health significance, changes in these and other systems might also be necessary to support a shift in the organism's energetic priorities (Figure 18-3), and, thus, might be viewed as components of an adaptive response to early environments. Although speculative, there are reasons to interpret the available data in this light (see Kuzawa, 2005). For instance, lower-birth-weight individuals end up smaller as adults and have reduced muscle mass (Kensara et al., 2005; Singhal et al., 2003). The number of muscle fibers present at birth is responsive to the nutritional milieu *in utero*, which helps determine lean mass and strength throughout life (Zhu et al., 2006). Although this reduction in insulin-sensitive tissue increases risk of diabetes, from an ecological perspective smaller bodies with less metabolically active tissue have reduced nutritional requirements. There is also evidence that prenatal undernutrition has the effect of reducing

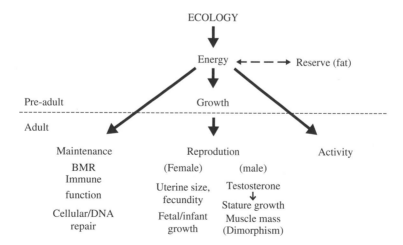

FIGURE 18-3 Organismal energy allocation. Organisms allocate a fraction of energy to growth, which is shunted into supporting reproduction upon cessation of growth. (Modified from Kuzawa, 2005.)

expenditures on other functions like reproduction and immunity (Galler et al., 1979; McDade et al., 2001; Moore et al., 2004), which might similarly be necessary to conserve resources when nutrition is scarce.

Some of the postnatal changes in the biology of specific tissues that are triggered by fetal undernutrition might further help the organism adapt to its environment. Compared to individuals of higher birth weight, the muscle of individuals born small appears to be relatively insensitive to the effects of insulin (Vaag et al., 2006), in part as a result of a reduction in the number of mitochondria (Park et al., 2003). Although insulin resistance is an important risk factor for the development of diabetes and thus CVD, this shift in glucose allocation can be viewed as a more conservative strategy of resource use. Insulin resistance in peripheral tissues has the effect of boosting delivery of glucose to non–insulin-sensitive tissues like the energy-demanding and fragile brain, perhaps at a cost to glycogen storage in muscle and thus physical endurance. Like the brain, the feto-placental unit during pregnancy also extracts glucose from the blood stream without the aid of insulin. A reduction in the use of glucose by the mother's muscle, as a result of reduced muscle insulin sensitivity established during her early development, would thus leave more glucose in the circulation to support fetal growth (see also Haig, 1993).

If such changes in energetic priorities are appropriate preparations for a marginal or less stable nutritional future, the developing organism might benefit by adjusting its strategy of metabolic partitioning in response to early life nutritional cues; that is, *if* the fetus has access to a cue that is an accurate predictor of future nutritional conditions. Given the elaborate strategy that the short-lived vole must use to predict its future, how plausible is a similar scenario of prediction in the comparatively long-lived human?

What Does Fetal Nutrition Signal About the Future in Humans?

Several questions must be considered when evaluating the potential for predictive signaling of this sort in humans. First, which resources cross the placenta and are sensed by the fetus? Second, with what, if anything, are these resources reliably correlated in the outside world? As with the vole, knowing the answer to these questions will provide a sense for what the fetus is potentially capable of "seeing" about its postnatal environment. Although assessing this is anything but straightforward, certain features of fetal biology create opportunities to evaluate this in a rough sense. During fetal life, growth rate is regulated by a different suite of hormones than during childhood and adolescence. Nutrients pass across the placenta to increase fetal insulin, which increases production of the insulin-like growth factors, which in turn stimulate skeletal growth at the growth plate and differentiation and proliferation of muscle cells (Gluckman & Pinal, 2003). Delivery of fuel substrate and insulin also drive fat deposition in the fetus during the third trimester (Symonds et al., 2003). Although an individual's growth potential is influenced by factors other than nutrition, this acute sensitivity of fetal growth to nutrition means that birth size serves as a useful, if rough, proxy for the stream of nutrients that the fetus received across the placenta. If we can identify the factors that predict birth weight, the fetus could evolve the capacity to achieve the same feat in reverse—much as the vole has done—and use intrauterine nutrition to infer these characteristics of the outside world.

So what predicts birth weight? Genetic factors generally account for at most 40% of birth-weight variation (Polani, 1974). Given the large variability in birth weight not accounted for by genetics, it is somewhat surprising that what a mother eats during pregnancy is also not a particularly strong predictor of birth weight. This is seen in the modest effects that maternal nutritional supplementation has on birth weight. Most trials increase birth weight on the order of 25 g for each 10,000 kcal of maternal supplementation (Institute of Medicine, 1990; Kramer, 2000). Given that 10,000 kcal is enough energy to build roughly 2 kg of new tissue (Waterlow, 1981), it is clear that only a small fraction of the supplement is passing across the placenta to augment fetal growth. The relatively modest effects of pregnancy supplementation on birth outcomes attest, in part, to the effectiveness of maternal buffering mechanisms. Maternal metabolism and physiology maintain a relatively constant supply of resources to the fetus, and this dampens the impact of changes in her intake or energy status on the fetus. When nutritionally stressed, the mother's body may mobilize fat stores while reducing metabolic expenditure on nonessential functions like thermogenesis and physical activity (see Dufour & Sauther, 2002). The minor effects of pregnancy supplementation trials show that this buffering works both ways: abrupt improvements in dietary intake in the form of supplements also fail to have large effects on fetal nutrition. This is not to suggest that supplementation does not benefit both mother and fetus—supplements *do* reduce the rates of fetal growth restriction, stillbirths and neonatal death (Kramer, 2000), and supplements may have larger effects on birth weight when high-risk women are targeted (Ceesay et al., 1997). Moreover, the balance of nutrients or the adequacy of specific micronutrients in the mother's diet can also influence fetal growth above and beyond any effects of gross macronutrient consumption (Institute of Medicine, 1990). However, for the purposes of the present discussion, the modest change in birth weight from most supplementation trials suggest that large fluctuations in what a mother consumes during pregnancy may often have comparably small effects on fetal nutrition, thus rendering these changes in the outside ecology relatively "invisible" to the fetus and its developing metabolism and biology (Kuzawa, 2005; Wells, 2003).

If large swings in the mother's dietary intake during pregnancy are not visible to the fetus, what features of the external ecology, if any, does intrauterine nutrition allow the fetus to see? Although energy intake during pregnancy is not a particularly strong predictor, weight gain during pregnancy is, because the weight of the feto-placental unit and amniotic fluid account for a large percentage of the gain (Institute of Medicine, 1990). What is perhaps more interesting is that nutritional status at the time of conception, or even before, predicts birth weight (Harding, 2003; Institute of Medicine, 1990; Rayco-Solon et al., 2005). A mother's nutritional status at conception in turn reflects her cumulative nutritional experiences in prior years. This provides important clues as to the type of information conveyed by fetal nutrition: if it serves as an ecological cue, it clearly must inform the fetus, in part, about conditions experienced by the mother in the *past*.

Additional evidence that fetal nutrition is a signal of the mother's nutritional history comes from studies that track the intergenerational predictors of birth weight. Although it is not surprising that larger mothers tend to give birth to bigger babies, studies find that different components of maternal stature predict birth weight with varying strength and that leg length tends to be a stronger predictor than trunk length (Lawlor et al., 2003). Studies that include measures of the mother's own growth show that her leg length measured during childhood is an even stronger predictor of offspring birth weight than is her leg length as an adult (Martin et al., 2004). Because childhood leg growth is among the most nutritionally sensitive components of skeletal growth (Scrimshaw & Béhar, 1965), these studies support the view that part of what the fetus sees in the stream of nutrition is a reflection of what the mother ate many years prior, during her own growth and development.

The intergenerational influences on fetal nutrition become particularly fascinating when we trace back even further to the mother's own intrauterine experiences as a fetus. Intergenerational correlations between maternal and offspring birth weight are high, with each kilogram increase in maternal birth weight predicting a 200-g increase in the birth weight of offspring (reviewed by Ramakrishnan et al., 1999). Several features of these correlations are worth noting. First, they tend to be independent of maternal stature or body size, suggesting that they are not merely a result of the fact that individuals born large end up as larger adults. Larger women do give birth to larger babies, but the intergenerational birth-weight correlation is independent of the mother's adult size. Second, the intergenerational correlation is strengthened after adjusting for gestational age, revealing that what is important is the nutritionally sensitive measure of fetal growth rate, rather than differences in the duration of prenatal growth (Alberman et al., 1992). Although some of this correlation is likely due to shared genes, there is also evidence for an environmentally induced component to these intergenerational effects on fetal nutrition. Women whose mothers experienced the Dutch famine winter of WWII during the first trimester of pregnancy gave birth to offspring (the grandoffspring of the original famine-exposed women) who were themselves smaller (Lumey, 1992). Thus, the intrauterine nutritional experiences of these women influenced the intrauterine nutritional environment that they provided their own offspring (Ounsted et al., 1986). The mechanisms that account for these intergenerational influences on nutrition and fetal growth remain poorly characterized, but likely involve changes in traits like placental perfusion and the size and blood flow to the uterus (Gluckman & Hanson, 2004).

Taken together, these studies provide a fascinating glimpse of what the intrauterine nutrient stream allows the fetus to "see," and, thus, what it might use this cue to infer about the world that it will be born into. Based upon the predictors of birth weight, fetal nutrition conveys information about the local nutritional ecology that stretches back into the mother's developmental past, all the way back to her own intrauterine experiences as a fetus. Because the mother's supply of nutrients to her current fetus is in part dependent upon the supply of nutrients that she received *in utero* from *her* mother, this implies that the fetus is partly seeing what the *grandmother* ate during her lifetime as well. Thus, although fetal nutrition is responsive to the mother's current nutrition and health, it is perhaps better described as a signal of her chronic intake, and one that provides something like an integrated, running average measure of the recent nutritional experiences of the matriline (Kuzawa, 2005).

THE ADAPTIVE SIGNIFICANCE OF INTERGENERATIONAL INERTIA

The preceding discussion highlights at least two interlocking processes that help link fetal nutrition with the past experiences of recent ancestors. The first is maternal buffering, which insulates fetal nutrition from acute changes in her current intake, thus decoupling the intrauterine nutritional signal from temporary, and thus potentially misleading, cues like an illness, a drought, or a particularly abundant season (or equivalently, supplementation). The second includes intergenerational mechanisms (discussed below) that link fetal nutrition with the nutritional and growth conditions experienced by the mother during her past, extending back to her own gestational experiences and thus to the nutritional history of recent matrilineal ancestors. The effect of these dual influences is to allow a recalibration of the nutritional signal in response to ecological change, but only gradually and with a lag resulting from the lingering influence of the past (Ounsted et al., 1986; Price & Coe, 1999).

Particularly striking evidence for this lag is seen in the gradual, intergenerational increase in birth weight documented in a troop of wild macaques that experienced an abrupt improvement in nutrition after being taken into captivity (Price and Coe, 1999; Price et al., 2000). The positive trend in birth weight had not stabilized after five generations, and there was an intergenerational component to the trend, with maternal birth weight predicting birth weight of female offspring (see also Ounsted et al., 1986). This shows how a population may require multiple generations of maternal–fetal transmission to recalibrate certain aspects of developmental biology to even abrupt ecological change. I have argued elsewhere that this type of gradual intergenerational response to change, or *phenotypic inertia* (Kuzawa, 2005), improves the reliability of fetal nutrition as a signal of typical ecological conditions (Figure 18-4). A strategy of ignoring transient changes while allowing intergenerational recalibration to more sustained change could allow the fetus to track ecological shifts that are longer-term and more stable, and thus more relevant to a long-lived species.

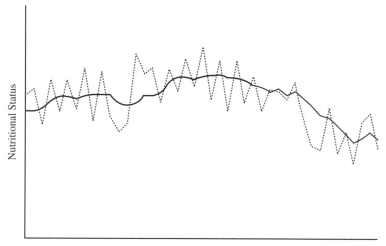

Time

FIGURE 18-4 The hypothesized capacity for fetal nutrition to be set to a running average signal of the nutritional experiences of recent ancestors. Maternal buffering of the effect of abrupt and transient changes in nutritional status (dotted line), combined with intergenerational influences on nutrition, allows the fetus to track more gradual but sustained ecological trends (solid line). (Adapted from Kuzawa, 2005.)

Mechanisms of Developmental Induction and Intergenerational Inertia

Although the specific pathways accounting for the intergenerational continuity of fetal nutrition and growth remain poorly understood, animal experiments provide important insights into how ecological information is conveyed across generations for similar traits and systems. The best documented mechanisms for the continuity of induced phenotypic states include heritable modifications in the molecular scaffolding from which the double helix of the DNA is built, such as the attachment of an extra methyl group to cytosine ("methylation") or other changes in the conformation of chromatin (reviewed by Jablonka & Lamb, 1995, 2005). These "epigenetic" changes can influence whether and how much a gene is expressed, while leaving the DNA itself unmodified. Epigenetic changes can be induced by an environmental stimulus like nutrition, can persist across a single life cycle, and in some cases also across generations.

As the list of examples of epigenetic effects, or "epigenetic inheritance systems," continues to grow (Jablonka & Lamb, 1995; 2005), their importance to the intergenerational transmission of environmental influences on biology and health is becoming clear (Drake & Walker, 2004). One study found that restricting the protein intake of pregnant rats changed the methylation of a gene that regulates lipid metabolism (PPARα) in offspring and that methylation status was correlated with the postweaning expression of mRNA at that particular locus (Lillycrop et al., 2005). Thus, changing the environment of one generation—the pregnant mother—leads to methylation and altered gene expression in offspring after birth. Another study exposed pregnant rats to a synthetic stress hormone (dexamethasone) and measured metabolism and growth in several generations of offspring (Drake et al., 2005). The female fetuses exposed *in utero* gave birth to offspring (the grandoffspring of the treated pregnant dams) who were themselves smaller and had impaired glucose tolerance. Interestingly, this effect was not limited to the offspring of exposed mothers. The *male* treated fetuses, when crossed with a control female later in adulthood, also sired smaller offspring who were glucose intolerant. In both patrilineal and matrilineal offspring, the effect on growth and metabolism lingered into the grandoffspring generation but was reversed in great-grandoffspring.

The patrilineal inheritance in this study helps clarify one type of epigenetic "memory" that may be transmitted across generations—in this case influencing how the body allocates and uses glucose. Unlike the female's contribution to the zygote, which includes not only genes but also the cytoplasm, chromatin, organelles, and enzymes present in the egg (Bonner, 1974), sperm are believed to donate nothing more than chromosomes to the zygote at conception. As such, the finding of an inherited paternal effect strongly suggests that environmental experiences can modify the pattern of gene expression of the germ line present at conception which is then transmitted to offspring (for review, see Chong & Whitelaw, 2004). Although the specific molecular details have yet to be described for this model, the findings are consistent with the known mechanisms of epigenetic inheritance: the genes themselves clearly are not changed, because the phenotype "washes out" and reverts to its preinduced state after two generations. Another recent study found that a different prenatal treatment—maternal protein restriction—had an effect on glucose metabolism that was transmitted across two generations of offspring, this time investigated only in females (Benyshek et al., 2006). In contrast to the results of the prenatal stress hormone protocol, not only the grand offspring but the *great*-grandoffspring of the pregnant dam exposed to protein restriction had glucose intolerance before the phenotype reverted to its preinduced state. Although not focused on early nutrition, another recent study showed that exposing pregnant rats to an endocrine disruptor around the time of sexual differentiation impairs spermatogenesis in male offspring for at least *four* generations of offspring (as many as were followed up) (Anway et al., 2005).

The early postnatal period of maternal–offspring interaction is a continued stage of plasticity and developmental induction, which gives rise to fascinating examples of epigenetic inheritance operating through distinct pathways. Michael Meaney and colleagues at McGill University have documented the molecular mechanisms underlying one such example in remarkable detail (Weaver et al., 2004). In this model, the stimulus is not nutrition, but how a mother rears her newborn pups. More nurturant mothers lick and groom their pups and also engage in a behavior called "arched back nursing" that encourages pup feeding. When compared to the pups of less nurturant mothers, the indulged pups show an attenuated physiological stress hormone response later in life when faced with a challenge or threat. Meaney's group has shown that the induced change in the stress hormone system involves changes in both the chromatin configuration and methylation status of the gene encoding the glucocorticoid receptor in a region of the brain (the hippocampus) that helps regulate stress hormone production (Weaver et al., 2004). This pattern of epigenetic inheritance occurs even when the young being raised by nurturant dams are the genetic offspring of the low nurturant dams, showing that the continuity of behavior is not merely a result of classic genetic inheritance, while an epigenetic basis for the effect is supported by the fact that the behavior is reversed by demethylation. Thus, rather than being a result of genetic inheritance or simple learning, this pattern of inheritance likely involves biological changes in gene expression in hippocampal neurons that influence how the stress hormone system is regulated. One trait that this change in stress reactivity influences is future rearing style, and amazingly, the indulged pups end up replicating a similar nurturant style when rearing their own young. Thus, in this model we have evidence for a mode of epigenetic inheritance that bypasses the zygote altogether, with an environmentally induced phenotype in one generation serving as a template for the construction of a similar phenotype in offspring.

It is highly unlikely that changes in chromatin and gene methylation in the hippocampus would result in a future rearing behavior that replicates the same chromatin and methylation changes in offspring purely by *chance*. This interpretation seems even less likely once other examples of maternal–fetal intergenerational transmission are considered, such as the lingering effect of the nutritional experiences of past generations on the intrauterine nutritional environment provided offspring. These observations, and the complexity of the epigenetic mechanisms that account for them, suggest that mammalian biology has been *designed* to allow certain nongenetic, environmentally induced phenotypic changes to be transmitted across generations (Jablonka and Lamb, 2005). As suggested above, such modes of nongenetic inheritance may have evolved to allow individuals to cope with changes that are too rapid to be tracked by the gradual process of natural selection operating on gene frequencies, but that are too slow, sustained, or extreme for our acutely responsive and reversible homeostatic processes to efficiently buffer given their limited range of response (Figure 18-5) (see Bateson, 1963).

Cycle duration			Adaptation	
Years			Mode	Process
0.00000001	Seconds			
0.0001	Hours		Physiological	Homeostasis
0.001	Days			
0.1	Months			Allostasis
1	Years		Developmental	Plasticity
10	Decades			
100	Centuries		Intergenerational	Inertia
1000	Millennia			
1000000	Millions		Genetic	Natural Selection

FIGURE 18-5 The spectrum of ecological change and the hypothesized role of intergenerational inertia as a mode of adaptation.

Intergenerational Inertia Versus Acute Effects as a Dimension of Developmental Adaptation

Each of these examples provides insight into the types of heritable epigenetic changes that allow the transfer of ecological information across generations, represented not in the specific sequence of DNA inherited, but in the pattern with which that DNA is expressed. The previously discussed examples of intergenerational birth-weight correlations, the effect of prenatal nutrition on the fetal growth of offspring, and the lag in the birth-weight response to nutritional change documented in the macaque population suggest that intrauterine nutrition provides the fetus with information about past ecologies, likely operating through similar, yet to be identified epigenetic pathways. At the same time, however, it is clear that a mother's gestational health or nutritional status, or stressors like smoking, have acute effects on her current birth outcome (Institute of Medicine, 1990). Thus, there are multiple influences on intrauterine signals, and the balance between them must influence the type and time depth of information that is encoded and communicated to the fetus.

It is interesting to consider how these inputs might converge to influence the signal received by the fetus. In this regard, maternal–fetal biological signaling might be analogous to the inheritance of cultural traditions, which vary markedly in their tendency to remain stable in the face of societal change. At one extreme are short-lived fads, which are selected for rapid turnover and novelty and may be learned at any stage in the life cycle. At the other are more deeply rooted traditions like language, linguistic accent, and religious belief, which have greater intergenerational staying power in the face of change. It is notable that the most stable cultural practices have a pattern of socialization dependent upon stimuli being experienced during early sensitive periods in neurocognitive development. Although humans have the ability to learn language throughout life, we are particularly efficient at learning grammatical structure and vocabulary during early childhood, when our brains are primed to latch onto and internalize what we hear (Pinker & Bloom, 1990). Our reliance upon prior generations at this age nearly ensures that we end up perpetuating linguistic patterns similar to those used in recent generations.

Thus, although language of course does change, the pace of that change is tempered by the fact that the critical period for language acquisition overlaps with the period of intergenerational dependence.

The biological and metabolic traits that are influenced by intergenerational epigenetic effects likely also vary in their relative sensitivity to current versus ancestral influences. Some plastic traits are sensitive to the mother's (or the neonate's) immediate experiences, while others have greater intergenerational stability because their mature state is—akin to our linguistic accent—established during early windows of development that overlap with, and are responsive to, the biology (or behavior) of the prior generation. The finding, reviewed above, that different experimental protocols induce phenotypic states that persist across two, three, or four generations of offspring before reverting to the preinduced state suggests that epigenetic information is not only transmitted across generations, but that the strength of inertia—the weighting of past versus current influences—is itself potentially modifiable. It seems likely that the number of generations across which an induced developmental effect lingers might itself be modified by natural selection, allowing information to be integrated, and a running average calculated, across different intergenerational time frames (Kuzawa, 2005).

To conclude this section, the minimum requirements for the evolution of a system of adaptive developmental plasticity, as outlined above, appear to be in place in humans: not only are humans confronted by different types of nutritional ecologies, but the biological effects of prenatal responses to nutrition could benefit the organism faced with this ecological variation. The fetus has access to a cue that is a reasonable indicator of the average, recent state of the ecology, boosting the likelihood that these adjustments will be well-matched to postnatal realities. Finally, there is a growing list of mechanisms to account for the intergenerational transfer of environmental information through nongenetic pathways, providing evidence that evolution has favored such strategies in mammals. Together these observations boost the plausibility that adaptive fetal plasticity could have evolved under the influence of natural selection.

INTERGENERATIONAL INERTIA AND HUMAN HEALTH

The vole and human illustrate two distinct strategies that species varying dramatically in life history and ecology have evolved to predict postnatal conditions from prenatal cues. The vole uses a combination of hormonal and chemical cues of maternal origin to predict its *future* position within a regular seasonal cycle of changing day length, temperature, and ecological productivity. This feat of forward-looking prediction is only possible because its dominant ecological cycle is not only regular, but also severe and prolonged relative to its life expectancy. The vole is not concerned with the nutritional experiences of ancestors during prior years, but instead with ensuring that its own single reproductive effort is well timed with respect to the present year's seasonal transitions. The vole uses at least three cues to achieve its sophisticated strategy of forward-looking prediction: it establishes whether day length is increasing or decreasing by calculating the change in photoperiod—first measured *in utero* via maternal melatonin signaling, and again after weaning. Starting before birth, it also senses the concentration of plant metabolites present in the maternal diet, which signal the presence of early spring vegetative growth.

Using this combination of cues, the vole manages to home in with reasonable precision on an appropriate developmental and reproductive strategy that helps ensure that its single shot at reproduction is well timed.

Unlike the vole, the human fetus will live through hundreds of seasons and has no comparable large-scale cycle to entrain its much longer life history to prior to birth. In many ways, the challenge faced by the human fetus is thus opposite that of the vole: to ignore the specific season of birth to a certain extent, and to minimize the impact of any extreme or unusual conditions that may be present during that particular gestation, such as might be expected during a particularly good or bad year or season. Humans have faced considerable ecological and nutritional variability, but unlike the forward-looking vole, the longer-term trends that we confront and must adapt to follow no predictable cycle. The human fetus is therefore forced to adopt the very different strategy of adjusting nutritional expectations on the basis of information reflecting conditions experienced by *past* generations. A "backward-looking" cue is likely the most useful strategy available to the human fetus, because there simply is no basis for predicting the future, other than by hedging that conditions will remain about the same as experienced by recent ancestors. By smoothing out the effect of any short-term seasonal or year-to-year perturbations, the buffering of fetal nutrition by maternal metabolism, combined with the intergenerational averaging of nutritional information conveyed to the fetus, should increase the fidelity of this signal, boosting its value as a guide when constructing the developing body and its future metabolic priorities.

It is not difficult to imagine how this same capacity to anchor metabolic expectations to a signal of average recent nutritional experiences could backfire, heightening risk for metabolic disease, when change is not only abrupt but sustained. Today, powerful ripples are sent through the global human nutritional ecology by institutions like industrial agriculture, which has increased the affordability of concentrated sources of calories like refined sugar and oil (Drewnowski & Popkin, 1997). Additional ripples come with the mechanization of our lives and changing patterns of activity. Human locomotion is increasingly powered by hydrocarbons rather than dietary energy, while employment options are often limited to sedentary occupations that require minimal physical exertion (Popkin & Gordon-Larsen, 2004). As a result of these changes, energy balance is shifting into the surplus column in many populations, and humankind is putting on extra body fat at an alarming rate (see Chapter 3). As emphasized in the introduction to this chapter, populations experiencing a particularly rapid pace of nutritional and lifestyle change are often predisposed to CVD. The model presented here outlines one adaptive feature of mammalian biology that may backfire when conditions change rapidly, thus helping explain some of this heterogeneity in the global CVD epidemic.

The now common finding that CVD risk is highest among individuals who were born small but later put on weight is consistent with the hypothesis of developmental mismatch, as it suggests that experiencing improved nutrition between birth and adulthood can exacerbate the effects of a compromised fetal environment (Fagerberg et al., 2004; Oken and Gillman, 2003). Developmental mismatch could help explain why stunting—a measure of early life undernutrition—is a risk factor for obesity in some populations experiencing rapid nutritional transition (Florencio et al., 2003; Popkin et al., 1996; Steyn et al., 1998). The model is also supported by the finding that poor gestational nutrition is *not* associated with elevated CVD risk in populations that remain marginally nourished in adulthood (Moore et al., 2001). If the mismatch hypothesis is correct, populations shifting rapidly from low to higher nutritional status would be expected to experience a period of transition marked by high CVD risk, followed by a gradual intergenerational recalibration of expectations to the new, more abundant nutritional plane (Gluckman & Hanson, 2005; Prentice and Moore, 2005). It has been argued that this type of gradual resetting of expectations could go some way towards explaining the recent decline in CVD in populations that already experienced peak rates of CVD earlier in the twentieth century, like the United States and western Europe (Barker, 1994).

Although a model of developmental adaptation predicts that transitional populations will eventually recalibrate and experience a reduction in CVD risk, there may be situations in which this does not occur. Diabetes relates to birth weight in a U-shaped fashion, and thus is more common among individuals who were either small *or* large at birth (Huang et al., 2006). This may lead to an unusual intergenerational pattern of disease transmission when nutritional environments change rapidly. An individual undernourished as a fetus is more prone to develop diabetes if nutrition improves and he or she gains weight. Gestational diabetes in the next generation of mothers, in turn, increases the flow of glucose and insulin across the placenta, leading to a fetus (grandoffspring) born with excessive body fat and altered glucose metabolism. Large or macrosomic babies have an increased risk of developing obesity and diabetes themselves, thus potentially setting in motion an intergenerational cycle of mutually reinforcing diabetic pregnancies and diabetic offspring. In this way, a particularly rapid pace of change may shift a population from a pattern of chronic undernutrition to an intergenerational susceptibility to obesity and diabetes. A mechanism of this sort has been proposed as an explanation for the very high rates of gestational diabetes among certain Native American populations in the United States, notably the Pima (Benyshek et al., 2001), and the emerging epidemic of metabolic disease on the Indian subcontinent (Yajnik, 2004).

Conditions such as poverty can also create a form of mismatch in the absence of rapid social change, and this can have an important, sustained influence on disease patterns in certain societies and demographic subgroups. In contrast to global trends in adult dietary intake and energy balance, the health and nutritional status of infants and young children remain tied to conditions that influence risk for infectious disease, including sanitation, crowding, and the availability of clean water. Many populations from developing nations that are experiencing weight gain as adults still have relatively high rates of early life undernutrition and growth stunting tracing to factors like childhood diarrhea and respiratory tract infections. If the developmental mismatch model is correct, there are dueling forces at work in these individuals, who enter a world that is nutritionally challenging, but gradually shift into positive energy balance and weight gain as they age. Because infant nutritional status remains tightly linked to poverty, while adult energy balance is increasingly decoupled from traditional economic barriers, this could also lead to mismatch, not because the ecology is changing, but because the *experience* of that ecology—poverty—differs by age. There is evidence for such patterns of concurrent early life undernutrition and adult overnutrition in the same populations, as suggested, for instance, in the finding of a co-occurrence of obese and malnourished individuals in the same household (e.g., Garrett & Ruel, 2005).

Revising the Model of Chronic Disease Epidemiology:
Genes, Environment, and Developmental Biology

The developmental processes reviewed in this chapter point to the need for an amended model of metabolic disease epidemiology. The traditional perspective, which views health as a product of our genome interacting with our own environment and lifestyle, is clearly not complete. Developmental and epigenetic processes also leave a lingering imprint on our biology that trace to formative environmental experiences during early life and are influenced to varying degrees by the historical experiences of ancestors prior to our own conception. The complexity of interactions generated by these influences is now becoming clear. As one example, genes that influence cholesterol metabolism have been shown to have effects on lipid profiles that depend upon the birth weight of the carrier of that allele (Garces et al., 2002; Infante-Rivard et al., 2003). Similar interactions with birth weight have been found for genes that influence insulin resistance (Cambien et al., 1998; Vu-Hong et al., 2006), bone mineral metabolism (Dennison et al., 2004), and blood pressure (te Velde et al., 2005), among others. As discussed in this chapter, birth weight, in turn, is a marker that partially reflects the historical nutritional experiences of *prior* generations. It thus seems clear that our health is a product of our genes interacting not solely with our *own* lived experiences, but also with the experiences of our immediate ancestors (Jablonka, 2004).

Although developmental responses to early environments may modify the effects of the genes that we inherit, they also reveal why it is no longer acceptable to uncritically assume that unexplained biological differences between populations trace to genes, even when those differences are already present at birth. This is particularly true when membership in a population or subgroup is established according to socially defined criteria, such as the labeling in the United States of individuals with any visible African ancestry as African American ("hypodescent"). I close this chapter with this example as it illustrates the power of a developmental model of adult health to challenge us with new ideas about the causes of social disparities in conditions like CVD. It is well established that African Americans have higher rates of hypertension, diabetes, and CVD mortality than their U.S. non-Hispanic white counterparts. When studies find that race is still a significant predictor of these conditions after adjusting for certain lifestyle and socioeconomic characteristics, it is not uncommon for researchers to suggest that the residual effect of race must indicate as-yet-undiscovered black–white differences in gene frequencies (see Cooper & Kaufman, 1998). This conflation of biological difference with genetics is one of the more pervasive errors committed in the modern study of biology and health, and in this case it is brought into question by the fact that U.S. blacks *also* have lower birth weights than their white counterparts (Alexander et al., 1999), which we now know is a risk factor for hypertension, diabetes, and CVD.

One may question whether black–white differences in birth weight and cardiovascular risk might both be the result of a common set of genetic differences between these groups. Although I am aware of no evidence to support this interpretation, recent research points to the power of developmental environments to shape these health disparities. In a study of birth records of recent immigrants to the United States, immigrants from the Caribbean and Africa, many of whom come from privileged socioeconomic positions in their home countries, were found to have a birth weight distribution nearly identical to that of U.S. whites upon arrival (David & Collins, 1998). This equivalence was short lived. Among subsequent generations born in the United States, the birth weight distribution of the offspring of African immigrants eventually shifted to the left, en route to a convergence with the lower African American mean (Collins et al., 2002). What is particularly fascinating is that the European immigrants in this study responded to the U.S. environment in opposite fashion: their birth weights were *lower* than the U.S. white mean upon arrival, but *increased* with each passing generation born in the United States.

These opposing biological responses were far too rapid to be the result of changes in gene frequencies (Boas, 1912). Instead, they reveal that living in the United States has different implications for the intrauterine environments that U.S. blacks and U.S. whites experience prior to birth. Whether from Europe or Africa, after several generations the birth-weight distributions of each group of immigrants and their descendents come to resemble those of their U.S. ethnic counterparts. If we believe the findings of this study, which had a sample in excess of 91,000, the widely documented black–white difference in birth weight is not likely the result of genes (David & Collins, 1997). Although the causes of the lower birth weights of African Americans and these offspring of African immigrants are not fully understood, factors associated with minority status, such as discrimination and racism, have been shown to increase the risk of prematurity and fetal growth restriction (e.g., Collins et al., 1998; Dole et al., 2004). This chapter, in turn, has reviewed evidence that this disparity in the gestational environment could help explain the prominent race-based U.S. health disparities in adult diseases like hypertension, diabetes, and CVD, all of which are more common in individuals born small. Indeed, a recent analysis of data from the biracial Bogalusa Heart Study cohort found that the black–white difference in hypertension in this sample was no longer significant after models adjusted for birth weight (Cruickshank et al., 2005; see also Fang et al., 1996).

Thus there is growing evidence, albeit indirect, for a developmental origin of some of the most prominent U.S. health disparities (Pike, 2005; see also Chapter 6). And yet, far more research continues to search for genetic explanations for these group differences (Cooper & Kaufman, 1998), despite the minor importance of racial categories or population membership as an explanation of human genetic variation (Serre & Paabo, 2004). I use this example not to question the influence of genetic structure on human biology and health, but to underscore why a model of disease that is limited to the inheritance of DNA base sequences, current environments, and the interaction between them is no longer complete or acceptable. Studies documenting developmental and intergenerational influences on health show how some seemingly hardwired and even inherited traits may be, at their core, the result of phenotypic strategies designed to maintain and transmit environmental information across life cycles and even generations. This can lead to mismatch when conditions change rapidly, as highlighted in this review. But these same mechanisms of intergenerational transmission could also amplify health disparities when unfavorable conditions, such as discrimination and stress, are chronically experienced (Figure 18-6). In the case of African American health disparities, the experience of stress during pregnancy and the passage of stress hormones across the placenta could initiate many of the same fetal responses as undernutrition and with similar long-term biological health risks for offspring (Seckl & Meaney, 2004; Worthman and Kuzara, 2005; see also Chapter 6).

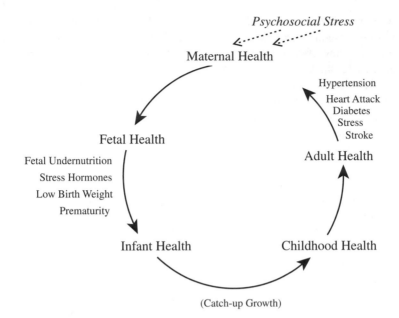

FIGURE 18-6 Model of the intergenerational amplification of health disparities in the absence of rapid social change.

Whether triggered by stress, nutrition, or other stimuli, the mechanisms of maternal—fetal signaling reviewed in this chapter are neither "genetic" nor "environmental" as traditionally defined. Although they involve potentially heritable changes in the expression of specific genes, these epigenetic changes are initiated in response to the environment. As such, they help blur the distinction between genetic and environmental influences on biology and health. The complex systems of inheritance that they undergird may have originally evolved to help organisms cope with environmental change that is beyond the narrow reach of homeostasis and its buffering capacity, but too abrupt to be visible to the more powerful, yet more gradual process of natural selection operating on gene frequencies. This chapter has reviewed evidence that even the capacity for developmental adaptation on this more rapid time scale may be outstripped by the contemporary pace of cultural and social change. In the case of nutrition, when early life signals are discordant with postnatal realities, the risk of metabolic disease may be elevated, thus linking the environmental experiences of recent ancestors with the diseases of the present.

On a more positive note, as the pace of environmental change attenuates, we can hope that the biology of future generations will recalibrate, having read the nutritional messages of the present and adjusted, over several generations, to the new nutritional world that we now inhabit. And our generation must help send this message to future generations by ensuring that today's pregnant mothers and their newborn offspring are well nourished. If the model presented in this chapter is correct, nutritional expectations are designed to shift in response to change that is sustained across multiple generations.

Nutritional interventions that target not only pregnant mothers, but also follow up with their nutritionally sensitive young, should help lift the nutritional expectations of off-spring generations, with health benefits that echo into the future.

ACKNOWLEDGMENTS

Warm thanks to Emma Adam, Alan Beedle, Peter Gluckman, Thom McDade, and the editors for helpful comments and to Terry Horton for references and for data used in Figure 18-2.

CHAPTER 19

An Evolutionary Perspective on the Causes of Chronic Diseases

Atherosclerosis as an Illustration

Paul W. Ewald

In his discussion of the possible role that a bacterial agent, *Chlamydia pneumoniae*, might play in the cause, degree, and expression of atherosclerosis (as well as multiple sclerosis and Alzheimer's disease), Ewald challenges us to think beyond "risk factors," stressing that we need to elucidate the cause of a disease in order to eliminate the disease rather than just reduce the chances of it being expressed. Moreover, he points out that nongenetic environmental factors and genetic factors are often presumed to be the causes of disease without consideration of the possible contribution made by infectious agents. He illustrates what might be considered the best that evolutionary medicine has to offer: questioning nonconscious ideologies about what constitutes health, what lines of evidence are useful, and what fundamental assumptions in medicine reflect far more our traditions or cultural orientations (recall Wiley's point about bioethnocentrism) than more sequential, complex thinking about "cause" that might better unravel, in this case, cumulative processes that cause disease. Perhaps one of the most important insights we gain, aside from understanding more fully the process of becoming atherosclerotic, is that he challenges us to think not in terms of what we might "know to be true," but what we "*know*" to be true that, in the words of Mark Twain' "*just ain't so*." Ewald is a long-time expert in assessing the dangers of the arms race occurring between infectious viruses and bacteria, on the one hand, and our species capacity to evolve immune responses capable of "keeping up," on the other. His message of conceptual reform is critical and an inherent part of the evolutionary way of thinking.

INTRODUCTION: CATEGORIES OF DISEASE CAUSATION

The three major categories of disease causation—genetic, parasitic, and (nonparasitic) environmental—have been recognized for over a century. Yet, as can be seen from any modern medical text, the relative importance of these categories is understood only for about half of all human diseases. This gap in our understanding is filled by quantification and accumulation of risk factors. To generate an accurate understanding of disease causation, however, the causal roles, if any, of these risk factors must be evaluated across the full spectrum of possible causes.

Nearly all of the diseases of uncertain cause are chronic, that is, diseases that develop slowly and persist over long periods of time. The actual causes of chronic human diseases are particularly difficult to resolve. The protracted course of chronic diseases often makes experimental manipulations difficult or impossible for ethical, logistical, or economic reasons. The protracted course also restricts the usefulness of animal models, which often have life spans shorter than the time over which human chronic diseases develop. When similar pathologies are generated in animal models over shorter time scales, their validity as anything more than analogs of human disease is open to question. For these reasons simple criteria for acceptance of disease causation, such as Koch's postulates, need to be replaced with a more comprehensive critical analysis to distinguish alternative hypotheses (Cochran et al., 2000).

Evolutionary medicine, defined as the study of medical problems that incorporates insights from evolutionary biology, may play an important role in this process. But to do so with scientific rigor, these studies must consider the array of feasible alternative hypotheses and test them with evidence (see Chapter 23). In this context, alternative mechanisms of disease causation are appropriately cast as alternative hypotheses that need to be distinguished by logical consistency and evaluation of evidence from ultimate as well as proximate perspectives. Evolutionary considerations offer structure for this process by identifying hypotheses that are consistent with evolutionary principles and therefore worthy of investigation. Evolutionary considerations can also stimulate needed research by drawing attention to fatal flaws in hypotheses that have been too readily accepted. The net effect of incorporating evolutionary insights should thus be a more efficient determination of actual causes of chronic diseases.

Although chronic diseases are often referred to as belonging to one of the three categories mentioned above, more than one of these categories of causal factors generally contribute to each disease (Figure 19-1). Cystic fibrosis, for example, is a genetic disease, but damage to the lungs and life-threatening crises have resulted largely from infections with respiratory pathogens, such as *Streptococcus pneumoniae* and *Pseudomonas aeruginosa*. All three categories of causal factors generally contribute to infectious diseases (defined broadly in this chapter to include all examples of internal parasitism); infections with *Mycobacterium tuberculosis*, for example, can range from asymptomatic to lethal, depending on genetic susceptibility and an individual's nutritional status. The important corollary of this generalization is that the identification of genetic or noninfectious environmental causes of disease cannot be used as evidence against infectious causation. Nevertheless, researchers and health professionals commit this logical error when they dismiss infectious causation on the basis of the evidence that implicates genetic causes or noninfectious environmental causes. This error is especially counterproductive when the evidence that is consistent with genetic causation is also consistent with infectious causation, as is the case, for example, with schizophrenia (Ledgerwood et al., 2003).

The tendency for candidate causes of chronic disease to be correlated with other variables has contributed to the tendency to cast discussions of chronic diseases in terms of

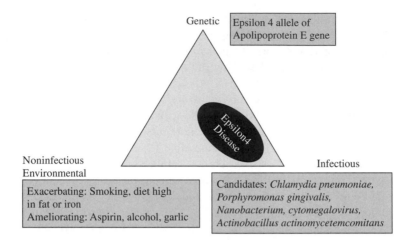

FIGURE 19-1 The triad of disease causation. The diagram depicts joint influences of the three categories of risk factors on disease using atherosclerosis as an illustration. The placement of a disease within the triangle corresponds to the relative importance of the three categories with regard to causation. The closest apex indicates the primary cause as defined in the text. The further from the vertex, the less the relative importance of the designated category as a primary cause. Boxed text specifies risk factors that may be primary or secondary causes of atherosclerosis. As discussed in the text, comprehensive consideration of evidence from all three categories favors placement of atherosclerosis and the other ε4-associated diseases close to the infectious causation vertex.

risk factors rather than causes. The term "risk factor" is safe because it implies only correlation and not causation, and correlation can be demonstrated much more definitively than causation. But focusing solely on risk factors can be misleading, because the accumulation of risk factors does not provide a conceptual framework for understanding the roles of the risk factors in disease causation. Some risk factors are primary causes, initiating the disease process, whereas others are secondary causes, exacerbating the disease process. Still other risk factors may not play a causal role at all, but may simply be correlated with primary or exacerbating causes. Unfortunately, although reference to risk factors is often made with sufficient care to avoid jumping from correlation to causation, the failure to integrate risk factors into a causal framework has left a vacuum that is filled by presuming a causal role for risk factors in subsequent discussions. These presumptions then influence the hypotheses that are evaluated. As a consequence, some risk factors are favored targets of research because their causal role is presumed without adequate evaluation of the full range of feasible causal hypotheses, as has been the case with schizophrenia (Ledgerwood et al., 2003).

The identification of primary causes is critical for the control of disease, because blocking a primary cause eliminates the disease, whereas blocking a secondary cause does not. The bacterium *M. tuberculosis* is the primary cause of tuberculosis, because tuberculosis cannot occur without *M. tuberculosis* infection. The reciprocal claim is not valid for host genetic or noninfectious environmental factors that exacerbate *M. tuberculosis* infections; tuberculosis can occur among people who are not particularly genetically susceptible to *M. tuberculosis* (as indicated by the moderate heritability of tuberculosis

[Vogel and Motulsky, 1997]) or who have not been exposed to particular environmental factors that exacerbate tuberculosis infection (e.g., poor nutrition). It is therefore appropriate to categorize *M. tuberculosis* as an infectious disease, even though genetic susceptibility and noninfectious environmental factors may influence the manifestations of *M. tuberculosis* infections. Analogously, it is appropriate to categorize cystic fibrosis as a genetic disease because mutations in the cystic fibrosis transmembrane conductance regulator gene are primary causes of cystic fibrosis, whereas *S. pneumoniae* and *P. aeruginosa* are exacerbating causes because elimination of *S. pneumoniae* or *P. aeruginosa* would not eradicate cystic fibrosis.

CAUSES OF ATHEROSCLEROSIS AND THE EPSILON 4 (ε4) ALLELE

Rich Diet Hypothesis

Nesse and Williams (1994) provided the first discussion of the causes of atherosclerosis in the context of evolutionary medicine. One part of their argument, echoed in Nesse's chapter in this volume, is that natural selection may design some body parts suboptimally. Applying this idea to the vulnerability of arteries to atherosclerosis, Nesse and Williams (1994) remark, "It is as if a Mercedes-Benz designer specified a plastic soda straw for the fuel line!" They then emphasize the inability of natural selection to design near-optimal solutions when the newness of the environment has not allowed sufficient to time for natural selection to act. Their hypothesis for the high prevalence of atherosclerosis in modern society applied this principle by suggesting risk factors that have arisen recently in our evolutionary history, particularly rich diets.

The mechanistic understanding of atherosclerosis has developed greatly since Nesse and Williams addressed this issue. In the first volume of *Evolutionary Medicine*, Gerber and Crews (1999) integrated some of these advancements in the context of dietary changes during the course of human evolution and the genetic susceptibility to atherosclerosis.They did not, however, evaluate alternative hypotheses. Currently available information allows such an evaluation, which is provided here as a paradigm for scientific inquiry into the causes of chronic disease.

Bad Allele Hypothesis

One of the alternatives to the rich diet hypothesis can be labeled the bad allele hypothesis. The epsilon 4 (ε4) allele of the apolipoprotein E (APOE) gene is the most important known genetic risk factor for atherosclerosis and thus heart attacks and stroke (Ilveskoski et al., 1999). Like the other alleles of the APOE gene, the ε4 allele codes for a protein that associates with fats and cholesterol and transports them between cells (Poirier et al., 1993). The ε4 allele is also an important risk factor for Alzheimer's disease and rapidly progressing multiple sclerosis (Evangelou et al., 1999; Hardy, 1995; Hogh et al., 2000; Ji et al., 1998; Love et al., 2003; Mahley and Huang, 1999; Pinholt et al., 2006; Saunders et al., 1993; Urakami et al., 1998). On the face of it, the ε4 allele looks like an inherently bad allele.

ε4-associated diseases have their greatest negative effects on health after direct reproduction; they therefore probably have had much of their negative effect on fitness through
reductions in aid and resources given to children and other relatives such as grandchildren. Still, a substantial portion of the negative effects of the ε4-associated diseases on
fitness occurs during reproductive periods, especially among males, because males
continue to have children into their sixth and seventh decades of life and because debilitating and lethal cases of ε4-associated diseases (particularly heart attacks, strokes, and
multiple sclerosis) often occur in the fifth decade of life or earlier.

The fitness cost (see Hamilton, 1964) of the ε4 allele due to the negative effects of
Alzheimer's disease, multiple sclerosis, atherosclerosis, and stroke is probably over 1%
(Cochran et al., 2000). Although 1% is a rough estimate, it is about two orders of magnitude greater than the maximal percentage that can be maintained solely by mutation without any compensating fitness benefit (Cochran et al., 2000). This estimate indicates that
there must be some compensating benefit of the ε4 allele, or that this disadvantage of the
ε4 allele has arisen relatively recently during the evolutionary history of humans.

The ε4 allele is present in all human populations at frequencies from about 5 to 40%
(Corbo & Scacchi, 1999; Fullerton et al., 2000). Phylogenetic analyses indicate that it is
the ancestral allele of *Homo sapiens* and of primates generally (Fullerton et al., 2000).

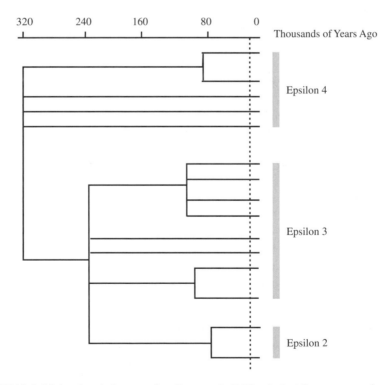

FIGURE 19-2 Molecular phylogeny of apolipoprotein E. The dashed line corresponds roughly to
the onset of agriculture. The figure shows how the diversification of ε alleles from ε4 occurred long
before the onset of agriculture. (Modified from Fullerton et al., 2000.)

Molecular data (Figure 19-2) suggest that it has been displaced in humans by ε2 and especially ε3 over the past 200,000 years (Fullerton et al., 2000). This evolutionary history is inconsistent with the hypothesis that ε4 is an inherently defective or damaging allele.

Longevity Hypothesis

A longevity hypothesis offers an explanation for the persistence of ε4 in early *Homo sapiens* and its apparent decline over the past 10,000 years. It proposes that humans have only recently lived long enough to experience the negative effects of the ε4-associated diseases, which often occur after the fourth decade of life. But multiple sclerosis occurs during or before the third decade of life. With a prevalence of up to 0.3%, it alone could have exerted a substantial selective pressure against ε4.

Another problem with the longevity hypothesis is that its fundamental assumption does not hold up to the evidence. Studies of hunter-gatherer societies have a high probability of survival into older age groups, contradicting the widely held but poorly supported belief that hunter-gatherers rarely lived past 40 years. The probability of surviving from the onset of reproduction to age 65 was about 50% among the !Kung San (Howell, 2000). Even among the more violent Ache of South America, survival over this interval was only slightly lower (Hill & Hurtado, 1996).

Thrifty Genotype Hypothesis

The rich diet hypothesis proposes that the disadvantage of ε4 is associated with the newness of food abundance in the human evolution. As applied to the ε4 allele, the rich diet hypothesis can be more narrowly cast as the "thrifty genotype" hypothesis, which was proposed by Neel (1962) to explain the maintenance of genotypes that predispose modern humans to diabetes. The thrifty genotype hypothesis suggests that the ε4 allele is too good for our own good when diets are rich. That is, its high efficiency at transporting fats and cholesterol was beneficial during times when food was scarce, but ε4 transports too much fat and cholesterol when diets are rich. The net effect could be the build-up of fats and cholesterol in cells, and thus the development of atherosclerosis.

The thrifty allele and longevity hypotheses are complementary rather than mutually exclusive. Both Nesse and Williams (1994) and Gerber and Crews (1999) integrated them by noting that natural selection may have been unable to select for resistance to atherosclerosis because rich diets and increased longevity may both have occurred relatively recently. According to this argument atherosclerosis may have resulted from the adverse effects of thrifty alleles that may have been manifested only in recent millennia when humans lived to older ages under conditions of rich diets.

Whether considered in isolation or in conjunction with the longevity hypothesis, the thrifty genotype hypothesis offers an explanation for the decline in ε4 during the last 10,000 years. Namely, rich diets associated with agriculture could have selected against the ε4 allele. The frequency of the ε4 allele is indeed lower in populations that have a long ancestry in agricultural settings, and this has been interpreted as support for the thrifty genotype hypothesis (Corbo & Scacchi, 1999). ε4 comprises only about 5–15% of the APOE alleles in China, Greece, Italy, and the Middle East, but about 20–40% in

TABLE 19-1 Frequencies of the ε4 Allele in Various Populations

Geographic region	Populaton	ε4 Frequency (%)
Mediterranean	Turks	7.9
	Greeks	6.8
	Italians	9.1
	Moroccans	8.5
Northern European	French	12.1
	British	14.1
	Finnish	17.4
	Sámi (Lapps)	31.0*
Sub-Saharan Africa	Ethiopian	14.3
	Sudanese	29.1
	San	37.0*
	Pygmies	40.7*
Americas	Mayan	8.9
	Yanomami	15.6*
	Inuit	21.4*

Denote peoples who have lived in isolated populations of low density largely if not exclusively as hunter-gatherers.
Source: Data from Corbo et al., 1999.

populations that lived as hunter-gatherers until the twentieth century (Table 19-1). This difference indicates that the allele has been declining with the rise of sedentary agriculture over the past 10,000 years.

A molecular phylogeny (Figure 19-2), however, indicates that the other two major epsilon alleles, ε3 and ε2, have increased in frequency over the past 200,000 years rather than just the past 10,000 years (Fullerton et al., 2000). This agricultural version of the thrifty allele hypothesis is therefore insufficient to explain the gradual decline in frequencies of the ε4 allele.

Another major problem with the thrifty allele hypothesis is that different defective functions must be envisioned for each ε4-associated disease. The thrifty allele hypothesis can offer a explanation for the association of rich diets with atherosclerosis and stroke, but it does not offer any obvious mechanism for the association between ε4 and both Alzheimer's and rapidly progressing multiple sclerosis, neither of which is attributed to excess deposition of fat and cholesterol within cells. To explain the association with Alzheimer's disease, Henderson (2004) hypothesized that ε4 damages the brain by a mechanism other than lipid deposition. He invoked the thrifty allele hypothesis, proposing that the negative effects of ε4 on Alzheimer's disease arose in response to the carbohydrate-rich diets associated with agriculture (Henderson, 2004). But the decline in the frequencies of ε4 long before the beginnings of agriculture argues against this application of the thrifty allele hypothesis, just as it argues against its application to atherosclerosis

Pathogen Vulnerability Hypothesis

The logic and evidence presented in the preceding section argue against the thrifty allele hypothesis as an explanation for the association between ε4 and atherosclerosis. ε4 must have conferred vulnerability to some cause of the ε4-associated diseases present when humans were still hunter-gatherers; this vulnerability may have increased during agricultural times to cause the accelerated decline in the ε4 prevalence during the agricultural period. The pathogen vulnerability hypothesis proposes that this genetic vulnerability is to one or more infectious agents (Ewald and Cochran, 2000). Genetic vulnerabilities to infectious agents appear to be a pervasive cause of allelic associations with disease (Abel and Dessein, 1997; Cochran et al., 2000). Such vulnerabilities could be more problematic as human populations become larger and denser and thus favor higher prevalences, dosages, and intensities of infection. This pathogen vulnerability hypothesis is consistent with the evidence mentioned earlier, because it suggests that the pathogen pressure would increase in agricultural societies but could have existed long before the onset of agriculture.

Chlamydia pneumoniae is the most obvious candidate for the pathogen vulnerability hypothesis, because it is the only infectious organism that is implicated as a cause of each of the ε4-associated diseases (Ewald and Cochran, 2000). Accordingly, a study of arthritis patients (Gérard et al., 1999) demonstrated that infection with *C. pneumoniae* is strongly associated with the ε4 allele (Figure 19-3). This finding suggests that ε4 somehow increases the vulnerability to *C. pneumoniae*. Densities of *C. pneumoniae* in cells from the brains of individuals with severe Alzheimer's diseases provide further support: *C. pneumoniae* replicated to the greatest density in people who were homozygous for ε4, to intermediate densities in ε4 heterozygotes, and to the lowest densities in people without any ε4 alleles (Gérard et al., 2005). Recent findings have revealed the mechanism of this vulnerability: *C. pneumoniae* attaches to the ε4 protein and rides it into its host cells as the ε4 protein first attaches to its receptor on the cell membrane and transports its lipid load into the cells (Gérard et al., 2006).

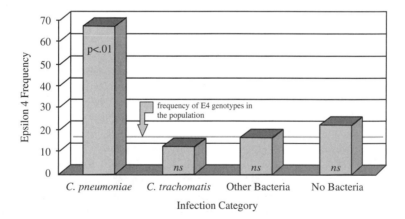

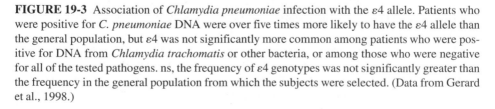

FIGURE 19-3 Association of *Chlamydia pneumoniae* infection with the ε4 allele. Patients who were positive for *C. pneumoniae* DNA were over five times more likely to have the ε4 allele than the general population, but ε4 was not significantly more common among patients who were positive for DNA from *Chlamydia trachomatis* or other bacteria, or among those who were negative for all of the tested pathogens. ns, the frequency of ε4 genotypes was not significantly greater than the frequency in the general population from which the subjects were selected. (Data from Gerard et al., 1998.)

These findings provide a theoretical basis for considering the ε4-associated illnesses as infectious diseases that share a common vulnerability to *C. pneumoniae* conferred by the ε4 allele (Figure 19-1). This pathogen vulnerability hypothesis offers a viable explanation for the association of ε4 with these diseases, because a given pathogen can cause very different pathologies in different tissues. The different ε4-associated diseases could therefore result from the different effects of the increased vulnerability to infection in different tissues. By this argument, *C. pneumoniae* in the brain causes damage that manifests itself as Alzheimer's disease (Balin et al., 1998). If brain damage occurs through an autoimmune mechanism triggered by *C. pneumoniae* (Lenz et al., 2001), it may be manifested as multiple sclerosis. Invasion of the endothelial lining of arteries and subsequent accumulation and oxidation of lipids is manifested as atherosclerosis (see Byrne and Kalayoglu, 1999; Kalayoglu et al., 1999).

The association between ε4 diseases and *C. pneumoniae* also offers a specific hypothesis to explain the pattern of ε4 allele frequency in human populations. Because *C. pneumoniae* is spread as a respiratory tract pathogen by coughing, the exposure should increase with increasing density of human populations. Those peoples who have been living in high densities and close quarters for more millennia should have had the greatest exposure to high frequencies and dosages of infection, and therefore should have experienced the strongest selective pressure against ε4. This hypothesis is consistent with the high ε4 frequencies among peoples who have until recently been hunter-gatherers (Table 19-1), and with the low frequencies of ε4 among people with a long ancestry in the Mediterranean and China (Corbo and Scacchi, 2000).

This hypothesis provides a basis for organizing our understanding of the ε4-associated diseases. Different forms of Alzheimer's disease, for example, are associated with different risk factors. Sporadic Alzheimer's disease (also known as late-onset Alzheimer's disease) appears to be an infectious disease for which *C. pneumoniae* is a primary cause and ε4 is an exacerbating cause (Balin et al., 1998). The less common familial Alzheimer's disease (also known as early-onset Alzheimer's disease) is a genetic disease in the traditional sense. Mutant alleles of at least three different genes contribute to three variants of early-onset Alzheimer's disease: the β-amyloid precursor protein gene on chromosome 21, the presenilin-1 gene on chromosome 14, and the presenilin-2 gene on chromosome 1 (Clark et al., 1996; Pastor et al., 2003). The ε4 allele exacerbates the subset of familial Alzheimer's disease that is attributable to mutations in the amyloid precursor protein. The influence of the ε4 allele on individuals with presenilin mutations is unclear—one large study (Pastor et al., 2003) indicates exacerbation, whereas smaller studies found no significant effect (Haan et al., 1994; Lendon et al., 1997; Romero et al., 1999; Sorbi et al., 1995; van Broeckhoven et al., 1994). Rural residence was associated with later onset of familial Alzheimer's disease (Pastor et al., 2003). This finding is consistent with an influence of *C. pneumoniae* infection on development of familial Alzheimer's disease, because the incidence of infections with respiratory pathogens is typically greater in urban environments where populations are more congested. Although *C. pneumoniae* has never been studied as an exacerbating cause of familial Alzheimer's disease, the association between ε4 and *C. pneumoniae* raises this possibility as a hypothesis for future study.

The emphasis on genetic vulnerability to infectious causes may also help clarify some confusion over infectious causation of multiple sclerosis. ε4 is positively associated with rapidly progressing multiple sclerosis in some study populations (Chapman et al., 1999;

De Stefano et al., 2004; Dousset et al., 1998; Enzinger et al., 2004; Evangelou et al., 1999; Fazekas et al., 2001; Hogh et al., 2000; Pinholt et al., 2006; Santos et al., 2004), but not in others (Niino et al., 2003; Savettieri et al., 2003; Sedano et al., 2006; Stevenson et al., 2000; Zakrzewska-Pniewska et al., 2004; Zwemmer et al., 2004) These differences argue against a direct negative effect of ε4; they suggest instead that the association between multiple sclerosis and ε4 depends on other causes that may vary in importance in different populations.

Infection with *C. pneumoniae* may be such a variable. Ever since the initial report of an association between *C. pneumoniae* and multiple sclerosis (Sriram et al., 1998), the existence of the association has been controversial (Gilden, 1999). Recently a second group of investigators found an association between *C. pneumoniae* and IgG positivity in two study populations but not in a third (Munger et al., 2003, 2004). A causal hypothesis is supported by the finding that a *C. pneumoniae*-specific peptide cross-reacts serologically with a portion of myelin basic protein (an antigen that stimulates the autoimmune response of multiple sclerosis) and causes a multiple-sclerosis-like disease in rats (Lenz et al., 2001).

In accordance with the tendency for ε4 to be associated with rapidly progressing multiple sclerosis, a study of the Nurses Health Study cohorts (Munger et al., 2003) showed that IgG positivity for *C. pneumoniae* was associated with progressive multiple sclerosis but not the less aggressive, relapsing-remitting forms. A similar association was found among participants in a medical care program (Munger et al., 2004). But no association was found among army personnel (Munger et al., 2004). These seemingly contradictory results make sense, however, when one considers that late-onset multiple sclerosis tends to be more severe (Confavreux et al., 1980; Evangelou et al., 1999). If this age-related increase results in part from a greater prevalence of ε4 in the late-onset patients, as is the case with Alzheimer's disease, then one could hypothesize that the lack of an association in the army population might be attributable to a higher frequency of early-onset multiple sclerosis in this population. The mean ages of onset were greater in the two studies in which *C. pneumoniae* was associated with multiple sclerosis: 39 for the nurses and 46 for medical care participants but only 27 for the army personnel. Evangelou et al. (1999) did not find a correlation between ε4 and age of onset, but their study population tended to be relatively young (mean age 30 years). An alternative hypothesis is that older individuals may be more vulnerable to infection and may therefore have more florid and hence more detectable and damaging *C. pneumoniae* infections than younger individuals. According to this alternative hypothesis, multiple sclerosis in older individuals would tend to be caused by *C. pneumoniae*, to which ε4 would confer vulnerability; the multiple sclerosis diagnosed among younger individuals would tend to be caused by something other than *C. pneumoniae*, and ε4 would therefore not be a significant risk factor.

Taken together, these arguments offer a broad causal perspective on ε4-associated chronic diseases. Rather than viewing ε4 as a deleterious allele that damages cardiovascular and neuronal tissue by disregulating the transport and reactivity of lipids and cholesterol, this new perspective considers ε4 to be an Achilles heel that makes the person vulnerable to *C. pneumoniae* infection. This argument thus casts *C. pneumoniae* infection, but not ε4, as a primary cause of the ε4-associated diseases (Figure 19-1)

Unlike the thrifty allele hypothesis, this pathogen vulnerability hypothesis is consistent with the available information on distribution of APOE alleles in different populations.

Whereas the thrifty allele hypothesis links the onset of a disadvantage associated with the ε4 allele with the onset of agriculture, the pathogen vulnerability hypothesis links the disfavoring of ε4 with events that that favor pathogen transmission. This disfavoring of ε4 could have arisen before the onset of agriculture if human populations were increasing, people were living increasingly in interior dwellings, or life span was increasing.

The epidemiology of *C. pneumoniae* fits this scenario especially well. It is a respiratory tract pathogen that appears to be present in all human populations; it therefore can persist across a broad range of population densities, technologies, and social structures. The persistence in small populations probably is attributable in part to its ability to cause persistent infections in humans. The intensity of exposure to *C. pneumoniae*, however, surely must have been low in hunter-gatherer societies where *C. pneumoniae* coughed into the outside air would be quickly diluted and destroyed by solar radiation. As population density increased, *C. pneumoniae* was probably transmitted to individuals more frequently and in higher doses. As is generally the case for pathogens, it would undoubtedly persist more continuously in larger human populations because the chance of local extinctions would decrease. These considerations suggest that increased population size and density should increase the negative effects of *C. pneumoniae* in vulnerable individuals and hence the fitness disadvantage associated with ε4. Any increase in human life span (e.g., see Caspari & Lee, 2004) would also tend to increase the negative fitness effects of *C. pneumoniae* on vulnerable people, because most of the life-threatening diseases for which *C. pneumoniae* is a suspect tend to occur after the fourth decade of life. With longer life spans, negative events that occur in these later decades of life would have a greater negative impact on the fitness of diseased individuals.

INTERPLAY OF ENVIRONMENTAL RISK FACTORS AND INFECTION IN ATHEROSCLEROSIS

The preceding overview illustrates the importance of considering genetic associations with disease in the context of infectious causes. Noninfectious environmental risk factors may similarly influence the expression of diseases in ways that seem paradoxical when taken in isolation, but make sense once the possibility of underlying infectious causation is considered. Atherosclerosis provides a particularly important example of this problem, because atherosclerosis is so damaging and because so much is known about its environmental risk factors. As is the case with the ε4 allele, noninfectious environmental risk factors for atherosclerosis may be not only consistent with infectious etiologies but difficult to explain without invoking infectious etiologies (Ewald & Cochran, 2000; Kinjo et al., 2003; Leinonen & Saikku, 1999; Saikku, 1995).

Smoking

Tobacco smoking is a risk factor for atherosclerosis (Berenson et al., 1998; Zieske et al., 1999). But is smoking a primary cause of cardiovascular disease or an exacerbating influence? It is reasonable to propose that harmful components of tobacco smoke directly damage the linings of arteries, causing them to accumulate fat and cholesterol. But smoking also contributes to pulmonary infection; it is, for example, associated with exacerbated pulmonary *C. pneumoniae* infection. In the lungs, *C. pneumoniae* infects macrophages that subsequently spread systemically (Mizooka et al., 2003; Saikku, 1995; von Hertzen, 1998).

The "direct-damage-from-smoke hypothesis," however, is problematic as an explanation for the increased risk for cardiovascular disease associated with exposure of nonsmokers to smoke from smokers. This exposure, termed "passive smoking," has been implicated as a risk factor for atherosclerosis (He et al., 1999) and atherosclerosis-associated diseases, such as stroke (Bonita et al., 1999). The increased risk for cardiovascular events that is associated with passive smoking amounts to about one third of the increased risk associated with smoking (He et al., 1999) even though passive smokers inhale only about 1% of the amount of smoke that is inhaled people who smoke 20 cigarettes per day (Pechacek & Babb, 2004). This risk associated with passive smoking seems far out of proportion to the small amount of smoke inhaled by passive smokers relative to smokers (Bailar, 1999). Lab tests have documented negative effects of small amounts of smoke on the functioning of platelets, vascular endothelium, myocardial exercise tolerance, antioxidants, and lipid metabolism (Howard and Thun, 1999; Valkonen & Kuusi, 1998). These findings lend some credence to the hypothesis that secondhand smoke could contribute directly to atherosclerosis. Still it is hard to imagine how disproportionately large negative effects of extremely small amounts of inhaled smoke would occur, especially in humans who have spent most of their evolutionary history in smoky environments.

This paradox vanishes, however, if the harmful effect among passive smokers is indirect, occurring through exacerbation of infectious causes of atherosclerosis. Smoking suppresses immune function and is associated with elevated rates and intensities of a variety of infectious diseases, as well as diseases suspected of being caused by infection (Sopori, 2002). Associations between exposure to secondhand smoke has been linked specifically with increased frequencies of respiratory tract infections (Arnold et al., 1993; Sorpori, 2002; Takala & Clements, 1992; Vadheim et al., 1992). By this argument the large risk to passive smokers arises could arise because of exposure to the more florid or more frequent *C. pneumoniae* infections of smokers rather than to secondhand smoke itself (Ewald and Cochran, 2000).

A similar argument applies to *Porphyromonas gingivalis*, which is a cause of gingivitis and periodontal disease and is present in atherosclerotic lesions (Eggert et al., 2001; Haraszthy et al., 2000; Kuroe et al., 2004; Stoltenberg et al., 1993). Smoking is strongly associated with periodontal disease, which in turn is strongly associated with stroke and myocardial infarction. Evaluations of associations between smoking and *P. gingivalis* have generated mixed results. Overall it appears that the prevalence of *P. gingivalis* at different sites in the mouth is greater among smokers than nonsmokers, even though the presence or absence of *P. gingivalis* differs little, if at all, between smokers and nonsmokers (Haffajee & Socransky, 2001). Nonsmoking partners of smokers are also more likely to have excacerbated periodontal disease (R. J. Genco, unpublished data), presumably because *P. gingivalis* and other causal organisms are transmitted by kissing or other salivary contact with the nonsmoking contacts of smokers.

A study of the relationship between smoking, infection, and the development of atherosclerosis showed that atherosclerosis was significantly associated with smoking only when an indicator of chronic infection, namely chronic obstructive pulmonary disease, chronic bronchitis, or periodontitis, was present (Kiechel et al., 2002). This finding raises the possibility that even among smokers the pathogens may be the main culprits, because these illnesses are associated with pathogens that are candidate causes of atherosclerosis: the pulmonary diseases are associated with *C. pneumoniae* and periodontitis is associated with oral bacteria, particularly *P. gingivalis*, *Actinobacillus actinomycetemcomitans*, and *Bacillus forsythus*.

Lipids

Lipid accumulation in atherosclerotic lesions has long been recognized as a hallmark of atherosclerosis. This association has led to the conclusion that high-fat diets contribute directly to atherosclerosis. Although this hypothesis is intuitive—too much input of fat leads to too much accumulation of fat in the arteries—it was accepted over the past 30 years with scanty evidence and little if any consideration of alternative hypotheses (Taubes, 2001). According to the lipid hypothesis, initiation of atherosclerotic lesions may involve reactive lipids, unstable intermediates in lipid reactions that can interact with other molecules and thereby damage the endothelium of arteries. But this idea raises other concerns about causality. If reactive lipids are important initiators of damage, why is there so much atherosclerosis that is not associated with lipid intake (Taubes, 2001)? And if the weakness of an association with lipids is the result of variation in the degree of vulnerability to damage caused by lipids, why is vulnerability so variable from person to person? An evolutionary perspective places considerable weight on these questions because people who are genetically vulnerable to lipids as a primary cause of atherosclerosis should have had this vulnerability weeded out by natural selection. Lipids must have been an important component of hunter-gatherer diets throughout human evolution. Ascribing a pathological effect to lipids therefore seems reasonable only if this effect results from an increased amount of lipids or a change in the kind of lipids in modern diets

The hypothesized role of dietary fat has been weakened by one of the most comprehensive experimental studies ever conducted on humans (Howard et al., 2006). The study tracked approximately 49,000 women between 50 and 79 years old for 8 years. Dietary fat was reduced by about one quarter in about half of these women. The reduced fat diet was not associated with a reduction in heart attacks or stroke. This study leaves open the possibilities that high-fat diets ingested at younger ages could contribute to cardiovascular disease, that reduction in the intake of certain kinds of fats could ameliorate cardiovascular disease, or that high caloric intake, even if low in fat, contributes to cardiovascular disease. It is also possible that even greater reductions in dietary fat could have a positive effect, although if this were the case one would expect to see at least some positive effect in response to the experimental reduction in dietary fat.

Any overarching causal explanation of atherosclerosis must be able to explain the pervasiveness of lipid accumulation in atherosclerotic lesions. The dietary fat hypothesis explains this accumulation by implicating greater lipids in the bloodstream. More lipids in the blood may favor greater lipid deposition in the arteries. This argument made sense when it was believed that the lipid accumulation was on the inside surface of the arteries. But it is now known that lipids accumulate within the wall of the arteries. This realization, together with the weakness of support for the dietary fats hypothesis, suggests that it would be wise to consider other explanations for the findings that at first glance seemed to implicate dietary fats. If dietary lipids play little role in the causation of atherosclerosis, how can one explain the lipid accumulation in atherosclerotic lesions? Infectious processes may resolve the matter if the primary causes of atherosclerosis are pathogens that foster increased accumulation of lipids within the arterial wall. *C. pneumoniae* and *P. gingivalis* are such pathogens because they induce lipid accumulation in macrophages, which can be transformed into foam cells by the lipid accumulation and can move into the artery wall (Belland et al., 2004; Kalayoglu et al., 1999, Miyakawa et al., 2004; Shor 2002). The transformation into foam cells is particularly important because the presence of foam cells in the arterial wall characterizes the early stages of atherosclerosis.

Alcohol

Another longstanding problem for the lipid hypothesis is that people in some areas have high-fat diets and low rates of cardiovascular disease. In France, for example, diets are high in fat, but cardiovascular disease is only approximately one-third the rate found in other Western countries with comparable fat intake (Gorinstein & Thrakhtenberg, 2003). This apparent anomaly is attributed to relatively high intake of wine in France. It was originally thought that wine might uniquely suppress development of atherosclerosis, but it is now clear that alcoholic beverages generally provide protection against atherosclerosis (Femia et al., 2006; Janszky et al., 2004; Li & Mukamal, 2004). The emerging view is that ethanol and perhaps some phenolic compounds found in wine and beer are responsible for the beneficial effects. Lipid researchers generally presume that effects of alcohol on atherosclerosis occur through effects on lipid metabolism (Gorinstein & Thrakhtenberg, 2003) even though infectious agents, such as *C. pneumoniae*, are known to alter lipid sequestration and metabolism. Immunologists focus on the anti-inflammatory effects of ethanol (Li & Mukamal, 2004), even though infectious agents are known to cause inflammation. Because alcohol has antimicrobial effects, a balanced perspective needs to consider effects of alcohol on microorganisms that may cause atherosclerosis, as well as direct effects of the alcohol on human physiology. It is important to assess, for example, whether the levels of ethanol that occur in the blood could inhibit the growth of *C. pneumoniae* in macrophages and affect the rate of the transformation of *C. pneumoniae*-infected macrophages into foam cells or the degree of inflammation induced by *C. pneumoniae*. These levels of ethanol might seem too low to have a beneficial effect, but even a slight inhibition *C. pneumoniae* might be sufficient to tip the balance in favor of host defenses.

Garlic

Garlic is another dietary component that appears to have beneficial effects on cardiovascular disease (Banerjee & Maulik, 2002). Researchers have investigated possible effects on serum lipids, blood pressure, and platelet aggregation (Banerjee & Maulik, 2002; Brace, 2002; Rahman, 2001). Although some studies have reported beneficial effects on these characteristics, results from different investigators have been contradictory (Brace, 2002). Most randomized, placebo-controlled studies, for example, have not supported the proposed suppressive effect of garlic on serum lipids, and evidence for suppressive effects on blood pressure and platelet aggregation remain inconclusive (Brace, 2002). Like alcohol, garlic is known to have powerful antibacterial effects (Ankri and Mirilman, 1999; Billing and Sherman, 1998; Harris et al., 2001; Lee et al., 2003).

Assessments of the value of garlic in protecting against atherosclerosis depend on the extent to which a mechanism of action can be demonstrated. The lack of supporting evidence for an effect of garlic on atherosclerosis through effects on lipid metabolism or other physiological characteristics may implicate an inappropriate focus. Research has not yet investigated effects of garlic on the infectious agents that are candidate primary causes of atherosclerosis. As is the case with studies of alcohol, such studies need to address whether pathogens are inhibited by in vivo concentrations of the active chemicals in garlic and whether inhibition in vivo could result in protection by allowing immune responses to better suppress the pathogens. Such studies also need to consider whether any physiological effects of garlic (e.g., on lipid levels) represent direct effects of garlic on human physiology or indirect effects that are brought about by suppressing the effects of lipid-altering pathogens.

Iron

High iron levels have also been associated with atherosclerosis (deValk & Marx, 1999). As is the case with garlic, most of the research on this association has investigated effects of iron on other biological molecules. One hypothesis suggests that iron ions oxidize lipids and the oxidized lipids damage arteries (deValk & Marx, 1999). Evolutionary considerations cast doubt on this hypothesis. Assessments of hunter-gatherer diets suggest that animal tissue comprised a large part of human diets prior to the development of agriculture (Cordain et al., 2002). Humans therefore should have evolved protective mechanisms against iron-induced oxidation of lipids. Iron supplementation is a recent event in the evolutionary history of humans. One could therefore question whether protective mechanisms can effectively control excess iron from vitamin pills or iron cookware. Physiological regulatory mechanisms, however, control iron from supplements more effectively than heme-associated iron, which is the primary form of iron from animal tissues (deValk & Marx, 1999).

Alternatively, iron may influence the progression of atherosclerosis indirectly by enhancing the growth of pathogens (Sullivan & Weinberg, 1999). Bacteria, like human cells, need iron. During infections, the host's iron-sequestering proteins bind the free iron, keeping it from the pathogens (Ratledge & Dover, 2000). Bacteria also produce iron-sequestering proteins to usurp iron for their own use before host sequestration mechanisms make the iron unavailable (Guerinot, 1994; Ratledge and Dover, 2000). If iron levels rise through excess iron in the diet, the ability of the body to sequester iron may be compromised, allowing the bacteria to acquire it, reproduce, and consequently cause elevated damage.

Inflammation

Associations between atherosclerosis and systemic indicators of inflammation, such as C-reactive protein (CRP), have led to an emphasis by some on the role of inflammation in the pathogenesis of atherosclerosis (Ridker et al., 2000). Although this association clarifies the pathogenesis of atherosclerosis, one of the most important parts of a full causal explanation is the mechanism by which the inflammatory process is switched on.

This mechanism is often glossed over, but it is central to an understanding of the primary causes of the atherosclerosis.

The initiating event is now often ascribed to collections of factors such as the oxidized lipoprotein–cholesterol complex, injury, and infection (Willerson & Ridker, 2004). Reference to "injury" does not resolve the problem of primary causation, but rather raises the question: "What causes the injury?" Similarly, reference to oxidized lipoprotein–cholesterol complexes raises the question: "What causes the oxidation, and why would oxidative damage be so variable from person to person?" Infection suggests a mechanism of primary causation, because infectious processes may cause injury, generation of oxidative molecules (e.g., see Byrne & Kalayoglu, 1999, for *C. pneumonia*), and elevation of biochemical correlates of atherosclerosis. CRP is, for example, elevated in persistent *C. pneumoniae* and *P. gingivalis* infections (Craig et al., 2003; Huittinen et al., 2003, Kuroe et al., 2004).

C. pneumoniae infection has been associated with elevated CRP in early and late phases of cardiovascular disease (Kaperonis et al., 2006). When *C. pneumoniae* is positively associated with CRP, the risk of cardiovascular events is elevated (Huittinen et al., 2003; Tasaki et al., 2003). These findings are consistent with the hypothesis that *C. pneumoniae* is a primary cause of atherosclerosis and of the inflammation that is associated with atherosclerosis.

Aspirin

Use of aspirin has been associated with protection against several chronic illnesses, including cardiovascular disease and Alzheimer's (Etminan et al., 2003; Nilsson et al., 2003). Although aspirin may ameliorate cardiovascular events through its blood-thinning effects, the therapeutic effects of aspirin on a variety of chronic diseases implicates a more general effect of aspirin on some aspect of pathology that is common to these diseases. Inflammation is the obvious candidate (Ridker et al., 1997).

If the inflammation associated with cardiovascular disease is a consequence of the immune system going wrong, it is easy to understand why aspirin would have a favorable effect—it is simply suppressing the part of the immune system that is malfunctioning. However, if inflammation is a response to infection, the beneficial effects of aspirin seem at first glance more surprising, because the inflammatory response is largely a response to control infection, and aspirin is known to exacerbate infections (Ewald, 1994). This apparent paradox is resolved through consideration of the difference between chronic and acute infectious diseases. Chronic infections tend to be chronic because the causal pathogen is not eliminated by the immune system. The immune system, however, does not simply shut down if it cannot eliminate a persistent pathogen. Aspects of the immune system, such as the inflammatory response, may still be triggered by the pathogen and will continue to cause damage to host cells that is inherent to immune function (i.e., "friendly fire"). When this continued immune response is ineffective at eliminating a pathogen—as is the case with persistent pathogens—its net effect may be negative. In such situations, turning down the response may have a net positive effect. Accordingly, effects of aspirin are generally beneficial for chronic diseases but generally detrimental for acute infectious disease (Ewald, 1994).

THE IMPORTANCE OF UNDERSTANDING CAUSATION

Disease causation is not well understood for about half of all human diseases. These diseases of uncertain cause include the most lethal and debilitating diseases in the United States: atherosclerosis, stroke, Alzheimer's disease, diabetes, and cancers. If infectious organisms cause even a few of these diseases and if these infections can be prevented or cured (as has been the case in the past through vaccination, anti-infective therapy, and hygienic improvements), such advancements would rank among the greatest achievements in the history of medicine. Expediting the discovery of any infectious causes of these diseases is therefore of great importance to public health. To foster this goal, it is critical that the range of feasible hypotheses be presented in a balanced and integrated manner. This need is perhaps greater now than ever because specialization among researchers has become so extreme. Even research on a single disease has become so detailed and data-rich that specialists on one aspect of the disease are unaware of relevant findings on another aspect. The various specialized areas of research on atherosclerosis illustrate this point; specialists on genetic predispositions, lipids, infectious causation, inflammation, stress, exercise, iron, smoking, garlic, aspirin, and alcohol will sometimes delve into the work in each others' areas of specialization, but integrated assessments have been lacking. The problem is compounded because clues may arise not only from the various aspects of a given disease but also from research on different diseases. The relationships among ε4-associated diseases detailed above offer a case in point.

Integrative assessments such as the one provided in this chapter are revealing that hypotheses of infectious causation have often been casualties of this specialization. The historical record reveals that researchers of chronic diseases have been on the trail of infectious causation repeatedly, but that the trail was lost for a variety of reasons that pertain more to the social aspects of science than to scientific rigor. Evidence supporting infectious causation of peptic ulcers, for example, was sufficiently strong by the mid-twentieth century to cause it to be accepted in some mainstream medical circles. Peptic ulcers were regularly cured with tetracycline in New York Hospital and Mount Sinai Hospital in the late 1940s, but this treatment was largely ignored and forgotten until Warren and Marshall rediscovered the spiral-shaped bacterium as the primary cause of peptic ulcers in the late 1970s. After over a decade of dismissiveness, and even ridicule, their hypothesis was accepted by mainstream medicine in the early 1990s. Similarly the link between schizophrenia and *Toxoplasma gondii* was reported in many research papers during the 1940s and 1950s, although the evidence was largely ignored by researchers in North America and western Europe until the last few years (Brown et al., 2005; Ledgerwood et al., 2003; Torrey & Yolken 2003). One of the recent advances in atherosclerosis research over the past two decades is the recognition that the pathogenesis of atherosclerosis involves inflammatory processes, but this idea can be traced back in the medical literature to the early 1800s (Nieto, 1998). Evidence for an association of atherosclerosis with what we now recognize as *Chlamydia* can be traced back to Chilean research published in the mid-twentieth century (Saikku, 1993).

These examples illustrate how progress in understanding disease causation is often slow and erratic, and sometimes even retrograde. By understanding the underlying reasons for this poor performance, we may be able to avoid repeating the mistakes of the past and thereby accelerate the rate at which we come to accurate understandings of disease causation. The lackluster record cannot be attributed solely to a lack of technological sophistication, although this factor does sometimes play an important role. Much of the slowness results from not asking the right questions, from not keeping all feasible hypotheses on the table when evaluating the promise of alternative lines of inquiry.

If potential effects of all the noninfectious risk factors for coronary artery disease are combined, only about half of the overall risk can be explained (Muhlestein, 2002). The association with ε4 has led some researchers to believe that a search for more genetic determinants was warranted. Similarly, the identification of noninfectious environmental risk factors led others to search for additional noninfectious environmental risk factors. The analysis presented in this chapter, however, indicates that ε4 and the known noninfectious environmental risk factors may affect the vulnerability to infectious causes of atherosclerosis. More generally, this analysis illustrates how a broadly based consideration of infectious, genetic, noninfectious environmental risk factors can offer an integrated and cohesive explanation of disease causation. Studies of disease have always implicated more than one of the three major categories of disease causation (and often all three) whenever diseases have been studied well enough to make a solid conclusion. As discussed in the introduction to this chapter, cystic fibrosis and tuberculosis offer instructive examples. Rigorous science demands that all three categories be kept under consideration until sufficient evidence warrants their rejection. This proposition is deceptively simple and has the ring of common sense. Yet it runs contrary to recent decades of medical research, probably because medical research has been increasingly specialized and disjointed, rather than broadly integrative.

Conceptual integration of medical information is a fundamental challenge for evolutionary medicine, because only evolutionary medicine focuses on both the how and the why questions, the proximate and ultimate mechanisms. Evolutionary medicine builds upon the most fundamental conceptual foundation of life sciences—evolution by natural selection—and then draws upon all disciplines of the health sciences to develop a cohesive understanding of any particular phenomenon. So far evolutionary medicine has not lived up to this challenge. It has tended to focus on particularly attractive hypotheses as explanations for states of disease, such as the thrifty allele hypothesis, rather than attempting to generate, integrate, and evaluate the full spectrum of alternative hypotheses. The analysis of atherosclerosis in this chapter illustrates how alternative hypotheses can be considered broadly and integratively within an evolutionary context. It is presented with the intent of raising the challenge of evolutionary medicine to all who are interested in forming an integrative, scientific perspective on issues of health and disease.

ACKNOWLEDGMENTS

The content of this chapter has benefited greatly from discussions with Greg Cochran, Alan Hudson, and Katie Scangos. Greg got me to recognize the scope and significance of focusing on infectious causation of chronic disease and drew my attention to ε4. Alan kept me abreast of his groundbreaking work on the relationship between ε4 and vulnerability to *C. pneumoniae*. Katie directed me to the work on ε4 frequencies of different human populations. Neal Smith provided valuable comments on an earlier draft of the manuscript.

CHAPTER 20

Genes, Geographic Ancestry, and Disease Susceptibility
Applications of Evolutionary Medicine
to Clinical Settings

Douglas E. Crews and Linda M. Gerber

Crews and Gerber ask in their chapter why it is that the "molecular revolution" in biology, so effective in providing new and powerful tools for profiling one's genetic risks for chronic degenerative diseases and for eventually understanding gene–environment and gene–culture interactions in predisposing individuals, families, and groups to specific conditions, has yet to be integrated into clinical settings and genetic counseling centers to improve human health and well-being. Reminiscent of Mysterud's appreciation of the significance of individual dietary needs and differences (Chapter 4), they argue that rather than emphasizing the value of using "ethnoracial" categories or descriptors to assess differences in geographically distinct people, clinicians should instead concentrate on very specific genotypes/DNA variants to specific phenotypes/diseases. Even for individuals sharing a common ancestry, they point out, there are important molecular variants other than "race" that are much more useful in predicting both disease susceptibility and the most effective therapy protocols when the disease is expressed. They suggest that along with obtaining a family history of all chronic degenerative diseases, clinicians should begin to produce genetic profiles of alleles that predispose a person to particular diseases known to be associated with each person's relatives. They suggest importantly that knowledge of a genetic predisposition for some ailment should never be used to discount the significant role of lifestyle and health conditioning in its expression or severity.

INTRODUCTION AND BACKGROUND

By developing new techniques for rapid analyses of DNA and identifying marker loci throughout the genome, the human genome project aided the search for DNA variants that predispose individuals and populations to chronic degenerative conditions (CDCs). Nowhere has this been more apparent than in cancer genetics (Eng et al., 2000). Multiple disease-predisposing alleles have been identified without regard to ethnicity, race, or geographic background (Crews and Williams, 1999; Narod and Offit, 2005). However, for multiple oncogenes (DNA variants that predispose to neoplasm), multiple founder mutations (newly arisen variants segregating within particular inbreeding groups or demes) specific to certain populations (e.g., Ashkenazi, Icelandic, Germanic) have been identified (Eng et al., 2000; Narod and Offit, 2005). Cross-populational variations in allele frequencies are associated with differences in frequencies of CDCs across such populations. Based upon these correlations, some propose that genetic variability in disease risk is structured by "race," "ethnicity," and "continental ancestry" (origins of some DNA alleles are from specific continents) and that such classifications are biological dimensions of disease and associated variability in physiological function (Carson et al., 1999; Crow, 2002; Risch et al., 2002; Sarich and Miele, 2003). Multiple authors have challenged the use of self-reported race for either sociopolitical or clinical decision making (Armelagos et al., 2005; Bloche, 2004; Cooper et al., 2003; Crews and Bindon, 1991; Dressler et al., 2005; Jones, 2001; Kaufman and Cooper, 1999; Kittles and Weiss, 2003) because of its poor definition, lack of biological reality in humans, and sociocultural construction. Independent of sociocultural and political debates on the nature of "race," geneticists are developing DNA profiles that identify the percentage of African, Asian, and/or European genetic ancestry of individuals for use as adjuncts for defining clinical risks for CDCs (Kittles and Weiss, 2003; Parra et al., 2001; Risch et al., 2002).

Today, multiple genetic markers, some showing large differences in observed frequencies between samples identified as African and European, are available for identifying the subgroup ancestry of individuals, admixture, and continent of ancestral origin (Chakraborty and Weiss, 1988; Parra et al., 2001; Risch et al., 2002). Highly informative markers are those that either show large differences in frequencies between populations of Africa, Asia, and Europe or have unique associations with specific populations. Easily identified and highly informative single nucleotide polymorphisms (SNPs) and Alu inserts (short stretches of DNA of about 300 base pairs, including an ALU1 recognition site, that are found throughout the human genome) provide fairly precise assessments of European, Asian, and African ancestry/admixture (percent of DNA from one or another continent of ancestry in a living population) (Parra et al., 2001; Risch et al., 2002). Using a set of 30–50 "highly selected" microsatellites (a simple sequence repeat that occurs n times; the number of repeats varies and each variant is a different allele), Risch et al. (2002) identified five "major racial groups" and distinguished their "continental ancestry" within a random sample of the U.S. population. One goal of research to document geographic/genetic ancestry of individuals is to provide clinicians and researchers with an improved basis for directing "race-based" clinical and pharmacological therapeutic interventions and research (Bloche, 2004; Risch et al., 2002). From anthropological and evolutionary medicine points of view, it is theoretically and diagnostically important that individual genetic profiles often document a lack of congruence between measured genetic ancestry and self-reported race and ethnic affiliations (Beal et al., 2006; Cooper et al., 2003); that is, the geographic ancestors of alleles carried by those reporting, for example, "European," "Asian," "South Pacific," or "African" origins, or "Italian," "Ebo," "German," "Aleut," "Yoruba," "Bantu," "American Indian," or "Irish" descent often are not from the areas reported by these individuals.

The molecular revolution has led to a bewildering array of "plans" for using genes, genomics (the array of DNA variation carried by an individual), and proteomics (the array of protein variants within a cell or individual) to improve public health, reduce disease burdens through gene therapy, and generally improve the health, diets, and well-being of modern humans. New fields using genetic analyses appear almost weekly, and dozens of gene corporations now litter the Internet and stock markets. Genes, genetic medicine, and evolutionary epidemiology are changing how biomedical research and clinical practice are being conducted. New subdisciplines combining genes with traditional epidemiological, medical, and public health concerns are being developed. Nutrogenetics (genetics of dietary metabolism and individual dietary guidelines), pharmacogenetics (genetics of drug metabolism within individuals), and obesogenic genes (genetics of energy metabolism and fat deposition) provide new ways to look at genes and health. A revolution in molecular oncology and cancer genetics also has occurred in recent decades (Eng et al., 2000; Hampel et al., 2003). At the same time, multiple researchers are examining "race-based" medicine, associations of "ancestral identity" with disease, and the genetic basis of "racial" classifications (Parra et al., 2001; Risch et al., 2002). Ongoing debates about the reality of races, specifically their cultural and biological constructions, continue. At the same time, applications of genetics in health research continue to bring up debate about "racially and ethnically" targeted pharmacological and clinical interventions and how to identify groups at higher risk for CDCs such as type 2 diabetes, coronary artery disease (CAD), or high blood pressure. Ethnicity and "race" continue to be used in research and clinical settings because their nominal identifiers are commonly reported on patients' medical records. This readily available information already is used when positing differential pathological mechanisms and treatment strategies across self-identified racial groupings, such as has occurred for at least one drug formulary in the United States (Bloche 2004; Kahn, 2004; Taylor et al., 2004). We have defined our usage of race and ethnicity elsewhere (Crews and Bindon,, 1991), as have others (Dressler et al., 2005; Risch et al., 2002). Herein, we use the term "ethnoracial" for these categories following Dressler et al.(2005). Ethnoracial terms used by other authors or those with which we are not in agreement are enclosed in quotation marks.

In this chapter, we examine briefly the historical and ongoing use of self-reported race and ethnicity in clinical medicine, epidemiology, and pharmacological research. To begin, we discuss how genetic applications to medicine and race-based therapeutics rely upon and apply principles of evolutionary medicine (see Trevathan et al., 1999). We then explore some advantages and disadvantages of using population-specific genetic variation to identify individual geographic ancestry as a parameter to replace the proxy of race/ethnicity. Last, potential applications of individual genetic profiles to clinical screening, counseling, evaluation, and individualized medicine are examined.

EVOLUTIONARY MEDICINE, CLINICAL PRACTICE, AND GENETICS

In a Darwinian model, continuous interactions among natural selection, genetic drift, mutation, migration, and assortative mating produce and restructure DNA variation within local populations. These processes leave their signatures on the DNA of populations and their descendents by introducing local allelic variants and unique population-specific genes, for example, the Duffy null allele in African populations. This commonality of alleles and frequencies shared by peoples of the same area is termed geographic ancestry. Individual DNA profiles reflect the signature of geographic ancestry. These DNA differences, not skin color or self-reported race, are sometimes associated with disease etiology and may produce differential individual and populational predispositions to disease susceptibility. Stratifying by individual ancestry in case-control studies may allow researchers to determine whether observed linkage disequilibrium (LD-genes and traits of interest being passed together more frequently than expected by chance) is due to genetic markers being causally related to disease prevalence across ancestrally related groups or to spurious associations resulting from genetic structure within a group (Parra et al., 2001). Some suggest a prevalence of the former option (Carson et al., 1999; Crow 2002; Risch et al., 2002; Sarich & Miele, 2003); others the latter (Armelagos et al., 2005; Bloche, 2004; Cooper et al., 2003; Crews & Bindon, 1991; Dressler et al., 2005; Jones, 2001; Kaufman & Cooper, 1999; Kittles & Weiss, 2003).

In the clinical setting, such debates take on a different meaning. Take for example the following two clinical scenarios:

1. A 40-year-old woman arrives at her gynecologist's office for her annual examination. She presents with a family history of breast cancer and says that she is of Ashkenazi Jewish background. There is strong evidence that specific mutations predisposing to breast cancer genes are more prevalent among Ashkenazi Jews (Sweet et al., 2002). Should this woman be advised to have genetic testing for the BRCA (breast cancer–promoting genes) mutations?

2. A 65-year-old African American male is suffering from congestive heart failure and does not seem to be responding to β-blocker treatment. There is new evidence that a specific polymorphism of the β_1AR genotype may be more responsive to a different β-blocker agent (Liggett et al., 2006) than the one he is currently taking. Should this patient be tested to see if he has the gene variant, β_1AR, which is responsive to a different β-blocker?

These are examples of the dilemmas facing clinicians on a daily basis as we move toward increased genetic applications in medicine and apply models of evolutionary medicine to the clinical setting. Does the fact that ethnoracial identifiers are available for patients alter the odds that they have these specific mutations? Do their self-reported ethnoracial identifiers indicate a need for genetic testing that is beyond the standard of care for these conditions? If such ethnoracial data were not available, might these patients not receive additional genetic testing? Persons of Ashkenazi Jewish ancestry (Ashkenazim) living in the United States carry BRCA1 and 2 mutant alleles at a frequency of about 1/50, compared to estimates between 1/150 and 1/800 among the wider North American population (Narod & Offit, 2005). Icelandic, Dutch, and Polish populations also show relatively high frequencies of specific BRCA 1 and 2 mutations (Eng et al., 2000; Narod & Offit, 2005). Among the Ashkenazim, multiple founder mutations have been reported in BRCA genes, but two in BRCA 1 and one in BRCA 2 account for 90% of all such mutations in this population (Eng et al., 2000; Narod & Offit, 2005). Knowing ancestry does indicate that different genetic-testing thresholds may be justified for this population group (Narod and Offit, 2005). BRCA mutations are rare, accounting for only 5% of all breast cancers in the general population. However, among the Ashkenazim 20–35% of breast–ovarian cancer is associated with one of these three founder mutations (Eng et al., 2000), and the likelihood that a person in this subgroup is a BRCA 1 or 2 mutation carrier approaches 2.5% (Hampel et al., 2003) or 1 of 40.

A major goal of epidemiological research is to determine behavioral, environmental (nongenetic), and biological (genetic) risks predisposing individuals and populations to disease. Evolutionary medicine suggests that the ancestry of individuals reflects long-term adaptations to specific environmental stressors, new mutations, and sociocultural factors such as inbreeding and isolation that have structured existing DNA variation into its current distribution. Elsewhere these have been described as "genetic clusters" or "population clusters" wherein the distribution of metabolic enzymes (DNA) differs from cluster to cluster (Risch et al., 2002). Clustering of genes is suggested to reflect divisions along geographical lines (Risch et al., 2002). However, associations of these gene clusters with preconceived ethnoracial categories based upon skin/hair color and other phenotypic categories is arbitrary and not likely to reflect variability in disease-promoting snippets of DNA. Similarly, clustering of reported ethnoracial categories with CDCs likely reflects shared nongenetic cultural behaviors, sociocultural environment, income, diet, or interpersonal relationships rather than "race-based" risks, particularly in U.S. samples (Cooper et al., 2003; Crews & Bindon, 1991; Dressler et al., 2005; Rogers, 1992). Rather than being due to "race" or variability secondary to geographic origin, observed associations may be due to nonbiological factors that cluster with these constructs.

"RACE-BASED" RESEARCH: CONTROVERSIES AND APPLICATIONS

The drive to tailor prevention and intervention efforts to specific "racial types" ("race-based" therapeutics) already is well under way (Bloche, 2004; Carson et al., 1999; Kahn, 2004; Kittles & Weiss, 2003). Current investigations of "race" obtain racial categorizations from a variety of sources—investigator-observed, self-reported, or genetically determined by ancestry informative markers (AIMs) (Kittles and Weiss, 2003). Today, home DNA-testing kits for determining one's own AIMs or cancer risks are available to retail consumers (Gray, 2003; McCabe & McCabe, 2004). Like "race," home-based DNA profiling is likely here to stay. Also, like "race," insufficient knowledge of interactions among genes, environment, culture, lifestyles, pathogenesis, senescence, medications, and degenerative diseases is available to make such tests accurate for predicting individual disease risks, or for endorsing specific lifestyles or personal nutritional programs. More important for epidemiology, public health, and clinical and evolutionary medicine is the use of ethnoracial categories, whether self-reported, investigator-/clinically determined, or determined via AIMs, to guide research, clinical interventions, and diagnosis. It has been widely accepted that "race" does not reflect any specific biological reality (Kittles & Weiss, 2003). The current question is whether clinicians can use what is known about the social construction of "race" and its representation of nongenetic factors to improve health care. Alternatively, should "race" not be used for biomedical research and clinical applications?

Use of observed, self-reported, and DNA-based "race" determinations to develop "race-based" clinical and pharmacological therapeutics generates debate across biological, sociocultural, medical, and clinical settings (Armelagos et al., 2005; Bloche, 2004; Crews & Bindon, 1991; Carson et al., 1999; Dressler at al., 2005; Gerber & Crews, 1999; Jones 2001; Jones et al., 1991; Kaufman & Cooper, 2001; Kittles & Weiss, 2003; Rosenberg et al., 2002; Sarich & Miele, 2003; Strohman, 1993; Wexler & Feldman, 2006; Wong et al., 2002). Many clinicians and biomedical scientists see "race" as an important dimension for determining the appropriateness of clinical interventions (Carson et al., 1999; Crow, 2002; Wong et al., 2002). Others suggest that although self-reported "racial" categories are inaccurate proxies for biological predispositions, medical research must accept that for some conditions "race-conscious" therapeutics better identify useful interventions and may improve outcomes (Bloche, 2004). However, the caution remains that "race" is not solely genetic, but represents multifactorial predispositions to disease (Bloche, 2004).

"Race-based" therapeutics carry the sociopolitical baggage of previous and continuing "racial" categorizations and discrimination in the United States and other nations. However, it seems likely that at least some "race-specific" interventions will appear to be clinically useful. The basis for this usefulness most likely will be found in the sociopolitical, sociocultural, and socioeconomic variability that "racial" categorizations structure in multiethnic societies where "racial minorities" are poor and marginalized (Armelagos et al., 2005; Crews, 2003; Crews & Bindon, 1991; Dressler et al., 2005). Numerous pharmacological agents reportedly show differential efficacy, disease responsiveness, metabolic properties, and toxicity in patients from different populations, of different ages, sexes, and body composition, and with variable comorbidities (Bloche, 2004; Gerber and Crews, 1999; Kittles & Weiss, 2003; Yang et al., 2006; Wexler & Feldman, 2006). After reviewing available data, Cooper et al. (2003) find that "race" is not an appropriate criterion for prescribing any pharmacological intervention. Differences in ecological, socioeconomic, diet/nutrition, and cultural settings and backgrounds, along with multiple additional physiological and demographic factors that extend well beyond variable ancestries, are what lead to differential responses to drugs and stressors (Crews & Bindon, 1991; Dressler et al., 2005).

Those promoting "race-based" therapeutics are suggesting that small or large differences in physiology, secondary to DNA/protein differences, produce "racial/ethnic" variability in chronic degenerative conditions (CDCs) such as diabetes, hypertension, obesity, and hyperlipidemia. This suggestion is the same as saying that specific risk alleles are in LD with other alleles that predispose to external morphology, for example skin color. One estimate is that as few as 6% of all CDCs are attributable to genetic differences between ancestrally related groups (Kittles & Weiss, 2003). Only a few loci appear to code for skin and hair color, hair texture, and other external traits identified as "racial." It is not likely that these few alleles are in LD with alleles at 1400 other loci (the 6% proposed by Kittles and Weiss, 2003, of the total 23,000 coding snippets of DNA) that produce differential risks for CDCs across populations. To suggest otherwise is to suggest either that disease-promoting alleles have been subjected to the same evolutionary pressures as the alleles for skin color or that many disease-promoting alleles are linked to those promoting skin color variation. Neither of these models is genetically realistic.

Many studies use self-reported "race" for research purposes. Although self-reported "race/ethnicity" has a longstanding history in clinical applications, drug-related research, and epidemiology (Jones et al., 1991), this usage has recently been challenged on multiple fronts (Beal et al., 2006; Jones, 2001; Kittles & Weiss, 2003; Parra et al., 2001). According to current sociocultural views of identity, "race" represents a situational reality that changes over one's lifetime and across environmental and sociocultural settings (see, Jones, 2001). Self-reported ethnicity and "race" are complex self-images of one's biological, social, and cultural self, and changes with the situation (Dressler et al., 2005; Jones, 2001). "Race" is a categorical or qualitative variable by definition, and one may change one's category over his or her lifetime.

Prior to the use of self-reported "race" and ethnicity in clinical medicine, epidemiology, and pharmacological research, researchers identified "race" based upon observations of skin color (Jones et al., 1991). "Self-reported race" was welcomed by epidemiology, public health, and census officials when first introduced into research and census reports because it was thought to assess a patients' ancestry and life ways more accurately. Use of "race" as a category in epidemiological and clinical research is pervasive (Dressler et al., 2005; Jones et al., 1991, 2001), as it is in human biology, physiology, and genetics (Crews & Bindon, 1991). When used for diagnostic or research purposes, poor agreement between "race" reported on a medical record and "self-reported race" from patients about themselves and their offspring may confound research (Beal et al., 2006). While examining risk factors for neonatal hyperbilirubinemia in mother–child pairs, Beal et al. (2006) found significant differences between "race" as reported on a medical record and that self-reported by mothers. Only 70% of mothers documented as "black" in the medical record self-identified themselves as "black," whereas 64% of mothers defined as "white" in the medical record self-identified as "white." Fourteen percent of mothers defined themselves as being of at least two "races" (Beal et al., 2006). Whether self- or researcher-identified, use of crude assessments of "race" in clinical and epidemiological research misinform the lay public and clinicians alike by assigning a biological reality to socioculturally and socioeconomic characterizations of modern human variation. Furthermore, "race" is a typological attribute that is renegotiated and differentially interpreted by its bearer, depending upon their situational and cultural context. In different situations, multiethnic persons may emphasize their skin color category ("black/white"), their familial/cultural background (Greek/Italian/Yoruban/Tongan), or their affiliation with a local tribal population (Sioux, Potawatomi).

"RACE-BASED" MEDICINE

Even within a single category such as "African American," broad genetic heterogeneity contributes to highly variable risks for CDCs across individuals and families (Bloche, 2004). In addition, most chronic disease categories encompass broad phenotypic and genotypic heterogeneity. For example, obesity includes those with visceral, subcutaneous, or hip/buttocks fat deposition, along with those suffering from a variety of additional CDCs such as diabetes, hyperinsulinemia, or metabolic syndrome, as well as those with specific obesity-inducing genetic, psychological, or physiological profiles. One estimate is that over 30 different obesity phenocopies, associated with 300–400 predisposing genetic markers, may be expressed in modern populations (Kaput & Rodriguez, 2006). Hypertension is another multifactorial condition wherein genes, environment, and culture, along with gene–environment, gene–gene, gene–culture, and gene–sex interactions, produce genetic and phenotypic heterogeneity that often remains unaccounted for in standard epidemiological analyses (Crews & Williams, 1999). Both conditions are observed more frequently among those identified as "African American" when compared to "European Americans" (Dressler et al., 2005). Both obesity and hypertension affect a large percentage of middle-aged and older adults in both ethnoracial groups. Certainly, allelic variants account for some amount of risk in each group. However, the alleles involved may not differ between the two groups in either their structure or their relative frequencies. Rather, the same alleles may be interacting with variable environments, sociocultural settings, and a different set of other alleles at the 23,000 or so known genetic loci. All major CDCs are multifactorial, and genetic variability underlies a component of their risk. The question in a clinical setting becomes: How well does the proxy variable "race/ethnicity" represent the underlying genetic risk, and how does one measure that risk?

Do "racial" categorizations provide any useful information to guide clinical applications and disease diagnosis in modern clinical, pharmacological, and public health settings? Ask a sample of practicing clinicians this question, and most will likely provide an affirmative response; however, see Cooper et al. (2003) for a negative response. This is in part because "self-reported race" in the United States doubles as a proxy variable for a number of factors linked to health and well-being. It also reflects how "racial" disparities in health care and knowledge are reported almost weekly by the print, radio, and TV media and are listed almost as often in requests for proposals by the National Institutes of Health. "Racial" disparities in health, well-being, and mortality are a current emphasis in public health and health services research. This emphasis continues even though all statistically significant "racial" variability in mortality between "white" and "black" residents of the United States may be accounted for by two sociocultural variables—income and household composition (Rogers, 1992, 2000); others suggest that such factors cannot account for the entirety of observed differences (Dressler et al., 2005). Still, results such as Rogers' (1992, 2000) suggest that underlying genetic differences between these two arbitrary groups for disease risks are not likely to be causally related to the observed disparities in CDCs. However, Wong et al. (2002) provide a contrary conclusion.

Major reasons for differences between "white" and "black" residents of the United States in mortality are income, which promotes better access to health care and health knowledge, and variability in living circumstances (Rogers, 1992, 2000). However, subtle genetic components of disease risk, secondary to geographic isolation, genetic drift, and adaptations of the ancestors of specific populations to variable environments, likely do account for a proportion of risks for CDCs across interbreeding groups of individuals. Still, aspects of allelic variation across all populations are unlikely to account for more than about 6% of total risks for common CDCs, while accounting for high proportions of morbidity and mortality from highly penetrant DNA variants (Kittles and Weiss, 2003). Gene-based measures of increased risk from such alleles are needed if we are to reduce the burden of the CDCs that produce health disparities across population subgroups today.

As stated earlier, continuing interactions between the forces of evolution and human culture structure allelic variability across populations. Therefore, geographic ancestry, more specifically the signature it leaves on the genomes of populations, is important for applying concepts from evolutionary medicine. Multiple examples exist; African-descended individuals are more likely to carry alleles promoting sickle cell anemia, have high frequencies of specific human leukocyte antigen (HLA) haplotypes, and have slightly greater overall nucleotide diversity than do those of European descent. They also show low frequencies of alleles predisposing to cystic fibrosis (CF) and phenylketonuria (PKU), conditions that are more common in European-descended populations (Kittles & Weiss, 2003). Given greater DNA variability and polymorphism frequencies in African samples, a larger number of alleles are available that may predispose to diseases, particularly senescent-related CDCs. Interesting questions arise from this greater genetic variation observed in African-derived populations. Are differences in response to treatment across population subgroups in the United States related to their greater genetic variability? For example, does a 5 mmHg drop in systolic blood pressure (SBP) that attenuates stroke mortality by about 14% in mainly European-derived samples (Wexler & Feldman, 2006) have the same, greater, or lesser effect across Africa- and Asia-derived populations? If the same dose-response pattern is observed, there is no need for "race-based" interventions. Both subgroups respond the same. However, given an observable and significant difference in responses between groups, there is a need for additional information on ancestry and ethnoracial assessments. In fact, it is widely known that some drugs work better in some populations. For example, finding the right drug *is* important to achieve blood pressure control in hypertensive patients, and variable responses to similar doses of specific drugs have been seen across Asian and European samples (reviewed in Gerber & Crews, 1999). Examination of the efficacy of enalapril (a drug formulary) therapy in patients with left ventricular dysfunction in reducing hospitalization for heart failure suggests significant reductions in "whites" (44% decline) compared to "blacks" (no significant reduction) (Exner et al., 2001). Such a large difference between ethnoracially defined groups of patients suggests that some underlying DNA variability reflecting geographic ancestry may be influencing the metabolism of enalapril.

GEOGRAPHIC ANCESTRY AS A SUBSTITUTE FOR RACE AND ETHNICITY

Analyses of geographic ancestry potentially go beyond "race-based" therapeutics. Based upon known genes and shared ancestry, AIMs may be used to estimate individual risk profiles for CDCs. This may be referred to as individual geographic ancestry (IGA) assessment. AIMs and geographic ancestry may aid in determining group-related and individual genetic risks for CDCs. However, large portions of risks for CDCs are secondary to lifestyle and environmental factors. These often are more important than genes in producing disease. Included here would be risks for obesity, hypertension, and hypercholesterolemia. Ultimately, use of AIMs/IGA may promote the goals of those advocating individualized medicine by allowing calculation of a patient's total ancestral (genetic) risk for a CDC without reference to any ethnoracial category (Bloche, 2004; Brasswer, 2006; Wexler & Feldman, 2006). This represents a complex undertaking. Today, most ancestry–disease linkages are studied in the absence of knowledge about specific disease-promoting alleles. LD with a CDC is often the clearest way of identifying a risk-increasing locus. The goal of candidate gene analyses is to determine LD between a segment of DNA and a condition/disease of interest. The goal of individual DNA profiling is to determine one's specific risk for a genetically influenced CDC or one's admixture and risks associated with AIMs (Kittles & Weiss, 2003; Parra et al., 2001). Individualized medicine based upon known genetic markers for CDCs is the goal of these analyses.

Populations of known geographic origin often show multiple loci where specific alleles are at high frequencies or even fixed (e.g., the Duffy null allele in many African populations). Such AIMs may be useful for estimating group, subgroup, and individual ancestry (Kittles & Weiss, 2003; Parra et al., 2001). AIMs provide a framework for designing risk-screening programs and examining LD between markers and disease phenotypes within ethnically and geographically defined groups (Kittles and Weiss, 2003). This allows one to determine if genetic factors linked to disease susceptibility differ sufficiently in their frequencies or types across geographic groups of ancestrally related persons. If they do, statistically specifiable patterns of disease and DNA sharing may be identified and may lead to improved risk assessment (Kittles & Weiss, 2003), such as in the case of a higher frequency of PKU in northern European populations. Most DNA variation is common to all groups (about 80%) with only about 10–20% of variation existing across groups. Multiple common DNA variants are likely to contribute to CDCs in polygenic and multifactorial ways within ancestrally related groups. Rather than being highly penetrant disease-causing alleles, such as those for Tay-Sachs or CF, which tend to be rare variants, alleles promoting CDCs are more likely to have small effects and to be more numerous, particularly in populations with greater genetic variation such as those of African ancestry. High frequencies of local variants, rare in the global population, also may have arisen in isolated populations via selection, drift, mutation, or founder effect, and today promote disease risks in new and altered environments (Kittles & Weiss, 2003). Some of these variants may be highly penetrant alleles such as those that cause recognized conditions (e.g., PKU, CF), while others may contribute only small effects to the multifactorial pattern of CDCs. These marker alleles are of interest to those seeking correlations between AIM/IGA and differential etiologies of disease across samples of ancestry-sharing individuals. Multiple common alleles, with frequencies ranging from 5 to 20%, predisposing to diabetes, hypertension, and obesity in populations with geographical ancestry in Africa, Europe, America, and Asia, have been identified (Crews & Williams, 1999; Kittles & Weiss, 2003). Some of these are unique to populations with specific geographic ancestry, but most are shared to some degree across populations albeit at highly variable frequencies.

APPLICATIONS OF GENETIC PROFILES TO CLINICAL SETTINGS

How will individual genetic profiles be useful as adjuncts to clinical evaluation and decision-making? Individual DNA profiles reflect the signatures of evolutionary forces, such as natural selection and genetic drift, that one's ancestors experienced. It is the DNA profile, not skin color, hair texture, or self-reported "race," that confers biological propensities to diseases, produces differential individual and populational predispositions to disease susceptibility, and interacts with environmental and sociocultural variables such as pathogens, toxins, diet, and socioeconomic status. We see three major areas of medical/clinical application for these new methods of genetic profiling: (1) screening, (2) counseling, and (3) development of pharmaceutical formularies and treatments for specific genetic variants that cause disease in individual patients.

SCREENING

Predisease screening for disease-promoting risk alleles is one of the least controversial applications of individual genetic medicine. Once high-risk alleles are identified, it is relatively simple with the use of today's high-throughput genetic processing to identify individuals as carriers or noncarriers of specific mutations. Once screened, targeted interventions may be aimed at those carrying specific risk-enhancing alleles. This would prevent interventions from being wasted on those of low risk. Such "DNA-predictive testing" is particularly effective when a mutant allele is highly penetrant and the condition is preventable or treatable by clinical intervention (Eng et al., 2000). Preventive efforts to reduce the burden of Tay-Sachs among Ashkenazim and nationwide testing for PKU and other highly penetrant single-locus conditions provide specific examples. In cases of less highly penetrant or later-acting age-related mutations (e.g., Huntington's disease, hereditary nonpolyposis colorectal cancer syndrome), a molecular diagnosis before disease presentation may be useful for early initiation of genetic counseling and disease prevention (Eng et al., 2000). Genetic screening of large representative samples from all geographic areas of the world have not been completed. To do so will be expensive. At least some large representative sampling is underway, and this should provide insights as to the distributions of some high-risk alleles across populations (Smith et al., 2006).

COUNSELING

Cancer prevention and care programs, where family history and predictive genetic testing are already being used to guide primary care efforts, best illustrate the clinical application of genetics and evolutionary medicine. Family history is similar to the concept of a genetic risk profile, but at the family rather than the individual level. This allows a familial focus for prevention efforts and assessment of those carrying the specific familial risk allele for a disease. Individual genetic profiles composed of AIM/IGA and high-risk alleles are more specific than family history. AIM/IGA, along with specific risk-promoting alleles, provide an array of susceptibility probabilities for individuals. These profiles may then be used to develop individually tailored prevention programs for a variety of CDCs and to develop prevention strategies that are most likely to reduce each individual's risk. In addition to the BRCA 1 and 2 loci, multiple additional mutations conferring increased susceptibility to both familial and nonfamilial forms of neoplastic disease have been identified (Eng et al., 2000; Narod & Offit, 2005; Offit et al., 2004). There are well-developed protocols for counseling those presenting with such hereditary forms of cancer that today constitute the current standard of clinical care (Eng et al., 2000). Many of these oncogenes show a penetrance of over 80%, are autosomal dominant, and show specific age-related patterns of clinical onset (Eng et al., 2000; Narod & Offit,

2005; Offit et al., 2004). Many oncogenes appear to have arisen as founder mutations, and their current distribution remains restricted to specific isolates and groups of inbreeding individuals. AIMs may be useful for identifying founder mutations because both are group specific. Still, identifying the actual risk-promoting alleles provides a more direct method of assessing disease risks. Once risk alleles are identified, geographic ancestry will likely become a trivial component of risk.

DRUG DEVELOPMENT AND TREATMENT

Pharmacogenetic and admixture/ancestry research pave the way toward developing individualized/personalized medicine and ancestry-based treatments for specific diseases (Kittles & Weiss, 2003). Currently, recommendations for the preferred initial agent in treating hypertension are the same for all patients (Chobanian et al., 2003, Wexler & Feldman, 2006). AIMs may aid in developing drug formularies that are more effective in treating particular segments of the population and for determining whether adverse drug reactions are specific to persons of a particular ancestry (such as with quinine in World War II, which led to hemolytic anemia in persons with a mutant form of glucose 6-phosphate dehydrogenase (G6PD). Although multiple methods and protocols have been used in attempts to identify population-specific interventions, ". . . race has never been shown to be an adequate proxy for use in choosing a drug; if you really need to know whether a patient has a particular genotype, you will have to do the test to find out" (Cooper et al, 2003; 1166–1167).

DISCUSSION

This chapter presented perspectives from evolutionary medicine that may contribute to a better understanding of how geographic ancestry, families defined by descent from common ancestors, and individuals defined by their own specific genetic profiles can inform clinicians of possible variability in disease risk. The molecular revolution has provided new and powerful tools for profiling one's genetic risks for CDCs and for understanding gene–environment and gene–culture interactions in predisposing individuals, families, and groups to specific conditions. As yet, these insights from molecular genetics and evolutionary biology have had only slight impact in clinical settings other than cancer genetics and counseling.

This review suggests that, along with obtaining a family history of all CDCs from every patient, clinicians also should begin to produce genetic profiles of alleles predisposing to the CDCs known to be segregating within each patient's family. Ideally, rather than ascribing etiological power to ethnoracial differences, applications of genetics to disease epidemiology should concentrate on relating specific genotypes/DNA variants to specific phenotypes/diseases regardless of the ethnoracial classifications of patients. Due to the relatively high frequencies of founder mutations observed in different ethnoracial groups by clinical cancer geneticists (Eng et al., 2000), there are likely to be multiple molecular variants that occur primarily or at much higher frequencies among individuals sharing ancestry. Moreover, although "race-based" therapeutics seems to be a goal of some pharmacological researchers, at present, techniques to determine "racial" differences in drug responses are inadequate at best and plain wrong at worst (e.g., Taylor et al., 2004). For better accuracy, new analyses with AIM and IGA should replace earlier analyses of "self-reported race." Neither alleles coding for superficial phenotypes of individuals such as skin color nor the cultural affiliations of patients need be linked to disease-promoting alleles that arose in the same geographic area as their ancestors. Persons categorized as "European American," "white," or "Caucasian" in self-reported or investigator-coded racial classifications may carry more alleles of predominately African origins than do others classified as "African American," "black," or "Negroid" (see Kittles & Weiss, 2003; Parra et al., 2001). People who classify themselves as socioculturally "black" in places like the United States may be identified as of European ancestry when AIMs are used.

Before concluding, a small aside based upon review of the literature on "race," "ethnicity," and "geographic ancestry" is indicated. When ethnoracial groups are being compared, it would help if researchers used the same taxonomic levels for their comparisons (such as geographic ancestry or skin color), along with providing complete descriptions of their categories (Crews, 2003; Crews & Bindon, 1991; Dressler et al., 2005). Samples for ethnoracial comparisons often label groups at different levels of specificity ("Caucasians" to "blacks"). For such comparisons, the researcher should use the same taxonomic level: white/black compares persons based upon attributed color and perceived associations with a specific sociocultural group. Conversely, African American/European American/Asian American/Native American compares groups on perceived geographical area of ancestry currently residing in the same area, but not color and sociocultural group. "Caucasian" is an old term that, along with other categories originally proposed by J. F. Blumenbach in 1789 ("Negroid," "Mongoloid"), should no longer be used because they have no specific meaning with reference to geographic ancestry (Crews, 2003; Crews & Bindon, 1991). Definitions for ethnoracial terms should be included whenever such are reported and the need for such groupings must also be articulated; possible definitions have been discussed elsewhere (Crews & Bindon, 1991; Dressler et al., 2005; Risch et al., 2002).

As with evolutionary medicine in general, individualized medicine, genetic epidemiology, clinical genetics, genomics-based personalized medicine, "race-based" therapeutics, and home-based DNA-testing kits are all the result of our growing knowledge of the human genome. Jointly, these activities represent two current trends in clinical medicine: (1) genes and genomics as predictors of disease risk and susceptibility, and (2) patient-centered self-management of health and disease. Genes have been so ingrained as causes for CDCs in our biomedical culture that many individuals presume their genes have a greater influence on health and morbidity than do more pervasive lifestyle risk factors. At the same time the Internet advertises the benefits of greater self-control of one's health and use of knowledge that previously had been only in the purview of those with formal medical training. Self-diagnosis and self-management of disease is promoted by television advertisements for prescription drugs and direct-to-consumer marketing of cancer gene testing kits to determine one's genetic propensities for selected neoplasms. The possible positive benefits of "race-based" therapeutics and drug formularies are undeniable when ethnoracial genetic differences in susceptibilities to CDCs are observed. This is currently most obvious for multiple hereditary cancers where treatment and counseling follow identification of a family proband with an inherited condition. The better the genetic models that underlie such research, the more useful for clinical applications they will be. However, the use of gene self-profiling from retail gene kits to determine one's dietary and nutritional requirements or to self-determine one's risks for breast cancer seems less practical at this time. The view from evolutionary medicine suggests that all individuals carry a unique set of susceptibility alleles for coronary artery disease, altered nutritional metabolism, cancers, dementias, and other CDCs. Although alleles for genetic susceptibility to conditions may continue to be identified, variation in disease risk conferred by lifestyle, socioeconomic status, diet, and other non-genetic factors will also continue to be better elucidated, and, in association with molecular propensities, may modify the causal web.

CHAPTER 21

From Ancient Seas to Modern Disease

Evolution and Congestive Heart Failure

E. Jennifer Weil

As do several other contributors to this volume, Weil makes the simple point that it is highly unlikely that our ancestors died from heart disease, and in particular, congestive heart failure (CHF).Her presentation delves far deeper into how and why both ultimate (i.e., evolutionary) factors can help, together with proximate ones, to understand why heart disease and CHF have become so prevalent for people living in Western, industrialized contexts. She explores how the vertebrate circulatory system first evolved, describing how functional anatomical homologues for distributing oxygen around an animal's body led eventually to the four-chambered heart characteristic of terrestrial mammals. She also describes the neural and hormonal modulators of the heart and circulatory system that evolved to handle gravity (e.g., the blood pressures associated with bipedalism), along with huge metabolic demands imposed by thermal regulation. The origins of what is referred to in the medical textbooks as the sympathetic nervous system, the renin–angiotensin–aldosterone system (RAAS) along with vasopressin from the brain, as Weil describes, provides the platform from which the human heart and circulatory system eventually came to sustain the needs of the most energy-needy creature of all: the human being. It is in the integrative aspect of her discussion where evolution and twenty-first century Western lifestyles meet that we understand how and why this ancient system can find itself at odds with a cultural system favoring a life style that makes this ancient otherwise effective system, dangerous, in some contexts.

INTRODUCTION

Congestive heart failure (CHF) is a life-threatening clinical syndrome that affects approximately 5 million patients in the United States and is increasing in prevalence both in the United States and worldwide. In order to understand CHF from an evolutionary perspective, one must first understand how neural and hormonal modulators of the cardiovascular system evolved. The sympathetic nervous system (SNS), the renin–angiotensin–aldosterone system (RAAS) and the vasopressin system evolved as critical adaptations for vertebrates, particularly in terrestrial environments. These neural and hormonal regulatory systems evolved to ensure the adequacy of circulation to vital organs when blood pressure or blood volume is compromised, and they remain adaptive today. However, these adaptations may also become maladaptations for modern humans living in postagricultural, postindustrial societies wherein heart disease is epidemic. Activation of neural and hormonal regulatory systems in CHF leads to substantial morbidity and mortality. An evolutionary understanding of CHF suggests prevention and treatment strategies that are strongly supported by clinical studies.

A MISMATCH BETWEEN OUR GENES AND OUR ENVIRONMENT

Darwin demonstrated long ago how heritable variations in anatomy and physiology are naturally selected, but medicine has been slow to recognize how successive adaptations have shaped the human body (Day, 1999). When Williams and Nesse applied the Darwinian paradigm to human health, they found that many adaptations, beneficial in our ancestral environment, have become maladaptations in our modern environment (Nesse & Williams, 1996; Williams & Nesse, 1991). Many human diseases result from or are worsened by anatomical and physiological adaptations to an environment that was markedly different from the one in which we now live.

CHF is a major public health problem that may result from any disease that impairs the heart's ability to circulate sufficient blood to the organs of the body. The most common cause of CHF is cardiac damage resulting from atherosclerotic coronary artery disease (CAD). Konner and Eaton explored concepts of Darwinian medicine as they relate to the epidemic of CAD (Eaton & Konner, 1985; Eaton, Eaton, & Konner, 1999). They identified modern nutrition as the primary reason why cardiovascular disease is the leading cause of death in the developed world and is increasing throughout the developing world. This paper will *not* re-examine CAD, but instead will explore concepts of Darwinian medicine as they relate to CHF (Harris 1983a, b, c, 1985; Nesse & Williams, 1996; Weil, 1993). To see how Darwinian medicine applies to CHF, I will (1) review how the heart and its neural and hormonal control systems evolved and how they were adaptive under ancestral conditions, and (2) how neural and hormonal modulators of the heart and circulation have become maladaptive in modern environments in which heart disease is epidemic.

EVOLUTION OF THE VERTEBRATE CIRCULATORY SYSTEM

The human circulatory system, including the heart, blood vessels, and blood, originated with the first vertebrates—jawless fish—nearly 500 million years ago (Figure 21-1). As marine fish gave rise to freshwater fish, which in turn gave rise to amphibians, reptiles,

Million Years Ago

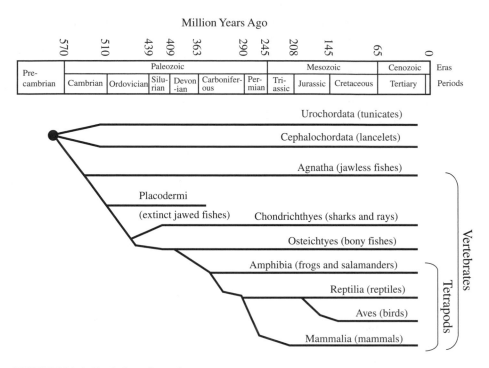

FIGURE 21-1 Evolution of vertebrates.

and ultimately to mammals, the vertebrate circulatory system also evolved. As each vertebrate class explored and conquered new environments, significant changes to the vertebrate circulatory system and the mechanisms that regulate it were required to meet new environmental demands.

The purpose of the heart is to perfuse organs, i.e., to drive blood through increasingly small blood vessels to capillaries, where nutrients and oxygen are transferred to tissues. Blood is composed mainly of water, sodium, and other minerals, including chloride, calcium, and potassium, and other chemicals along with the blood cells. The first vertebrates evolved in a marine environment where most of the components of blood are readily available and where circulation does not require much complexity. The fishes have single-circuit circulatory systems in which a low-pressure, two-chambered heart pumps blood first through the gills for oxygenation, and then through arteries to the internal organs. After delivery of nutrients and oxygen to organs and tissues, veins return blood to the heart. In comparison, the circulatory system of amphibians is more complex and is characterized by a three-chambered heart and partially divided circulation (Bishopric, 2005). Divided circulation, with one low-pressure circuit going from the heart to the lungs and a second high-pressure circuit going from the heart to the organs of the body, is an important adaptation to life on land. High pressures in the systemic circulation allow the force of the heart to overcome the effect of gravity on the blood volume as occurs in terrestrial environments (Farrell, 1991; Lillywhite, 1995). Most reptiles also have three-chambered hearts, and mammals have four-chambered hearts, thought to have evolved in part to meet the increasing metabolic demands imposed by physiological regulation of body temperature (Bennett, 1991).

Even more important than the evolution of cardiac anatomy, however, is the evolution of the neural and hormonal systems, which regulate the heart and blood vessels. Three physiological systems that first evolved in the seas became critical for life on land: the SNS, the RAAS, and the vasopressin system.

EVOLUTION AND PHYSIOLOGY OF THE SYMPATHETIC NERVOUS SYSTEM

The autonomic nervous system reflexively controls circulation by modulating the heart and the blood vessels over short periods of time—on the order of seconds—to exert fine control over the circulation. The autonomic nervous system has two different anatomical and physiological components that balance one another. The parasympathetic nervous system (PNS) is the source of nerves that decrease heart rate, thereby decreasing cardiac output (measured in liters of blood per minute) and lowering blood pressure. The SNS is the source of nerves that increase heart rate, increase the contractile force of the heart, and constrict arteries thereby raising blood pressure (Guyton, 1986). The SNS increases secretion of sympathetic mediators including epinephrine from the adrenal medulla and norepinephrine from sympathetic nerve endings on target organs and blood vessels (Guyton, 1986).

Sensory receptors that detect pressure or stretch (baroreceptors) in the large arteries and in the heart provide information to the brain about blood volume and blood pressure, both within the heart, as it fills between each contraction, and within the blood vessels. If blood decreases in volume, either as a result of blood loss or pooling within the veins, blood pressure drops. Baroreceptors send information to the brain that excites sympathetic nerves that, in turn, constrict blood vessels and increase the rate and force of contraction of the heart. These responses restore arterial pressure towards normal despite decreased blood volume and ensure adequate delivery of nutrients and oxygen to organs and tissues (Guyton, 1986). By returning blood pressure and organ perfusion towards normal the PNS and SNS maintain homeostasis in the circulation, i.e., a constant internal state necessary for life.

Depending on the environment or the physiological demands on an organism, blood pressure may vary considerably. The gravitational effect on blood circulation is completely different in water and on land. Because the effect of gravity on blood volume is offset by buoyancy in an aquatic environment, the distribution of blood volume is not changed when an aquatic organism changes position, and blood remains fairly well distributed over the entire circulatory system. On land, however, the density of water and air are markedly different, so blood has a tendency to pool in dependent regions of a terrestrial organism's body. If blood, under the influence of gravity, does not return to the heart, it decreases amount of blood the heart can pump, and cardiac output (defined above) declines. Over the course of vertebrate evolution, the SNS evolved as a significant countermeasure to gravitational stress on terrestrial vertebrates (Lillywhite, 1995). Physiological stresses have also shaped the evolution of the SNS. Organisms that run or fly have complex organ perfusion needs. The SNS allows all vertebrate organisms to increase blood flow to exercising muscle while decreasing flow to the digestive tract and other organs (Morris & Nilsson, 1994).

The most archaic of living vertebrates, the hagfish, has no anatomical evidence of sympathetic nerves (Augustinsson, Fange, Johnels, & Ostlund, 1956). Other primitive fishes, including cyclostomes (e.g., lampreys), cartilaginous fish (e.g., sharks and rays) and dipnoans (e.g., lungfish), have sympathetic nerves, but they do not have nerve endings that reach the heart. Instead, they have specialized (chromaffin) cells located within or near the heart, which release norepinephrine, thereby promoting cardiac excitation (Morris & Nilsson, 1994). The evolutionarily more recent teleosts (bony fish, e.g., salmon) have sympathetic nerves that modify both the heart and the blood vessels in response to stimuli such as oxygen deprivation and exercise (Morris & Nilsson, 1994). The SNS of amphibians, reptiles, and mammals generally follow the anatomical pattern evolved in the teleost fishes (Morris & Nilsson, 1994).

Because vertebrates are extraordinarily diverse and live in marine, freshwater, and terrestrial environments, the SNS and the mechanisms that regulate it have evolved among the different classes of vertebrates and even among species to meet specific ecological or environmental demands. The SNS has unique properties among species that are subject to particular gravitational stresses, like tree snakes (Lillywhite, 1996), giraffes (Hargens, Millard, Pettersson, & Johansen, 1987), and perhaps humans, because of our upright posture (Mathias, 2002; Pawelczyk & Levine, 2002). In general, SNS evolution is characterized by increasing sympathetic innervation of the heart and veins over time (Morris & Nilsson, 1994), increasing the flexibility of organisms to respond to diverse environmental challenges (Gibbins, 1994).

As in other vertebrates, appropriate activation of the SNS allows our circulatory systems to function effectively under a wide array of circumstances. If we change position from supine to standing, blood volume is redistributed as gravity draws blood toward our feet and less blood returns to the heart. Baroreceptors sense decreased filling of the heart and large blood vessels and activate the SNS to preserve perfusion of vital organs by increasing the rate and force of contraction of the heart and constricting arteries to increase blood pressure. Similarly, if blood volume is reduced as a result of actual blood loss (hemorrhage), baroreceptors signal the SNS, which modulates the heart and blood vessels so that organs continue to receive nutrients and oxygen. There are many other ways in which blood volume and blood pressure may become diminished, including loss of fluids from the body (as a result of vomiting, diarrhea, or profuse sweating) or impaired access to sodium (a key component of blood plasma) and water. In sum, the SNS is a critical adaptation that helps humans and other vertebrates whenever blood volume or blood pressure drops.

EVOLUTION AND PHYSIOLOGY OF THE RAAS

Present in the blood vessels of the kidneys are nonneural receptors that differ from baroreceptors described above. These receptors are present on juxtaglomerular (JG) cells and measure the stretch and pressure within the kidneys' blood vessels to assess blood volume. Instead of sending nervous impulses to the brain, however, they regulate a hormonal system known as the RAAS (Guyton, 1986). The RAAS is also modulated by chloride-sensing cells in the kidney (the so-called macula densa), which measure the rate of urine production, and by the SNS directly (Guyton, 1986). In concert with the SNS, the RAAS helps vertebrates survive loss of blood pressure and blood volume by restoring perfusion of vital organs.

The RAAS has several component proteins (Figure 21-2). Renin is an enzyme secreted by JG cells in the blood vessels of the kidneys, which cleaves off a portion of the circulating protein angiotensinogen to create angiotensin I. Angiotensin I (ATI) is then cleaved by another enzyme, angiotensin-converting enzyme (ACE), to create angiotensin II (ATII). ATII has many powerful effects on the circulation. When it binds to AT1 receptors located within arteries, blood vessels constrict and dramatically increase blood pressure. When ATII binds to AT2 receptors in the brain, it increases thirst, thereby increasing blood volume. ATII also acts in the brain by increasing SNS activity. Finally, ATII stimulates the adrenal gland to synthesize and release aldosterone, a steroid hormone that acts in the kidneys to increase the return of sodium from urine to blood. The effects of ATII are rapid, taking place in the order of minutes, whereas stimulation of aldosterone takes more time (Guyton, 1986). Thus the RAAS complements the rapid action of the SNS— which acts in the order of seconds—with actions that increase blood volume and blood pressure over minutes, hours, and days.

Perfusion of the kidneys is normally under the tight control of both the SNS and the RAAS to ensure adequate glomerular filtration (glomerular filtration rate [GFR] is the rate of filtration of the blood plasma by the filters in the kidneys). The SNS and RAAS also regulate the two most important components of blood volume—sodium and water retained—as they are filtered by the kidneys when they make urine. The RAAS is activated whenever the blood volume or blood pressure drops. When the RAAS is activated, the kidneys reabsorb sodium and water from the urine and raise the volume of the liquid component of blood, i.e., the plasma. By returning blood volume, blood pressure, and GFR towards their normal levels, the RAAS serves a homeostatic function (Guyton, 1986).

The RAAS probably first evolved to help fish navigate waters of variable salinity. The proteins of the RAAS are found in one primitive fish, the lamprey (Brown, Cobb, Frankling, & Rankin, 2005), in sharks and rays (Hazon, Tierney, & Takei, 1999), and in teleost fishes (Nishimura, 1980, 2001). These animals survive in both salt and freshwater. As they transition from a high-sodium to a low-sodium environment, activation of the RAAS allows them to retain sodium (Galli & Phillips, 1996). The RAAS is not present in the most archaic of living vertebrates, the hagfish (Cobb et al., 2004). This suggests that evolutionary pressure for sodium conservation occurred later in the history of

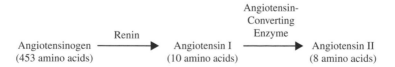

FIGURE 21-2 The enzyme renin cleaves angiotensinogen into angiotensin I. The angiotensin-converting enzyme cleaves angiotensin I into angiotensin II. Angiotensin II has powerful vasoconstrictive effects and increases blood volume via stimulation of sodium and water reabsorption in the kidneys.

fishes, probably as an adaptation to life in freshwater, where sodium, a key component of blood, is scarce.

Proteins of the RAAS are also present in all tetrapod vertebrates (Nishimura, 1980, 2001), reflecting the scarcity of sodium and water in the terrestrial environment and the threat thereby posed to blood volume and blood pressure. In addition, ATII has species-specific effects that appear to correlate with unique environmental pressures placed upon the organisms. Toads, for example, respond to decreasing blood volume with increasing concentrations of ATII (Konno, Hyodo, Takei, Matsuda, & Uchiyama, 2005), which stimulates water absorption through their skins (Goldstein, Hoff, & Hillyard, 2003). In mammals, ATII regulates blood volume independent of sodium and water concentrations individually.

The adrenal glands of most species respond to ATII by increasing production of steroid hormones (Nishimura, 1980). In lower vertebrates, steroid hormones are variable and have multiple effects, including sodium reabsorption in the kidneys. In mammals, however, the steroid hormone activated by the RAAS is exclusively aldosterone, and it has only one function, sodium conservation. Nishimura (1980) has speculated that aldosterone represents a more recent adaptation in vertebrate evolution that occurred when mammals explored environments characterized by scarcity of sodium.

In all vertebrate species, the RAAS reacts to reductions in blood volume and low blood pressure (Nishimura, 1980). Another response to RAAS activation common to all vertebrates is increased GFR (Nishimura & Bailey, 1982). More filtration by the kidneys allows removal of unnecessary minerals and waste blood even as sodium and water are returned from the urine to the blood. While the RAAS evolved to help fish manage sodium concentrations, it has become a key homeostatic system for maintenance of blood volume and blood pressure in terrestrial vertebrates.

EVOLUTION AND PHYSIOLOGY OF VASOPRESSIN

Another hormone with important effects on the circulation is vasopressin, a short peptide synthesized in the hypothalamus and secreted by the posterior part of the pituitary gland. Secretion of vasopressin occurs when specialized receptors in the brain determine that the blood is lacking sufficient water and has become too concentrated (Guyton, 1986). Another stimulus for vasopressin release is decreased blood volume, as sensed by barore-ceptors in the large arteries of the neck and heart (Guyton, 1986). Vasopressin has two major effects in the body mediated by two different receptors. First, vasopressin raises blood pressure via V1a receptors in the smooth muscles of arteries (Koshimizu et al., 2006). Second, vasopressin increases blood volume by increasing water reabsorption from urine, an effect mediated by V2 receptors, in the kidneys (Hayashi et al., 1994).

The origin of vasopressin dates back a billion years to the evolution of coelenterates (jellyfish) (Grimmelikhuijzen, Dierickx, & Boer, 1982). Peptides similar to vasopressin are found among various invertebrate species including annelids (worms), mollusks (shellfish), and arthropods (crustaceans, insects) (Mizuno & Takeda, 1988). In fish species, the molecular ancestor of vasopressin is called vasotocin and is a critical adaptation for those fish that tolerate waters of variable salinity. Vasotocin and its receptor increase only the water component of plasma, not the sodium, a useful adaptation in waters of high sodium concentration. This effect would be particularly useful to fish such as salmon, which migrate from freshwater to saltwater as they mature (anadromy). Vasotocin is also found in amphibians (Konno et al., 2005) and in reptiles (Bradshaw & Bradshaw, 2002), where it regulates blood pressure and blood concentration via water reabsorption in the kidney. Vasopressin itself is found only in mammals, along with several different receptors (Mohr, Meyerhof, & Richter, 1995). Despite the amino acid substitutions between vasotocin and vasopressin, however, the effect of these peptides on their receptors is to increase blood pressure and water within the body.

Whether its release is triggered by osmoreceptors in the brain or by baroreceptors in arteries of the chest, neck, and heart, vasopressin serves a homeostatic function by raising blood pressure and increasing plasma volume when an organism becomes dehydrated. Although vasopressin and its receptors have a long evolutionary history, clearly they were critical adaptations for life on land where fresh water is scarce.

THE NATRIURETIC PEPTIDES:
A COUNTERREGULATORY SYSTEM

In balance with systems that raise blood pressure and blood volume (the SNS, RAAS, and vasopressin system), natriuretic peptides and their receptors evolved to lower blood pressure and blood volume. These hormones constitute an adaptive system for the rare instances in which sodium concentration, blood pressure, or blood volume becomes excessive.

Atrial natriuretic peptide (ANP) and brain natriuretic peptide (BNP) are synthesized in and secreted by the heart, and c-type natriuretic peptide (CNP) is synthesized and secreted in the brain and other organs (Farrell & Olson, 2000). ANP and BNP are secreted in response to stretch of the cardiac muscle, a result of excessive blood volume in the circulation (McGrath & de Bold, 2005). The function of C-type natriuretic peptide remains somewhat unclear in mammals, but is active in vascular tissue (Anand-Srivastava, 2005). These hormones bind to receptors in the brain, arteries, and kidneys, where they inhibit thirst, relax blood vessels, and stimulate sodium and water excretion in the urine. These are useful adaptations in situations where the sodium concentrations are too high or blood volumes are excessive.

The natriuretic hormones and their receptors are ancient within vertebrate evolution, while closely related hormones are found in invertebrates, including mollusks (Bystrova, Parfenov & Marynova, 2002) and insects (Kim et al., 1994). The hagfish possesses a unique natriuretic peptide, and sharks and rays have only CNP (Kawakoshi, Hyodo, Yasuda, & Takei, 2003). Teleosts have four natriuretic peptides: ANP, BNP CNP, and a related hormone, ventricular natriuretic peptide (VNP) (Kawakoshi, Hyodo, Yasuda, & Takei, 2003). These play a particularly important role when a euryhaline fish (a fish that adapts to waters of variable salinity, e.g., eel) moves from freshwater to saltwater (Toop & Donald, 2004). The natriuretic peptides are released from the heart and act on the kidney to unload sodium as blood volume increases (Takei & Hirose, 2002).

The natriuretic hormones are thought to have initially evolved to regulate sodium concentration, because fish may navigate waters of variable salinity due to anadromy, catadromy, or euryhalinity (migration or tides) (Loretz & Pollina, 2000). In terrestrial environments, however, where there are no sources for great quantities of sodium, total blood volume (i.e., sodium and water together) is more important. Consequently, the natriuretic peptides have less of an effect on sodium concentration and more of an effect on blood pressure and blood volume in amphibians, reptiles, and mammals (Takei, 2001). In the rare event that the blood pressure and blood volume becomes excessive, the natriuretic peptides decrease blood pressure and allow sodium and water to be eliminated in urine.

DEFINITION OF CONGESTIVE HEART FAILURE

CHF is a clinical syndrome that arises when the heart and blood vessels cannot effectively deliver sufficient blood to organs of the body to meet their metabolic needs. Without adequate blood flow, tissues do not function properly. Cardiomyopathies are diseases that weaken the heart, thereby initiating CHF. Some of the most common cardiomyopathies are caused by damaged cardiac valves, ischemia (decreased blood flow through coronary arteries to the muscle of the heart), hypertension, diabetes, and alcohol (Collucci, 2006a). CHF occurs when the heart's pumping function is impaired and the cardiac output declines (so-called high output heart failure will not be discussed here).

Risk factors for CHF include obesity, hypertension, hyperlipidemia (together creating "metabolic syndrome"), diabetes, and tobacco and alcohol abuse. Each of these risk factors may cause cardiomyopathy directly. More commonly, patients have multiple risk factors, especially for CAD. In CAD, atherosclerotic plaque (composed of cholesterol, calcium, and fibrous tissue) is deposited in the arteries of the heart, thereby limiting flow of blood to the muscle of the heart, resulting in impaired cardiac contraction. A myocardial infarction (heart attack) occurs when deposits of cholesterol in the arteries of the heart rupture, causing a blood clot to completely block the flow of blood through the vessel. The heart muscle that would normally receive blood through the now clotted coronary artery dies, and a scar forms in its place. A scarred heart does not contract properly and delivers too little nutrients and oxygen to the organs and tissues of the body. After CAD, the most common single cause is alcohol abuse, which has a direct toxic effect on the muscle cells of the heart. Whatever the cause, the impairment in cardiac pumping function is the common denominator of low output CHF.

Patients with any form of advanced CHF develop edema, defined as an accumulation of fluid in the tissues. When edema is present, the patient is said to have "cogestion." The site of edema in the body depends on the part of the heart that is dysfunctional (Figure 21-3). Diseases affecting the left ventricle cause pulmonary edema (fluid accumulation in the lungs), resulting in hypoxia (low oxygen tension in the blood). Patients with left heart failure feel short of breath in the extreme, and pulmonary edema is a life-threatening condition (Colucci, 2006a). Diseases affecting principally the right ventricle cause peripheral edema, or fluid accumulation in the lower extremities and torso. Patients with peripheral edema may accumulate a considerable amount of fluid, which, although not immediately life threatening, may result in discomfort and skin ulceration. Most patients with CHF eventually experience both left and right ventricular failure and therefore both pulmonary and peripheral edema.

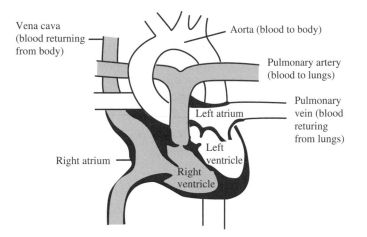

FIGURE 21-3 Left heart failure: the left side of the heart is weak and cannot pump out as much blood as it receives from the right side of the heart. As a result, blood backs up in the lungs. Right heart failure: the right side of the heart cannot pump as much blood to the lungs as it receives from the body. As a result, fluid backs up in the body tissues.

EPIDEMIOLOGY OF HEART FAILURE

CHF is a major public health problem in the United States (Levy et al., 2002), other developed nations (Cowie et al., 1997), and increasingly in South America (Cubillos-Garzon, Casas, Morillo, & Bautista, 2004), Africa (Cooper, Amoah, & Mensah, 2003), and Asia (Reddy, 2004; Sanderson, 2004). CHF affects men and women approximately equally, and its incidence increases with age (Thom et al., 2006). According to the American Heart Association 2006 update on heart disease, 4–5 million Americans are believed to have symptomatic heart failure, and many more have left ventricular dysfunction that will likely progress to CHF (Thom et al., 2006). Heart failure is the leading hospital admission diagnosis in the United States. In 2001, there were over 500,000 hospital admissions primarily for heart failure in women and over 400,000 in men (Young, 2004). This number represents about an eightfold increase from the 200,000 admissions for CHF tallied in 1970 (Young, 2004).

Nearly 15 million individuals are affected with heart failure worldwide (Wilson, 2003; Young, 2004), and that prevalence is expected to increase as populations undergo transition in their economies from agriculture to industry (Mendez, 2001). In the United States, 50% of heart failure patients are over the age of 65 years, and the prevalence increases with increasing age (Young, 2004). These statistics reflect the underlying diseases causing heart failure. It takes years for obesity, hypertension, hyperlipidemia, diabetes, tobacco abuse, and alcohol abuse to cause CHF. In the rest of the world, valvular cardiomyopathy is a more common cause of CHF, which is caused by an infection with streptococcus and affects younger patients (Mendez, 2001). However, the increasing prevalence of heart failure worldwide reflects an epidemiological transition that mirrors economic transition, with prevalence of valvular heart disease remaining stable, but prevalence of ischemic, hypertensive, diabetic, and alcoholic cardiomyopathies increasing. The fact that CHF results from diseases more prevalent in aging is important from an evolutionary perspective and will be discussed below.

Heart failure is deadly. Data from the Framingham Heart Study demonstrate that the 5-year mortality for men diagnosed with CHF between 1990 and 1999 was 59%, an improvement over mortality in previous decades (Levy et al., 2002). Despite the decline in mortality rates secondary to better therapy, however, the increased incidence and prevalence of CHF in the United States and worldwide will still result in an increasing death toll in the years to come.

NEUROHORMONAL ACTIVATION IN CONGESTIVE HEART FAILURE

CHF develops with any disease that impairs cardiac function, but progresses because of neurohormonal activation—activation of the SNS, RAAS, and other hormones in CHF. Neurohormonal activation is paradoxical in CHF, because it results in a further increase in blood volume and vasoconstriction even though initial blood volume is already normal or increased. The severity of CHF is best judged by symptoms, such as shortness of breath, which a patient experiences as a result of neurohormonal activation (Francis et al., 1990; Swedberg, Eneroth, Kjekshus, & Wilhelmsen, 1990). Prognosis in CHF is also closely associated with the degree of neurohormonal activation.

SNS activation occurs early in the natural history of CHF and results in blood vessel constriction and faster heart rate (Grassi, Seravalle & Cattaneo, 1995; Rundqvist et al., 1997). SNS activation should also increase the force of contraction of the heart, but in CHF the heart is less capable of responding to the SNS on account of its intrinsic disease. The exact mechanisms that lead to neurohormonal activation in CHF are not well understood. Activation of the SNS is likely due, at least in part, to reduced control by barore-ceptors in the heart and large arteries. These receptors normally limit SNS activity, but they seem to function abnormally in CHF, thereby removing their restraining influence.

SNS activation is, to a degree, homeostatic because it constricts arteries and maintains blood pressure. This allows the limited cardiac output to be distributed in such a way as to maintain perfusion of vital organs, i.e., the heart and brain, but often at the expense of other organs, i.e., the skin, the gut and the kidneys. However, SNS activation contributes to the worsening of CHF because of its vasoconstrictive effect on arteries. The heart must over-come the resistance load placed on it by the constriction of the vessels it is trying to fill. Over time, the extra work required to overcome this resistance further weakens the heart. Elevated levels of circulating norepinephrine and epinephrine, secreted respectively from the sympa-thetic nerves and from the adrenal medulla, give quantitative evidence of SNS activation in CHF (Benedict, 1996). Effects of the SNS on the cardiovascular system lead to "the vicious cycle" of CHF (Figure 21-4). The weaker the heart, the greater the activation of the SNS, which in turns weakens the heart further. The more activated the SNS (as reflected by blood concentration of norepinephrine), the worse the prognosis (Benedict, 1996).

The RAAS is also activated in CHF, and it too appears to have a homeostatic function. Although kidneys normally receive 25% of the cardiac output, renal perfusion is greatly diminished when heart function is impaired and GFR declines. Receptors in the kidneys located on JG cells and in the macula densa detect the decrease in perfusion and urinary

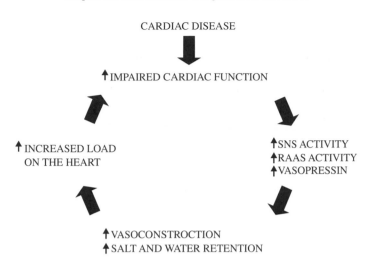

CARDIAC DISEASE

↑IMPAIRED CARDIAC FUNCTION

↑INCREASED LOAD
ON THE HEART

↑SNS ACTIVITY
↑RAAS ACTIVITY
↑VASOPRESSIN

↑VASOCONSTROCTION
↑SALT AND WATER RETENTION

FIGURE 21-4 The vicious cycle of heart failure. Each adjustment by the nervous and hormonal systems that regulate the heart in CHF increases the load on the heart and further weakens it.

filtrate and activate both the SNS and RAAS, which together restore blood flow to the kidneys by increasing blood pressure and blood volume. The normalization of kidney function, however, comes at a great price. The RAAS contributes to the vicious cycle of CHF by expanding blood volume and increasing the load on the heart (Parmley, 1992) (Figure 21-4).

Vasopressin secretion occurs in severe CHF when baroreceptors in the heart and large arteries of the neck signal a decreased blood volume. Vasopressin levels rise, raising blood pressure and increasing water reabsorption from urinary filtrate. Consequently the blood becomes excessively dilute and concentrations of the minerals in the blood, particularly sodium, can drop to dangerously low levels (Chaterjee, 2005). Vasopressin too contributes to the vicious cycle of CHF. Elevated vasopressin and low sodium concentrations in the blood herald a very poor prognosis (Lee & Packer, 1986; Leier, Dei Cas, & Metra, 1994).

The final component of neurohormonal activation in heart failure is the natriuretic peptides. Natriuretic peptide levels, which are secreted by the heart in response to increased blood volume, rise early and progressively in heart failure (Lee, Miller, Edwards, & Burnett, 1989). Since natriuretic peptides evolved to cause arterial relaxation and a decrease in blood volume, it remains one of the central paradoxes of CHF why the kidneys respond more vigorously to the SNS and RAAS than they do to the natriuretic peptides. This may have some important implications for an evolutionary understanding of CHF, as will be addressed below.

TREATMENT OF CONGESTIVE HEART FAILURE

Therapy for CHF has advanced over the last 25 years, reflecting our increasing understanding of how neurohormonal activation drives progression of CHF. New treatments have focused on blocking neurohormonal activation, a detail that will become important in the conclusions below.

Prior to these advances, therapy for heart failure consisted mainly of digoxin, an agent thought to reverse heart muscle weakness by increasing the contractile force of the heart, and diuretics, medicines that decrease reabsorption of sodium and water from the urine. While diuretics relieve the body of volume overload, they have the additional effect of *activating* the neural and hormonal systems that lead to congestion in the first place.

In the late 1970s, drugs developed to antagonize the RAAS were first used in patients with CHF (Turini, Brunner, Gribic, Waebaer, & Gavras, 1979). Angiotensin-converting enzyme (ACE) inhibitors, agents that block the conversion of ATI to ATII, both relieve symptoms and prolong life in patients with heart failure (CONSENSUS Trial Study Group, 1987; SOLVD Investigators, 1991). In the early 1990s, angiotensin receptor blockers (ARBs), which block the binding of ATII to the AT1 receptor, were found to have effects similar to ACE inhibitors on morbidity and mortality in heart failure while avoiding some of the side effects of ACE inhibitors (Gottlieb et al., 1993; Pitt et al., 1999a).

β-Blockers (BBs) are agents that block the SNS. They were developed in the 1960s but for many years were thought to be contraindicated in CHF, since blocking the SNS was believed to decrease the contractile force of an already weakened heart. Some researchers maintained, however, that by antagonizing the SNS, BBs could block the vicious cycle of heart failure (Waagstein, Hjalmarson, Varnausakas, & Wallentin, 1975). BBs seem to improve cardiac performance over the long term by decreasing heart rate, altering the way the heart fills, and by improving muscle metabolism. As the importance of blocking the SNS became fully appreciated in the mid-1980s (Anderson et al., 1985) the rationale for avoidance of BBs was abandoned and BBs emerged as critical drugs for the treatment of heart failure. The COPERNICUS study of carvedilol (Packer et al., 1996, 2002) and the MERIT-HF study of metoprolol (Hjalmarson & Fagerberg, 2000) confirmed that BBs relieve symptoms and reduce mortality in patients with CHF.

Because ATII is the major stimulus for aldosterone secretion from the adrenal gland, it was believed for many years that RAAS inhibition with ACE inhibitors or ARBs would be sufficient for blocking aldosterone release and therefore sodium reabsorption in the kidney. There are, however, several other stimuli for aldosterone release, and aldosterone concentrations may actually rise after initiation of therapy with RAAS inhibitors, a phenomenon known as "aldosterone escape" (Struthers, 1996). Spironolactone, a selective blocker of aldosterone, was found to add benefits in CHF beyond blockade of the RAAS with ACE inhibitors and ARBs in the RALES trial (Pitt et al., 1999b). Blocking aldosterone removes a major stimulus to sodium retention in the body in heart failure, so blood volume does not increase.

Although the kidneys fail to excrete sodium and water in response to elevated levels of BNP released by the heart in CHF, it was found that high doses of synthetic BNP can overwhelm the kidneys' reluctance. Nesiritide, a recombinant BNP given by intravenous administration, is used to treat CHF in patients with severe edema. It has both vasodilator and sodium-excreting (natriuretic) effects.

The newest agents for potential treatment of CHF are the vasopressin antagonists called vaptans. These drugs have not yet undergone extensive clinical testing and are not yet approved by the U.S. Food and Drug Administration for the therapy of CHF. One large multicenter, randomized, double-blind, placebo-controlled study is underway to determine if tolvaptan is efficacious and if it will reduce mortality of patients with CHF (Gheorghiade et al., 2005).

Finally, it is worth mentioning that digitalis, a drug originally derived from the foxglove plant and used for centuries in the treatment of CHF, was thought to act by improving the force of contraction of the heart. It now appears that digitalis and its derivatives may act mainly by decreasing SNS activity, thereby decreasing neurohormonal activation and blocking the vicious cycle of heart failure (Teruya, 1997).

Patients with CHF do not receive all of these drugs simultaneously. Rather, they are usually started first on a diuretic and an ACE inhibitor or an ARB, and then a BB or an aldosterone antagonist completes the regimen. Additional medicines are added as needed. A "cocktail" of medication works best, since multiple physiological systems are activated in CHF. In addition to drugs, recommendations for the treatment of CHF include treatment of underlying heart disease and lifestyle modification. Reduction of salt intake and cessation of alcohol are critically important in the treatment of heart failure (Colucci, 2006b).

GENETIC AND ENVIRONMENTAL MISMATCH: CHF IN THE MODERN WORLD

The adaptations we inherited from our vertebrate ancestors when we became human, approximately 100,000 years ago, protect us from threats posed by our environment and have served us well for the better part of our history as a species. Since the emergence of *Homo sapiens* in the late Paleolithic period, we have spent the majority of our time making our living by hunting and gathering. Foraging for food presents many challenges: running, climbing, pursuing game into hostile environments, and encountering savage predators. Imagine one of your ancestors who, while foraging, encounters a bear. The bear attacks and wounds your relative, but then ambles off. Now your ancestor must make his or her way back to camp, perhaps a long distance away, sweating and bleeding. Adaptations to upright posture, hard exercise, and an environment with an unpredictable supply of sodium and fresh water are crucial for your ancestor's survival. Despite the bleeding, your ancestor's blood pressure is maintained because three physiological systems—the SNS, RAAS, and vasopressin—are all activated in this situation. In addition, the SNS keeps your relative upright so he or she can walk, the RAAS preserves kidney function and restores plasma volume lost through bleeding, and vasopressin conserves water. Your ancestor returns safely to camp, eats, drinks and restores the lost volume of blood. His or her blood pressure rises, and the three systems return to baseline levels of activity. Although life in the Paleolithic period was accompanied by many hardships, we survived because our bodies were well adapted to the challenges of that environment.

It is highly unlikely your ancestor died of CHF. Epidemic heart disease was certainly not commonplace in the evolutionary history of the vertebrates or in our past as a species. The reason our ancestors did not develop CHF is that the modern risk factors for heart diseases were all but absent in our ancestral environment. The Paleolithic diet was high in protein, fiber, and unrefined carbohydrates from fruits and vegetables and low in fat, simple sugars, and sodium. It included no milk after weaning and no alcohol (Eaton & Konner, 1985; Eaton, Eaton, & Konner, 1999). Our Paleolithic ancestors did not smoke tobacco. Moreover, our ancestors expended a lot of energy to obtain food, and when prey became scarce, they trekked long distances in search of better hunting (Eaton, 2003). Our ancestral dietary and exercise patterns were protective against heart disease.

While there are no Paleolithic humans available for physiological measurements, hunter-gatherers still living in remote parts of the world are our best available surrogates for determining our ancestors' health (Eaton, Eaton, & Konner, 1999). Many of the risk factors for heart disease are not present in hunter-gatherers. Among the !Kung San hunter-gatherers of Botswana, for example, there is no obesity. The mean body mass index (BMI, a measure of obesity) for women is $19.1\,kg/m^2$ and for men, $19.4\,kg/m^2$. According to World Health Organization standards, the !Kung San are at the low end of normal for BMI (Kirchengast, 1998). Another important risk factor for heart disease is high blood pressure. Like BMI, the mean blood pressure of modern hunter-gatherers is low and does not rise with age (Stamler, 1997). The ingestion of sodium in these societies is very low. The cholesterol levels of hunter-gatherers are likewise low, and hunter-gatherers exhibit very low risk for type 2 diabetes, a disease in which many of the risk factors for CHF are clustered together (Joffe et al., 1971; Merimee et al., 1972). Members of these communities do not drink alcohol or smoke tobacco unless they are brought in by colonizers or by trade with the outside world. Hunter-gatherers die of many different causes (mainly infectious), but not heart disease (Eaton, Eaton, & Konner, 1999).

In the last 10,000 years (a blink of an eye in the history of human evolution) our species has experienced both the agricultural and industrial revolutions. We have, through our cultural attainments, shaped our environment so rapidly that our genome has not kept up. Our modern environment, complete with industrial agriculture, burdens our bodies in ways never expected based on our evolutionary history. We are adapted to a meager diet and strenuous activity, and now we eat excessively and exercise too little. We are adapted to a low-salt environment, and yet we now eat excessive amounts of salt. We are adapted to eating lean game, and instead fatten our domesticated animals and then fry our food in yet more fat. We are adapted to eating high fiber and no simple sugars, and yet now we eat processed foods loaded with high-fructose corn syrup. We are not adapted to drinking alcohol, and yet many of us drink to excess. We have easy access to cheap tobacco, and many of us smoke it. A consequence of becoming fat, hypertensive, diabetic, hypercholesterolemic drinkers and smokers is the epidemic of heart disease we now face (Figure 21-5).

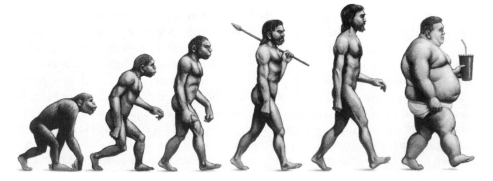

FIGURE 21-5 Human evolution in postagricultural, postindustrial societies. (Reprinted with permission from www.jonberkeley.com)

CONCLUSIONS

Now, having abandoned our ancestral ways of life, we face epidemics of both heart disease and CHF. The CHF epidemic has come about because of a convergence of two factors: (1) increasing amounts of heart disease and (2) ancestral adaptations to gravity and a low sodium and water environment. The hypothesis presented in this chapter is that the SNS, RAAS, and vasopressin evolved early in our vertebrate history in response to threats upon the blood volume, particularly in terrestrial environments. Neurohormonal activation as a result of hemorrhage, vomiting, diarrhea, or profuse sweating is homeostatic and returns circulatory function towards normal. Neurohormonal activation in CHF, however, is pathological, increasing both the load on the heart as well as the blood volume, and driving the vicious cycle of heart failure.

Why do the natriuretic peptides fail to reverse or even significantly modify the clinical state of heart failure, even when levels of these hormones are increased 100-fold above normal in CHF? In contrast to the seas from which vertebrates originally came, the terrestrial environment is sodium poor. The need to reduce sodium in the blood has therefore been unusual throughout most of the history of the tetrapods. Similarly, our species has suffered from limited access to sodium for most of our history (Kurlansky, 2002; Laszlo, 2001; Pliny the Elder). Therefore, evolutionary pressure to develop robust systems to promote sodium excretion has not existed throughout vertebrate history, whereas pressure for development of systems that ensure sodium retention has been intense. Now that salt is commonly available, however, it plays a significant role in human disease (Law, 2000). Accordingly in CHF, when the SNS, RAAS, vasopressin, and the natriuretic peptides are *all* activated, the natriuretic peptides are overwhelmed by the other more robust neurohormonal systems, reflecting the far greater importance of the SNS, the RAAS, and vasopressin to our survival throughout most of our evolutionary history.

Because CHF occurs too late in our individual life histories to affect our success at reproduction, we will never evolve a way to turn off the 500-million-year-old adaptations that help us survive episodes of decreased blood pressure and blood volume. Instead, we must use an evolutionary understanding CHF to enlighten our clinical approach to the prevention and treatment of heart failure. To reverse the epidemic of heart disease and CHF, an evolutionary perspective suggests that we should mimic, if not recreate, ancestral conditions. As Eaton, Konner, and Shostak recommend in their book, *The Paleolithic Prescription* (1989), we can eat and exercise more like our ancestors did, despite living in a postagricultural and postindustrial society. Indeed, the American Heart Association (AHA) also recommends changes in diet and exercise as primary prevention for heart disease (American Heart Association, 2006; Thom et al., 2006). The AHA does not use an evolutionary rationale for its guidelines, but relies on studies of many thousands of patients to show that reduction of key risk factors associated with our postagricultural, postindustrial lifestyle—obesity, hypertension, hyperlipidemia, and diabetes, tobacco abuse and alcohol abuse—reduces the risk of cardiovascular disease and CHF. For patients who *do* develop CHF, an evolutionary perspective suggests that the best way to alleviate suffering and prolong life is to block the ancient adaptations, which lead to neurohormonal activation and the vicious cycle of CHF, using medications. Studies of drugs developed to treat heart failure, outlined above, validate precisely such an approach.

ACKNOWLEDGMENTS

The author wishes to acknowledge editorial assistance by Marc D. Thames, M.D. and Robert G. Nelson, MD, PhD. Their suggestions have improved the clarity of this chapter. This research was supported, in part, by the Intramural Research Program of the National Institute of Diabetes and Digestive and Kidney Diseases.

CHAPTER 22

Evolution at the Intersection of Biology and Medicine

Stephen Lewis

In his review of the various intellectual and practical applications and limitations of evolutionary medicine, including its potential weaknesses but its promise, too, Lewis observes that so far much of the work in evolutionary medicine has concentrated on disease rather than on health. He reveals here why he worries that the title "evolutionary" or "Darwinian" medicine suggests that while the emphasis falls on "medicine," biology has as much to gain as does medicine, and he laments that the application of evolutionary principles to defining and sustaining health has inadvertently been centered outside of biology. His ability to support and criticize from a historical point of view has the potential to further guide research in this emerging field away from being too comfortable with what he calls the simplicity yet deceptiveness of the evolutionary interpretation. He suggests that evolutionary medicine will do well to be a bit circumspect "when offering its explanations." What it brings to the conceptual area, however, are profoundly new questions, new kinds of analyses, and new ways to look at old problems. He is wise to remind us that the "practical impact of evolutionary medicine cannot be expected to be the same for every ailment," at least for this relatively early phase of evolutionary medicine. Furthermore, the field continues to pick up new insights and theoretical and methodological refinements (illustrated throughout this volume), not the least of which includes learning where evolutionary medicine can help, and where it cannot, just as the doctor ordered.

> Science is seeing what everyone else can see, but thinking what no one else thinks.[1]

OLD KNOWLEDGE, NEW CONTEXT

Many general medicine textbooks now tend to be so large and structured in such a way that no one can realistically be expected to read one from cover to cover. Yet, at the same time, there is a strong onus on the author—or, frequently, team of authors—to include, as

399

far as is possible, everything of practical relevance. Certainly nothing of vital importance can afford to be excluded. Typically "[c]urrent textbooks summarize what is known about a disorder under traditional headings: signs and symptoms of the disease, laboratory findings, differential diagnosis, course, complications, epidemiology, aetiology, pathophysiology, treatment, and outcome" (Nesse & Williams, 1994, p. 237). Medical textbooks have arguably become little more than catalogues of clinically relevant information rather than explications of what that information reveals about the organism affected. Furthermore, in practice, a dichotomy exists between what must be included and what can be assimilated even by the brightest minds. Access to that information previously confined to medical textbooks is increasingly being made available in portable electronic form. However easy access to information becomes, a certain sense of explication is missing; while the "whats" and "hows" abound, the "whys" and "wherefores" are relatively few. If the latter constitute the framework within which the detail can be better understood and remembered, then it is questionable whether the way in which medical information is currently approached is ideal. After all, it is much easier remembering a narrative than a catalogue. Certainly having the right intellectual framework within which to understand something is one of the best aids to mastering a subject. The best teachers are not necessarily those who know the most about a given subject; rather, they are the ones who, among other things, can reveal meaning amid a mass of data.

Although the content of medical textbooks is already extensive, it has been suggested that they, in fact, "fall one category short... [a] comprehensive discussion of a disease must also provide an evolutionary explanation" (Nesse & Williams, 1994, p. 37). Thus, a new category that seeks to augment clinical medicine has come into being in order to fill this gap. Variously called "Darwinian medicine" or "evolutionary medicine," this new category of biomedical study may be set to add to the burden of medical information or, alternatively, to liberate it by offering a framework within which disease and health may be understood. Evolutionary medicine is now past its infancy and reaching such a stage that some critical questions can now be asked in a timely and constructive fashion that may help guide it as it evolves into a more mature discipline.

WHAT'S IN A NAME?

The term "Darwinian medicine" was coined by George Williams and Randolph Nesse (Williams & Nesse, 1991), although they were not the first to see a role for evolutionary theory in understanding human ailments. Although in their subsequent book *Why We Get Sick*,[2] they refer to what they describe as Estabrooks' largely "eugenicist tract" (p. 263), *Man, The Mechanical Misfit* (Estabrooks, 1941), as prefiguring the notion of maladaptation to some extent, they omit reference to other works such as Haldane's paper "Disease and Evolution" (Haldane, 1949) and Krogman's *Scientific American* article "Scars of Evolution" (Krogman, 1951). Indeed, in her combined review of *Why We Get Sick* and Niles Eldredge's *Reinventing Darwin: The Great Debate at the High Table of Evolutionary Theory*, Sharon Kingsland (1996)[3] makes the point that "[e]volutionary medicine has not been as neglected as [Williams and Nesse] imply, for it has had some prominent champions in the past century." In many respects, Williams and Nesse did not so much create a new discipline as bring together and provide a name for a somewhat dispersed set of ideas that were already extant but lacking academic coherence. This act was, in itself, a significant step. By drawing people's attention to an association between the objects of medicine and biology's central thesis, they gave particular focus and impetus to new ways in which medical issues might be understood—a new intellectual framework no less—and how they might be explored in future.

However, there is a sense in which the title "Darwinian medicine" is a little baffling. Clearly, it harkens back to Charles Darwin (1809–1882) and the theory of evolution by natural selection, but it was not until Darwin's ideas could be fused with those of genetics in the second quarter of the twentieth century, in what was called "Neo-Darwinism" or the new or modern synthesis, that they really began to have any significant influence on biological thinking. It is this synthesis upon which Darwinian medicine draws. Accordingly, as a beneficiary of that legacy, it might have been more accurate—although certainly less catchy—to have chosen the term "Neo-Darwinian medicine."[4] For some, the term "Darwinian" simply conjures up the whole notion of evolution. However, for others, the implications are more limited; drawing attention primarily to those processes described by Darwin—in particular, natural selection and adaptation. Certainly, these are important processes, but there are others that contribute to evolution. Thus, the terms "Darwinian medicine" and "evolutionary medicine" are not, strictly speaking, synonymous. The former, if limited to the processes associated with Darwin, would, in fact, form a subset of the latter. The term of choice here is "evolutionary medicine," because it offers greater inclusivity by allowing all evolutionary processes admittance, as our knowledge of them continues to develop.

Although it has been Williams and Nesse's form of evolutionary medicine with its strong adaptationist stance that has largely set the agenda for what has ensued, theirs was not the only expression or conception of the discipline. In the same year that *Why We Get Sick* was published in the United States, Marc Lappé (1994) also published *Evolutionary Medicine—Rethinking the Origins of Disease*. The styles of the two books were quite different. Lappé's grew out of a course[5] he had given many years before and sought to keep the relationship between humans and the environment very much in evidence. Significantly, he limited himself to considering somatic conditions, in particular, infection, those associated with the immune system and cancer.

But it is Lappé who gives the most concise (even axiomatic) description of the aims of a medicine that has fully assimilated evolutionary theory when he suggests that: "[w]e need to understand the evolutionary origins of disease in order to fully comprehend their prevention" and "[w]e need to incorporate evolutionary models of disease in order to treat them effectively" (p. 9).

Lappé's choice of topics is quite specific, when compared to that of Nesse and Williams (1994). Their choice of topics is taken from clinical medicine. Their position is that all that concerns clinical medicine also concerns evolutionary medicine—at least, they introduce no specific boundaries or limitations, and we find, for example, that psychiatric conditions are considered in much the same way as somatic conditions. Indeed, in a paraphrase of the title of Theodosius Dobzhansky's (1973) famous article, they tellingly conclude *Why We Get Sick* with the statement "nothing in *medicine* makes sense except in the light of evolution" (my emphasis).

One must question, however, the extent to which the ideas that launched evolutionary medicine are now the same as those propelling the discipline. Certainly, as any discipline develops, fewer and fewer workers tend to read the seminal texts. How many evolutionary biologists, for example, have read Darwin's *Origin of Species* all the way through? It is now more likely to be a core text on a course in the history of science than of evolutionary biology. We are now at a point of transition in the development of evolutionary medicine where, as Stearns and Ebert (2001) have noted, we are "moving from an initial phase dominated by speculation and hypothesis formation into a more rigorous phase of experimental testing of explicit alternatives." The point that evolutionary theory has a place in understanding the objects of medicine has been made—even though the medical establishment has been slow to take this onboard. As the publication of various reviews (Stearns 1999; Trevathan, Smith, & McKenna, 1999) demonstrates, the topics currently being studied under the banner of evolutionary medicine are being investigated largely by nonclinicians. Increasingly, it appears that evolutionary medicine is becoming related to medicine only in so far as it concerns human conditions, not because it is being conducted within a primarily medical context. The discipline is clearly now taking on an agenda of its own, rather than a medically directed one. One now sees, perhaps, more similarities with older, more established disciplines such as human biology and anthropology and fewer similarities with the medicine it was originally supposed to augment. For example, medicine tends to see conditions that are characteristic of different stages throughout life—from infancy to senescence via adolescence and sexual maturity—in isolation, devoting separate departments and clinics to each. This could have been the approach adopted by evolutionary medicine. However, we find that evolutionary medicine is less prone to this form of compartmentalization, and work in the aforementioned areas tries to understand the nature of these life stages and how they fit into the strategy our species has evolved for living. In this respect, evolutionary medicine does not focus exclusively on the conditions associated with these stages but is aware of a wider context. Here one sees perhaps a shaping influence being exerted by human biology and biological anthropology. These disciplines have traditionally been concerned with the study of the varieties of human existence. Until the advent of evolutionary medicine, this had included the question of disease to only a limited extent. Now, by taking the question of disease on board more fully, human biology and biological anthropology together appear to be shifting evolutionary medicine away from the initial medical focus and towards a wider human perspective.

BIOLOGY AND MEDICINE—A MEETING OF MINDS?

It is generally assumed that biology and medicine are closely allied disciplines. Of the two, it should be remembered that biology is the much younger discipline. Indeed, the very term "biology" is little more than two centuries old, having been coined at the turn of the nineteenth century,[6] whereas medicine, in one form or another, has been in existence for as long as people have relieved each other's ailments. When biology emerged, it was into a world already colored by a variety of medical and nonmedical metaphysical ideas. For example, bloodletting, itself associated with the theory of the humors, was commonly practiced, and the idea that there was a vital force that animated living creatures was still prevalent. Although medicine has always dealt with a biological being, it has not always understood him in wholly modern biological terms. The assumption implicit in evolutionary medicine is that biology is a basic science which underpins and forms a foundation for medicine. There is certainly some truth in this; biology does contribute to medicine in a variety of technical ways in that it has developed numerous laboratory techniques and procedures that medicine has been able to co-opt for its own use in obtaining information about the physical states of patients. However, the idea that because humans are biological entities, medicine, in dealing with them, therefore, rests on biology as a fundamental science, is a little too simplistic. Biology and medicine meet within the ethical and metaphysical confines of a social and cultural context. It is one thing for biology to contribute to medicine in a technical way; it is quite another for it to contribute in a conceptual way. Any conceptual contribution that biology might make can only be made within the prevailing social and cultural context. For example, if that context is one of religious fundamentalism, medicine would continue to draw on the practical and technical contributions that biology might offer, but it would be unlikely to adopt biology's explanatory framework should the latter be at odds with the prevailing theological view. This is no hypothetical scenario. There are certainly many in the medical profession who, for religious reasons, do not accept the theory of evolution and are, therefore, likely to be impervious to the conceptual aspects of evolutionary medicine.

Despite these different worldviews, one characteristic that is constant is medicine's aim of alleviating suffering. The history of medicine is, in effect, the history of people's individual suffering and the attempts that have been made to alleviate that suffering. An important lesson from the history of medicine is that explanation and treatment often go hand in hand. There have been numerous, sometimes fanciful, explanations offered as to what caused a particular form of suffering, accompanied by some often quite bizarre treatments meted out as a consequence. In a real sense, the explanations proffered by evolutionary medicine are the latest in a long line of such offerings. But whereas medicine began with magico-religious explanations, it is now in a position to adopt the full force of scientific thinking. To clearly demarcate them from the fanciful notions of the past, the explanations offered by evolutionary medicine should be carefully tested before they are allowed general acceptance.

One cannot assume that because two different disciplines deal with the same objects, they do so in the same way. When suggesting that medicine should adopt, albeit in part, an intellectual perspective associated with biology, one must look at how medical and biological thinking differ to see if that perspective can be transposed unproblematically. While sciences like biology tend to think that they operate in a value-free way without moral or ethical encumbrances, is this really true? Medicine clearly does not operate in this way and gives considerable attention to the motives and effects of its actions. There is a strong ethical element inherent in medicine that simply does not exist in biology.

This raises an important issue that needs to be mentioned, if only in passing. The ethical consequences of the application of evolutionary theory to medicine in the form of evolutionary medicine are not as yet clear, and although, so far, none seem to have been raised, this does not exclude the possibility that some issues might arise in the future. It is not enough to deplore the eugenics of the past (as Nesse & Williams [1994, p. 263] do in response to Estabrooks [1941]) and state that we are not proposing a new form of the same. This time the reasons for applying evolutionary theory to medicine must be absolutely beyond reproach. All ideas, especially those pertaining to humans, have consequences. Some of these consequences may be quite subtle and unexpected. Medical practice is much more than the mere application of biological ideas. As evolutionary medicine moves from its infancy to a phase where it seeks clinical application in order to help establish itself, there is now a need for the involvement of ethicists in an appraisal of the potential consequences of ideas expressed within evolutionary medicine. Otherwise, there would always be the danger that the whole enterprise could become tarnished.

There are other, perhaps more fundamental, intellectual differences between biology and medicine. Biology frequently deals with populations, their statistical norms and averages, whereas medicine, notwithstanding the activities of epidemiologists and the move towards "evidence-based medicine," deals primarily with individuals and their unique, usually problematic, experiences of living. In biology, there is a tendency to think of what is *generally* the case. We tend to think in terms of populations rather than individuals. Sometimes it is even convenient to think simply of "gene pools," and we often go so far as to limit ourselves to consideration of the frequencies of just one gene. We even, at times, seem to forget that sexually reproductive species are composed of a male form and a female form, each leading sometimes very different lives. In particular, evolutionary biology is often concerned with the characteristics of species continuity via reproduction, whereas medicine is concerned with the survival of the individual, that is, with organismal survival. Here, despite various attempts (Bertalanffy, 1950a, b, 1969; Mesarovic, Sreenath, & Keene, 2004), both biology and medicine can be said to lack a thoroughly worked-out theory of the organism as a unified whole.

Notwithstanding the move towards health promotion, for a long time medicine has been closely associated with disease, whereas biology has been more closely associated with the "normal"—that is, with species design and with the taxonomy of the typical. As a result, it can be argued that biology has not dealt fully with the lives of individuals; as the study of life, it has not, thus far, included all that pertains to life, as a *lived* phenomenon. Disease, for example, has been largely excluded in any sense of it being a typical aspect of living. There is a real sense in which the phenomenon of "life" and the activity of "living" have been separated, with biology dealing primarily with the former and medicine with the problems associated with the latter.

Furthermore, biology is described as a science, whereas medicine is often described as an art. Certainly there is legitimate scope for an individual clinician to exercise judgment based upon experience and even intuition when evaluating a patient's condition and trying to assess the exact treatment to offer. These are qualities that would be frowned upon were biologists to rely on them for the description and reporting of their findings.

A FUSION OF IDEAS?

Whether a genuine fusion of evolutionary ideas with those prevailing within the medical profession can be achieved is a largely unexplored question. From the inception of evolutionary medicine, the assumption has always been that such a fusion is possible. However, the case proposed in *Why We Get Sick* was a biological one and did not address, in any depth, the institutional issue of how a medical establishment might be made to take on ideas from evolutionary biology. While there is a biological case for studying the objects of medicine from an evolutionary angle, the acceptability of the project at an institutional level, within the prevailing social and cultural context, has yet to be established.

Some have sought to have evolutionary medicine taught in medical schools (Charlton, 1996; Downie, 2004a, b; Nesse, 2001; Nesse & Schiffman, 2003; Nesse & Williams, 1997). Whether teaching evolution in medical schools in this way will have the desired effect of having evolutionary ideas accepted into medical practice is a question that educationalists might be best suited to investigate. However, given the modern trend for courses to be built up from self-contained taught modules, it cannot be assumed that offering a module on evolutionary medicine—least of all an optional one—will necessarily lead to a general acceptance or use of evolutionary ideas within the medical profession.

It is possible that evolutionary medicine may currently be operating on two different, perhaps distinct, levels. As noted by Stearns and Ebert (2001), when reviewing the first 10 years of evolutionary medicine, more of the new ideas that have been generated have implications for medical research than for clinical practice. This leaning towards medical research rather than clinical practice and a readiness by academic departments to develop courses in evolutionary medicine suggests that it is possible that a *de facto* research or academic version of evolutionary medicine and a smaller *de facto* clinical version may be emerging, with each maintaining their innate professional distinctions. It is even possible that evolutionary medicine may be in the process of dividing into two distinct forms along these lines, each with their own respective agendas. Perhaps the picture will become clearer over the next 10 years or so. However, the existence of nonclinical academic courses in evolutionary medicine allows an alternative model for the adoption of evolutionary ideas by medicine to be suggested. Rather than add courses in evolutionary medicine to clinical education, one might allow courses in academic departments to flourish in their own right by increasingly allowing clinical topics to be studied from a nonclinical perspective. Given what this reveals, medicine may then wish to take onboard what it can use, picking and choosing as it sees fit. So far, this approach does not seem to have been very productive in terms of getting evolutionary ideas a prominent place in medicine, which does not mean that it will not prove to have a useful role in the long term.

A CONFUSION OF TERMS

It generally goes unnoticed that, at this meeting point between biology and medicine, key terms such as *sickness, illness, disease,* and *health,* which both use, are words taken from ordinary language (Nordenfelt, 2001), that is, they are nontechnical terms belonging to everyday speech. Indeed, terms such as these represent notions used freely by medicine, the general public and various sections of academic biology, not least evolutionary medicine. As a result, these terms have the practical usefulness of allowing information to be conveyed from patient to clinician and vice versa. But although each knows what the other is talking about, this does not mean that clear definitions of these terms are necessarily easy or obvious. There is often a lack of precision when these terms are used. Some terms are even used interchangeably. If evolutionary medicine is to be a scientific enterprise, it needs a scientifically rigorous way of understanding the terms it uses; it cannot be allowed to tolerate the lack of precision and interchangeability that exists elsewhere. If evolutionary medicine is to use the same words, it must use them with a certain exactitude. Being drawn from ordinary language, words such as *sickness, illness, disease*, and *health* come to be used in a variety of ways as language usage changes. Sometimes *sickness, illness*, and *disease* can even be used interchangeably. While it is not inappropriate to use these words in a scientific context, they must not be used in the same conceptually imprecise or variable fashion. Instead, their meanings must be distinct and not interchangeable, otherwise the scientific explanations that evolutionary medicine seeks to provide would also be imprecise.

Of the terms mentioned above, "sickness" and "illness" have technical meanings about which there is general agreement. Describing different forms of what he called "unhealth," Marinker (1975) gives a concise definition of sickness as "... the external and public mode of unhealth. Sickness is a social role, a status, a negotiated position in the world, a bargain struck between the person henceforward called 'sick,' and a society which is prepared to recognise and sustain him" (p. 83). Illness he described as "... a feeling, an experience of unhealth which is entirely personal, interior to the person of the patient" (p. 82).

Of these terms, illness is probably the most easily understood, because of its very subjectivity: we all have some form of direct experience of illness upon which to draw. We all know what it is like to be ill to some degree and can transfer this experience onto others. However, the situation is not so clear with regard to "disease," which has proved to be a particularly problematic term (Boorse, 1997; Nordenfelt, 1997, 2001; Twaddle & Nordenfeldt, 1993). However, despite various nuances of opinion, two main schools of thought about the definition of disease exist. One school argues that disease can be understood objectively as statistically subnormal biological functioning for a given species and that such a definition is uninfluenced by prevailing human values. The other school of thought argues that there is a strong subjective element to defining disease and that this differs between cultures and through history and that, as a result, our notion of what constitutes a disease is not fixed.

What is more, one also finds "disease" and the more technical term "pathology" to be used interchangeably. For example, Wade and Halligan (2004), writing in the *British Medical Journal*, go so far as to refer to "disease (pathology)." As noted above, one also finds both "disease" and "illness" to be used interchangeably. If "disease" can be used interchangeably with both "illness" and "pathology," then it must follow that "illness" and "pathology" are equivalent to each other in some way. But this is clearly not the case. The term "pathology" usually applies to some tangible lesion, whereas "illness"—being a subjective experience—clearly does not. It is perhaps only when it is spelled out in this way that can one begin to see the nature of the problem. It appears that there is something about the concept of "disease" that can imply "illness" and something about it that can also imply "pathology." Thus, the term "disease" is clearly less precise than one usually assumes, and one needs to be very careful about its use. If one claims to be engaged in trying to understand a disease scientifically, is one's main concern the behavior of pathological lesions or the state of the individual as a whole? Furthermore, is one sure that a disease as named by the medical profession constitutes a biological reality? One of the ways in which the notion of disease works, in the clinical setting, is as a medical construct—a convenient label—that allows clinicians a framework within which to practice. Here, more important than the accuracy, or even the reality, of the label is the question of whether the patient can be made better. "Drapetomania" and "Dysaesthesia Æthiopsis," for example, were two medically defined "diseases" prevalent in the United States in the mid-nineteenth century. The former was a disease that made black slaves run away, the latter a disease that made them damage their master's property. "Sufferers" who caused damage could be made better by anointing them with oil and having this slapped into their skins with leather straps. Needless to say, these "diseases" can no longer be found in any medical textbook. However, this example raises an important question: Are there any modern diseases—somatic or psychiatric—like "Drapetomania"? That is, are there any conditions that are medically defined—and for which we might be tempted to seek evolutionary explanations—but which are biologically fatuous?

Surprising as it may seem, the question of the definition of disease does not appear to be particularly problematic for medicine. This is probably because, when dealing with patients, a clinician is able to address the experiential and subjective "illness" component as described by the patient separately from the objective "pathological" component. In effect, the "illness" component fits into the category of a patient's symptoms and the "pathological" component into that of their signs.[7] The situation is not so simple for evolutionary medicine because the fundamental aim is that of "trying to find evolutionary explanations for vulnerabilities to disease."[8] As such, the concept of disease is central to the whole enterprise. If we do not know precisely what constitutes a disease, then we can hardly expect to offer accurate evolutionary explanations for our vulnerabilities to them. Furthermore, the explanations that are offered for our vulnerabilities will be affected by the way in which we use the term "disease." If we use it in a sense interchangeable with illness, we would be intent on explaining vulnerabilities to the subjective experience of symptoms. Subjective experience relates to the whole organism and reflects how comfortable it is at a given moment in time within its environment. If it is not comfortable, its ability to survive and/or reproduce may be impaired. If we use the term in a sense interchangeable with pathology, we would be intent on explaining vulnerabilities to the physical manifestations that can be observed.

That the definition of disease has not so far caused a problem for evolutionary medicine is perhaps unsurprising. First, as noted above, "disease" is an ordinary language term, and we do not tend to worry about the definitions of words in everyday parlance. Second, if medicine does not appear to have cause to worry about the definition of this word, there would appear to be no obvious reason for evolutionary medicine to do otherwise.

A full discussion of how the term "disease" should best be used in the context of evolutionary medicine is not possible here. However, signs and symptoms form a set of objective and subjective parameters to which the term "disease" may be applied as a label[9] or brief descriptor of the biological state of the individual as a whole. In medicine, where the aim is to effect a cure, a disease label is convenient in managing a patient's condition. In effect, that label indicates what the clinician is to expect under the "traditional headings" noted above. Although the idea of disease as a label is not an unreasonable suggestion, if we are clear that that is how we use the term, this is not perhaps how disease is most frequently understood.

THE REIFICATION OF DISEASE

It is not uncommon for someone to be described as "having a disease." To talk in this way implies that the disease is something that can be possessed; that it is, in some way, distinct from the person who "has it." In this way the disease becomes reified, taking on the identity of a real and distinct entity with an existence of its own. This is often referred to as the ontological model of disease and has an interesting and surprisingly recent history (Tavassoli, 1987). At least part of the responsibility for our current way of thinking the psychiatrist Frederick Kräupl Taylor (1980) traces back to the German pathologist Rudolf Virchow (1821–1902). Taylor notes how "Virchow . . . towards the latter part of his life, was most outspoken in . . . declaring that a disease was a living physical entity, an *ens morbi*." In particular, he cites Virchow as stating:

> In my view the disease entity is an altered part of the body; in principle, an altered cell or cell aggregate . . . In this sense I am a thoroughgoing ontologist and have always regarded it as a merit to have brought into line with genuine scientific knowledge the old and essentially justified assertion that disease is a living entity . . . [which has] a parasitic relationship with the otherwise healthy body to which it belongs and at the expense of which it lives (Virchow quoted in Taylor, 1980, p. 420).

Virchow seems to be referring to localized lesions and following the trend in identifying "disease" with "lesion," an idea that appears to have been a product of nineteenth-century Parisian medical thinking (Porter, 1997). Before then it was not uncommon for the whole person to be considered as "dis-eased" in the sense of having "lost ease." For Giovanni Battista Morgagni (1682–1771), lesions were only the "seats" of disease,[10] the locations from which the loss of ease emanated. The problem with speaking of diseases as if they are distinct entities is that it colors our thinking in subtle ways. In particular, diseases as distinct entities can appear to have a separate, almost independent, existence. Nesse and Williams (1994) state that "[w]e know more and more about why individuals *get* specific diseases but still understand little about why diseases *exist* at all" (p. 3) (my emphases) and, again a few pages later, that "[e]xperts on various diseases often ask themselves why a particular disease *exists* at all" (p. 8) (my emphasis). Even if unintended, this way of referring to disease allows it to be interpreted as if it were something distinct from the person in whom it can be found to reside.

Upon reflection, there should appear to be something inherently wrong with talking about "having a disease" when it is, in fact, the very stuff of which we are made that is affected; when we are, in effect, physically "at one" with the telltale signs and symptoms. The signs and symptoms that result are the products of our own bodies reacting to given stimuli. Importantly, a disease is not a biologically distinct or separate entity; there is no one thing that can be pinned down and exposed as being the disease per se. Instead, a disease is better seen as a label that characterizes a particular way in which different signs and symptoms are exhibited by a patient. As such, a disease term is a medical construct that brings multiple observations under a convenient heading. As a medical construct, there is a sense in which a disease cannot, therefore, be the product of biological evolution. That said, all that is biologically associated with this construct—not least the signs and symptoms—has an evolutionary context. Thus, evolutionary medicine can only provide "evolutionary explanations for vulnerabilities to disease" in terms of the associated signs and symptoms that a body has the capacity to express.

TOWARDS AN EVOLUTIONARY CONCEPT OF "DIS-EASE"

One of the most striking statements to come out of evolutionary medicine when it was first popularized was the suggestion that certain unpleasant phenomena characteristic of illness could, in fact, be beneficial to the individual and that trying to quell something simply because it was unpalatable could do more harm than good. Indeed, one U.K. review of *Why We Get Sick* (as *Evolution and Healing*) was even entitled *Sickness Can Be Good For You*.[11] Although perhaps missing the technical meaning of "sickness," the sense of surprise, even irony, was clear. Included among these potentially beneficial, although unpleasant, phenomena were fever, vomiting, diarrhea, coughing, nausea, fatigue, pain, and anxiety, which, it has been suggested (Nesse & Williams 1994), might be considered as "defenses." Although there is a certain energetic cost associated with each, when exhibited they could be explained as conferring a net benefit on the sufferer. However, medicine has been typically concerned with making the patient feel better. As a result, the effect has sometimes been to target the body's own defenses and in so doing nullify the benefits the body is trying to confer upon itself.

As such, these "defense" mechanisms contribute, first and foremost, to individual survival. As a consequence, there are potential reproductive (evolutionary) benefits of a prolonged life in that the number of mating opportunities and potential offspring is increased. It was suggested that these "defenses" have been shaped by natural selection. However, what we can observe with regard to each of these defenses is likely to be only the "tip of the iceberg." When it comes to such mechanisms, we must remember that the physiological processes that combine to produce them are quite complex. The list of "defenses" offered by Nesse and Williams (1994) consists of some of the more striking physical responses we are able to mount. Other equally important but less obvious responses may be in need of identification lest they too be misunderstood and mismanaged. What is clear is that we have traditionally seen such responses in the wrong light and are only now beginning to see them for what they really are. Because of evolutionary medicine, no reaction—no sign or symptom—expressed by the body can now be safely viewed in the traditional way but must be re-evaluated in terms of its net costs and benefits to the survival of the individual.

A PLACE FOR MIND AND BODY

Nesse and Williams' (1994) position that all that concerns clinical medicine also concerns evolutionary medicine means that evolutionary theory comes to be applied in a similar way to both physical and mental conditions. This is not necessarily wrong; there may well be valid evolutionary explanations for certain mental phenomena and behaviors. However, it should not be forgotten that some find such positions difficult to accept (Rose & Rose, 2001). Academically, "mind" and "body" are usually studied in different departments—sometimes even in different faculties or schools—which may rarely, if ever, meet to share ideas. Even medicine, while dealing with problems of both mind and body under the same professional umbrella, does so via quite distinct specialties. There may be good reasons for dealing with certain conditions in this way. However, a particularly serious criticism of the Western biomedical model is that a patient's state of mind—or, at least, their experience of themselves during illness—is not given sufficient attention when considering the state of their body. It is frequently argued that a patient's predicament cannot be fully understood unless all that pertains to them is taken into account (Engel, 1977, 1981, 1997). Evolutionary medicine has the option of following one or other of the current approaches—or of forging a "third way." It can take an approach that is academic in style and for research and/or teaching purposes separate mind and body or it can take the approach, evident in medicine, of including mind and body under the same umbrella, that of evolutionary medicine, while still keeping a union of mind and body at a discrete distance. Alternatively, it can seek a different path that avoids the criticisms currently leveled at the biomedical model by finding a way of allowing mind—or at least self-experience—and body to be considered concurrently. If that were possible, instead of simply squeezing an extra evolutionary category into medicine's already extensive array of information, evolutionary medicine may have something distinctive to offer to the way in which medicine is practiced. This is likely to require further research into the ways in which an individual's self-experience and his or her physical state interrelate. However, knowing what that self-experience brings to an individual's condition—how that experience inclines one to react and the effect this has on the root cause of one's ailment—might then be reinforced as part of the treatment offered.

A noticeable feature of the "defenses" listed above is that, as a group, they do not fit neatly into a single category of sign or symptom. Fever, vomiting, diarrhea, and coughing, being discernable by an independent observer, have an objective element about them and so properly belong to the category of signs, whereas nausea, fatigue, pain, and anxiety are subjective and so properly belong to the category of symptoms. Thus, within this group of "defenses," we find both signs and symptoms working to the same biological end: that of individual survival. If the defenses which the body brings to its own aid belong to both subjective and objective—that is, experiential and physical—categories, it is questionable whether medicine can help the body achieve maximum benefit if aspects of both are not taken into account and used in concert for what each can bring to the well-being of the whole. This may also have ramifications at a conceptual level. Ten Have (1995) has suggested that for medicine—or for that matter, evolutionary medicine—to "evolve into a science of the human person, it should overcome the usual distinction between the objective and subjective" (p.10).

AND WHAT OF HEALTH?

So far, evolutionary medicine has tended to concentrate upon disease rather than health. This is in contradistinction to Lappé's first "axiom," given above, that we "need to understand the evolutionary origins of disease in order to fully comprehend their prevention." That is not to say that the promotion of health has been entirely devoid of attention. Eaton and colleagues, for example, have suggested how this may be approached from an evolutionary perspective (Eaton, Cordain, & Eaton, 2001; Eaton, Cordain, & Lindeberg, 2002; Eaton, Shostak, & Konner, 1988). However, to be health orientated requires an understanding of what health is. If, as the World Health Organization would have it, "health is not merely the absence of disease,"[12] then health must have its own particular characteristics. But, like "disease," the definition of "health" has caused considerable conceptual difficulties. For example, is being healthy much the same as being average (or "normal")—an approach that has been described as "naïve normalism" (Sadegh-Zadeh, 2000)—or is it a more idealized state that few, if any, ever attain?

Evolutionary medicine may not be able to solve this problem completely, but it may have something quite new to add that is in need of careful attention. As noted above, one of the most novel and striking ideas to come out of evolutionary medicine has been the suggestion that certain unpleasant phenomena that we associate with illness are, in fact, beneficial to the body. That being the case, it may be argued that the ability to mount a defensive response is a positive characteristic; a feature, one might suggest, of being healthy. Thus, a lesson that evolutionary medicine may teach is that certain aspects of illness may actually be a part of being healthy in that the body is acting in a self-preserving fashion. A healthy individual may be one who—among other things—can mount a defensive response that can help ensure individual survival. In short, certain aspects of what we have called illness may be characteristic of being healthy. A corollary of this lesson is that for the whole of human history up until now, we have used how "good" or "bad" we feel as a way of assessing the state of our bodies. Now we are coming to the realization that feeling "bad" can have positive connotations. A body that is able to mount a successful defense is surely a good thing even if it "feels bad" in doing so. Indeed, the experience of "feeling bad"[13] may itself confer benefits in terms of the behavioral modifications that often ensue. A case in point is the tendency to withdraw from the normal round of daily life. In so doing, the below-par individual removes himself from encounters that, in his weakened state, become potentially hazardous to survival. In humankind's original habitat, this would include having to deal with potentially life-threatening situations.

MORE THAN MEDICINE

Biologists interested in clinical problems have not tended to give the concepts of disease and health due consideration, but neither have the vast majority of clinicians. Applying evolutionary theory to the question of disease and health via evolutionary medicine, while keeping to standard medical perspectives, is unlikely to offer much conceptual advancement in understanding the biological significance and meaning of clinical phenomena. Indeed, mixing evolutionary theory's dynamic and often sophisticated ideas with lax or outmoded thinking about disease and health may be more likely to generate misconceptions than solutions. For example, if the prevailing medical view still held that disease was a product of an imbalance in the four bodily humors, then, if evolutionary medicine were to offer explanations couched in the same terms, those explanations would not only be false, they would further compound the misconceptions that that theory of disease promulgates.

Furthermore, there may be a downside to the use of the terms "Darwinian medicine" and "evolutionary medicine" in that, whichever term one uses, one finds that the emphasis falls on "medicine," which, in turn, implies the preserve of a sometimes exclusive medical profession. While medicine has much to gain from the application of evolutionary theory to its objects of interest, biology has much to gain from the enterprise too. As noted above, for a long time medicine has been closely associated with disease, whereas biology has been more closely associated with the "normal." By introducing disease as a concept that must be understood into biology, a more complete understanding of human biology is possible. Evolutionary medicine is an intellectual discipline that belongs to both medicine and biology and forms a point of common interest where both sides can meet in rigorous debate. It, therefore, occupies a unique and potentially privileged position where an exchange of ideas can pass in both directions. That this has not been a particularly prominent feature of the relationship between biology and medicine in the past may be due to the absence of the sort of bridge that evolutionary medicine now offers. One way of fostering a more open intellectual exchange between both sides is via conferences and periodicals that are specifically targeted at mixed audiences of clinicians, health workers, and nonclinical academics. Indeed, there exists a broader notion of an "evolutionary health science" where a much wider range of health professionals and allied workers can engage with evolutionary medicine. For example, as the role of nurses continues to change and they take on responsibilities formerly restricted to clinicians, they too will be in need of an evolutionary perspective within which to practice.

Applying evolutionary ideas to the objects of medicine should expand not only the clinical perspective but the biological perspective also. In so doing, we must be willing to go beyond considering only human beings. Already some key notions in evolutionary medicine have been derived from animal studies. A case in point is our current evolutionary perspective on fever (Kluger 1978, 1979, 1991). Fever, it has been suggested, is a mechanism whereby homeotherms (so-called warm-blooded animals) are able to raise their body temperature in response to infection. This has the benefit of impeding the activity of infectious agents and so has a clear adaptive advantage. Poikilotherms (so-called "cold-blooded" animals), who cannot do this physiologically, have adopted a different strategy. In response to infection, they increase their body temperature by seeking out warm places from which they can absorb heat. Conversely, an extension of evolutionary medicine for veterinarians has also been suggested (LeGrand & Brown 2002). Boaz (2002) goes further and provides an attempt at relating our present ailments to key points in our phylogenetic history. In so doing, he not only draws attention to the consequences of our evolutionary heritage, but implies that there are commonalities in pathophysiology associated with commonalities in structure and process. One striking example of this may be seen in museums displaying dinosaur skeletons. It is not uncommon to see in these exhibits evidence around the joints that demonstrates that, like us, dinosaurs experienced osteoarthritis. There may be numerous characteristics that we share with organisms to which we are only distantly related that can inform our understanding of not only our own ailments but those of other members of the animal kingdom.

A SPECIAL ROLE FOR BIOLOGISTS

The philosopher William Stempsey (2000), who had received residency training in pathology before turning to philosophy, suggested that the major task of pathologists was "to find morphological correlates and biological explanations of phenomena that clinicians and patients call disease." They did not, he argued, make fine distinctions between the theoretical and practical aspects of medicine. Where such distinctions were necessary in order to support various conceptual notions concerning disease,[14] someone better was needed. Biologists, he suggested, "would be the most likely candidates." In saying this, he implied something very subtle. If the role of pathologists is as he suggested, then there must be something extra that biologists should be able to contribute. In the present context, clearly one such "extra" is an evolutionary perspective. However, in suggesting a possible role for biologists, Stempsey also suggests that this "has the implausible consequence of holding that disease is best understood by people who are not physicians." I do not find this in the least bit implausible. In fact, I would argue to the contrary; it is biologists, I believe, who are potentially best situated to deal with these fine distinctions between the theoretical and practical aspects of medicine. Biologists may not have day-to-day clinical experience upon which to draw, but this is not necessarily a shortcoming that cannot be remedied. It is the biologist who is best suited to interpret human phenomena in terms of the characteristics demonstrated by animal life in general. It is the biologist who is able to take a more dispassionate view of the conceptual biological basis of the human physical condition. But they must be careful to do just that and not be affected by the ethical and moral concerns of medicine. Biologists need to apply evolutionary theory to questions of disease and health from a purely biological perspective and express their findings accordingly. Some conditions for which evolutionary medicine has been able to offer explanations are quite harrowing and concern issues of life and death. Sufferers from conditions such as cystic fibrosis and sickle cell anemia, for example, have limited life expectancies and a number of other difficulties to endure in the meantime. In describing these conditions from an evolutionary perspective, evolutionary medicine has been able to avoid any implication that the value of the lives of such individuals differs in any way from that of others. To do so would be to speak in terms that do not belong to biology, whose aim is, first of all, to understand.

Textbooks of general medicine, if written by people such as these, would be no smaller given the weight of the information that they would be compelled to convey, but they would not be the same as before, nor would they necessarily have a separate section on evolutionary explanations added to the "traditional headings." Instead, they would be described from the perspective of evolutionary biology, which would provide the guiding intellectual framework within which different states of the individual as an integrated organism could be understood.

EVOLUTIONARY MEDICINE AS A GUIDING HEURISTIC

Although evolution by natural selection is a relatively simple idea that many find instantly compelling, one should not overlook the fact that there are also aspects that are conceptually complex. If evolutionary ideas are to gain a foothold in medicine, perhaps it is advisable to emphasize the general picture before elaborating upon the less intuitive aspects. There is certainly a general evolutionary picture that can be usefully portrayed, one that health workers and laypeople alike can understand. In that sense, evolutionary medicine can be used as a heuristic or commonsense rule serving as a useful guide to understanding.

Evolutionary ideas do indeed appear to be creeping into everyday medical thinking. In the British media, it is not uncommon for one to encounter discussions of certain conditions given with an evolutionary nuance. Certainly, there is now an appreciation that there is a mismatch between our present environment and that within which our ancestors evolved. Furthermore, in the waiting rooms of British general practitioners, one can now find leaflets about the dangers of antibiotic resistance and how the patient has an important role in combating this, described in implicitly evolutionary terms. These are perhaps small beginnings, but the ultimate success of evolutionary medicine may not be that it will be cited at all turns but that it will form the unstated heuristic by which the biological bases of medicine are understood.

However, evolution's simplicity and beauty can be deceptive. It should not be forgotten that there is a vastness about evolution in that it applies to all living things. Indeed, it is what makes biology make sense (Dobzhansky, 1973). We are aware of a number of the mechanisms involved in bringing about evolutionary change, but we can never be sure that we know them all or that we have ever understood those of which we are aware fully. Arguably, there is something transcendent[15] about evolution in that it goes beyond our ordinary range of experience and understanding. Indeed, there may yet be new ways of understanding the richness of biological evolution that our current intellectual framework does not fully allow us to recognize. It is perhaps inevitable that different workers will adopt different intellectual perspectives as they grapple with different facets of evolution. Thus, evolutionary medicine will do well to adopt a circumspect attitude when offering its explanations. Furthermore, just as we should be careful not to reify disease, we should also be careful not to reify evolution as some kind of force when it is better understood as an emergent phenomenon that is evident when certain conditions apply (Ridley, 2004).

THE END OF A BEGINNING

Nesse and Williams (1994, p. 11) were right to point out that:

> [A]n evolutionary perspective on disease does not change the ancient goals of medicine carved on a statue honouring physician E. L. Trudeau's work at Saranac Lake: "To cure, sometimes, To help, often, To console, always." The goal of medicine has always been (and, in our belief, always should be) to help the sick, not the species.

Clearly, it is the practical outworking of medical knowledge that concerns clinicians. However, one still detects that many in the medical profession also have nagging doubts about evolutionary medicine. Questions such as "What is its practical use?" and "What improvements to treatment follow from it?" are typical. Given the breadth of medical specialties that exist, answering these questions is not straightforward. Simply providing lists of known or speculated benefits offers some useful illustrations, but does not provide a complete answer to such questions. The practical impact of evolutionary medicine cannot be expected to be the same for every human ailment. Furthermore, some clinical specialties may benefit more than others—perhaps some will not benefit at all. Perhaps we should be ready to accept that while evolutionary medicine may be able to contribute to important advances in certain areas of human suffering, it may also reveal that we are limited in what we can do in others. But while some areas have attracted particular attention, as yet, nothing like an "audit" of where evolutionary medicine best applies appears to have been performed. While evolutionary medicine may have a role with regard to the treatment of infectious conditions, cancer, and some immune conditions, it is harder to see how much practical impact it might have on orthopedics or orthodontics, for example.

However, apart from these practical concerns, it is possible that what evolutionary medicine brings to the conceptual arena in understanding, not only notions of disease and health, but of the human being as an organism, will be that which proves to be of particular and wide-ranging significance. It proposes new ways of looking at old familiar issues. Some of these have been highlighted here. In so doing, new perspectives have begun to emerge. Evolutionary medicine helps us take a different view of disease and health within a biological context—and in so doing, we may begin to understand life and living in new and quite different ways.

ACKNOWLEDGMENTS

I would like to give particular thanks to the trustees and fellows of the Konrad Lorenz Institute, Altenberg, Austria, where, as a Visiting Fellow, I was able to explore some of the ideas expressed in this chapter. I would also like to thank Annette Lewis for her help in preparing the manuscript for this chapter.

CHAPTER 23

The Importance of Evolution
for Medicine

Randolph M. Nesse

As one of the "fathers" of evolutionary medicine, Nesse's sense of confidence
can be seen as he assesses from the perspective of a more mature discipline
the potential sticking points and inherent differences between clinical practice and basic medical research, medical culture, theories, and practice. His
analysis of the "state of the field" helps to establish in this chapter a realistic
and critical perspective on the early years of evolutionary thinking and moves
to offering advice on what can be done better and, more generally, what can
be done to assure expansion, integration, and growth toward the future of
the field. He provides some advice about how to assure that research itself
will continue and directs his comments to what in the future, from the framing of an evolutionary medicine curriculum to pedagogy to a teaching
point of view, needs yet to be done. That he ends his chapter and, not coin-
cidentally, this volume with a concrete curriculum for the teaching of
Darwinian medicine is one significant indicator that, as this volume hopes
also to assure, the next wave of this new application of evolutionary principles to sustaining and improving human health is not just around the corner
but is already here.

INTRODUCTION

The importance of evolutionary biology for medicine should be obvious. Medicine is
based on biology and biology is based on evolution, so you would think that medicine
would long ago have applied evolutionary principles in every possible way. Would that it
were so! Instead, nearly a century and a half after publication of *The Origin of Species*
(Darwin, 1859), medicine is just beginning to make full use of evolutionary biology.
The chapters in this book illustrate the rapid progress and substantial promise of evolutionary medicine. Each examines a particular problem or bodily system and shows how
an evolutionary perspective can deepen understanding. In conjunction with other recent
and forthcoming publications, they document the many specific ways that evolution is
important for medicine.

This chapter does not attempt to review these specific contributions, but instead steps back to address several more general questions. What is evolutionary medicine? Should it be a distinct field? What is its history? How can it be useful? How can evolutionary hypotheses about disease be tested? And, what is needed to move work forward faster at the intersection of evolution and medicine? The theme throughout is that quickly trying to meet demands for direct clinical applications now may limit the scope of the field in the long run. While evolutionary medicine has some useful applications, its greater promise arises from its ability to pose new research questions and to offer a solid framework for integrating much medical knowledge about why our bodies are so vulnerable to disease.

WHAT IS EVOLUTIONARY MEDICINE?

Evolutionary medicine is the enterprise of using evolutionary biology to address the problems of medicine. Some areas of medicine, such as infectious disease and genetics, have long been grounded in evolutionary biology. For them, the main question is how they can best incorporate and contribute to new advances in evolutionary biology. Many of the more recent applications of evolution in medicine address somewhat different questions about the adaptive significance of aspects of the body that make it vulnerable to diseases. This emphasis on adaptive functions has long been at the center of physiology, where such questions are so intrinsic to the discipline that they sometimes are not even recognized as evolutionary. Anatomy is also inherently based on evolution, although time pressures in the medical curriculum have greatly reduced its ability to provide a comparative perspective. Other topics, however, such as nutrition, pharmacology, and even developmental biology, are often still researched and taught with little attention to evolutionary principles. Opportunities for progress are plentiful.

It is easy to offer a few specific examples of how evolution can help in the clinic today, such as how a deeper understanding of host–pathogen co-evolution can assist in managing antibiotic resistance, or the need to consider the utility of defenses such as fever and cough before prescribing medication. However, the great benefits of evolution in medicine will emerge from new research and from the framework evolution provides for understanding why organisms are vulnerable to disease.

Why We Get Sick (Nesse & Williams, 1994) ends with the famous Dobzhansky quotation, "Nothing in biology makes sense except in the light of evolution" (1973). The quotation is not, however, entirely correct. While evolution is essential to make complete sense of any trait, much biology proceeds without much attention to evolution. Examples include studies of drug outcomes, endocrine mechanisms, epidemiology, and research that identifies new genetic variations. Most work in biology is, however, connected to evolution; in medicine, most is not. This should not be surprising. Medicine is not a science, it is a profession. To prevent and treat disease it uses tradition and empirical studies along with basic science. Setting a bone, doing a colonoscopy, treating acne, or treating diabetes, depression, or hypertension is mostly a matter of technical knowledge and routine. Doctors do not need to know why the appendix persists in order to treat appendicitis or why modern humans are prone to atherosclerosis to treat heart failure.

The best doctors are wary of grand theories, and for good reason. Consider homeopathy. This long-standing alternative medicine recommends infinitesimal doses of drugs that cause symptoms similar to the patient's complaints, using the rationale of Samuel Hahnemann's principle *Similia Similibus Curentur* (like cures like) (Hahnemann, 1916). Dozens of similarly simple theories entrance patients and physicians alike. Many attribute most diseases to one cause, whether sugar, imbalances in energy flow, misalignment of the spine, or stress. Such factors do contribute to disease; the problem is the human tendency to simplify by overemphasizing one cause. Likewise, it is attractive to think that one treatment can work for the vast majority of diseases. Practitioners understandably recommend the kind of treatment they provide. Surgeons recommend surgery, internists recommend medications, nutritionists recommend dietary change, and psychotherapists recommend whatever kind of psychotherapy they offer. Theories tend to be too simple, and patients are often shortchanged.

In short, good doctors are justifiably wary of theories in general. They will embrace evolutionary biology as a foundation for medicine only after they recognize evolutionary biology as a basic science for medicine. In contrast to other theories, evolutionary medicine does not overemphasize one cause or one treatment. Most important of all, it does not does not make direct clinical recommendations and should not be the basis for a special kind of medical practice. Instead, it suggests new research questions whose answers, carefully validated, will improve clinical care. It also provides a framework for deeper understanding of every disease and every patient. The importance of these two benefits is addressed below at length.

Concerns that evolutionary medicine will distort clinical practice are premature at best. The growth of the field has been almost entirely in research institutes and basic science classrooms. While many undergraduates now get an introduction to evolution as a basic science for medicine, no medical school has a systematic course on the applications of evolutionary biology in medicine. Only a handful of medical schools have any evolutionary biologists on the faculty (Nesse & Schiffman, 2003). Every month several well-qualified physicians and researchers contact me to ask where they can get specialized training to pursue research in Darwinian medicine; so far no such program exists. While it would be wonderful if evolution was already recognized as the foundation for medicine, we are far from that goal; the idea of evolutionary or Darwinian medicine remains essential in order to develop work in the field.

The above paragraphs emphasize some difficulties encountered in bringing evolutionary biology to bear more fully on the problems of medicine. Why not just focus on the many positive recent developments? Because the above difficulties and related obstacles are keeping medicine from making full use of evolutionary biology. Recognizing and overcoming them will speed progress. Another important principle is to promise only what we can deliver, taking care not to overstate the practical benefits that evolutionary medicine offers now. Evolutionary medicine is not focused on a specific clinical problem or one aspect of the body's mechanisms; its contributions are more like those of embryology, biochemistry, and other basic sciences.

NOMENCLATURE

What should we call work at the interface of medicine and evolutionary biology? A brief historical review may help minimize the distraction about the matter. This volume and its predecessor use the phrase "evolutionary medicine" (Trevathan, McKenna, & Smith, 1999). The other major overview edited volume, also published by Oxford University Press, is titled *Evolution in Health and Disease* (Stearns, 1998). In our 1991 article and 1994 book, Williams and I used the phrase "Darwinian medicine" (Nesse & Williams, 1994; Williams & Nesse, 1991). A brief note is in order to explain why we chose "Darwinian medicine" instead of "evolutionary medicine."

I argued for calling the field "evolutionary medicine," on the belief that this would speed acceptance by staying away from any "ism," by dissociating the field from the negative connotations that Darwin has for many people, and by not associating the field too closely with one scientist. George Williams argued for a more exacting approach, noting that "evolution" refers to any gradual change over time and does not necessarily refer to natural selection or even biology. He noted that "Darwinism" signals close attention to natural selection, and that we should not shy away from crediting the great man whose work inspired us. He convinced me. While "Darwinian medicine" is more exact, on practical grounds it has disadvantages because so many people associate the term "Darwinism" with ruthless competition. The designation "evolutionary medicine" reduces these concerns, but only modestly. The search term "Darwinian medicine" yields more specific results than "evolutionary medicine," but neither locates all relevant research. After talking with many people about the alternatives, my main conclusion is that debate about nomenclature is not especially useful. In order to provide a designation as general and inclusive as possible, I now call the field "evolution and medicine." This avoids any possible misunderstanding about the field being excessively circumscribed and emphasizes the intersection between the basic science of evolutionary biology and the applied profession of medicine. The web site EvolutionAndMedicine.org strives for the broadest possible coverage of work in the field.

THE HISTORY OF EVOLUTIONARY MEDICINE

The first mention of the potential utility of evolution for medicine is found in Darwin, not Charles, but his grandfather, the physician and poet Erasmus Darwin. The preface to his 1796 philosophical poem, *Zoonomia*, contains a remarkably prescient description of evolution, as well as its potential as a foundation for medicine (Darwin, 1796, pp. vii-viii; italics and capitalization as in original):

> The purport of the following pages is an endeavor to reduce the facts belonging to ANIMAL LIFE into classes, orders, genera, and species; and, by comparing them with each other, to unravel the theory of diseases. It happened, perhaps unfortunately for the inquirers into the knowledge of diseases, that other sciences had received improvement previous to their own; whence, instead of comparing the properties belonging to animated nature with each other, they, idly ingenious, busied themselves in attempting to explain the laws of life by those of mechanism and chemistry; they considered the body as an hydraulic machine, and the fluids as passing through a series of chemical changes, forgetting that animation was its essential characteristic.
>
> The great CREATOR of all things has infinitely diversified the works of his hands, but has at the same time stamped a certain similitude on the features of nature, that demonstrates to us, that the whole is one family of one parent. On this similitude is

founded all rational analogy; which, so long as it is concerned in comparing the essential properties of bodies, leads us to many and important discoveries; but when with licentious activity it links together objects, otherwise discordant, by some fanciful similitude; it may indeed collect ornaments for wit and poetry, but philosophy and truth recoil from its combinations.

The want of a theory, deduced from such strict analogy, to conduct the practice of medicine is lamented by its professors; for, as a great number of unconnected facts are difficult to be acquired, and to be reasoned from, the art of medicine is in many instances less efficacious under the direction of its wisest practitioners; and by that busy crowd, who either boldly wade in darkness, or are led into endless error by the glare of false theory, it is daily practiced to the destruction of thousands; add to this the unceasing injury which accrues to the public by the perpetual advertisements of pretended nostrums; the minds of the indolent become superstitiously fearful of diseases, which they do not labour under; and thus become the daily prey of some crafty empyric.

A theory founded upon nature, that should bind together the scattered facts of medical knowledge, and converge into one point of view the laws of organic life, would thus on many accounts contribute to the interest of society. It would capacitate men of moderate abilities to practice the art of healing with real advantage to the public; it would enable every one of literary acquirements to distinguish the genuine disciples of medicine from those of boastful effrontery, or of wily address; and would teach mankind in some important situations the knowledge of themselves.

There are some modern practitioners, who declaim against medical theory in general, not considering that to think is to theorize; and that no one can direct a method of cure to a person labouring under disease without thinking, that is, without theorizing; and happy therefore is the patient, whose physician possesses the best theory.

These lines are remarkable on several counts. In the first paragraph, Erasmus Darwin notes the need for a theoretical foundation for medicine, he chides those who think of the body as only a machine, and he presages the distinction between proximate and evolutionary explanations. In the second paragraph, he anticipates the origin of species, with the phrase, "*the whole is one family of one parent*." He concludes by arguing in support of my main thesis: that the theory can "bind together the scattered facts of medical knowledge," providing a framework that "would capacitate men of moderate abilities to practice the art of healing with real advantage." Unfortunately, little has changed. Many physicians still see the body as a designed machine instead of an evolved organism, and myriads of medical facts remain unconnected, awaiting a scientific framework.

Of course, there was no real theory to justify Erasmus Darwin's vision until his grandson Charles Darwin and Alfred Wallace discovered natural selection. In the century and a half since the publication of *The Origin of Species* (1859), one would think that these ideas would have been applied to medicine in every possible way, but it now appears that we are still just getting started. Why it has taken so long is a good question for historians; the one available history of Darwinian medicine is not yet available in English (Zampieri, 2006).

While we wait for historians to address the issue, some reasons for the delay seem straightforward. One is the slow acceptance of Darwinism in general. Opposition from religious quarters is part of the picture. Some doctors are creationists, and a remarkable number of physicians think intelligent design is a viable alternative to evolution. They are too few to constitute a major obstacle in themselves, but together with community sentiment, they make deans and other leaders wary of public commitments to evolution that may arouse controversy.

A more significant impediment has been skepticism among scientists. At the end of the nineteenth century, many scientists thought natural selection was a theory whose time had passed (Richards, 1987). In particular, Darwin's notion of hereditary transmission from generation to generation via "gemmules" was recognized as incorrect. Also, many scientists believed the critique of the leading physicist of the time, Lord Kelvin, who used the laws of heat radiation to calculate that the earth could not possibly be older than 20,000 years or it would be merely a cold rock (Kelvin, Tait, & Darwin, 1883). This bit of physics was, for many scientists, sufficient to outweigh all Darwin's arguments and the accumulating fossil evidence. The rediscovery of genetics in the first years of the twentieth century eventually provided the foundation for new work on evolution, but early on it was more often seen as proof that Darwin's theory of heredity was wrong than as evidence that his theory of natural selection was right.

Another reason for delay was the timing of the great curricular reforms in medicine instituted by Flexner (1910). He proposed adding basic science education during the early decades of the twentieth century, just when evolutionary biology was in maximum eclipse (Richards, 1987). Not until the synthesis with population genetics in the 1930s and 1940s was evolutionary theory widely accepted (Mayr, 1982). Even then, however, applications to medicine developed slowly save for a few exceptions. Population genetics quickly became sophisticated; its initial focus on single gene mutations with medical effects emphasized the role of selection in eliminating deleterious mutations and the power of random factors to influence gene prevalence. The study of adaptation became a foundation for physiology (Schmidt-Nielsen, 1990) and inspired the emergence of modern animal behavior from its precursors in ethology (Alcock, 2001). However, an effective attack on excesses of "adaptationism" (Gould & Lewontin, 1979) got such wide attention that even today, despite many rebuttals (Queller, 1995) and reliable methods (Reeve & Sherman, 1993), many medical researchers remain wary about studying evolutionary questions about function.

The increasing use of antibiotics in the mid-twentieth century was followed quickly by recognition of antibiotic resistance (Cohen, 1992). Here, finally, was an example of natural selection in action. This was not, however, "nice" natural selection shaping wonderful adaptations; instead, it adapts bacteria so our antibiotics can no longer kill them. Perhaps this is why antibiotic resistance is often described as "change" or "adaptation" without explicit mention of evolution. Nonetheless, antibiotic resistance demonstrates that selection can take place before our eyes with profound clinical consequences.

As already noted, microbiology and population genetics are the established elders in the evolutionary medicine family. Their progress is increasingly fast as they make use of newly available genetic information. The question is whether they might advance yet faster if they incorporated evolutionary principles more systematically. In infectious disease, fundamental advances (Anderson & May, 1979; May & Anderson, 1979) and the synthesis offered in Ewald's book (Ewald, 1994), as well as more recent advances (Anderson, 2004; Ebert, 1998; Levin & Bull, 1994), suggest that there is much more to come. Genetics is quickly getting past the technical problems of genotyping and on to evolutionary questions about genes that predispose to disease (Lewontin, Singh, & Krimbas, 2000; Maynard Smith, 1998).

Many recent efforts to further develop the field of evolution and medicine have addressed somewhat different questions. Instead of studying the actions of selection on

TABLE 23-1 Tinbergen's Four Questions

Proximate Questions
    1. *Mechanism*—What is structure and composition of the trait and
       how does it work?
    2. *Ontogeny*—How does the trait develop in an individual?

Evolutionary Questions
    3. *Phylogeny*—What is the evolutionary history of this trait?
    4. *Selective Advantage*—What selection forces shaped this trait?

genes and pathogens directly, this new emphasis begins from the principle that all biological phenomena need evolutionary, as well as separate proximate explanations (Tinbergen, 1963). Proximate explanations are about the body's mechanisms, how they work, and how they develop from a strand of DNA. Evolutionary explanations are about the phylogeny of the body's components and what selection forces shaped them to their present form. Both kinds of explanations are needed for every aspect of the body. Full recognition of the value of this distinction has been slow in medicine. It was advocated effectively by Niko Tinbergen (1963) and Ernst Mayr (1982, 2004), but so far medical research has made full use of only the proximate half of biology; many physicians have not even heard of Tinbergen's "four questions." There is not room here to describe them in detail, but Table 23-1 summarizes them as two kinds of questions (proximate and evolutionary) about two different objects of explanation (a trait at one time and the series of events that create a trait).

Williams and I began by trying to find evolutionary explanations for diseases. We soon recognized that this was a mistake; with a few exceptions, natural selection does not shape diseases. Progress came when we shifted the focus to shared traits that leave all members of a species vulnerable to a disease—traits such as the appendix, the narrow pelvic outlet, and the limitations of the immune response. We began posing questions about vulnerability to disease in the form: "Why has natural selection left this species vulnerable to this disease?" The potential explanations can be sorted into the six categories listed in Table 23-2.

These six categories have been discussed at length elsewhere (Nesse, 2005; Nesse & Williams, 1994, 1998), so they will not be described in detail here. It is important to recognize that multiple factors may contribute to vulnerability to one disease. For instance, vulnerability to atherosclerosis arises from a mismatch with the modern environment and also from trade-offs involving the endothelium's ability to protect against infection. These causes can be subdivided and categorized in other ways. In the definitive review of the growth of evolutionary contributions to medicine, Stearns and Ebert offer a more differentiated list of possible factors (Stearns & Ebert, 2001). Most categories in the first part of their list correspond to one of the six factors in Table 23-2, but they treat genetic variations separately, offering a very useful taxonomy of reasons for the origins and maintenance of variations that may be associated with disease.

The development of evolutionary medicine was advanced by conferences as well as publications. Several major gatherings in the 1990s brought together scientists working on topics in evolution and medicine, but the most influential was the conference organized by Stephen Stearns. The resulting edited volume, *Evolution in Health and Disease* (Stearns, 1998), was pivotal for connecting work in the field with established lines

TABLE 23-2 Six Categories of Reasons for Vulnerability to Disease

---

Natural selection is slow

1) **Mismatch:** Our bodies were shaped for environments far different from those we live in, and the mismatch gives rise to much disease. This explanation is emphasized in this volume and its predecessor.

2) **Co-evolution with fast-evolving pathogens:** Because their generation times are so much shorter, pathogens evolve much faster than we can, so evolution cannot provide perfect protection against infection.

There are limits to what selection can shape

3) **Constraints:** There is much that selection simply cannot do, such as starting a design from scratch to fix a design defect such as the vessels in the eyeball running between the light and the retina, or creating a gene replication method that never makes mistakes.

4) **Trade-offs:** Inevitable trade-offs make every trait suboptimal; for instance, if our vision was as acute as that of the eagle, our color vision and field of vision would be worse.

Common difficulties in understanding what selection shapes

5) **Reproduction at the expense of health:** Natural selection increases the frequency of genes that yield a net increase in reproduction even if they compromise health and longevity.

6) **Defenses:** Defenses such as pain, fever, nausea, vomiting, and fatigue are not problems, but useful responses shaped by natural selection.

---

of medical research. Published about the same time, the first edition of *Evolutionary Medicine* (Trevathan et al., 1999) instead emphasized connections with anthropology and topics such as child development, reproductive health, diet, and changes in the environment. The limited overlap of the topics covered in these two volumes reflects differences between preexisting disciplines. Whether the disciplinary barriers will lead to speciation or continued exchange and hybrid vigor remains uncertain.

HOW CAN EVOLUTIONARY BIOLOGY BE USEFUL FOR MEDICINE?

On first hearing about the field of Darwinian medicine, every news reporter and most doctors and medical school deans ask, "How can Darwinian medicine help doctors practice better today?" One is tempted to reply, as Benjamin Franklin did upon being asked about the utility of the just-invented hot air balloon, "What good is a newborn baby?" The question of the practical utility of evolutionary biology for medicine is, however, sincere and deep. We should be grateful to those who want to apply every advance as quickly as possible. However, probing questions are an appropriate response to those who demand practical benefits before they will invest in learning, supporting, or teaching an established body of knowledge that has such utility for medicine. Examples of such short-sightedness are legion. To take one, as the Rockefeller Institute was being organized, some argued that a large investment was not justified because biochemistry had not proven its practical utility. Genomic research, by contrast, is now generously funded, probably because so many diseases are caused by specific genes and because many other diseases show large genetic influences. So far, however, the billions of dollars invested in genetic research have provided remarkably little benefit in day-to-day clinical treatment. That will likely soon change. But if 5% of the investment in genetic research was put towards investigating evolutionary questions about disease, the benefits would likely be

TABLE 23-3 Contributions Evolution Can Make to Medicine

1. Expanding evolution's contribution to existing research enterprises that rely on it (e.g., genetics, infectious disease, and research on aging)
2. Providing a theoretical foundation for epidemiology and public health
3. Heuristic value: formulating new questions about disease that motivate new studies
4. Unifying research from different disciplines
5. Providing a framework for understanding disease from the perspective of evolutionary as well as proximate biology

as large as those we have seen so far from the genomic revolution. Among a hundred other valuable projects, it would be relatively inexpensive to find out whether lowering fever slows recovery from influenza, whether uric acid levels are correlated with rates of tissue aging, whether there are benefits to high bilirubin immediately after birth, and whether the capacity for depressed mood is sometimes useful. The results of such investigations would have immediate clinical utility.

Citing examples of how evolution motivates research that will improve clinical care is worthwhile, but it is important to emphasize that finding quick fixes is not the main goal. As in the case of other basic sciences, many benefits will emerge only after years of research. In addition, some of the most profound benefits may arise, not from specific research findings, but from the secure framework evolution provides for synthesizing knowledge from every area of medicine into a more organic understanding of disease.

Lists of contributions evolution can make to medicine tend to jumble very different kinds of things. The categories in Table 23-3 help to differentiate some of the ways in which evolutionary medicine can be useful.

1. Expanding Evolution's Contribution in Research Enterprises That Already Rely on It

Most scientists who study genetics or infectious disease already ground their work in evolutionary biology. Infectious disease and genetic researchers with a background in evolutionary biology tell me, however, that evolutionary theory is by no means fully utilized in their fields and many of their colleagues have outmoded notions about natural selection. The levels at which selection works, for instance, remains a major stumbling block; many otherwise well-educated scientists are unaware of the revolution in biology initiated by recognition that selection rarely acts for the good of the species (Williams, 1966).

Interestingly, many studies of antibiotic resistance do not describe the process as natural selection, and very few systematically analyze the trade-offs between better protection against infection and the risks of damage from protective mechanisms (Anderson, 2004). The notion that pathogens and hosts co-evolve is widespread, but not all scientists recognize the ubiquity of arms races and how selection for defenses and counterdefenses leaves both host and pathogen vulnerable to new problems. Mathematical models of pathogen evolution are becoming more sophisticated, and their conclusions can have immediate applications. For instance, some hospitals have tried to prevent antibiotic resistance by shifting to a different preferred antibiotic every 6 months or so. Evolutionary-based mathematical modeling demonstrates, however, that such regimes may hasten development of antibiotic resistance; using multiple agents may be a better strategy (Bergstrom, Lo, & Lipsitch, 2004). The implications of influenza evolution for vaccine design are increasingly considered systematically, with models now even making predictions about which strain of influenza is likely to evolve next; the public health implications are obvious and valuable (Ghedin et al., 2005; Smith, 2006).

While all genetics is based on evolutionary biology, simple models of mutation–selection balance and drift predominate in many texts, and there is a tendency, especially in medical research, to presume that genes associated with diseases are defects. For instance, the ApoE4 allele is associated with atherosclerosis and Alzheimer's disease, but it is not a new mutation but the universal genotype in our primate ancestors (Finch & Sapolsky, 1999). On the other hand, criteria for assessing possible selection advantages associated with such genes remain weak. For instance, it is very difficult to tell if ApoE4 offers benefits that help to maintain its prevalence in the gene pool.

New techniques for measuring the signals of natural selection are identifying genes that have been subject to recent positive selection (Ronald & Akey, 2005; Sabeti et al., 2006). The organizer of a meeting at Cold Spring Harbor, Douglas Wallace, has proposed calling work in this field "evolutionary medicine" (Olson, 2002). Studies of "knockout genes," whose function has been eliminated in certain lines of mice, rats or fruit flies, are fundamentally evolutionary studies about the adaptive significance of genes, but they are often described with little reference to natural selection. For instance, the finding that as many as 30% of genes can be knocked out with no observable effect is sometimes interpreted to mean that many genes are not necessary; an evolutionary view suggests that many genes are selected for because they provide benefits in the face of certain environmental challenges such as starvation, infection with a certain organism, or mating competition.

2. Providing a Theoretical Foundation for Epidemiology and Public Health

Environmental factors that increase disease vulnerability are the focus of public health and anthropology. This volume emphasizes such factors, especially those that are novel in modern environments. Public health has made remarkable strides without a foundational theory, but work like that reported in this volume suggests that evolutionary biology could provide a unifying framework. For instance, an evolutionary perspective on common chronic diseases of adult life, such as hypertension and atherosclerosis, focuses suspicion on novel aspects of our modern environment, such as the new availability of a wonderful diversity of delicious foods we cannot resist. Novel aspects of the environment are immediate suspects for any common disease that is vastly more prevalent now than it was for hunter gatherers, and for any condition with high heritability that causes early death.

Many genetic contributions to vulnerability are not defects but "quirks"; they cause little harm in the natural environment, but cause disease when they interact with aspects of the modern environment. In contrast, rare genetic diseases are far more likely to arise from mutations. Geographical differences in the prevalence of some diseases appear to arise in part from differences in gene frequencies resulting from natural selection. For instance, the prevalence of different alleles of the GNB3 gene vary in a latitudinal gradient and strongly predict vulnerability to high blood pressure (Young et al., 2005).

3. Heuristic Value

A third way evolution can be useful to medicine is by suggesting new questions. Asking why body is the way it is, and why it is vulnerable to disease, is not new. In fact, it was a theme of William Paley's book *Natural Theology* (Paley, 1970 [1802]). This book originated the analogy of the body with a watch, whose intricacies demonstrated, Paley said, the hand of a designer. Paley was, however, an astute observer who found much in the body that seemed preposterously designed, such as the wandering path of the recurrent laryngeal nerve, descending to below the neck before coming back up to the vocal cords. In a classic example of staying true to the evidence and shifting the theory to fit, he suggested that God placed all manner of such anomalies in the body for scientists to study and wonder at. His examples make good reading today, as they did for Darwin. They also illustrate the seductive appeal of intelligent design.

While the body's flaws are no longer presented as evidence for design, they remain a staple of conversations in the medical lunchroom. "Why," one doctor will ask another jokingly, "did the good Lord create one passage for both food and air, thus making choking possible?" What is new is not the questions, but the opportunity to take them seriously, formulating alternative hypotheses, and testing them. This was facilitated by increasing recognition of the need for both proximate and evolutionary explanations as suggested by Tinbergen and Mayr and by the work of Williams (1992), Hamilton (1995), Trivers (2002), and others who posed evolutionary questions about traits such as senescence, sexual reproduction, and menopause. While debates about the scientific study of adaptation set back the study of functions in biology (Gould & Lewontin, 1979), they also called much attention to such questions and encouraged greater rigor (Segerstråle, 2000).

The core idea that we should seek reasons for the body's vulnerability to every disease now seems relatively well accepted in evolutionary medicine. A hundred examples are possible, but relatively few are strongly supported and even fewer have major practical implications. For instance, it seems likely that human vulnerability to gout results from the trade-off antioxidant benefits of high levels uric acid, but this by no means proven (Ames, Cathcart, Schwiers, & Hochstein, 1981; Moe, 2006), and I doubt that it has influenced clinical recommendations. Likewise, the antioxidant properties of bilirubin are well documented (Stocker, Yamamoto, McDonagh, Glazer, & Ames, 1987) and the oxidative stress on newborns emerging into the atmosphere is clear, but whether this should influence criteria for putting infants with mild bilirubin increases under lights to reduce bilirubin levels has not been considered as far as I know.

As demonstrated by the chapters in this book, evolutionary thinking encourages asking new research questions. Is menstruation necessary? Why does mountain sickness exist? Do conditions in early life influence later ovarian function in ways that are generally useful even though they increase the risk of cancer? Evolution is not the method for answering these questions, but it is essential to inspire asking them in the first place. An evolutionary perspective also suggests scores of studies that should have been done long ago. Does taking drugs to reduce fever speed or slow recovery from influenza and other common infections? Is menopause explained because taking care of grandchildren increases one's genes in the next generation more than having more children (Hawkes,

2004; Williams, 1957)? Do genes compete with each other within the individual in ways that cause disease (Haig, 1993)? Are negative emotions like anxiety and depression useful (Nesse, 1999)? Is crying by infants useful aside from signaling the need for something (Barr, 1990)? The list of good questions could go on for pages. Without an evolutionary perspective, no one would think to ask them.

4. Unifying Research from Different Disciplines

Evolutionary studies of infection, genetic diseases, novel environmental causes, and reasons for the bodies' vulnerability have proceeded along relatively separate tracks. Each may benefit from closer contact with the others. For instance, it increasingly appears that genetic contributions to disease often arise from otherwise harmless genetic variations interacting with novel environmental factors. A genetic polymorphism may even influence vulnerability to lead toxicity (Kelada, Shelton, Kaufmann, & Khoury, 2001). Some genetic variations that moderate the effects of environmental factors are products of selection. Sickle cell anemia is the exemplar. The allele that causes sickle cell disease was selected for in Africa where it protects against malaria (Livingstone, 1971). A variety of other genetic variations also protect against malaria (Kwiatkowski, 2005), such as absence of the Duffy antigen (Hamblin & Di Rienzo, 2000). At least one genotype, $\alpha +$ thalassemia, may offer protection by increasing the risk of getting a mild form of malaria in childhood, which provides immunological protection against severe malaria later (Weatherall, 1997). The mutation that protects against HIV infection is present more frequently in northern Europe (Martinson, Hong, Karanicolas, Moore, & Kostrikis, 2000), although the explanation for this remains elusive.

Will researchers in areas as diverse as genetics, epidemiology, child development, and vaccine development see a benefit to extending their identities to evolution and medicine more generally instead of just their core disciplines? The pressures to keep up in any specialized area are severe, but evolutionary biology offers a simple and secure framework to allow meaningful collaborations across diverse disciplines.

5. Developing a Framework for Understanding Disease

This section began with the refrain, "How is evolutionary medicine useful in the clinic right now?" Given the many ways evolution can contribute to medicine, such narrow practicality is frustrating. Students learn thousands of important things in medical school that contribute to their overall understanding, even though they do not directly influence clinical care. Many concepts from embryology, biochemistry, physiology, genetics, and histology are in the curriculum not because they tell doctors what to do, but because doctors need a scientific framework that makes sense of what is otherwise a hodgepodge of unconnected facts. From this point of view, evolutionary biology should be at the very center of the medical curriculum. It is the ultimate foundation for all other basic sciences in the curriculum; it is the only one that can unify the rest into a consilient whole (Wilson, 1998).

Those who devote their careers to medical education are all too aware that their curricula cannot present all the knowledge medical students need, much less ensure that students learn it. Their first response to the suggestion of adding a new course on evolution is to describe the impossibility of adding one more hour to the curriculum. Given that most medical schools do not have even one evolutionary biologist on the faculty, the outlook for getting future doctors up to speed in the basic medical science of evolution would seem dim. However, the very frustration with the current system, and recognition that it consists of thousands of poorly connected facts, provides an opportunity to start from scratch in a way that natural selection never can. Sometime soon, a student who studied evolution and medicine as an undergraduate will be in charge of the curriculum at a major medical school and will have the opportunity to create a learning experience that makes more sense. On a larger scale, medical schools would quickly bolster their teaching of evolution if medical certification examinations included questions on evolutionary biology, as they do for every other basic medical science. How can it be that we do not test students on the basic principles of evolutionary biology?! Many medical students never learn about proximate and evolutionary explanations, kin selection, levels and speed of selection, the importance of drift, pleiotropy, parent–offspring conflict, the evolutionary origins of sexual reproduction, or even the evolution of virulence. We insist that engineers learn physics. We should insist that doctors learn evolution. (Nesse, Stearns, & Omenn, 2006)

A FEELING FOR THE ORGANISM

The above many specific benefits of evolution for medicine may be less important than the ability of an evolutionary perspective to give physicians and researchers a deeper feeling for the organism. At present, many see the body as a machine—a machine that fails and often needs repair. This incorrect analogy gives rise to false beliefs. For instance, many physicians think there is a normal human genome. Exposure to evolutionary thinking helps most to realize that genes increase or decrease in frequency depending on the reproductive success of the phenotypes they make. There is no normal human genome, there are just genes that are less or more successful in gaining representation in the gene pool.

Doctors also find it easy to think of pathogens as evil intruders who threaten us instead of small bits of DNA that replicate themselves at our expense. It seems as if pathogens should become more benign after long-term association with a host, but this is incorrect; selection shapes virulence up as well as down to whatever level maximizes the pathogen's spread (Ewald, 1994; Frank, 1996).

Descartes is widely cited for fostering mischievous mind body dualism (Rozemond, 1998), but in the seventeenth century he was a radical for suggesting that the body could be understood as a machine. The analogy served well to extricate biology from religion and metaphysics. It is, however, fundamentally inaccurate. Machines are created from plans made by designers. Bodies were not designed. Bodies arise from interactions between genetic codes and environments. They exist in an unbroken continuity from the first living cells billions of years ago. We are only now beginning to grasp the severity of constraints imposed because nothing in a body can be redesigned from scratch. The body has to work well in every single generation, so big sudden changes are impossible. There is no way selection can turn the eyeball right side out, or route childbirth through the abdominal wall instead of through the narrow pelvic opening. Some of the body's most marvelous adaptations are compensations for fundamental design flaws; for instance, the tiny constant eye movements that give us a complete field of vision unobstructed by the blind spot or shadows of blood vessels would be unnecessary if the nerves and vessels ran on the outside of the eyeball instead of the inside.

Machines inevitably wear out and break, and organisms age and die, but the reasons are fundamentally different. Machines cannot replicate their parts, so eventually things break. Bodies can make new parts; lizards grow new tails, and we can replace damaged skin and liver cells. But we cannot regrow a severed finger, nor can we replace heart or brain cells to any extent. The explanations are evolutionary. Rates of aging, abilities to replace damaged cells and organs, rate of growth, age at sexual maturity, and life span are all life history traits that are shaped by natural selection (Stearns, 1992). Why doesn't natural selection do a better job so we can live longer with fewer diseases? Table 23-2 lists six specific reasons. But the global reason is that organisms are not machines shaped for some purpose by a designer. Organisms are, instead, in Dawkins's memorable metaphor, vehicles for genes to maximize the transmission of genetic information regardless of the impact on individuals or society (Dawkins, 1989). Some genes that cause aging are never exposed to selection; others may offer benefits earlier in life when selection is stronger. Evolution's greatest contribution to medicine may be replacing the analogy of body as machine with a feeling for the organism as a product of natural selection.

OBSTACLES

The application of evolutionary principles to the problem of medicine is slowed by several factors: first is general ignorance about how natural selection works, even among medical researchers, second is difficulty grasping the distinction between proximate and evolutionary explanations, and third is the lack of agreed-upon methods for testing evolutionary hypotheses.

How Natural Selection Works

Many readers of this book have never had a course in evolutionary biology, and some will never have read a book describing natural selection in depth. Like other volumes on evolution and medicine, this one provides no overview of how selection works for the very good reason that there is too much to cover. However, without the basics, confusion is inevitable. Little can be done about the problem here except to note it and to recommend reading an engaging authoritative text (e.g., Bell, 1997; Futuyma, 2005; Stearns & Hoekstra, 2005).

Well, perhaps one recommendation may be worthwhile. Many students learn about natural selection by memorizing answers to exam questions. The currently popular mnemonic is VIST (variation, inheritance, selection, time). This static approach does little to impart a feeling for the dynamic process that is evolution. It is far better to encourage students to look for nonbiological examples of selection (such as what television shows persist and which are dropped) and examples of breeding (everyone knows breeds of dogs). Then, after the general principle of selection is vividly illustrated with many examples, students are ready to grasp natural selection with the help of dozens of examples from the natural world.

The Need for Both Proximate and
Evolutionary Explanations

It is as difficult as it is essential to get across the idea that every biological trait needs an evolutionary as well as proximate explanation. Students have spent years thinking there is only one explanation for one phenomenon, and many suffer from the misconception that all explanation involves reduction. Here again, examples and discussion prove more helpful than lists and lectures. One student names a trait such as the do not explain the behavior, instead explain how squirrel's tale or the dog's ears or the firefly's glow, and others are invited to propose proximate and evolutionary explanations. I spend a full hour on this exercise in my classes with undergraduates and doctors in training, which is enough for only about half the students to get a secure grasp of these crucial concepts.

How to Test an Evolutionary Hypothesis About Disease

Discussions about evolutionary explanations tend to generate wild speculations. One student may suggest that nearsightedness exists so that that some members of the group stay home to make tools, another that diabetes is useful to keep blood sugar levels elevated to increase energy, and another may hypothesize that cancer cells are reproducing for their own advantage. While these wild ideas are disturbing to listen to, they also provide a valuable reminder about how difficult it is to think clearly about evolution and disease. I have tried to forestall such excesses by emphasizing experimental and comparative methods, the need to test alternative hypotheses, and the scientific method. Students dutifully listen, but this approach does little to make their thinking more critical. Instead, I now encourage students to consider one aspect of the body that makes it vulnerable to disease, and to come up with as many hypotheses as possible. We then go through possible explanations, one by one, showing why most are false, and discussing what it would take to assess the rest. Most proposals are incorrect because the student has either formulated the hypothesis incorrectly or misunderstood a core concept. Correcting these and other errors in example after example is frustrating, but it helps students to develop their critical skills. It encourages a deep feeling for science in general, as well as better understanding of evolutionary principles.

Developing these critical skills is by no means easy, however. If the task is left half-finished, students are liable to leave a class on Darwinian medicine with severely mistaken notions about evolution and disease. In an attempt to provide secondary prevention, I give students explicit instructions on how to test an evolutionary hypothesis about disease (Tables 23–4 and 23–5). This cookbook set of guidelines helps to encourage clear thinking about how to assess hypotheses about why selection has left the body vulnerable to a disease.

CONCLUSION

Evolution is important for medicine. Its full range of possible applications is, however, just now being appreciated. The value of evolutionary medicine in providing direct clinical advice is real, but limited so far. It heuristic value is enormous, as is its potential to offer a framework for deeper understanding of bodily systems, as documented by the chapters in this volume. However, its greatest contribution may be to foster a deeper feeling for the organism as a bundle of trade-offs that emerges from varying environments interacting with those genes that have given rise to individuals who have had the most offspring in past generations. From so simple a beginning in the principle of natural selection, endless ideas most beautiful and most wonderful have been, and are being, applied to medicine.

ACKNOWLEDGMENTS

Thanks to Neal Smith for extensive and helpful comments that greatly improved the manuscript.

TABLE 23-4 How to Test an Evolutionary Hypothesis About Disease

1. Define the object of explanation with great specificity.
    a. A trait shaped by natural selection will usually be the object of explanation.
    b. A disease is an appropriate object only if the hypothesis is that the "disease" is actually a defense, or otherwise increases fitness.
    c. Usually the object is a trait that is universal in the species and that makes an organism vulnerable to a disease.
    d. If the object is not a universal trait, justify the exception.
        i. The most common exceptions are traits that reflect genetic differences in subpopulations responding to local environment, e.g., sickle cell alleles that protect against malaria.
        ii. Other exceptions are facultative adaptations that explain individual differences, e.g., the number of sweat glands increases as a function of early exposure to high temperatures.
        iii. If the trait is a behavior, do not explain the behavior, instead explain how selection shaped the behavior regulation system.
    e. Do not propose an evolutionary explanation for why one individual gets a disease and another does not. Evolutionary explanations are about populations. They may however, predict who get a disease.
    f. Evolutionary explanations are not alternatives to proximate explanations. Evidence about proximate mechanisms is often useful in assessing a hypothesis, however, especially when the hypothesis is that vulnerability to disease results from constraints or trade-offs.
2. Specify all possible alternative hypotheses for why the trait is apparently suboptimal. There are six main possibilities (see Table 23-2):
    a. The environment has changed faster than selection and the disease results from this *mismatch*.
    b. The relevant environmental factor is a *pathogen* that evolves faster than host defenses.
    c. *Constraints*, e.g., natural selection's limited ability to clear mutations or correct a fundamentally defective design, leave the organism vulnerable.
    d. The trait offers *trade-off* compensatory benefits that account for apparently suboptimal features.
    e. The trait offers *benefits to reproduction or to kin* that are greater than the costs to the individual.
    f. The trait is not a disease at all, but a useful protective response such as pain or fever.
3. Make explicit predictions from each possible hypothesis.
    a. If relevant data from other species can be obtained and analyzed, use the comparative method.
    b. Otherwise, try to make predictions about aspects of the trait or its regulation, preferably previously unrecognized and quantitative.
    c. Other useful predictions may be made about the relative fitness of individuals with and without the trait in different environments.
    d. Predictions about proximate aspects of the trait may be possible.
4. Use all available evidence to test the predictions from all alternative hypotheses to arrive at a judgment about the contributions of different factors.
    a. Note that multiple factors often operate together to explain an apparently suboptimal trait. This is quite different from proximate explanations where evidence for one alternative usually weighs against others.
    b. Many hypotheses can be falsified because they are inconsistent with evolutionary theory.
    c. Others can be falsified by experiments that show that a trait does not serve the proposed function.
    d. Assess the overall plausibility of the proposal and the relative viability of alternative hypotheses.

TABLE 23-5 Some Common Mistakes in Testing Evolutionary Hypotheses About Disease

The guidelines in Table 23-4 tacitly describe a variety of possible errors, some of which are made explicit below.

1. Attempting to explain a disease: Instead, reformulate the question as an explanation for vulnerability to a disease.
2. Proposing an explanation based on what is good for the species: This is group selection, an elementary error. Almost all evolutionary explanations must be based on advantages to genes or individuals.
3. Proposing adaptive functions for rare genetic conditions: There are sometimes evolutionary reasons why deleterious mutations stay in the gene pool, but the explanation is hardly ever some useful function of the disease itself.
4. Confusing proximate and evolutionary explanations: This is a common and serious mistake. Knowledge about how the body works can be very useful in assessing an evolutionary hypothesis, but it is no substitute for an evolutionary explanation.
5. Thinking that evidence for learning influencing a trait indicates that no evolutionary explanation is needed: Learning is a capacity shaped by natural selection, and the pathologies that arise from learning mechanisms, such as phobias, are likely to harm fitness.
6. Thinking that evidence for environmental or cultural differences in a trait is evidence against evolutionary influences: Natural selection shaped the behavioral mechanisms that give rise to culture, and environments and culture influence human behavior and fitness strongly. An evolutionary approach to behavior does not imply that behavior is somehow "determined by the genes," only that the mechanisms that give rise to behavior and culture were shaped by natural selection. These mechanisms obviously are capable of profound flexibility, with attendant major benefits and costs.
7. Confusing genetic explanations, especially behavioral genetic explanations, with evolutionary explanations: Traits need evolutionary explanations whether or not individual variations arise from genetic variations.
8. Failing to consider all of the alternative hypotheses: This is very common and very serious. All too often an author will propose one possibility without making the alternatives explicit
9. Assuming that evidence for one hypothesis is evidence against another: Multiple factors may all contribute to a complete explanation and they may interact in complex ways. Correct explanations often incorporate multiple explanatory factors.
10. Presenting all the evidence in favor of a pet hypothesis and all of the evidence against other hypotheses, instead of offering a balanced consideration of all evidence for and against all hypotheses: This is rhetoric, not science. It is observed commonly, for good reasons arising from human nature, not just in testing evolutionary hypotheses but across the range of sciences. Nonetheless, such advocacy should be avoided.

NOTES

Chapter 1

1. We should note that this transmission works both ways and that exposure to humans has resulted in novel diseases for many animal species.

2. See Trevathan, 1987, for a review of labor and delivery in human and nonhuman primates.

3. One of the design constraints on human infants is that they must suckle and breathe at the same time. Adult humans are unable to perform these two feats simultaneously because the developmental modifications for speech have moved the tracheal opening farther back in the throat. For the first few months of life, human infants can breathe and drink at the same time. During breastfeeding the larynx is elevated so that the epiglottis can slide behind the soft palate and larynx all the way to the nasopharynx. Food actually passes in two channels (faucium channels) around the epiglottis (Crelin & Scherz, 1978).

4. The evolution of parental investment (resources given to offspring that reduce the parents' ability to invest in future offspring) (Trivers, 1972) directly affects our decisions in the cases described above. One of the problems that organisms face, particularly in the context of parental care, is whether to base continued investment in an offspring upon the amount of past investment (Arkes & Ayton, 1999; Curio, 1987; Coleman & Gross, 1991; Gross, 2005; Sargent & Gross, 1985). Hence, continuing to invest based on the past is a poor way to allocate resources, and parents should look to other factors to determine optimal investment strategies.

5. Metabolic syndrome X is a combination of medical disorders that affect as many as 25% of the U.S. population. Symptoms include fasting hyperglycemia (diabetes mellitus type 2), hypertension, visceral obesity, elevated triglycerides, decreased HDL cholesterol, and elevated uric acid levels.

6. More appropriately called "adolescent subfecundity."

7. Hippocrates was the first to apply the idea that there were bodily fluids that were associated with the four basic elements of nature. An imbalance in these fluids was thought to affect an individual's personality. Each of the fluids was linked to a specific personality type.

Elements of nature	Spring	Autumn	Summer	Winter
Humours	Blood	Black bile	Yellow bile	Phlegm
Organ	Liver	Gall bladder	Spleen	Brain/lungs
Characteristics	Courageous/ amorous	Despondent/ sleepless	Easily angered	Calm/ restrained
Temperament	Sanguine	Melancholic	Choleric	Phlegmatic

8. Modern-day psychiatry has done an outstanding job of identifying various phobias that we experience. The following table summarizes fears that humans experience:

Name	Fear of	Name	Fear of
Agoraphobia	Open places	Erythorophobia	Blushing
Acrophobia	Heights	Hematophobia	Blood

Aerophobia	Flying	Mysophobia	Dirt and germs
Ailurophobia	Cats	Panophobia	Everything
Algophobia	Pain	Pathophobia	Disease and suffering
Claustrophobia	Confined spaces	Xenophobia	Strangers

Source: Nicholi, 1999, p. 35.

9. Asian and Pacific Islanders.

Chapter 4

1. Sunnanå U. En syk, syk nasjon ... Aftenposten, March, 1999. These data are based on numbers from patient organizations in Norway. We have not been able to obtain reliable public statics on this.

2. The Norwegian Association of Pharmaceutical Manufacturers, "Facts and Figures 2006," Oslo 2006. www.lmi.no.

NTB. Medisiner for 3500 kr. hver. Aftenposten, January 29, 2007: 18.

3. Celiac disease is an autoimmune disorder that affects the small intestine and is genetically determined. In affected individuals there is an abnormal reaction to gliadin, a gluten protein found in wheat. Exposure to gliadin cause the immune system to cross-react with the enzyme tissue transglutaminase, causing a flattening of the villi of the small intestine, thus inhibiting the absorption of nutrients.

4. Today's wheat varieties are based on genetic crossing of three primitive species. There is a continuous genetic selection going on mainly involving criteria such as yield and other agricultural considerations and, to a lesser extent, nutrients. Such genetic changes are generally taking place at a much faster rate than the capacity for change in the human genome. As many as 50,000 Norwegians suffer from gluten intolerance, and many more may have immune reactions in the gut from wheat ingestion. Norwegian researchers have found that primitive wheat varieties (spelt, kamut), which are still grown in remote areas in the Middle East, cause fewer immune reactions than modern varieties when exposed to cells from the small intestine of celiac patients (Molberg, Uhlen, Flæte, Fleckenstein, Arentz-Hansen, Raki, Lundin, & Sollid, 2005).

5. USDA National Nutrient Database sr17abxl.zip may be downloaded or accessed at www.nal.usda.gov/fnic/foodcomp/search.

6. Exorphines (opioid peptides) are normally broken down into amino acids by digestion enzymes, but in some individuals are not. Exorphins mimic the effects of opiates and therefore influence the mind.

7. http://www.shdir.no/ernaering/fakta_mat/positive_forandringer___men_fortsatt_ern_ ringsmessige_svakheter_i_norsk_kosthold_5842 and http://www.medisin.ntnu.no/ism/nofe/norepid/ 2000(1)%2005-Johansson.pdf#search = %22fettinnhold%20i%20tradisjonelt%20norsk% 20kosthold%22.

8. This may be achieved by sprouting (eliminates lectins and increases vitamin content), fermentation (reduces phytates) and supplementing with kelp flour (increases mineral content), deficient amino acids (increases protein quality), ω-3 fatty acids (improves the ω-3:ω-6 ratio) and fats (e.g., coconut fat, which is heat resistant). If the bread is baked several hours at low temperature (80–90°C), minimal destruction of nutrients will take place.

9. http://www.who.int/mediacentre/factsheets/fs138/en/

10. http://www.healthierus.gov/dietaryguidelines/index.html and http://www.sante.gouv.fr/ htm/pointsur/nutrition/1nbis.htm.

11. http://www.shdir.no/vp/multimedia/archive/00006/IS-1325_6097a.pdf.

12. Such new standards should be based on individual needs for optimal physiological and mental function, i.e., a level that in principle would prevent most illnesses resulting from increased nutrient needs. One such example may be schizophrenia, which can be seen as a niacin-deficiency

disease, which would be more or less eradicated if sufficient amounts of niacin were added to common foods (Hoffer, 2005).

Chapter 5

1. Individuals with the C nucleotide at a locus in the 13th intron or a G in the 9th intron (these two introns being eight kilobases apart) within a neighboring gene about 14 kilobases upstream from the lactase gene were found to be lactase impersistent, while those with T or A at these same loci were lactase persistent. Although the exact mechanism by which these loci regulate lactase production remains unclear, current evidence points to their action at the level of gene transcription, as most studies demonstrate variation in mRNA levels between those who are lactase persistent or impersistent, a pattern that becomes evident during childhood (Wang et al., 1998).

2. As Durham (1991) noted, fortifying milk with vitamin D is unnecessary in lactase-persistent populations, as the lactose in the milk can substitute for vitamin D as a calcium-absorption mechanism in the small intestine.

3. Milk from cows treated with rbGH does not have to be labeled as such in the United States, and so it is difficult to know how much milk that is consumed is from treated cows.

4. Stunting was defined in this study as having reached less than the 90th percentile of the standard. The standard used was the Harvard 50th percentile (Waterlow, 1972).

Chapter 7

1. During WW II, the Netherlands became one of the main western battlefields, and the western part of the country was occupied by the Nazis and subject to a food embargo that lasted until November 1944. During the winter of 1944–1945, which became known as the *Hongerwinter* (hunger winter), approximately 30,000 Dutch people starved to death. A number of factors combined to starve the Dutch people: the winter itself was unusually harsh, and together with the widespread dislocation and destruction of the war, the retreating German army destroyed locks and bridges to flood the country and impede the Allied advance, which ruined much agricultural land and made the transport of existing food stocks difficult. The official food rations dropped below 1000 kcal (4200 J) per person per day, and although pregnant women were allocated some additional food rations, the extent to which redistribution of these additional rations occurred within families is not known. The famine ceased immediately with liberation in May 1945, when Allied food supplies became abundant.

Chapter 9

1. Created by Barr Pharmaceuticals to both prevent pregnancies and reduce the number of yearly menstrual cycles, Seasonale® was approved by the U.S. Food and Drug Administration in September 2003. The active ingredients in Seasonale are 0.15 mg levonorgestrel, a synthetic progestin, and 0.03 mg of ethinyl estradiol, a synthetic estrogen (Anderson and Hait 2003; FDA 2003). The same active ingredients are found in other oral contraceptives. Lybrel™ manufactured by Wyeth Pharmaceuticals, is awaiting approval from the U.S. FDA, Health Canada, and authorities in Finland (for marketing in the European Union). Lybrel is a low dose oral contraceptive that will eliminate menstruation altogether (Babinski, 2005). The active ingredients in Lybrel are 90 mcg levonorgestrel and 20 mcg ethinyl estradiol.

2. See, for example, *Maclean's* (George, 2005), *The New York Times* (Kelley, 2003), *Newsday* (Rabin, 2004), *Time* (Gorman, 2000), and CBS News (2003).

3. There is, actually, a surprising degree of variation in the length of menstrual cycles (Treloar, Boynton, Behn, & Brown 1967), but a 28-day cycle continues to be the textbook norm. This

allows for a fairly even division between the follicular and luteal phases on either side of ovulation on day 14.

4. A blastocyst develops from a fertilized egg. It is a sphere of cells—the outer layer of cells (trophoblast) will form the placenta, an inner cluster of cells will form the embryo.

5. The role of hypoxia in menstruation is somewhat controversial (Jabbour et al., 2006).

6. The amount of iron lost in menstrual blood is a topic of some contention and of relevance to the topic of menstrual suppression. Sullivan (1989, 1996) argues that cyclic iron depletion has cardiovascular benefit, and Rako (2003) uses this argument to oppose menstrual suppression. In contrast, Profet (1993, p. 337) notes that the human body has developed "exquisite mechanisms" to store, recycle, and regulate iron levels, and that "if cyclic bleeding functioned to eliminate iron, one would expect it to occur in both sexes." Gosden et al. (1999) note that in the evolutionary past, menstruation was relatively rare, and the diet was probably sufficient for replacing iron. Even with repeated cycling, iron loss is slight except when menstrual bleeding is unusually frequent or heavy.

7. In other words, women who gave the signal earlier (during adolescent subfertility), more regularly (every 28 days), and later (during the peri-menopausal period) were selected for by natural selection through higher reproductive success.

8. The first advertisement to appear after FDA approval emphasized the use of Enovid to postpone menstruation "for convenience, for peace of mind, for full efficiency on critical occasions" (Watkins, 1998, p. 37).

9. The Seasonale web site provides an interactive Personal Planner to help women "plan events like vacations, business travel, romantic encounters, and family reunions based on your inactive Pill dates" (www.seasonale.com).

10. As a contraceptive, Seasonale is just as effective as other combination pill oral contraceptives, with a failure rate of, theoretically, 0.1%. Actual failure rates are somewhat higher (3%) because of human error, illness, and drug interactions (Speroff et al., 1999).

11. During the first year, a 39-year-old nonsmoker experienced a pulmonary embolism (Anderson and Hait, 2003). No thromboembolic events were reported during the study extension, although there was one report of cholecystits and one report of bile duct stone that may have been related to the use of Seasonale (Anderson et al., 2006).

12. The deleterious effects of hormone therapy after menopause took decades to document (Grady et al., 2002; Manson et al., 2003; Rossouw et al., 2002; Wassertheil-Smoller et al., 2003).

Chapter 15

1. Optimality theory examines the trade-offs in costs and benefits for behaviors in local environments using quantitative data to determine the optimal solution for investing time and effort in particular behaviors. Evolutionary stable strategies extend optimality analysis to examine the best possible strategy for populations, where no other adaptive strategy can successfully compete in that population and environment due to consistently lower pay-offs (benefits vs. costs). Since addiction obviously involves a lower pay-off than could be optimal for the individual, human behavioral ecology is limited in its theoretical applicability.

2. Behavioral biology—given its functional approach—is compatible with evolutionary theory, and this section focuses on this area. Nevertheless, social factors do play a role in substance abuse and should not be forgotten even though they are not discussed in this section.

3. Dopamine is a neurotransmitter that stimulates neurons with dopamine receptors. Mesolimbic systems are located in the limbic area of the brain, where many emotional and motivational processes are mediated. The prefrontal cortices are at the front of the brain, are much larger in humans than in nonhuman primates, and play a central role in abstract reasoning, symbolic thought, and self-control. Web sites that provide informative tutorials (with visuals) on the neurobiology of addiction include: http://www.nida.nih.gov/pubs/Teaching/ and http://www.sfn.org/index.cfm?pagename = brainBriefings_main

Chapter 18

1. An organism inherits a specific set of genes that comprise its *genotype*. The genotype interacts with the environment to determine the development of its *phenotype*, which can refer to the flesh and blood characteristics of the body as a whole or more narrowly to a specific trait or characteristic.

2. There are notable exceptions of convergent evolution in which complex adaptations, such as the eye, have developed independently in distantly related taxa (see Dawkins, 1996).

Chapter 22

1. This is purported to have been suggested by a Hungarian scientist by the name of Saint George.

2. In the United Kingdom, this book was published as Nesse, R. & Williams, G. (1995). *Evolution and Healing—The New Science of Darwinian Medicine*. London, Weidenfeld and Nicolson.

3. For a transcript, see also: http://www.chester.ac.uk/~sjlewis/DM/Texts/text4.htm

4. To some, the term "Neo-Darwinian medicine" might also have implied that some older "Darwinian medicine" had been supplanted by this form.

5. This course was entitled "Ecosystem Disruption and Disease" and was taught at Berkeley between 1968 and 1970.

6. The term "biology" was first used with its current meaning in 1802 by Gottfried Treviranus (1776–1837) in *Biologie* and by Jean-Baptiste Lamarck (1744–1829) in *Hydrogéologie*. Both were reacting against the cataloguing tendencies of the natural historians of the previous century by naming a new field of study directed at a more dynamic scrutiny of life.

7. Signs and symptoms are also terms that are confused and used interchangeably. Throughout, I use the terms "signs" and "symptoms" in the strict sense of referring to objectively observable and subjectively experienced bodily phenomena, respectively. It is, therefore, possible for a clinician or other observer, including the patient, to report on physical signs but only the patient can describe their symptoms.

8. See: http://www.chester.ac.uk/~sjlewis/DM/Texts/text1.htm

9. See: http://www.chester.ac.uk/~sjlewis/DM/BrownBag.htm

10. Morgagni famously related what he noted in his patients while alive to their postmortem findings in "De Sedibus et Causis Morborum per Anatomen Indagatis" *(On the Seats and Causes of Disease Investigated by Anatomy)*, 1761.

11. This review appeared in *The Times Higher Education Supplement*, June 9, 1995. For a transcript, see also: http://www.chester.ac.uk/~sjlewis/DM/Texts/text2.htm

12. Extract taken from WHO (1948) Preamble to the Constitution of the World Health Organization as adopted by the International Health Conference, New York, June 19–22, 1946; signed on July 22, 1946, by the representatives of 61 States (Official Records of the World Health Organization, no. 2, p. 100) and entered into force on April 7, 1948.

13. To such expressions as "feeling bad" may be added "feeling under the weather," "feeling off-color," etc.

14. In particular, Stempsey had Christopher Boorse's *Biostatistical Theory* (1997) in mind. However, I believe the general notion that there is a need for certain professionals who can make fine distinctions between the theoretical and practical aspects of medicine (and evolutionary medicine) applies.

15. Here, "transcendent" is used in the nonreligious sense of surpassing ordinary human understanding.

REFERENCES

Aaby, P. (1995). Soc Sci Med, 41(5):673–686.

Aamodt, A. H., Borch-Iohnsen, B., Hagen, K., Stovner, L. J., et al. (2004). Cephalalgia, 24(9):758–762.

Aas, V., Kase, E. T., Solberg, R., Jensen, J., et al. (2004). Diabetologia, 47(8):1452–1461.

Abad, V. C., & Guilleminault, C. (2005). Dialogues Clin Neurosci, 7(4):291–303.

Abbasi, F., McLaughlin, T., Lamendola, C., Kim, H. S., et al. (2000). Am J Cardiol, 85(1):45–48.

Abbout, D. H., Barnett, D. K., Bruns, C. M., & Dumesic, D. A. (2005). Hum Reprod Update, 11(4):357–374.

Abel, L., & Dessein, A. J. (1997). Curr Opin Immunol, 9(4):509–516.

Abou Zahr, C., Wardlaw, T. M., World Health Organization Reproductive Health and Research, United Nations Population Fund, et al. (2004). Maternal Mortality in 2000: Estimates Developed by WHO, UNICEF, and UNFPA. Geneva: Department of Reproductive Health and Research, World Health Organization.

Abrahams, P. W., & Parsons, J. A. (1996). Geogr J, 162(1):63–72.

Adair, L. S., & Politt, E. (1985). Am J Clin Nutr, 41(5):948–978.

Adair, L. S. (2001). Pediatrics, 107(4):e59–e65.

Adair, L. S., Kuzawa, C. W., & Borja, J. (2001). Circulation, 104(9):1034–1039.

Adair, L. S., & Cole, T. J. (2003). Hypertension, 41(3):451–456.

Adair, L. S., & Dahly, D. (2005). Annu Rev Nutr, 25:407–434.

Adams, O., Besken, K., Oberdorfer, C., MacKenzie, C. R., et al. (2004). J Virol, 78(5):2632–2636.

Adams, P. F., & Barnes, P. M. (2004). Nat Vital Stat Rep, 10(229):1–104.

Ademec, R. E., Blundell, J., & Burton, P. (2005). Neurosci Biobehav Rev, 29(8):1225–1241.

Ader, R., Felten, D. L., & Cohen, N. (eds.). (2006). Psychoneuroimmunology. San Diego, CA: Academic Press.

Adler, N. E., Boyce, W. T., Chesney, M. A., Folkman, S., et al. (1993). J Am Med Assoc, 269(24):3140–3145.

Adlercreutz, H. (2002). Lancet Oncol, 3(6):364–373.

Adolfsson, O., Meydani, S. N., & Russell, R. M. (2004). Am J Clin Nutr, 80(2):245–256.

Adolphs, R. (2003). Nat Rev Neurosci, 4(3):165–178.

Adolphson, S., & Westphal, O. (1981). Pediatr Res, 15(1):82.

Agarwal, A. K., & Shah, A. (1997). J Asthma, 34(6):539–545.

Ahima, R. S., Qi, Y., & Singhal, N. S. (2006). Prog Brain Res, 153:155–174.

Ahmad, N., Pollard, T. M., & Unwin, N. (2002). Cancer Epidemiol Biomarkers Prev, 11(1):147–151.

Ahmed, A. A., Osman, H., Mansour, A. M., Musa, H. A., et al. (2000). Am J Trop Med Hyg, 63(5–6):259–263.

Ahnert, L., Gunnar, M. R., Lamb, M. E., & Barthel, M. (2004). Child Dev, 75(3):639–650.

Aho, K., Pyhala, R., & Visakropi, R. (1980). Tissue Antigens, 16:310–313.

Ahren, I. L., Williams, D. L., Rice, P. J., Forsgren, A., et al. (2001). J Infect Dis, 184:150–158.

Aiello, L. C. (1992). Body size and energy requirements. In: The Cambridge Encyclopedia of Human Evolution, S. Bunney, S. Jones, R. Martin, & D. Pilbeam (eds.). Cambridge, UK: Cambridge University Press, pp. 41–45.

Aiello, L. C., & Wheeler, P. (1995). Curr Anthropol, 36(2):199–221.

Aiello, L. C. (1997). Rev Bras Genet, 20(1).

Aiello, L. C., & Wells, J. C. K. (2002). Ann Rev Anthropol, 31:323–338.

Alan Guttmacher Institute. (1958). Into a New World: Young Women's Sexual and Reproductive Lives. New York: Alan Guttmacher Institute.

Alberman, E., Emanuel, I., Filakti, H., & Evans, S. J. (1992). Paediatr Perinat Epidemiol, 6(2):134–144.

Albina, J. E., & Reichner, J. S. (2003). Wound Repair Regen, 11(6):445–451.

Alcock, J. (2001). The Triumph of Sociobiology. New York: Oxford University Press.

Alexander, G. R., Tompkins, M. E., Allen, M. C., & Hulsey, T. C. (1999). Matern Child Health J, 3(2):71–79.

Alexander, J., Andersen, S. A., Aro, A., Becker, W., et al. (2004). Nordic Nutrition Recommendations 2004. Copenhagen: Nordic Council of Ministers.

Alexander, R. D. (1987). The Biology of Moral Systems. New York: Aldine de Gruyter.

Alexander, R. D. (1989). Evolution of the human psyche. In: The Human Revolution: Behavioural and Biological Perspectives on the Origins of Modern Humans, P. Mellars & C. Stringer (eds.). Princeton, NJ: Princeton University Press, pp. 455–513.

Alexander, R. D. (2005). Evolutionary selection and the nature of humanity. In: Darwinism and Philosophy V. Hösle, & C. Illies (eds.). South Bend, IN: University of Notre Dame Press, pp. 301–348.

Allaert, F.-A., & Urbinelli, R. (2004). CNS Drugs, 18(Suppl 1):3–7.

Allan, C. B., & Lutz, W. (2000). Life Without Bread: How a Low-Carbohydrate Diet Can Save Your Life. Los Angeles, CA: Keats Publishing.

Allison, A. C. (1953). Man, 53:23–24.

Allison, A. C. (1954). Trans R Soc Trop Med Hyg, 48:312–318.

Allison, A. C. (1954). Ann Hum Genet, 19:39–57.

Allison, A. C. (1954). BMJ, 1:290–294.

Allison, A. C., Ikin, E. W., & Mourant, A. E. (1954). J Roy Anthro Inst Great Brit Ireland, 84(1–2):158–162.

Allison, T., & Cicchetti, D. V. (1976). Science, 194:732–734.

Allman, J. M. (1999). Evolving Brains. New York: Scientific American Library.

Allman, J. M., Hakeem, A., Erwin, J. M., Nimchinsky, E., et al. (2001). Ann NY Acad Sci, 935:107–117.

Allsworth, J. E., Weitzen, S., & Boardman, L. A. (2005). Ann Epidemiol, 15(6):438–444.

Alm, B., Lagercrantz, H., & Wennergren, G. (2006). Acta Paediatr Scand, 95(3):260–262.

Al–Mobireek, A. F., Darwazeh, A. M. G., & Hassanin, M. B. (2000). Dentomaxillafac Radiol, 29(5):286–290.

Al–Shammri, S., Rawoot, P., Azizieh, F., AbuQoora, A., et al. (2004). J Neurol Sci, 222(1–2):21–27.

Alvares–da–Silva, M. R., Fancisconi, C. F. M., & Waechter, F. L. (2000). J Viral Hepat, 7(1):84–86.

American Academy of Pediatrics. (1985). Pediatrics, 76(4):635–643.

American Academy of Pediatrics Task Force on Sudden Infant Death Syndrome. (2005). Pediatrics, 116(5):1245–1255.

American College of Gastroenterology (2004), Food Intolerance, http://www.acg.gi.org/patients cgp/pdf/food_i.pdf

American Diabetes Association. (2004a). Diabetes Care, 27(Suppl 1):5S–10.

American Diabetes Association (2004b), What is Prediabetes?, http://aww.diabetes.org diabetes-prevention/prediabetes.jsp

American Diabetes Association. (2006). Diabetes Care, 29(Suppl 1):S43–48.

American Psychiatric Association. (2000). Diagnostic and Statistical Manual of Mental Disorders: DSM-IV-TR, 4th ed. Washington, DC: American Psychiatric Association.

Ames, B. N., Cathcart, R., Schwiers, E., & Hochstein, P. (1981). Proc Natl Acad Sci USA, 78(11):6858–6862.

Ames, B. N., Elson–Schwab, I., & Silver, E. A. (2002). Am J Clin Nutr, 75(4):616–658.

Amin, H., Singhal, N., & Suave, R. S. (1997). Acta Paediatr, 86(3):306–314.

Anand–Srivastava, M. B. (2005). Peptides, 26(6):1044–1059.

Anders, T. (1979). Pediatrics, 63(6):860–864.

Anderson, F. D., & Hait, H. (2003). Contraception, 68(2):89–96.

Anderson, F. D., Gibbons, W., & Portman, D. (2006). Am J Obstet Gynecol, 195(1):92–96.

Anderson, G. C., Moore, E., Hepworth, J., & Bergman, N. (2003). Birth, 30(3):206–207.

Anderson, G. H. (1995). Am J Clin Nutr, 62(1 [Suppl 1]):195S–202S.

Anderson, J. J. B. (2001). J Am Coll Nutr, 20(2):186S–191S.

Anderson, J. L., Lutz, J. R., Gilbert, E. M., Sorensen, S. G., et al. (1985). Am J Cardiol, 55(4):471–475.

Anderson, J. L., Carlquist, J. F., Muhlestein, J. B., Horne, B. D., et al. (1998). J Am Coll Cardiol, 32(1):35–41.

Anderson, R. M., & May, R. M. (1979). Nature, 280(5721):361–367.

Anderson, W. (2004). Osiris, 19:39–61.

Andersson, R. E., Olaison, G., Tysk, C., & Ekbom, A. (2003). Gastroenterology, 124(1):40–46.

Andreas, H. (1961). Z Arztl Fortbild, 55:1344–1349.

Andrews, J. C., Ator, G. A., & Honrubia, V. (1992). Arch Otolaryngol Head Neck Surg, 118(1):74–78.

Andrist, L. C., Hoyt, A., Weinstein, D., & McGibbon, C. (2004). J Am Acad Nurse Pract, 16(1):31–37.

Aney, M. (1998). AAP News, 14(4):1–2.

Ang, S. O., Chen, H., Gordeuk, V. R., Sergueeva, A. I., et al. (2002). Blood Cells Mol Dis, 28(1):57–62.

Angold, A., & Worthman, C. W. (1993). J Affect Disord, 29(2–3):145–158.

Angold, A., Costello, E. J., & Worthman, C. M. (1998). Psychol Med, 28(1):51–61.

Anim–Nyame, N., Domoney, C., Panay, N., Jones, J., et al. (2000). Hum Reprod, 15(11):2329–2332.

Ankel–Simons, F. (2007). Primate Anatomy, 3rd ed. San Diego, CA: Academic Press.

Ankri, S., & Mirelman, D. (1999). Microbes Infect, 1(2):125–129.

Anonymous. (1980). J Am Med Assoc, 243(6):519–520.

Anonymous. (1991). N Engl J Med, 325(5):293–302.

Anonymous. (1993). The Economist, 326(7799):79–80.

Anonymous. (1994). MMWR Morb Mortal Wkly Rep, 43(5):77–81.

Anonymous (2004). America's obesity crisis. Time, June 7, p. 89.

Anonymous (2005). Obesity. Time, December 5, p. 75.

Anthony, J. (1952). Ann Paléon, 38:71–79.

Anthony, J. C., Warner, L. A., & Kessler, R. C. (1994). Exp Clin Psychopharmacol, 2(3):244–268.

Antonio, A., & Gonyea, W. J. (1993). Med Sci Sports Exerc, 25(12):1333–1345.

Apter, D. L., & Vikho, R. (1985). Clin Endocrinol, 22(6):753–760.

Apter, D. L., Reinila, M., & Vikho, R. (1989). Int J Cancer, 44(5):783–787.

Apter, D. L., & Vihko, R. (1990). J Clin Endocrinol Metab, 71(4):970–974.

Apter, D. L. (1996). Eur J Cancer Prev, 5(4):476–482.

Apter, D. L. (1997). Clin Endocrinol, 47(2):175–176.

Arcari, C. M., Gaydos, C. A., Nieto, J., Krauss, M., et al. (2005). Clin Infect Dis, 40(8):1123–1130.

Arenz, S., Ruckerl, R., Koletzko, B., & von Kries, R. (2004). Int J Obes Relat Metab Disord, 28(10):1247–1256.

Arkes, H. R., & Ayton, P. (1999). Psychol Bull, 125(5):591–600.

Armelagos, G. J. (1987). Biocultural aspects of food choice. In: Food and Evolution, M. Harris & E. Ross (eds.). Philadelphia: Temple University Press, pp. 579–594.

Armelagos, G. J. (1990). Health and disease in prehistoric populations in transition. In: Disease in Populations in Transition: Anthropological and Epidemiological Perspectives, A. C. Swedlund & G. J. Armelagos (eds.). New York: Bergin and Garvey, pp. 127–144.

Armelagos, G. J., Goodman, A. H., & Jacobs, K. H. (1991). Popul Environ, 13(1):9–22.

Armelagos, G. J. (1998). Sciences, 38(1):24–29.

Armelagos, G. J., & Brown, P. J. (2002). The body as evidence; the body of evidence. In: The Backbone of History: Health and Nutrition in the Western Hemisphere, R. Steckel & J. C. Rose (eds.). New York: Cambridge University Press, pp. 593–602.

Armelagos, G. J. (2004). Evol Anthropol, 13(2):53–55.

Armelagos, G. J., Brown, P. J., & Turner, B. (2005). Soc Sci Med, 61(4):755–765.

Armelagos, G. J., & Harper, K. N. (2005a). Evol Anthropol, 14(2):68–77.

Armelagos, G. J., & Harper, K. N. (2005b). Evol Anthropol, 14(3):109–121.

Armstrong, B. K., Brown, J. B., Clarke, H. T., Crooke, D. K., et al. (1981). J Natl Cancer Inst, 67(4):761–767.

Armstrong, E. (1990). Brain Behav Evol, 36(2–3):166–176.

Arnbjornsson, E. (1982). Surg Gynecol Obstet, 155(5):709–711.

Arnbjornsson, E. (1984). Surg Gynecol Obstet, 158(5):464–466.

Arnold, C., Makintube, S., & Istre, G. R. (1993). Am J Epidemiol, 138(5):333–340.

Arosio, M., Ronchi, C. L., Gebbia, C., Cappiello, V., et al. (2003). J Clin Endocrinol Metab, 88(2):701–704.

Arslanian, S. (1996). Nutritional disorders: Integration of energy metabolism and its disorders in childhood. In: Pediatric Endocrinology, M. Sperling (ed.). New York: Elsevier, pp. 523–548.

Ashina, M., Bendtsen, L., Jensen, R., & Olesen, J. (2000). Brain, 123(9):1830–1837.

Aspray, T. J., Mugusi, F., Rashid, S., Whiting, D., et al. (2000). Trans R Soc Trop Med Hyg, 94(6):637–644.

Astrup, A., Toubro, S., Raben, A., & Skov, A. R. (1997). J Am Diet Assoc, 97(Suppl 7):S82–S87.

Astrup, A., & Finer, N. (2000). Obes Rev, 1(2):57–59.

Atkins, R. C. (1992). Dr. Atkins' New Diet Revolution. New York: M. Evans and Company, Inc.

Atkins, R. C. (2001). Dr. Atkins Nye Slankerevolusjon [Dr. Atkins' New Diet Revolution]. Oslo, Norway: Forlaget WEM3.

Audette, R. V., & Gilchrist, T. (1995). NeanderThin: Eat Like a Caveman to Achieve a Lean, Strong, Healthy Body. Dallas, TX: Paleolithic Press.

Aufderheide, A. C., Rodríguez-Martín, C., & Langsjoen, O. (1998). The Cambridge Encyclopedia of Human Paleopathology. Cambridge, UK: Cambridge University Press.

Augustinsson, K. B., Fange, R., Johnels, A., & Ostlund, E. (1956). J Physiol, 131(2):257–276.

Austin, S. B., Melly, S. J., Sanchez, B. N., Patel, A., et al. (2005). Am J Public Health, 95(9):1575–1581.

Avonts, D., Sercu, M., Heyerick, P., Vandermeeren, I., et al. (1989). J R Coll Gen Pract, 39(327):418–420.

Babcock, G. T. (1999). Proc Natl Acad Sci USA, 96(23):12971–12973.

Babinski, R. (2005). Obstet/Gynecol News, 40(22):2.

Backhed, F., Ding, H., Wang, T., Hooper, L. V., et al. (2004). Proc Natl Acad Sci USA, 101(44):15718–15723.

Baddock, S. A., Galland, B. C., Bolton, D. P. G., Williams, S. M., et al. (2006). Pediatrics, 117(5):1599–1607.

Badiani, A., & Robinson, T. E. (2004). Behav Pharmacol, 15(5–6):327–339.

BaHamman, A. (2003). Sleep Hyp, 5(4):165–174.

Baierlein, J. L., & Foster, J. M. (1968). Blood, 32(3):412–422.

Bailar 3rd, J. C. (1999). N Engl J Med, 340(12):958–959.

Bailey, D. M., & Davies, B. (2001). High Alt Med Biol, 2(1):21–29.

Bailey, D. M. (2003). Adv Exp Med Biol, 543:201–221.

Bailey, D. M., Davies, B., Castell, L. M., Collier, D. J., et al. (2003). High Alt Med Biol, 4(3):319.

Bailey, D. M., Kleger, G.-R., Holzgraefe, M., Ballmer, P., et al. (2004). J Appl Physiol, 96(4):1459–1463.

Bailey, D. M., Roukens, R., Knauth, M., Kallenberg, K., et al. (2006). J Cereb Blood Flow Metab, 26(1):99–111.

Bailey, R. C., Jenike, M. R., Ellison, P. T., Bentley, G. R., et al. (1992). J Biosoc Sci, 24(3):393–412.

Baird, D. T., Collins, J., Egozcue, J., Evers, L. H., et al. (2005). Hum Reprod Update, 11(3):261–276.

Baird Jr., J. N. (1981). Am J Obstet Gynecol, 141(3):345–346.

Baker, I. A., Elwood, P. C., Hughes, J., Jones, M., et al. (1980). J Epidemiol Community Health, 34(1):31–34.

Baker, P. T., & Mazess, R. B. (1963). Science, 142:1466–1467.

Balandraud, N., Roudier, J., & Roudier, C. (2004). Autoimmun Rev, 3(5):362–367.

Balen, A. (1999). Lancet, 354(9183):966–967.

Balin, B. J., Gerard, H. C., Arking, E. J., Appelt, D. M., et al. (1998). Medical Microbiol Immunol, 187(1):23–42.

Ball, H. L., Hooker, E., & Kelly, P. J. (1999). Am Anthropol, 10(1):143–151.

Ball, H. L., & Panter-Brick, C. (2001). Child survival and the modulation of parental investment: Physiological and hormonal considerations. In: Reproductive Ecology and Human Evolution, P. T. Ellison (ed.). New York: Walter de Gruyter, pp. 249–266.

Ball, H. L. (2002). J Reprod Infant Psychol, 20(4):207–222.

Ball, H. L. (2003). Birth, 30(3):181–188.

Ball, H. L. (2006). Hum Nat, 17(3):301–318.

Ball, H. L., Ward–Platt, M., Heslop, E., Leech, S. J., et al. (2006). Arch Dis Child, 91:1005–1010

Ballesteros, M. N., Cabrera, R. M., Saucedo, M., & Fernancez, M. L. (2004). Am J Clin Nutr, 80(4):855–861.

Banerjee, S. K., & Maulik, S. K. (2002). Nutr J, 1(4):1–14.

Bangham, C., Anderson, R., Baquero, F., Bax, R., et al. (1999). Evolution of infectious diseases: The impact of vaccines, drugs, and social factors. In: Evolution in Health and Disease, S. C. Stearns (ed.). Oxford, UK: Oxford University Press, pp. 152–160.

Bankovi, G., Forrai, G., & Tauszik, T. (1993). Acta Biol Hung, 44(2–3):303–309.

Banting, W. (1864). Letters of Corpulence. London: Harrison.

Barker, D. J. P., Osmond, C., Golding, J., Kuh, D., et al. (1989). BMJ, 298(6673):564–567.

Barker, D. J. P., Hales, C. N., Fall, C. H., Osmond, C., et al. (1993). Diabetologia, 36(1):62–67.

Barker, D. J. P. (1994). Mothers, Babies, and Disease in Later Life. London: BMJ Publishing Group.

Barker, D. J. P. (1995). BMJ, 311(6998):171–174.

Barker, D. J. P., Winter, P. D., Osmond, C., Phillips, D. I. W., et al. (1995). Lancet, 345(8957):1087–1088.

Barker, D. J. P. (1997). Br Med Bull, 53(1):96–108.

Barker, D. J. P. (1998a). Clin Sci, 95(2):115–128.

Barker, D. J. P. (1998b). Mothers, Babies, and Health in Later Life, 2nd ed. Edinburgh, UK: Churchill Livingstone.

Barker, D. J. P. (1999). Ann Intern Med, 130(4 [Pt 1]):322–324.

Barker, D. J. P. (2004a). J Am Coll Nutr, 23(Suppl 6):588S–595S.

Barker, D. J. P. (2004b). Acta Paediatr Suppl, 93(446):26–33.

Barker, D. J. P. (2005). Horm Res, 64(Suppl 3):2–7.

Barker, D. J. P. (2006). Clin Obstet Gynecol, 49(2):270–283.

Barker, L. M. (1982). Building memories for foods. In: The Psychobiology of Human Food Selection, L. M. Barker (ed.). Westport, CT: AVI Publishing Company, Inc, pp. 85–99.

Barker, M., Robinson, S., Osmond, C., & Barker, D. (1997). Arch Dis Child, 77(5):381–383.

Barnes, K. C., Armelagos, G. J., & Morreale, S. C. (1999). Darwinian medicine and the emergence of allergy. In: Evolutionary Medicine, W. R. Trevathan, E. O. Smith, & J. J. McKenna (eds.). New York: Oxford University Press, pp. 209–243.

Barnes, S. (1998). Proc Soc Exp Biol Med, 217(3):386–392.

Barr, R. G., & Elias, M. F. (1988). Pediatrics, 81(4):529–536.

Barr, R. G. (1990). Hum Nat, 1(4):355–389.

Barr, S. I., Janelle, K. C., & Prior, J. C. (1994). Am J Clin Nutr, 60(6):887–894.

Barry, P. W., & Pollard, A. J. (2003). BMJ, 326(7395):915–919.

Barsalou, L. W. (1999). Behav Brain Sci, 22(4):577–660.

Barsalou, L. W., Niedenthal, P. M., Barbey, A., & Ruppert, J. (2003). Social embodiment. In: Psychology of Leaning and Motivation: Advances in Research and Theory, B. Ross (ed.). New York: Elsevier Science, pp. 43–92.

Bartolomucci, A., Palanza, P., Sacerdote, P., Panerai, A. E., et al. (2005). Neurosci Biobehav Rev, 29(1):67–81.

Bartsch, P., Maggiorni, M., Schobersberger, W., Shaw, S., et al. (1991). J Appl Physiol, 71(1):136–143.

Bartsch, P., & Roach, R. C. (2001). Acute mountain sickness and high-altitude cerebral edema. In: High Altitude: An Exploration of Human Adaptation, T. F. Hornbein, & R. B. Schoene (eds.). New York: Marcel Dekker, Inc., pp. 731–776.

Bartsch, P., Bailey, D. M., Berger, M. M., Knauth, M., et al. (2004). High Alt Med Biol, 5(2):110–124.

Basheer, R., Strecker, R. E., Thakkar, M. M., & McCarley, R. W. (2004). Prog Neurobiol, 73(6):379–396.

Basnyat, B., & Murdoch, D. R. (2003). Lancet, 361(9373):1967–1974.

Basso, O., Wilcox, A. J., & Weinberg, C. R. (2006). Am J Epidemiol, 164(4):303–311.

Bates, C. (1987). Essential Fatty Acids and Immunity in Mental Health. Tacoma, WA: Life Science Press.

Bates, S. L., Sharkey, K. A., & Meddings, J. B. (1998). Am J Physiol, 274(3 [Pt 1]):G552–G560.

Bateson, G. (1963). Evolution, 17(4):529–539.

Bateson, P. (2001). Int J Epidemiol, 30(5):928–934.

Bateson, P., Barker, D., Clutton–Brock, T., Deb, D., et al. (2004). Nature, 430(6998):419–421.

Bauer, R. L. (1998). Am J Epidemiol, 127(1):145–149.

Bayless, T. M., & Rosensweig, N. S. (1966). J Am Med Assoc, 197(12):968–972.

Bayless, T. M., & Rosensweig, N. S. (1967). Johns Hopkins Med J, 121(1):54–64.

Bdolah, Y., Sukhatme, V. P., Karumanchi, S. A., Bdolah, Y., et al. (2004). Semin Nephrol, 24(6):548–556.

Beal, A. C., Chou, S. C., Palmer, R. H., Testa, M. A., et al. (2006). Pediatrics, 117(5):1618–1625.

Beale, C. L. (2000). Food Rev, 23(1):16–22.

Beardsworth, A., & Keil, T. (1997). Sociology on the Menu: An Invitation to the Study of Food and Society. London: Routledge.

Beauchamp, G. K. (1989). Appetite, 12:72.

Beauchamp, G. K., Bachmanov, A., & Stein, L. J. (1998). Ann NY Acad Sci, 855:412–416.

Bechara, A., Damasio, H., & Damasio, A. R. (2000). Cereb Cortex, 10(3):295–307.

Begley, S. (1993). Newsweek, 121(19):62–63.

Beidler, L. M. (1982). Biological basis of food selection. In: The Psychobiology of Human Food Selection, L. M. Baker (ed.). Westport, CT: AVI Publishing Company, Inc, pp. 1–15.

Bekker, A., Holland, H. D., Wang, P. L., Rumble 3rd, D., et al. (2004). Nature, 427(6970):117–120.

Bel Aiba, R. S., Dimova, E. Y., Gorlach, A., & Kietzmann, T. (2006). Expert Opin Ther Targets, 10(4):583–599.

Bell, C. (1997). Ritual: Perspectives and Dimensions. New York: Oxford University Press.

Bell, D. S. (2000). Endocr Pract, 6(3):272–276.

Bell, G. (1997). Selection: The Mechanism of Evolution. New York: Chapman, & Hall.

Belland, R. J., Ouellette, S. P., Gieffers, J., & Byrne, G. I. (2004). Cell Microbiol, 6(2):117–127.

Bellanger, T. M., & Bray, G. A. (2005). J La State Med Soc, 157 (Spec No 1):S42–S49.

Bellisle, F. (1999). Neurosci Biobehav Rev, 23(3):423–438.

Belsky, J., Steinberg, L., & Draper, P. (1991). Child Dev, 62(4):647–670.

Belsky, J. (1997). Hum Nat, 8(4):361–381.

Belsky, J. (2005). The developmental and evolutionary psychology of intergenerational transmission of attachment. In: Attachment and Bonding: A New Synthesis, C. S. Carter, L. Ahnert, K. E. Grossmann, S. B. Hrdy, M. E. Lamb, S. W. Porges, & N. Sachser (eds.). Cambridge, MA: MIT Press.

Belsky, J., Jaffee, S. R., Sligo, J., Woodward, L., et al. (2005). Child Dev, 76(2):384–396.

Ben Shaul, D. M. (1962). Int Zoo Yearbook, 4:333–342.

Benedict, C. R., Shelton, B., Johnstone, D. E., Francis, G., et al. (1996). Circulation, 94(4):690–697.

Benjamin, N. (1999). Lancet, 353(9149):256–257.

Bennett, A. F. (1991). J Exp Biol, 160:1–23.

Bennett, J. W., & Klich, M. (2003). Clin Microbiol Rev, 16(3):497–516.

Ben-Shlomo, Y., Holly, J. M. P., McCarthy, A., Savage, P., et al. (2003). Clin Endocrinol, 59(3):366–373.

Ben-Shlomo, Y., Holly, J. M. P., McCarthy, A., Savage, P., et al. (2005). Cancer Epidemiol Biomarkers Prev, 14(5):1336–1339.

Bentley, G. R., Harrigan, A. M., & Ellison, P. T. (1990). Am J Phys Anthropol, 81(2):193–194.

Bentley, G. R., Harrigan, A. M., & Ellison, P. T. (1998). Eur J Clin Nutr, 52(4):261–270.

Bentley, G. R., Vitzthum, V. J., Caceres, E., Spielvogel, H., et al. (2000). Am J Hum Biol, 12:279.

Benyshek, D. C., Martin, J. F., & Johnston, C. S. (2001). Med Anthropol, 20(1):25–64.

Benyshek, D. C., Johnston, C. S., & Martin, J. F. (2006). Diabetologia, 49(5):1117–1119.

Berenson, A. B., Wiemann, C. M., Rickerr, V. I., & McCombs, S. L. (1997). Am J Obstet Gynecol, 176(3):586–592.

Berenson, G. S., Srinivasan, S. R., Bao, W. H., Newman, W. P., et al. (1998). N Engl J Med, 338(23):1650–1656.

Bergemann, N., Parzer, P., Nagl, I., Salbach, B., et al. (2002). Arch Womens Ment Health, 5(3):119–126.

Berger, P. J., Negus, N. C., Pinter, A. J., & Nagy, T. R. (1992). Can J Zool, 70(3):518–522.

Berger, R. J., & Phillips, N. H. (1995). Behav Brain Res, 69(1–2):65–73.

Bergeron, C., Ferenczy, A., & Shyamala, G. (1988). Lab Invest, 58(3):338–345.

Bergstrom, C. T., Lo, M., & Lipsitch, M. (2004). Proc Natl Acad Sci USA, 101(36):13285–13290.

Berkey, C. S., Frazier, A. L., Gardner, J. D., & Colditz, G. A. (1999). Cancer, 85(11):2400–2409.

Berkey, C. S., Gardner, J. D., Frazier, A. L., & Colditz, G. A. (2000). Am J Epidemiol, 152(5):446–452.

Berkey, C. S., Rockett, H. R. H., Willett, W. C., & Colditz, G. A. (2005). Arch Pediatr Adolesc Med, 159(6):543–550.

Bernardino, M. E., & Lawson, T. L. (1976). Digest Dis, 21(6):503–506.

Bernhardt, W. M., Schmitt, R., Rosenberger, C., Münchenhagen, P. M., et al. (2006). Kidney Int, 69(1):114–122.

Bernstein, I. L. (1999). Nutrition, 15(3):229–234.

Bernstein, L., & Ross, R. K. (1993). Epidemiol Rev, 15(1):48–65.

Bernstein, L. (2002). J Mammary Gland Biol Neoplasia, 7(1):3–15.

Bernstein, L., Teal, C. R., Joslyn, S., & Wilson, J. (2003). Cancer, 97(Suppl 1):222–229.

Berridge, K. C. (2003). Comparing the emotional brain of humans and other animals. In: Handbook of Affective Sciences, R. J. Davidson, H. H. Goldsmith, & K. Scherer (eds.). New York: Oxford University Press, pp. 25–51.

Berthoud, H. R. (2004). Physiol Behav, 81(5):781–793.

Better Homes and Gardens. (1965). Baby Book. New York: Bantam.

Beyers, J. M., Toumbourou, J. W., Catalano, R. F., Arthur, M. W., et al. (2004). J Adolesc Health, 35(1):3–16.

Beylin, A. V., & Shors, T. J. (2003). Horm Behav, 43(1):1124–1131.

Biegert, J. (1957). Morph Jahr, 98:77–199.

Biegert, J. (1963). The evaluation of characteristics of the skull, hands, and feet for primate taxonomy. In: Classification and Human Evolution, S. L. Washburn (ed.). Chicago: Aldine Publishing Co, pp. 116–145.

Billing, J., & Sherman, P. W. (1998). Q Rev Biol, 73(1):3–49.

Bilton, R. L., & Booker, G. W. (2003). Eur J Biochem, 270(5):791–798.

Bingham, C. R., Miller, B. C., & Adams, G. R. (1990). J Adolesc Res, 5(1):18–33.

Binkin, N. J., Yip, R., Fleshood, L., & Trowbridge, F. L. (1988). Pediatrics, 82(6):828–834.

Biong, A. S., Veierød, M. B., Ringstad, J., Thelle, D. S., et al. (2006). Eur J Clin Nutr, 60(2):236–244.

Birch, L. L. (1987). The acquisition of food acceptance patterns in children. In: Eating Habits: Food, Physiology and Learned Behaviour, R. A. Boakes, D. A. Popplewell, & M. J. Burton (eds.). Chichester, UK: John Wiley, & Sons, pp. 107–130.

Birch, L. L., & Fisher, J. A. (1996). The role of experience in the development of children's eating behavior. In: Why We Eat What We Eat: The Psychology of Eating, E. D. Capaldi (ed.). Washington, DC: American Psychological Association, pp. 113–141.

Bishopric, N. H. (2005). Ann NY Acad Sci, 1047:13–29.

Biss, K., Ho, K.–J., Mikkelson, B., Lewis, L., et al. (1971). N Engl J Med, 284(13):694–699.

Bjorklund, D. F., & Pellegrini, A. D. (2002). The Origins of Human Nature: Evolutionary Developmental Psychology. Washington, DC: American Psychological Association.

Bjorkland, D. F., & Bering, J. M. (2003). Big brains, slow development and social complexity: The development and evolutionary origins of social cognition. In: The Social Brain: Evolution and Pathology, M. Brüne, H. Ribbert, & W. Schiefenhövel (eds.). New York: Wiley, pp. 113–151.

Bjorklund, D. F., & Rosenberg, J. S. (2005). The role of developmental plasticity in the evolution of human cognition: Evidence from enculturated, juvenile great apes. In: Origins of the Social Mind: Evolutionary Psychology and Child Development B. J. Ellis & D. F. Bjorklund (eds.). New York: Guilford Press, pp. 45–75.

Björntorp, P. (1990). Atherosclerosis, 10(4):493–496.

Björntorp, P. (1991). J Intern Med, 230(3):195–201.

Björntorp, P., & Eden, S. (1996). Hormonal influences on body composition. In: Human Body Composition, A. F. Roche & S. B. Lohman (eds.). Champaign, IL: Human Kinetics, pp. 329–344.

Björntorp, P. (1997). Hum Reprod, 12(Suppl 1):21–25.

Black, M. M., Hutcheson, J. J., Dubowitz, H., & Berenson–Howard, J. (1994). J Pediatr Psychol, 19(6):689–707.

Black, P. H. (2006). Med Hypotheses, 67(4):879–891.

Black, R. E., WIlliams, S. M., Jones, I. E., & Goulding, A. (2002). Am J Clin Nutr, 76(3):675–680.

Black, R. E., Morris, S. S., & Bryce, J. (2003). Lancet, 361(9376):2226–2234.

Blair, P. S., Fleming, P. J., Smith, I. J., Ward Platt, M., et al. (1999). BMJ, 319(7223):1457–1461.

Blair, P. S., & Ball, H. L. (2004). Arch Dis Child, 89(12):1106–1110.

Blair, S. N., LaMonte, M. J., & Nichaman, M. Z. (2004). Am J Clin Nutr, 79(5):913–920.

Blass, E. M., Shide, D. J., & Weller, A. (1989). Appetite, 12:75.

Bledsoe, E. R., O'Rourke, M. T., & Ellison, P. T. (1990). Am J Phys Anthropol, 81(2):195–196.

Bloche, M. G. (2004). N Engl J Med, 351(20):2035–2037.

Bloom, G., & Sherman, P. W. (2005). Evol Hum Behav, 26(4):301–312.

Bloom, P. D., & Boedeker, E. C. (1996). Semin Gastrointest Dis, 7(3):151–166.

Blum, K., Cull, J. G., Braverman, E. R., & Comings, D. E. (1996). Am Sci, 84(2):132–145.

Blurton Jones, N. G. (1987). Soc Sci Inf, 26(1):31–54.

Blurton Jones, N. G., Hawkes, K., & O'Connell, J. F. (2002). Am J Hum Biol, 14(2):184–205.

Blurton Jones, N. G., & Marlowe, F. W. (2002). Hum Nat, 13(2):199–238.

Boas, F. (1912). Am Anthropol, 14(3):530–562.

Boaz, N. (2002). Evolving Health: The Origins of Illness and How the Modern World Is Making Us Sick. New York: John Wiley, & Sons, Inc.

Bock, J. A. (2005). Farming, foraging, and children's play in the Okavango Delta, Botswana. In: The Nature of Play: Great Apes and Humans, A. D. Pellegrini, & P. K. Smith (eds.). New York: Guilford Press, pp. 254–281.

Bodaghi, B., Goureau, O., Zipeto, D., Laurent, L., et al. (1999). J Immunol, 162(2):957–964.

Bode, L., Dietrich, D. E., Stoyloff, R., Emrich, H. M., et al. (1997). Lancet, 349(9046):178–179.

Bode, L., Reckwald, P., Severus, W. E., Stoyloff, R., et al. (2001). Mol Psychiatry, 6:481–491.

Boehm, C. (1978). Am Anthropol, 80(2):265–296.

Boehm, C. (1999). Hierarchy in the Forest: The Evolution of Egalitarian Behavior. Cambridge, MA: Harvard University Press.

Bogaert, A. F. (2005). J Adolesc, 28(4):541–546.

Bogin, B. (1994). Acta Paediatr, 406:29–35.

Bogin, B., & Smith, B. H. (1996). Am J Hum Biol, 8(6):703–716.

Bogin, B. (1998). Evolutionary and biological aspects of childhood. In: Biosocial Perspectives on Children, C. Panter-Brick (ed.). Cambridge, UK: Cambridge University Press, pp. 10–44.

Bogin, B. (1999). Patterns of Human Growth, 2nd ed. Cambridge, UK: Cambridge University Press.

Bogin, B., & Marela–Silva, M. I. V. (2003). J Child Health, 1:149–173.

Boncristiano, M., Paccani, S. R., Barone, S., Ulivieri, C., et al. (2003). J Exp Med, 198(12):1887–1897.

Bongaarts, J. (1980). Science, 208(4444):564–569.

Bonilla, J. (2001). Executive Summary: A Demographic Profile of Hispanics in the U.S. Washington, DC: Population Resource Center.

Bonita, R., Duncan, J., Truelsen, T., Jackson, R. T., et al. (1999). Tob Control, 8(2):156–160.

Bonjour, J.–P., Carrie, A.–L., Ferrari, S., Clavien, H., et al. (1997). J Clin Invest, 99(6):1287–1294.

Bonjour, J.–P., Chevalley, T., Ammann, P., Slosman, D., et al. (2001). Lancet, 358(9289):1208–1212.

Bonner, J. T. (1965). Size and Cycle: An Essay on the Structure of Biology. Princeton, NJ: Princeton University Press.

Bonner, J. T. (1974). On Development: The Biology of Form. Cambridge, MA: Harvard University Press.

Bonnet, M. H., & Arand, D. L. (1995). Sleep, 18(10):908–911.

Bonnet, M. H. (2000). Sleep deprivation. In: Principles and Practice of Sleep Medicine, M. H. Kryger, T. Roth & W. C. Dement (eds.). Philadelphia: W.B. Saunders, pp. 53–71.

Boon, B., Stroebe, W., Schut, H., & Jansen, A. (1998). Br J Health Psychol, 3(1):27–40.

Bøorresen, B. (1994a). Tidsskr Nor Lægeforen, 114(1864).

Bøorresen, B. (1994b). Tidsskr Nor Lægeforen, 114(3501).

Boorse, C. (1997). A rebuttal on health. In: What Is Disease? J. Humber & K. Almeder (eds.). Totowa, NJ: Humana Press, pp. 3–134.

Booth, D. A. (1987). Cognitive experimental psychology of appetite. In: Eating Habits: Food, Physiology and Learned Behaviour, R. A. Boakes, D. A. Popplewell, & M. J. Burton (eds.). Chichester, UK: John Wiley, & Sons, pp. 175–209.

Booth, F. W., Chakravarthy, M. V., & Spangenburg, E. E. (2002). J Physiol, 543(2):399–411.

Booth, K. M., Pinkston, M. M., & Poston, W. S. (2005). J Am Diet Assoc, 105(5 [Suppl 1]):S110–117.

Borbély, A. A., & Achermann, P. (2000). Sleep homeostasis and models of sleep regulation. In: Principles and Practices of Sleep Medicine, M. H. Kryger, T. Roth, & W. C. Dement (eds.). Philadelphia: W.B. Saunders, pp. 377–390.

Borch–Johnsen, K., Colagiuri, S., Balkau, B., Glumer, C., et al. (2004). Diabetologia, 47(8):1396–1402.

Borgerhoff Mulder, M. (1992). Reproductive decisions. In: Evolutionary Ecology and Human Behavior, E. A. Smith, & B. Winterhalder (eds.). Hawthorne, NY: Aldine de Gruyter, pp. 339–374.

Bouchard, C., & Johnston, F. E. (eds.). (1988). Fat Distribution During Growth and Later Health Outcomes: A Symposium Held at Manoir St–Castin, Loc Beauport, Quebec, June 9–11. 1987. New York: John Wiley and Sons.

Bourgois, P. (2003). In Search of Respect: Selling Crack in El Barrio, 2nd ed. New York: Cambridge University Press.

Bowlby, J. (1969a). Attachment and Loss: Volume 1. Attachment. New York: Basic Books.

Bowlby, J. (1969b). Attachment and Loss: Volume 2. Separation Anxiety and Anger. New York: Basic Books.

Boyer, D., & Fine, D. (1992). Fam Plann Perspect, 24(1):4–11.

Boyer, P., & Lienard, P. (2006). Behav Brain Sci, 29(6):635–650.

Boys, A., & Marsden, J. (2003). Addiction, 98(7):951–963.

Bozza, S., Fallarino, F., Pitzurra, L., Zelante, T., et al. (2005). J Immunol, 174(5):2910–2918.

Brabin, L. (2001). BMJ, 323(7309):394–395.

Brace, L. D. (2002). J Cardiovasc Nurs, 16(4):33–49.

Bradshaw, S. D., & Bradshaw, F. J. (2002). Gen Comp Endocrinol, 126(1):7–13.

Braly, J., & Hoggan, R. (2002). Dangerous Grains: Why Gluten Cereal Grains May Be Hazardous To Your Health. New York: Penguin Putman Inc.

Brandt, I., Sticker, E. J., & Lentze, M. J. (2003). J Pediatr, 142(5):463–468.

Bratberg, G. H., Nilsen, T. I., Holmen, T. L., & Vatten, L. J. (2005). Eur J Pediatr, 164(10):621–625.

Braun, B., Butterfield, G. E., Dominick, S. B., Zamudio, S., et al. (1998). J Appl Physiol, 85(4):1966–1973.

Bray, G. A. (1987). Nutr Rev, 45(2):33–43.

Bray, G. A., Bouchard, C., & James, W. P. T. (eds.). (1998). Handbook of Obesity. New York: Marcel Dekker.

Brehm, B. J., Seeley, R. J., Daniels, S. R., & D'Alessio, D. A. (2003). J Clin Endocrinol Metab, 88(4):1617–1623.

Brenner, B. M., Garcia, D. L., & Anderson, S. (1988). Am J Hypertens, 1(4 [Pt 1]):335–347.

Breslau, N., Roth, T., Rosenthal, L., & Andreski, P. (1996). Biol Psychiatry, 39(6):411–418.

Brett, J., & Niermeyer, S. (1999). Is neonatal jaundice a disease or an adaptive process? In: Evolutionary Medicine, W. R. Trevathan, E. O. Smith, & J. J. McKenna (eds.). New York: Oxford University Press, pp. 7–26.

Brillat–Savarin, J. A. (1995). The Physiology of Taste, or Meditations on Transcendental Gastronomy. Washington, DC: Counterpoint.

Brindley, D. N., & Rolland, Y. (1989). Clin Sci, 77(5):453–461.

Broadhurst, C. L. (1997). Altern Med Rev, 2:378–399.

Brocks, J. J., Love, G. D., Summons, R. E., Knoll, A. H., et al. (2005). Nature, 437(7060):866–870.

Bronner, M. P. (2004). Semin Diagn Pathol, 21(2):98–107.

Broocks, A., Pirke, K. M., Schweiger, U., Tuschl, R. J., et al. (1990). J Appl Physiol, 68(5):2083–2086.

Brook, I. (2002). Pediatr Emerg Care, 18(5):358–359.

Brook, J. S., Brook, D. W., de la Rosa, M., Duque, L. F., et al. (1998). J Am Acad Child Adolesc Psychiatry, 37(7):759–766.

Brothers, L. (1990). The social brain: A project for integrating primate behavior and neurophysiology in a new domain. In: Concepts in Neuroscience, Anonymous (ed.). Teaneck, NJ: World Scientific, pp. 27–51.

Brown, P. J., & Konner, M. J. (1987). Ann NY Acad Sci, 499:29–46.

Brown, A. S., Begg, M. D., Gravenstein, S., Schaefer, C. A., et al. (2004). Arch Gen Psychiatry, 61(8):774–780.

Brown, A. S., Schaefer, C. A., Quesenberry Jr., C. P., Liu, L., et al. (2005). Am J Psychiatry, 162(4):767–773.

Brown, J. A., Cobb, C. S., Frankling, S. C., & Rankin, J. C. (2005). J Exp Biol, 208(2):223–232.

Brown, M. A. (1997). Lancet, 349(9048):297–298.

Brown, W. D. (2006). Insomnia: Prevalence and daytime consequences. In: Sleep: A Comprehensive Handbook, T. L. Lee-Chiong (ed.). Hoboken, NJ: John Wiley, pp. 93–98.

Brownell, K. D., & Horgen, K. B. (2004). Food Fight: The Inside Story of the Food Industry, America's Obesity Crisis, and What We Can Do About It. Chicago, : Contemporary Books.

Bruinsma, J., Alexandratos, N., Schmidhuber, J., Bödeker, G., et al. (2003). World Agriculture: Toward 2015/2030—An FAO Perspective. London, UK: Earthscan Publications Ltd.

Brundtland, G. H., Liestøl, K., & Walløoe, L. (1975). Tidsskr Nor Lægeforen, 95:79–83.

Brundtland, G. H., Liestøl, K., & Walløoe, L. (1980). Ann Hum Biol, 7:307–322.

Brunner, E. (1997). BMJ, 314(7092):1472–1476.

Brunvand, L., Henriksen, C., & Haug, E. (1996). Tidsskr Nor Lægeforen, 116:1585–1587.

Bruset, S., & Henriksen, J. (1996). Slank på Steinaldermat: Følg Jon fra Overvekt til Jaktvekt [Slim on Paleolithic Diet: Follow Jon From Overweight to Hunting Weight]. Oslo, Norway: Gyldendal.

Bucala, R., Cerami, A., & Vlassara, H. (1995). Diabetes Rev, 3(2):258–268.

Buckley, N. (2004). Finding the taste for profit: Obesity forces food companies to rethink their recipes. London: Financial Times, Aug. 31, 1.

Buckley, T., & Gottlieb, A. (1988). A critical appraisal of menstrual symbolism. In: Blood Magic: The Anthropology of Menstruation, T. Buckley, & A. Gottlieb (eds.). Berkeley, CA: University of California Press, pp. 1–50.

Buemi, M., Cavallaro, E., Floccari, F., Sturiale, A., et al. (2003). J Neuropathol Exp Neurol, 62(3):228–236.

Buka, S. L. (2000). Potential Applications of the National Collaborative Perinatal Project for the Study of Toxoplasma Infections and Psychiatric Disease, Presented at the Stanley

Symposium, Toxoplasma Infection and Schizophrenia. Johns Hopkins University, Baltimore, MD.

Buka, S. L., Tsuang, M. T., Torrey, E. F., Klebanoff, M. A., et al. (2001). Arch Gen Psychiatry, 58(11):1032–1037.

Bulbrook, R. D. (1991). Oxf Rev Reprod Biol, 13:175–202.

Buljevac, D., Verkooyen, R. P., Jacobs, B. C., Hop, W., et al. :2003). Ann Neurol, 54(6):828–831.

Bullen, B. A., Skrinar, G. S., Beitins, I. Z., von Mering, G., et al. (1985). N Engl J Med, 312(21):1349–1353.

Buller, D. J. (2005). Adapting Minds: Evolutionary Psychology and the Persistent Quest for Human Nature. Cambridge, MA: MIT Press.

Burkhart, C. G., Burkhart, C. N., & Lehmann, P. F. (1999). Postgrad Med J, 75(884):328–331.

Burkitt, D. P., & Eaton, S. B. (1989). Nutrition, 5(3):189–191.

Burkman, R. T. (2001). Clin Obstet Gynecol, 44(1):62–72.

Burrows, R., Hofer, H., & East, M. L. (1995). Proc R Soc Lond B Biol Sci, 262(1364):235–245.

Burton, J. L., Cartlidge, M., & Shuster, S. (1973). Acta Derm Venereol, 53(2):81–84.

Bushuev, V. I., Miasnikova, G. Y., Sergueeva, A. I., Polyakova, L. A., et al. (2006). Haematologica, 91(6):744.

Buskila, D., Shnaider, A., Neumann, L., Zilberman, D., et al. (1997). Arch Intern Med, 157(21):2497–2500.

Buskila, D. (2000). Curr Opin Rheumatol, 12(2):113–123.

Butler, T., Pan, H., Epstein, J., Protopopescu, X., et al. (2005). Neuroreport, 16(11):1233–1236.

Butte, N., & Jensen, C. B. (1992). Pediatr Res, 32(5):514–519.

Butte, N., Wong, W., & Hopkinson, J. (2001). J Nutr, 131(1):53–58.

Butterfield, G. E., Gates, J., Fleming, S., Brooks, G. A., et al. (1992). J Appl Physiol, 72(5):1741–1748.

Buwalda, B., Kole, M. H. P., Veenema, A. H., Huininga, M., et al. (2005). Neurosci Biobehav Rev, 29(1):83–97.

Buxton, K. E., Gielen, A. C., Faden, R. R., Brown, C., H., et al. (1991). Am J Prev Med, 7(2):101–106.

Buysse, D. J. (2005). J Psychiatr Pract, 11(2):102–115.

Byard, R. W. (1994). J Paediatr Child Health, 30(3):198–199.

Byard, R. W. (1998). J Paediatr Child Health, 34(5):418–419.

Byrne, G. I., & Kalayoglu, M. V. (1999). Am Heart J, 138(5 [Part2]):S488–490.

Byrne, R. W., & Whiten, A. (eds.). (1988). Machiavellian Intelligence: Social Expertise and the Evolution of Intellect in Monkeys, Apes, and Humans. New York: Clarendon Press/Oxford University Press.

Byrne, R. W. (2002a). The primate origins of human intelligence. In: The Evolution of Intelligence, R. J. Sternberg, & J. C. Kaufman (eds.). Mahwah, NJ: Lawrence Erlbaum Associates, pp. 79–95.

Byrne, R. W. (2002b). Social and technical forms of primate intelligence. In: Tree of Origin: What Primate Behavior Can Tell Us About Human Social Evolution, F. B. M. de Waal (ed.). Cambridge, MA: Harvard University Press, pp. 145–172.

Bystrova, O. A., Parfenov, V. N., & Martynova, M. G. (2002). Tsitologiia, 44(2):115–119.

Cacioppo, J. T., Hawkley, L. C., Berntson, G. G., Ernst, J. M., et al. (2002). Psychol Sci, 13(4):384–387.

Cadogan, J., Eastell, R., Jones, N., & Barker, M. E. (1997). BMJ, 315(7118):1255–1260.

Cahill, G. F., & Veech, R. L. (2003). Trans Am Clin Climatol Assoc, 114:149–161.

Cambien, F., Leger, J., Mallet, C., Levy-Marchal, C., et al. (1998). Diabetes, 47(3):470–475.

Cameron, N. (2002). Human Growth and Development. New York: Academic Press.

Cameron, N., & Demerath, E. W. (2002). Yearb Phys Anthropol, 45:159–184.

Cameron, N. M., Champagne, F. A., Parent, C., Fish, E. W., et al. (2005). Neurosci Biobehav Rev, 29(4–5):843–865.

Campbell, B. C., & Cajigal, A. (2001). Med Hypotheses, 57(1):64–67.

Campbell, B. C., Leslie, P., & Campbell, K. I. (2006). Am J Hum Biol, 18(1):71–82.

Campbell, D. I., Elia, M., & Lunn, P. G. (2003). J Nutr, 133:1332–1338.

Campbell, J., Hauser, M., & Hill, J. (1991). Nutritional Characteristics of Organic, Freshly Stone-Ground, Sourdough and Conventional Breads. Quebec, Canada: McGill University.

Cannon, C. M., & Bseikri, M. R. (2004). Physiol Behav, 81(5):741–748.

Cannon, W. B. (1914). J Philos Psychol Sci Meth, 11:162–165.

Capaldi, E. D. (1996). Conditioned food preferences. In: Why We Eat What We Eat: The Psychology of Eating, E. D. Capaldi (ed.). Washington, DC: American Psychological Association, pp. 53–80.

Capaldi, V. F., Handwerger, K., Richardson, E., & Stroud, L. R. (2005). Behav Sleep Med, 3(4):177–192.

Capellini, I., Barton, R. A., McNamara, P., & Nunn, C. L. (in press). J Expe Biol.

Caplan, P. (ed.) (1997). Food, Health and Identity. New York: Routledge.

Cardinal, R. N., Parkinson, J. A., Hall, J., & Everitt, B. J. (2002). Neurosci Biobehav Rev, 26(3):321–352.

Cardinal, R. N., & Everitt, B. J. (2004). Curr Opin Neurobiol, 14(2):156–162.

Carey, W. B. (1975). J Pediatr, 87 (2):327.

Carpenter, R. G., Irgens, L. M., Blair, P. S., England, P. D., et al. (2004). Lancet, 363(9404):185–191.

Carroll, R. L. (1997). Patterns and Processes of Vertebrate Evolution. New York: Cambridge University Press.

Carskadon, M. A., & Dement, W. C. (2000). Normal human sleep: An overview. In: Principles and Practice of Sleep Medicine, M. H. Kryger, T. Roth, & W. C. Dement (eds.). Philadelphia: W.B. Saunders, pp. 15–25.

Carskadon, M. A. (ed.) (2002). Adolescent Sleep Patterns: Biological, Social, and Psychological. Cambridge, UK: Cambridge University Press.

Carson, P., Ziesche, S., Johnson, G., & Cohn, J. N. (1999). J Card Fail, 5(3):178–187.

Carson, R. (1962). Silent Spring. London: Penguin.

Carter, C. S. (2005). Biological perspectives on social attachment and bonding. In: Attachment and Bonding: A New Synthesis, C. S. Carter, L. Ahnert, K. Grossmann, S. B. Hrdy, M. E. Lamb, S. Porges, & N. Sachser (eds.). Cambridge, MA: MIT Press, pp. 85–100.

Cartmill, M. (1974). Arboreal adaptations and the origins of the Order Primates. In: The Functional and Evolutionary Biology of Primates, R. H. Tuttle (ed.). Chicago, : Aldine Atherton, pp. 97–122.

Case, A. M., & Reid, R. L. (1998). Arch Intern Med, 158(13):1405–1412.

Case, A. M., & Reid, R. L. (2001). Compr Ther, 27(1):65–71.

Casey, R., & Rozin, P. (1989). Appetite, 12(3):171–182.

Caspari, R., & Lee, S. H. (2004). Proc Natl Acad Sci USA, 101(30):10895–10900.

Caspi, A., & Moffitt, T. E. (1991). J Pers Soc Psychol, 61(1):157–168.

Casserly, I., & Topol, E. (2004). Lancet, 363(9415):1139–1146.

Castelo-Branco, C., Reina, F., Montivero, A. D., Colodron, M., et al. (2006). Gynecol Endocrinol, 22(1):31–35.

Catanese, D. M., Koetting O'Byrne, K., & Poston, W. S. C. (2001). The epidemiology of obesity in developed countries. In: Obesity, Growth and Development, F. Johnston, & G. Foster (eds.). London: Smith-Gordon, pp. 69–90.

CBS News (2003). New pill stops women's periods. Washington, DC.

Ceesay, S. M., Prentice, A. M., Cole, T. J., Foord, F., et al. (1997). BMJ, 315(7111):786–790.

Centers for Disease Control and Prevention (2003), Get Smart: Know When Antibiotics Work, http://www.cdc.gov/drugresistance/community/media/Virtual_Press_Kit Complete_ABR_VPK.pdf

Centers for Disease Control and Prevention (2004a), Malaria Facts, http://www.cdc.gov/ malaria facts.htm

Centers for Disease Control and Prevention. (2004b). MMWR Morb Mortal Wkly Rep, 53(36):844–847.

Centers for Disease Control and Prevention (2005a). Chronic Disease Prevention: Preventing Heart Disease and Stroke. Atlanta, GA: CDC.

Centers for Disease Control and Prevention (2005b). National Diabetes Fact Sheet, http: www.cdc.gov/diabetes/pubs/estimates05.html

Centers for Disease Control and Prevention. (2005c). MMWR Morb Mortal Wkly Rep, 54(37):933.

Centers for Disease Control and Prevention (2006a). U.S. Physical Activity Statistics: 2005 State Summary Data. Atlanta, GA: CDC.

Centers for Disease Control and Prevention. (2006b). National Program of Cancer Registries Invasive Cancer Incidence Request, http://wonder.cdc.gov/cancer.html

Centers for Disease Control and Prevention (2006c). Health Disparities in Cancer: Cancer Among Women. Atlanta, GA: Centers for Disease Control and Prevention.

Centers for Disease Control and Prevention (2006d). Health Disparities in Cancer: Cancer Among Men. Atlanta, GA: Centers for Disease Control and Prevention.

Cerhan, J. R., Habermann, T. M., Vachon, C. M., Putnam, S. D., et al. (2002). Cancer Causes Control, 13(2):131–136.

Ceriello, A., & Pirisi, M. (1995). Diabetologia, 38(12):1484–1485.

Chagnon, N. A., Barlow, G. W., & Silverberg, J. (1980). Kin-selection theory, kinship, marriage and fitness among the Yanomamö indians. In: Sociobiology: Beyond Nature/Nurture? Reports, Definitions, and Debate, G. W. Barlow & J. Silverberg (eds.). Boulder, CO: Westview Press, pp. 545–571.

Chagnon, N. A. (1992). Yanomamö: The Last Days of Eden. San Diego, CA: Harcourt Brace Jovanovich.

Chakraborty, R., & Weiss, K. M. (1988). Proc Natl Acad Sci USA, 85(23):9119–9123.

Chakravarthy, M. V., & Booth, F. W. (2004). J Appl Physiol, 96(1):3–10.

Chaline, J., David, B., Magniez-Jannin, F., Malasse, A. D., et al. (1998). C R Acad Sci II, 326(4):291–298.

Chaline, J. (2003). J Reprod Immunol, 59(2):137–152.

Challis, B. G., Pinnock, S. B., Coll, A. P., Carter, R. N., et al. (2003). Biochem Biophys Res Commun, 311(4):915–919.

Challis, J. R., Bloomfield, F. H., Bocking, A. D., Casciani, V., et al. (2005). J Obstet Gynaecol Res, 31(6):492–499.

Champagne, F. A., Francis, D. D., Mar, A., & Meaney, M. J. (2003). Physiol Behav, 79(3):359–371.

Chan, G. M., Hoffman, K., & McMurry, M. (1995). J Pediatr, 126(4):551–556.

Chandler, M. H. H., Schuldheisz, S., Phillips, B. A., & Muse, K. N. (1997). Pharmacotherapy, 17(2):224–234.

Chandra, R. K. (2003). Nutrition, 19(11–12):978–979.

Chang, C. L., Donaghy, M., & Poulter, N. (1999). BMJ, 318(7175):13–18.

Chang, E. T., Smedby, K. E., Hjalgrim, H., Schöllkopf, C., et al. (2005). Am J Epidemiol, 162(10):965–974.

Chang, K.-L., Hung, T.-C., Hsieh, B.-S., Chen, Y.-H., et al. (2006). Nutrition, 22(5):465–474.

Chaouat, G., Ledee-Bataille, N., & Dubanchet, S. (2005). Am J Reprod Immunol, 53(5):222–229.

Chapman, C. A., & Chapman, L. J. (1990). Primates, 31(1):121–128.

Chapman, D. J., & Perez-Escamilla, R. (1999). J Am Diet Assoc, 99(4):450–454.

Charlton, B. G. (1996). Q J Med, 89(3):233–236.

Charnov, E. L., & Berrigan, D. (1993). Evol Anthropol, 1:191–194.

Charnov, E. L. (2001). Evol Ecol Res, 3(5):521–535.

Chatoor, I., Ganiban, J., Colin, V., Plummer, N., et al. (1998). J Am Acad Child Adolesc Psychiatry, 37(11):1217–1224.

Chatterjee, K. (2005). Am J Cardiol, 95(9A):8B–13B.

Chaudhari, N., Landin, A. M., & Roper, S. D. (2000). Nat Neurosci, 3(2):113–119.

Cheer, S. M., & Allen, J. S. (1997). Am J Hum Biol, 9(2):233–246.

Chehab, F. F., Mounzih, K., Lu, R., & Lim, M. E. (1997). Science, 275(5296):88–90.

Chen, A., & Rogan, W. J. (2004). Pediatrics, 113(5):e435–e439.

Chen, K. (2003a). Dairy firms churn out milk products in China, http://www.tschang.net/ articles 20030301.htm

Chen, K. (2003b). Got Milk? The new craze in China is dairy drinks. New York: Wall Street Journal, February 28.

Chen, N. G., Azhar, S., Abbasi, F., Carantoni, M., et al. (2000). Atherosclerosis, 152(1):203–208.

Chen, S. T. (1989). Asia Pac J Pub Health, 3(1):19–25.

Chesley, L. C. (2000). Am J Obstet Gynecol, 182(1 [Pt 1]):249–250.

Chevalley, T., Rizzoli, R., Hans, D., Ferrari, S., et al. (2005). J Clin Endocrinol Metab, 90(1):44–51.

Chiappe, D., & MacDonald, K. (2005). J Gen Psychol, 132(1):5–40.

Chisholm, J. S. (1993). Curr Anthropol, 34(1):1–24.

Chisholm, J. S. (1996). Hum Nat, 7(1):1–38.

Chisholm, J. S. (1999). Death, Hope, and Sex: Steps to an Evolutionary Ecology of Mind and Morality. Cambridge, UK: Cambridge University Press.

Chisholm, J. S. (2003). Uncertainty, contingency and attachment: A life history theory of theory of mind. In: From Mating to Mentality: Evaluating Evolutionary Psychology, K. Sterelny & J. Fitness (eds.). Hove, UK: Psychology Press, pp. 125–155.

Chisholm, J. S., Quinlivan, J. A., Petersen, R. W., & Coall, D. A. (2005). Hum Nat, 16(3):233–265.

Chivers, D. J., & Hladik, C. M. (1980). J Morphol, 166(3):337–386.

Chobanian, A. V., Bakris, G. L., Black, H. R., Cushman, W. C., et al. (2003). Hypertension, 42(6):1206–1252.

Choi, A. H., Kang, S. B., & Joe, S. H. (2001). Psychosom Med, 63(5):822–829.

Choi, H. K., Willett, W. C., Stampfer, M. J., Rimm, E., et al. (2005). Arch Intern Med, 165(9):997–1003.

Chong, S., & Whitelaw, E. (2004). Curr Opin Genet Dev, 14(6):692–696.

Church, A. J., Dale, R. C., Lees, A. J., Giovannoni, G., et al. (2003). J Neurol Neurosurg Psychiatry, 74(5):602–607.

Cizza, G., Skaarulis, M., & Mignot, E. (2005). Sleep, 28(10):1217–1220.

Claman, H. N. (1993). Recurrent pregnancy loss, immunologic and nonimmunologic aspects. In: The Immunology of Human Pregnancy, H. N. Claman (ed.). Totowa, NJ: Humana Press, pp. 171–212.

Clark, A. (1996). Being There: Putting Brain, Body, and World Together Again. Cambridge, MA: MIT Press.

Clark, D. H. (1953). BMJ, 1(4882):1254–1257.

Clark, R. F., Hutton, M., Talbot, C., Wragg, M., et al. (1996). Cold Spring Harb Symp Quant Biol, 61:551–558.

Clarke, A. S. (1993). Dev Psychobiol, 26(8):433–446.

Clarke, J. (1994). Hum Reprod, 9(7):1204–1207.

Clavel–Chapelon, F. (2002). Br J Cancer, 86(5):723–727.

Cleave, T. L. (1975). The Saccharine Disease. New Canaan, CT: Keats Publishing.

Cleeman, J. I. (2001). J Am Med Assoc, 285(19):2486–2497.

Clemens, L. E., Siiteri, P. K., & Stites, D. P. (1979). J Immunol, 122(5):1978–1985.

Clements, M. S., Mitchell, E. A., Wright, S. P., Esmail, A., et al. (1997). Acta Paediatr, 86(1):51–56.

Clydesdale, F. M. (1993). Crit Rev Food Sci Nutr, 33(1):83–101.

Coall, D. A., & Chisholm, J. S. (2003). Soc Sci Med, 57(10):1771–1781.

Cobb, C. S., Frankling, S. C., Thorndyke, M. C., Jensen, F. B., et al. (2004). Comp Biochem Physiol B Biochem Mol Biol, 138(4):357–364.

Cochran, G. M., Ewald, P. W., & Cochran, K. D. (2000). Perspect Biol Med, 43(3):406–448.

Coe, C. (1999). Psychosocial factors and psychoneuroimmunology within a lifespan perspective. In: Developmental Health and the Wealth of Nations: Social, Biological, and Educational Dynamics, D. P. Keating, & C. Hertzman (eds.). New York: Guilford Press, pp. 201–219.

Coe, C. L., & Shirtcliff, E. A. (2004). Pediatr Res, 55(6):914–920.

Cohen, G. J. (ed.) (1999). American Academy of Pediatrics: Guide to Your Child's Sleep. New York: Villard.

Cohen, M. A., Ellis, S. M., Le Roux, C. W., Batterham, R. L., et al. (2003). J Clin Endocrinol Metab, 88(10):4696–4701.

Cohen, M. L. (1992). Science, 257(5073):1050–1055.

Cohen, M. N. (1977). The Food Crisis in Prehistory. New Haven, CT: Yale University Press.

Cohen, M. N., & Armelagos, G. J. (eds.). (1984). Paleopathology at the Origins of Agriculture. Orlando, FL: Academic Press.

Cohen, M. N. (1987). The significance of long-term changes in human diet and food economy. In: Food and Evolution: Toward a Theory of Human Food Habits, M. Harris, & E. B. Ross (eds.). Philadelphia: Temple University Press, pp. 261–283.

Cohen, M. N. (1989). Health and the Rise of Civilization. New Haven, CT: Yale University Press.

Cohen, S., Doyle, W. J., Turner, R. B., Alper, C. M., et al. (2003). Psychosom Med, 65(4):652–657.

Cohn, G. J. (ed.) (1999). The American Academy of Pediatrics Guide to Your Child's Sleep: Birth Through Adolescence. New York: Random House.

Colditz, G. A., Willett, W. C., Stampfer, M. J., Rosner, B., et al. (1987). Am J Epidemiol, 126(5):861–870.

Cole, L. C. (1954). Q Rev Biol, 29(2):103–137.

Cole, T. J. (2000). Proc Nutr Soc, 59(2):317–324.

Coleman, R. M., & Gross, M. R. (1991). Trends Ecol Evol, 6(12):404–406.

Colin Bell, A., Adair, L. S., & Popkin, B. M. (2002). Am J Epidemiol, 155(4):346–353.

Collaborative Group on Hormonal Factors in Breast Cancer. (1996). Lancet, 347(9017):1713–1727.

Collins Jr., J. W., David, R. J., Symons, R., Handler, A., et al. (1998). Epidemiology, 9(3):286–289.

Collins Jr., J. W., Wu, S. Y., & David, R. J. (2002). Am J Epidemiol, 155(3):210–216.

Colpo A. (2006). The Great Cholesterol Con: Why Everything You've Been Told About Cholesterol, Diet And Heart Disease Is Wrong! Morrisville, NC: Lulu.

Colson, E. (1979). J Anthropol Res, 35(1):18–29.

Colucci, W. S. (2006a). Patient Information: Overview of Heart Failure. In: UpToDate, B. D. Rose (ed.). Waltham, MA: UpToDate.

Colucci, W. S. (2006b). Overview of therapy of heart failure due to systolic dysfunction. In: UpToDate, B. D. Rose (ed.). Waltham, MA: UpToDate.

Compton, W. M., Thomas, Y. F., Conway, K. P., & Colliver, J. D. (2005). Am J Psychiatry, 162(8):1494–1502.

Condon, J. (1993). Br J Psychiatry, 162:481–486.

Confavreux, C., Aimard, G., & Devic, M. (1980). Brain, 103(2):281–301.

Conger, R. D., Ge, X., Elder Jr., G. H., , Lorenz, F. O., et al. (1994). Child Dev, 65(2):541–561.

Conroy, G. C. (1990). Primate Evolution. New York: Norton.

CONSENSUS Trial Study Group. (1987). N Engl J Med, 316(23):1429–1435.

Constantine, G., Arundell, L., Finn, K., Lowe, P., et al. (1988). Br J Obstetr Gynecol, 95(5):493–496.

Cook, J., Irwig, L. M., Chinn, S., Altman, D. G., et al. (1979). J Epidemiol Community Health, 33(3):171–176.

Cook, P. J., Davies, P., Tunnicliffe, W., Ayres, J. G., et al. (1998). Thorax, 53(4):254–259.

Cooper, C., Kuh, D., Egger, P., Wadsworth, M., et al. (1996). Br J Obstet Gynaecol, 103(8):814–817.

Cooper, M. L., Frone, M. R., Russell, M., & Mudar, P. (1995). J Pers Soc Psychol, 69(5):990–1005.

Cooper, R. S., & Kaufman, J. S. (1998). Hypertension, 32(5):813–816.

Cooper, R. S., Amoah, A. G., & Mensah, G. A. (2003). Ethn Dis, 13(2 [Suppl 2]):S48–S52.

Cooper, R. S., Kaufman, J. S., & Ward, R. (2003). N Engl J Med, 348(12):1166–1170.

Copley, M. S., Berstan, R., Dudd, S. N., Docherty, G., et al. (2003). Proc Natl Acad Sci USA, 100(4):1524–1529.

Corbo, R. M., & Scacchi, R. (1999). Ann Hum Genet, 63(4):301–310.

Cordain, L., Gotshall, R. W., & Eaton, S. B. (1997). World Rev Nutr Diet, 81:49–60.

Cordain, L., Gotshall, R. W., Eaton, S. B., & Eaton III, S. B. (1998). Int J Sports Med, 19(5):328–335.

Cordain, L. (1999). World Rev Nutr Diet, 84:19–73.

Cordain, L., Brand Miller, J., Eaton, S. B., Mann, N., et al. (2000). Am J Clin Nutr, 71(3):682–692.

Cordain, L., Watkins, B. A., & Mann, N. J. (2001). World Rev Nutr Diet, 90:144–161.

Cordain, L. (2002). The Paleo Diet: Lose Weight and Get Healthy by Eating the Food You Were Designed to Eat. New York: John Wiley, & Sons.

Cordain, L., Eaton, S. B., Miller, J. B., Mann, N., et al. (2002). Eur J Clin Nutr, 56(Suppl 1):S42–52.

Cordain, L., Eades, M. R., & Eades, M. D. (2003). Comp Biochem Physiol A Mol Integr Physiol, 136(1):95–112.

Cordain, L., Eaton, S. B., Sebastian, A., Mann, N. J., et al. (2005). Am J Clin Nutr, 81(2):341–354.

Cordain, L., & Friel, J. (2005). The Paleo Diet for Athletes: A Nutritional Formula for Peak Athletic Performance. Emmaus, PA: Rodale.

Cordain, L. (2006). Saturated fat consumption in ancestral human diets: Implications for contemporary intakes. In: Phytochemicals: Nutrient-Gene Interactions, M. S. Meskin, W. R. Bidlack, & R. K. Randolph (eds.). Boca Raton, FL: CRC/Taylor, & Francis, pp. 115–126.

Corrao, G., Tragnone, A., Caprilli, R., Trallori, G., et al. (1998). Int J Epidemiol, 27(3):397–404.

Cosgrove, K. P., Hunter, R. G., & Carroll, M. E. (2002). Pharmacol Biochem Behav, 73(3):663–671.

Cosmides, L., & Tooby, J. (1997), Evolutionary psychology: A primer, http: //www.psych.ucsb.edu/research/cep/primer.html

Costantini, A. V., Wieland, H., & Qvick, L. I. (1998). The Garden of Eden Longevity Diet. Freiburg, Germany. Johann Friedrich Oberlin Verlag.

Côté, A. (2006). J Paediatr Child Health, 11(Suppl A):34A–38A.

Cottingham, J., & Hunter, D. (1992). Genitourin Med, 68(4):209–216.

Counihan, C. M. (1999). The Anthropology of Food and Body: Gender, Meaning, and Power. New York: Routledge.

Counihan, C. M. (ed.) (2002). Food in the USA. New York: Routledge.

Coutinho, E. M., & Segal, S. J. (1999). Is Menstruation Obsolete? New York: Oxford University Press.

Couturier, E. G. M., Bomhof, M. A. M., Knuistingh Neven, A., & van Duijn, N. P. (2003). Cephalalgia, 23(4):302–308.

Cowie, M. R., Mosterd, A., Wood, D. A., Deckers, J. W., et al. (1997). Eur Heart J, 18(2):208–225.

Crabbe, J. C. (2002). Annu Rev Psychol, 53:435–462.

Craig, R. G., Yip, J. K., So, M. K., Boylan, R. J., et al. (2003). J Periodontol, 74(7):1007–1016.

Cravchik, A., & Goldman, D. (2000). Arch Gen Psychiatry, 57(12):1105–1114.

Crawford, M., & Marsh, D. (1989). The Driving Force: Food, Evolution and the Future. London: Heinemann.

Crawley, J. N., & Corwin, R. L. (1994). Peptides, 15(4):731–755.

Crelin, E. S., & Scherz, R. G. (1978). Patient Care, 12(5):234–241.

Crespi, E. J., & Denver, R. J. (2005). Am J Hum Biol, 17(1):44–54.

Cresswell, J. L., Egger, P., Fall, C. H., Osmond, C., et al. (1997). Early Hum Dev, 49(2):143–148.

Crews, D. E., & Bindon, J. R. (1991). Ethn Dis, 1(1):42–49.

Crews, D. E., & Williams, S. R. (1999). Hum Biol, 71(4):475–503.

Crews, D. E. (2003). Human Senescence: Evolutionary and Biocultural Perspectives. Cambridge, UK: Cambridge University Press.

Crimmins, E. M., & Finch, C. E. (2006). Proc Natl Acad Sci USA, 103(2):498–503.

Critchley, H. O. D., Kelly, R. W., Brenner, R. M., & Baird, D. T. (2001). Clin Endocrinol, 55(6):701–710.

Critchley, H. O. D., Kelly, R. W., Brenner, R. M., & Baird, D. T. (2003). Steroids, 68(10–13):1061–1068.

Crombag, H. S., & Robinson, T. E. (2004). Curr Dir Psychol Sci, 13(3):107–111.

Cromer, B. A. (2003). Curr Opin Obstet Gynecol, 15(5):353–357.

Cronin, C. C., & Shanahan, F. (2001). Perspect Biol Med, 44(3):342–352.

Crow, J. F. (2002). Daedalus, 131(1):81–88.

Crow, T. J. (1995). Int Clin Psychopharmacol, 10(Suppl. 3):49–56.

Cruickshank, J. K., Mzayek, F., Liu, L., Kieltyka, L., et al. (2005). Circulation, 111(15):1932–1937.

Crystal, S. R., Bowen, D. J., & Bernstein, I. L. (1999). Physiol Behav, 67(2):181–187.

Cubillos-Garzon, L. A., Casas, J. P., Morillo, C. A., & Bautista, L. E. (2004). Am Heart J, 147(3):412–417.

Cummings, D. E., Purnell, J. Q., Frayo, R. S., Schmidova, K., et al. (2001). Diabetes, 50(8):1714–1719.

Cunnane, S. C., Harbige, L. S., & Crawford, M. A. (1993). Nutr Health, 9(3):219–235.

Cunningham, A. S. (1995). Breastfeeding: Adaptive behaviour for child health and longevity. In: Breastfeeding: Biocultural Perspectives, P. Stuart–Macadam, & K. Dettwyler (eds.). Hawthorne, NY: Aldine de Gruyter, pp. 243–263.

Curio, E. (1973). Experientia, 29(9):1045–1058.

Curio, E. (1987). Trends Ecol Evol, 2(6):148–152.

D'Adamo, P., & Whitney, C. (1996). Eat Right 4 Your Type: The Individualized Diet Solution to Staying Healthy, Living Longer, & Achieving Your Ideal Weight. New York: G.P. Putnam's Sons.

D'Adamo, P., & Whitney, C. (1998). Cook Right 4 Your Type. New York: G.P. Putnam's Sons.

D'Adamo, P. J., & Whitney, C. (1999). Blodtypedietten [The Blood Group Diet]. Oslo: WEM3.

D'Adamo, P., & Whitney, C. (2001). Live Right 4 Your Type: The Individualized Prescription for Maximizing Health, Metabolism, and Vitality in Every Stage of Life. New York: G.P. Putnam's Sons.

Dahl, O. P., Aarseth, J. H., Myhr, K. M., Nyland, H., et al. (2004). Acta Neurol Scand, 109(10):378–384.

Dahl, R. E. (2002). The regulation of sleep-arousal, affect, and attention in adolescence: Some questions and speculations. In: Adolescent Sleep Patterns: Biological, Social, and Psychological Influences, M. A. Carskadon (ed.). New York: Cambridge University Press, pp. 269–284.

Dahl, R. E. (2006). J Adolesc Health, 38(6):641–642.

Dalal, S., & Zhukovsky, D. S. (2006). J Support Oncol, 4(1):9–16.

Dale, R. C., Church, A. J., Surtees, A. H., Lees, A. J., et al. (2004). Brain, 127(Pt 1):21–33.

Dallman, M. F., Akana, S. F., Strack, A. M., Hanson, E. S., et al. (1995). Ann NY Acad Sci, 771:730–742.

Dallman, M. F., Pecoraro, N., Akana, S. F., La Fleur, S. E., et al. (2003). Proc Natl Acad Sci USA, 100(20):11696–11701.

Dalton, K. (1994). Once a Month, 5th ed. Alameda, CA: Hunter House Inc.

Daly, A. (1994). Diabetes Educ, 20:156, 162.

Daly, M., & Wilson, M. I. (1999). Anim Behav, 57(3):509–519.

Dal-Zatto, S., Marti, O., & Armario, A. (2003). Psychoneuroendocrinology, 28(8):992–1009.

Damasio, A. R. (2003). Looking for Spinoza: Joy, Sorrow, and the Feeling Brain. Orlando, FL: Harcourt.

Dambricourt Malasse, A. (1987). Ontogenèses, Paléontogenèses et Phylogenèse du Corps Mandibulaire Catarhinien. Nouvelle Interprétation de la Mécanique Humanisante (Théorie de la Foetilisation, Bolk, 1926). Paris: Museum National d'Histoire Naturelle.

Dambricourt Malasse, A. (1988). C R Acad Sci II, 307(2):199–204.

Dambricourt Malasse, A., & Deshayes, M. J. (1992). Modeling of the craniofacial architecture during ontogenesis and phylogenesis. In: The Head-Neck Sensory Motor System, A. Berthoz, W. Graf, & P. P. Vidal (eds.). New York: Oxford University Press, pp. 36–46.

Dambricourt Malasse, A. (1993). Quat Int, 19:86–98.

Dambricourt Malasse, A., Deshayes, M. J., Marchand, D., & Chaline, J. (1999). Hum Evol, 14:277–300.

Dambricourt Malasse, A. (2006). C R Palevol, 5(1–2):109–117.

Danbrot, M. (2004). The New Cabbage Soup Diet. New York: St. Martin's Press.

Danutra, V., Turkes, A., Read, G. F., Wilson, D. W., et al. (1989). J Endocrinol, 121(2):375–381.

Darwin, E. (1794–1796). Zoonomia; or, The Laws of Organic Life, 2nd Corrected ed. London: Printed for J. Johnson [Available from Project Gutenberg, http: www.gutenberg.org/files/15707/15707–h/15707–h.htm].

Darwin, C. R. (1859). On the Origin of the Species by Means of Natural Selection, or, The Preservation of Favoured Races in the Struggle for Life. London: J. Murray.

Darwin, C. R. (1871). The Descent of Man, and Selection in Relation to Sex. London: John Murray.

Davey Smith, G., Shipley, M. J., & Rose, G. (1990). J Epidemiol Community Health, 44(4):265–270.

Davey Smith, G., Neaton, J. D., Wentworth, D., Stamler, R., et al. (1996). Am J Public Health, 86(4):486–496.

Davey Smith, G., Wentworth, D., Neaton, J. D., Stamler, R., et al. (1996). Am J Public Health, 86(4):497–504.

David, B., & Laurin, B. (1992). Procrustes: An Interactive Program for Shape Analyses Using Landmarks, Version 2.0. Dijon, France: Paléontologie Analytique.

David, R. J., & Collins Jr., J. W. (1997). N Engl J Med, 337(17):1209–1214.

Davidson, A. (1999). The Oxford Companion to Food. New York: Oxford University Press.

Davidson, R. J., Putnam, K. M., & Larson, C. L. (2000). Science, 289(5479):591–594.

Davidson, R. J., Jackson, D. C., & Kalin, N. H. (2001). Psychol Bull, 126(6):890–906.

Davies, M. J., & Norman, R. J. (2002). Trends Endocrinol Metab, 13(9):386–392.

Dawkins, R. (1989). The Selfish Gene. Oxford, UK: Oxford University Press.

Dawkins, R. (1996). Climbing Mount Improbable. New York: Norton.

Dawood, M. Y., McGuire, J. L., & Demers, L. M. (1985). Premenstrual Syndrome and Dysmenorrhea. Baltimore, MD: Urban, & Schwarzenberg.

Dawson, D., & Reid, K. (1997). Nature, 388(6639):235.

Dawson, D. A. (1990). Fam Plann Perspect, 22(4):169–172.

Day, M. H. (1999). Forward. In: Evolutionary Medicine, W. R. Trevathan, E. O. Smith, & J. J. McKenna (eds.). New York: Oxford University Press, pp. vii–ix.

de Angelis, M., Coda, R., Silano, M., Minervini, F., et al. (2006). J Cereal Sci, 43(3):301–314.

de Araujo, I. E., Rolls, E. T., Kringelbach, M. L., McGlone, F., et al. (2003). Eur J Neurosci, 18(7):2059–2068.

de Bellis, M., Chrousos, G. P., Dorn, L. D., Burke, L., et al. (1994). J Clin Endocrinol Metab, 78(2):249–255.

de Bruin, J. P., Dorland, M., Bruinse, H. W., Spliet, W., et al. (1998). Early Hum Dev, 51(39–46.

de Chateau, P., & Wiberg, B. (1977). Acta Paediatr Scand, 66(2):145–151.

de Kloet, E. R. (1991). Front Neuroendocrinol, 12(2):95–164.

de Kloet, E. R., Oitzl, M. S., & Joels, M. (1999). Trends Neurosci, 22(10):422–426.

de Kloet, E. R., Sibug, R. M., Helmerhorst, F. M., & Schmidt, M. (2005). Neurosci Biobehav Rev, 29(2):271–281.

de Lauzon–Guillian, B., Basdevant, A., Romon, M., Karlsson, J., et al. (2006). Am J Clin Nutr, 83(1):132–138.

de Luca Brunori, I., Battini, L., Simonelli, M., Clemente, F., et al. (2000). Hum Reprod, 15(8):1807–1812.

de Moura, E. G., & Passos, M. C. F. (2005). Biosci Rep, 25(3–4):251–269.

de Onis, M., & Blossner, M. (2000). Am J Clin Nutr, 72(4):1032–1039.

de Ronchi, D., Faranca, I., Forti, P., Ravaglia, G., et al. (2000). Int J Psychiatry Med, 30(2):173–183.

de Valk, B., & Marx, J. J. M. (1999). Arch Intern Med, 159(14):1542–1548.

de Waal, F. B. M. (1989). J Hum Evol, 18(5):433–460.

de Waal, F. B., Luttrell, L. M., & Canfield, M. E. (1993). Am J Primatol, 29(1):73–78.

Deepa, M., Farooq, S., Datta, M., R., D., et al. (2007). Diabetes Metab Res Rev, 23(2):127–134.

Defay, R., Papoz, L., Barny, S., Bonnot-Lours, S., et al. (1998). Int J Obes (Lond), 22(9):927–934.

DeJong, W. (1994). Int J Addict, 29(6):681–705.

Dekker, G. A., Robillard, P. Y., & Hulsey, T. C. (1998). Obstet Gynecol Surv, 53(6):377–382.

Dekker, G. A., & Robillard, P. Y. (2005). Curr Pharm Des, 11(6):699–710.

Delattre, A. (1952). Rev Sci, 3315:239–245.

Delattre, A., & Fenart, R. (1954). C R Acad Sci II, 239(11):676–678.

Delattre, A., & Fenart, R. (1956). C R Acad Sci II, 243:429–431.

Delattre, A. (1958). La formation du crâne humain. In: Les Processus de l'Hominisation, Colloques Internationaux du Centre National de la Recherche Scientifique (ed.). Paris: Centre National de la Recherche Scientifique, pp. 37–57.

Delattre, A., & Fenart, R. (1960). L'hominisation du Crâne. Paris: Centre National de la Recherche Scientifique.

Delcourt–Debruyne, E. M. C., Boutigny, H. R. A., & Hildebrand, H. F. (2000). J Periodontol, 71(5):816–824.

Deliège, R. (1996). Anthropologie de la Parenté. Paris: A. Colin/Masson.

den Tonkelaar, I., & Oddens, B. J. (1999). Contraception, 59(6):357–362.

Deniker, J. (1886). Arch Zool Exp, 2:1–265.

Dennison, B. A., Erb, T. A., & Jenkins, P. L. (2002). Pediatrics, 109(6):1028–1035.

Dennison, E. M., Syddall, H. E., Rodriguez, S., Voropanov, A., et al. (2004). J Clin Endocrinol Metab, 89(10):4898–4903.

Denver, R. J. (1999). Ann NY Acad Sci, 897:46–53.

Derimanov, G. S., & Oppenheimer, J. (1998). Ann Allergy Asthma Immunol, 81(3):243–246.

Deroche-Gamonet, V., Belin, D., & Piazza, P. V. (2004). Science, 305(5686):1014–1017.

Des Marais, D. J. (2005). Nature, 437(7060):826–827.

Deshayes, M.-J. (1986). Croissance Cranio-Faciale et Orthodontie. Paris: Masson.

Deshayes, M.-J. (1988). Rev Orthop Dento Faciale, 22(11):283–298.

Deshayes, M.-J., & Dambricourt Malasse, A. (1990). Rev Stomatol Chir Maxillofac, 91(4):249–258.

Deshayes, M.-J. (1991). Rev Orthop Dento Faciale, 25(3):353–365.

Desjarlais, R. R., Eisenberg, L., Good, B., & Kleinman, A. (1995). World Mental Health: Problems and Priorities in Low-Income Countries. New York: Oxford University Press.

Després, J.–P., Lamarche, B., Mauriege, P., Cantin, B., et al. (1996). N Engl J Med, 334(15):952–957.

Després, J.-P. (2006). Ann Med, 38(1):52–63.

Dettwyler, K. A. (1994). Dancing Skeletons. Prospect Heights, IL: Waveland Press.

Dettwyler, K. A. (1995a). Beauty and the breast: The cultural context of breastfeeding in the United States. In: Breastfeeding: Biocultural Perspectives, P. Stuart-Macadam & K. A. Dettwyler (eds.). New York: Aldine de Gruyter, pp. 167–216.

Dettwyler, K. A. (1995b). A time to wean: The hominid blueprint for the natural age of weaning in modern human populations. In: Breastfeeding: Biocultural Perspectives, P. Stuart-Macadam & K. A. Dettwyler (eds.). New York: Aldine de Gruyter, pp. 39–73.

Deurenberg-Yap, M., Chew, S. K., & Deurenberg, P. (2002). Obes Rev, 3(3):209–215.

Deuster, P. A., Adera, T., & South-Paul, J. (1999). Arch Fam Med, 8(2):122–128.

Deutsch, J. A. (1987). Signals determining meal size. In: Eating Habits: Food, Physiology and Learned Behaviour, R. A. Boakes, D. A. Popplewell, & M. J. Burton (eds.). Chichester, UK: John Wiley, & Sons, pp. 155–173.

Devine, C. M., Conners, M. M., Sobal, J., & Bisogni, C. A. (2003). Soc Sci Med, 56(3):617–630.

DeWalt, B. R. (1998). The political ecology of population increase and malnutrition. In: Building a New Biocultural Synthesis: Political-Economic Perspectives on Human Biology, A. H. Goodman, & T. L. Leatherman (eds.). Ann Arbor, MI: The University of Michigan Press, pp. 295–316.

DeWalt, K. M. (1981). Fed Proc, 40(11):2606–2610.

Dewey, K. (1997). Annu Rev Nutr, 17:19–36.

Dhabbar, F. S., & McEwen, B. S. (2001). Bidirectional effects of stress and glucocorticoid hormones on immune function: possible explanations for paradoxical observations. In: Psychoneuroendocrinology, R. Ader, D. L. Felten, & N. Cohen (eds.). San Diego, CA: Academic Press, pp. 301–338.

Di Cagno, R., De Angelis, M., Lavermicocca, P., De Vincenzi, M., et al. (2002). Appl Environ Microbiol, 68(2):623–633.

Di Cagno, R., De Angelis, M., Auricchio, S., Greco, L., et al. (2004). Appl Environ Microbiol, 70(2):1088–1096.

Di Cagno, R., De Angelis, M., Alfonsi, G., De Vincenzi, M., et al. (2005). J Agric Food Chem, 53(11):4393–4402.

Diamond, J. M. (1997a). Guns, Germs, and Steel: The Fates of Human Societies. New York: Norton.

Diamond, J. M. (1997b). Why Is Sex Fun? The Evolution of Human Sexuality. New York: Harper Collins.

Diamond, J. M. (2000). Le Troisième Chimpanzé. Paris: Gallimard.

Diamond, J. M. (2003). Nature, 423(6940):599–602.

Dibba, B., Prentice, A., Ceesay, M., Stirling, D. M., et al. (2000). Am J Clin Nutr, 71(2):544–549.

Dickerson, F. B., Boronow, J. J., Stallings, C., Origoni, A. E., et al. (2003). Arch Gen Psychiatry, 60(5):466–472.

Dickerson, L. M., Mazyck, P. J., & Hunter, M. H. (2003). Am Fam Physician, 67(8):1743–1752.

Dickerson, S. S., Gruenewald, T. L., & Kemeny, M. E. (2004). J Pers, 72(6):1191–1216.

Dickerson, S. S., & Kemeny, M. E. (2004). Psychol Bull, 130(3):355–391.

DiGirolamo, A. M., Grummer-Strawn, L. M., & Fein, S. B. (2001). Birth, 28(2):94–100.

Diliberti, N., Bordi, P. L., Conklin, M. T., Roe, L. S., et al. (2004). Obes Res, 12(3):562–568.

Dillard, C. J., & German, J. B. (2000). J Sci Food Agric, 80(12):1744–1756.

Dillon, K., & Brooks, D. (1992). Psychol Rep, 70(1):35–39.

Ding, E. L., Song, Y., Malik, V., & Liu, S. (2006). J Am Med Assoc, 295(11):1288–1299.

Dobzhansky, T. (1973). Am Biol Teach, 35(3):125–129.

Doctor's Associates Inc. (2006), Subway Around the World, http://www.subway.com subwayroot/ AroundTheWorld/index.aspx

Dole, N., Savitz, D. A., Siega-Riz, A. M., Hertz-Picciotto, I., et al. (2004). Am J Public Health, 94(8):1358–1365.

Doll, R., & Hill, A. B. (1950). BMJ, 2(4682):739–748.

Dominiak, B. J., Oxberry, W., & Chen, P. C. (2003). Ultrastruct Pathol, 27(4):271–283.

Dominy, N. J., & Lucas, P. W. (2001). Nature, 410(6826):363–366.

Dominy, N. J., & Lucas, P. W. (2004). Am J Primatol, 62(3):189–207.

Donald, M. (1991). Origins of the Modern Mind: Three Stages in the Evolution of Culture and Cognition. Cambridge, MA: Harvard University Press.

Donaldson, B. F. (1961). Strong Medicine. London: Cassell, & Company Ltd.

Donati, D., Akhyani, N., Fogdell–Hahn, A., Cermelli, C., et al. (2003). Neurology, 61(10):1405–1411.

dos Santos Silva, I., de Stavola, B., Mann, V., Kuh, D., et al. (2002). Int J Epidemiol, 31(2):405–412.

Douglas, M. (1966). Purity and Danger; An Analysis of Concepts of Pollution and Taboo. New York: Praeger.

Douglas, M., & Bolo, P. F. C. (1979). Communications, 31(145–170.

Douglas, M., & Gross, J. (1981). Soc Sci Inf, 20(1):1–35.

Douglas, M. (1984). Food in the Social Order: Studies of Food and Festivities in Three American Communities. New York: Russell Sage Foundation.

Dousset, V., Gayou, A., & Brochet, B. (1998). Mult Scler, 4(4):357.

Downie, J. R. (2004a). Biosci Ed, 4(3). http://www.bioscience.heacademy.ac.uk/journal/

Downie, J. R. (2004b). Lancet, 363(9415):1168.

Doyle, J. A. (1998), The Exercise and Physical Fitness Web Page. http://www2.gsu.edu ~wwwfit/

Drago, D. A., & Dannenberg, A. L. (1999). Pediatrics, 103(5):1–8.

Drake, M., Grant, K. A., Gage, H. D., Mach, R. H., et al. (2002). Nat Neurosci, 5(2):169–174.

Drake, A. J., & Walker, B. R. (2004). J Endocrinol, 180(1):1–16.

Drake, A. J., Walker, B. R., & Seckl, J. R. (2005). Am J Physiol Regul Integr Comp Physiol, 288(1):R34–R38.

Dressler, W. W., Oths, K. S., & Gravlee, C. C. (2005). Annu Rev Anthropol, 34(231–252).

Drewnowski, A. (1989). Appetite, 12(1):71.

Drewnowski, A., Krahn, D. D., Demitrack, M. A., Nairn, K., et al. (1992). Physiol Behav, 51(2):371–379.

Drewnowski, A. (1995). Am J Clin Nutr, 62(Suppl 5):1081S–1085S.

Drewnowski, A., & Popkin, B. M. (1997). Nutr Rev, 55(2):31–43.

Drewnowski, A. (1997a). Annu Rev Nutr, 17:237–253.

Drewnowski, A. (1997b). J Am Diet Assoc, 97(Suppl 7):S58–S62.

Drewnowski, A. (2004). Am J Prev Med, 27(Suppl 3):154–162.

Drewnowski, A., & Specter, S. E. (2004). Am J Clin Nutr, 79(1):6–16.

Drotar, D. (1991). Am J Orthopsychiatry, 61(1):23–34.

Du, X., Zhu, K., Trube, A., Zhang, Q., et al. (2004). Br J Nutr, 92(1):159–168.

Dudley, R. (2000). Q Rev Biol, 75(1):3–15.

Dudley, R. (2002). Addiction, 97(4):381–388.

Dudley, R. (2004). Integr Comp Biol, 44(4):315–323.

Duffy, V. B., & Bartoshuk, L. M. (1996). Sensory factors in feeding. In: Why We Eat What We Eat: The Psychology of Eating, E. D. Capaldi (ed.). Washington, DC: American Psychological Association, pp. 145–172.

Dufour, D. L. (1995). A closer look at the nutritional implications of bitter cassava use. In: Indigenous Peoples and the Future of Amazonia, L. Sponsel (ed.). Tucson,: University of Arizona Press, pp. 149–165.

Dufour, D. L., Staten, L. K., Reina, J. C., & Spurr, G. B. (1997). Am J Phys Anthropol, 102(1):5–15.

Dufour, D. L., & Sauther, M. L. (2002). Am J Hum Biol, 14(5):584–602.

Duleba, A. J., Spaczynski, R. Z., & Olive, D. L. (1998). Fert Ster, 69(2):335–340.

Dunaif, A. (1997). Endocr Rev, 18(6):774–800.

Dunbar, R. I. M. (1998). Evol Anthropol, 6(5):178–190.

Duncan, G. E. (2006). Arch Pediatr Adolesc Med, 160(5):523–528.

Duncan, M. J., Nakao, S., Skobe, Z., & Xie, H. (1993). Infect Immun, 61(5):2260–2265.

Duncan, S., Read, C. L., & Brodie, M. J. (1993). Epilepsia, 34(5):827–831.

Dunford, R. E. (2002). The Grapefruit and Apple Cider Vinegar Combo Diet. McKinney, TX: The Magni Company.

DuPuis, E. M. (2002). Nature's Perfect Food: How Milk Became America's Drink. New York: New York University Press.

Durham, W. H. (1991). Coevolution: Genes, Culture, and Human Diversity. Stanford, CA: Stanford University Press.

Durmer, J. S., & Dinges, D. F. (2005). Semin Neurol, 25(1):117–129.

Durnin, J. V. (1991). Acta Paediatr Scand Suppl, 373:33–42.

Dweik, R. A., Laskowski, D., Abu-Soud, H. M., Kaneko, F., et al. (1998). J Clin Invest, 101(3):660–666.

Dzoljic, E., Sipetic, S., Vlajinac, H., Marinkovic, J., et al. (2002). Headache, 42(3):185–193.

Eade, J., Peach, C., & Vamplew, T. (1996). The Bangladeshis: The encapsulated community. In: Ethnicity in the 1991 Census. The Ethnic Minority Populations of Great Britain, C. Peach (ed.). London: Her Majesty's Stationery Office, pp. 150–160.

Eaton, S. B., & Konner, M. J. (1985). N Engl J Med, 312(5):283–289.

Eaton, S. B., & Konner, M. J. (1986). ASDC J Dent Child, 53(4):300–303.

Eaton, S. B., Konner, M. J., & Shostak, M. (1988). Am J Med, 84(4):739–749.

Eaton, S. B., Shostak, M., & Konner, M. J. (1988). The Paleolithic Prescription: A Program of Diet & Exercise and A Design for Living. New York: Harper & Row.

Eaton, S. B. (1990). Fibre intake in prehistoric times. In: Dietary Fibre Perspectives: Reviews and Bibliography, A. R. Leads (ed.). London: John Libbey, pp. 27–40.

Eaton, S. B., & Nelson, D. A. (1991). Am J Clin Nutr, 54(Suppl 1):281S–287S.

Eaton, S. B. (1992). Lipids, 27(10):814–820.

Eaton, S. B., Pike, M. C., Short, R. V., Lee, N. V., et al. (1994). Q Rev Biol, 69(3):353–367.

Eaton, S. B., Eaton III, S. B., & Konner, M. J. (1997). Eur J Clin Nutr, 51(4):207–216.

Eaton, S. B., Eaton III, S. B., Sinclair, A. J., Cordain, L., et al. (1998). World Rev Nutr Diet, 83:12–23.

Eaton, S. B., Eaton III, S. B., & Konner, M. J. (1999). Paleolithic nutrition revisited. In: Evolutionary Medicine, W. R. Trevathan, E. O. Smith, & J. J. McKenna (eds.). New York: Oxford University Press, pp. 313–332.

Eaton, S. B., & Eaton III, S. B. (1999a). Breast cancer in evolutionary context. In: Evolutionary Medicine, W. R. Trevathan, E. O. Smith, & J. J. McKenna (eds.). New York: Oxford University Press, pp. 429–442.

Eaton, S. B., & Eaton III, S. B. (1999b). The evolutionary context of chronic degenerative diseases. In: Evolution in Health, & Disease, S. C. Stearns (ed.). Oxford, UK: Oxford University Press, pp. 251–259.

Eaton, S. B., & Eaton III, S. B. (2000). Eur J Nutr, 39(2):67–70.

Eaton, S. B., Cordain, L., & Eaton III, S. B. (2001). World Rev Nutr Diet, 90:5–12.

Eaton, S. B., Cordain, L., & Lindeberg, S. (2002). Prev Med, 34(2):119–123.

Eaton, S. B., Eaton III, S. B., & Cordain, L. (2002). Evolution, diet, and health. In: Human Diet: Its Origin and Evolution, P. S. Ungar & M. F. Teaford (eds.). Westport, CT: Bergin & Garvey, pp. 7–17.

Eaton, S. B., Strassman, B. I., Nesse, R. M., Neel, J. V., et al. (2002). Prev Med, 34(2):109–118.

Eaton, S. B., & Eaton III, S. B. (2003). Comp Biochem Physiol A Mol Integr Physiol, 136(1):153–159.

Ebert, D. (1998). Science, 282(5393):1432–1435.

Edgerton, R. B. (1992). Sick Societies: Challenging the Myth of Primitive Harmony. New York: The Free Press.

Eeg-Larsen, N. (1971). Ernæringslære [Textbook of Nutritional Science]. Oslo: Landsforeningen for kosthold og helse.

Eeg-Olofsson, O., Bergström, T., Andermann, F., Andermann, E., et al. (2004). Acta Neurol Scand, 109(3):169–174.

Eggert, F. M., McLeod, M. H., & Flowerdew, G. (2001). J Periodontol, 72(9):1210–1220.

Eilam, D., Zor, R., Szechtman, H., & Hermesh, H. (2006). Neurosci Biobehav Rev, 30(4):456–471.

Eisenberger, N. I., & Lieberman, M. D. (2004). Trends Cogn Sci, 8(7):294–300.

Ekirch, A. R. (2005). At Day's Close: Night in Times Past. New York: Norton.

Ekman, J., & Rosander, B. (1992). Theor Pop B, 42(2):117–129.

Elenkov, I. J., Wilder, R. L., Bakalov, V. K., Link, A. A., et al. (2001). J Clin Endocrinol Metab, 86(10):4933–4938.

Elgar, M. A., Pagel, M. D., & Harvey, P. H. (1988). Anim Behav, 36(5):1407–1419.

Elias, M. F., Nicolson, N. A., Bora, C., & Johnston, J. (1986). Pediatrics, 77(3):322–329.

Elias, S. G., van Noord, P. A., Peeters, P. H., den Tonkelaar, I., et al. (2005). Hum Reprod Update, 20(9):2483–2488.

Ellis, B. J., Essex, M. J., & Boyce, W. T. (2005). Dev Psychopathol, 17(2):303–328.

Ellison, P. T. (1981a). Hum Biol, 53(4):635–643.

Ellison, P. T. (1981b). Am J Phys Anthropol, 54(2):216.

Ellison, P. T. (1982). Hum Biol, 54(2):269–281.

Ellison, P. T., & Lager, C. (1986). Am J Obstet Gynecol, 154(5):1000–1003.

Ellison, P. T., Peacock, N. R., & Lager, C. (1986). Hum Biol, 58(4):473–483.

Ellison, P. T., Peacock, N. R., & Lager, C. (1989). Am J Phys Anthropol, 78(4):519–526.

Ellison, P. T. (1990). Am Anthropol, 92(4):933–952.

Ellison, P. T., Lipson, S. F., O'Rourke, M. T., Bentley, G. R., et al. (1993). Lancet, 342(8868):433–434.

Ellison, P. T., Panter–Brick, C., Lipson, S. F., & O'Rourke, M. T. (1993). Hum Reprod, 8(12):2248–2258.

Ellison, P. T. (1994a). Hum Nat, 5(2):155–165.

Ellison, P. T. (1994b). Ann NY Acad Sci, 709:287–298.

Ellison, P. T. (1995). Understanding natural variation in human ovarian function. In: Human Reproductive Decisions: Biological and Social Perspectives, R. I. M. Dunbar (ed.). New York: St. Martin's Press, pp. 22–51.

Ellison, P. T. (1996). Am J Hum Biol, 8(6):725–734.

Ellison, P. T., Lipson, S. F., & Sukalich, S. (1996). Am J Phys Anthropol, 22(Suppl):102.

Ellison, P. T. (1999). Reproductive ecology and reproductive cancers. In: Hormones, Health and Behaviour. A Socio-Ecological and Lifespan Perspective, C. Panter–Brick, & C. Worthman (eds.). Cambridge, UK: Cambridge University Press, pp. 184–209.

Ellison, P. T. (2001). On Fertile Ground: A Natural History of Human Reproduction. Cambridge, MA: Harvard University Press.

Ellison, P. T. (2003). Am J Hum Biol, 15(3):342–351.

Ellison, P. T. (2005a). Am J Hum Biol, 17(1):113–118.

Ellison, P. T. (ed.) (2005b). Wiley-Liss Plenary Symposium: Evolutionary Perspectives on the Fetal Origins Hypothesis. Am J Hum Biol, 17 (1), 1–125.

Elson, D. A., Ryan, H. E., Snow, J. W., Johnson, R., et al. (2000). Cancer Res, 60(21):6189–6195.

Elwood, P. C., Pickering, J. E., Hughes, J., Fehily, A. M., et al. (2004). Eur J Nutr, 58(5):718–724.

Embry, A. F. (2004). J Nutr Environ Med, 14(4):307–317.

Enattah, N. S., Sahi, T., Savilahti, E., Terwilliger, J. D., et al. (2002). Nat Genet, 30(2):233–237.

Eng, C., Hampel, H., & de la Chapelle, A. (2001). Annu Rev Med, 52(371–400.

Engel, G. L. (1977). Science, 196(4286):129–136.

Engel, G. L. (1981). J Med Philos, 6(2):101–123.

Engel, G. L. (1997). Psychomatics, 38(6):521–528.

Engelbregt, M. J. T., van Weissenbruch, M. M., Lips, P., van Lingen, A., et al. (2004). Bone, 34(1):180–186.

Enig, M. (2000). Know Your Fats: The Complete Primer for Understanding the Nutrition of Fats, Oils and Cholesterol. Silver Springs, MD: Bethesda Press.

Enig, M., & Fallon, S. (2005). Eat Fat, Lose Fat: Lose Weight and Feel Great with Three Delicious, Science-Based Coconut Diets. New York: Hudson Street Press.

Ensom, M. H. H. (2000). Pharmacotherapy, 20(5):523–539.

Enzinger, C., Ropele, S., Smith, S., Strasser–Fuchs, S., et al. (2004). Ann Neurol, 55(4):563–569.

Epstein, S. S. (1996). Int J Health Serv, 26(1):173–185.

Epstein, S. S. (1998). The Politics of Cancer Revisited. New York: East Ridge Press.

Epstein, W. W., Rowsemitt, C. N., Berger, P. J., & Negus, N. C. (1986). J Chem Ecol, 12(10):2011–2020.

Erasmus, U. (1993). Fats That Heal: Fats That Kill. Burnaby, British Columbia, Canada: Alive Books.

Erens, B., Primatesta, P., & Prior, G. (2001), Health Survey for England: The Health of Ethnic Minority Groups, http://www.doh.gov.uk/public/hse99.htm

Eriksson, J. G., Forsen, T., Tuomilehto, J., Osmond, C., et al. (2001). Int J Obesity Relat Metab Disord, 25(5):735–740.

Eriksson, J. G., Forsen, T., Tuomilehto, J., Jaddoe, V. W., et al. (2002). Diabetologia, 45(3):342–348.

Esmail, A., Lambert, P. C., Jones, D. R., & Mitchell, E. A. (1995). J Public Health Med, 17(3):282–289.

Essex, M. J., Klein, M. H., Cho, E., & Kalin, N. H. (2002). Biol Psychiatry, 52(8):776–784.

Estabrooks, G. (1941). Man, the Mechanical Misfit. New York: Macmillan.

Etminan, M., Gill, S., & Samii, A. (2003). BMJ, 327(7407):128.

Ettinger, B., Sidney, S., Cummings, S., Libanati, C., et al. (1997). J Clin Endocrinol Metab, 82(2):429–434.

Etzel, R. A. (2002). J Am Med Assoc, 287(4):425–427.

Euser, A. M., Finken, M. J., Kejzer–Veen, M. G., Hille, E. T., et al. (2005). Am J Clin Nutr, 81(2):480–487.

Evangelou, N., Jackson, M., Beeson, D., & Palace, J. (1999). J Neurol Neurosurg Psychiatry, 67(2):203–205.

Eveleth, P. B., & Tanner, J. M. (1990). Worldwide Variation in Human Growth, 2nd ed. Cambridge, UK: Cambridge University Press.

Everitt, B. J., & Robbins, T. W. (2005). Nat Neurosci, 8(11):1481–1489.

Ewald, P. W. (1991a). Hum Nat, 2:1–30.

Ewald, P. W. (1991b). Epidemiol Infect, 106(1):83–119.

Ewald, P. W. (1994). Evolution of Infectious Disease. New York: Oxford University Press.

Ewald, P. W. (1999a). Evolutionary control of HIV and other sexually transmitted viruses. In: Evolutionary Medicine, W. R. Trevathan, E. O. Smith, & J. J. McKenna (eds.). New York: Oxford University Press, pp. 271–312.

Ewald, P. W. (1999b). Using evolution as a tool for controlling infectious disease. In: Evolutionary Medicine, W. R. Trevathan, E. O. Smith, & J. J. McKenna (eds.). New York: Oxford University Press, pp. 245–270.

Ewald, P. W., & Cochran, G. M. (2000). J Infect Dis, 181(Suppl 3):S394–401.

Exner, D. V., Dries, D. L., Domanski, M. J., & Cohn, J. N. (2001). N Engl J Med, 344(18):1351–1357.

Expert Committee on the Diagnosis and Classification of Diabetes Mellitus. (2003). Diabetes Care, 26(Suppl 1):S5–20.

Ezzell, C. (1993). J NIH Res, 5:64–66.

Ezzo, G., & Bucknam, R. (1998). On Becoming Babywise. Simi Valley, CA: Parent-Wise Solutions Inc.

Faas, M., Bouman, A., Moes, H., Heineman, M. J., et al. (2000). Fertil Steril, 74(5):1008–1013.

Færgeman, O. (2003). Coronary Artery Disease: Genes, Drugs, and the Agricultural Connection. Amsterdam: Elsevier.

Fagerberg, B., Bondjers, L., & Nilsson, P. (2004). J Intern Med, 256(3):254–259.

Fainardi, E., Castellazzi, M., Casetta, I., Cultrera, R., et al. (2004). J Neurol Sci, 217(2):181–188.

Fajardo, R. V. (1981). Philipp J Ophthalmol, 13(1):19–21.

Falk, D. (1990). Behav Brain Sci, 13(2):333–381.

Falk, R. T., Fears, T. R., Hoover, R. N., Pike, M., et al. (2002). Br J Cancer, 87(1):54–60.

Falkowski, P. G., Katz, M. E., Milligan, A. J., Fennel, K., et al. (2005). Science, 309(5744):2202–2204.

Falkowski, P. G. (2006). Science, 311(5768):1724–1725.

Fallon, S., & Enig, M. G. (1999). Nourishing Traditions: The Cookbook That Challenges Politically Correct Nutrition and the Diet Dictocrats. Winona, IN: New Trends Publishing.

Fang, J., Madhavan, S., & Alderman, M. H. (1996). N Engl J Med, 335(21):1545–1551.

Farb, P., & Armelagos, G. J. (1980). Consuming Passions: The Anthropology of Eating. Boston: Houghton Mifflin and Company.

Farb, P., & Armelagos, G. J. (1982). The wisdom of cuisine. In: Food and People, D. Kirk, & E. K. Eliason (eds.). San Francisco: Boyd and Fraser, pp. 40–46.

Farmer, P. (2003). Pathologies of Power: Health, Human Rights, and the New War on the Poor. Berkeley, CA: University of California Press.

Farrell, A. P. (1991). Circulation of body fluids. In: Comparative Animal Physiology, C. L. Prosser (ed.). New York: John Wiley and Sons, pp. 509–558.

Farrell, A. P., & Olson, K. R. (2000). Physiol Biochem Zool, 73(1):1–11.

Fayon, M., Just, J., Vu Thien, H., Chiba, T., et al. (1999). Acta Paediatr, 88(11):1216–1222.

Fazekas, F., Strasser-Fuchs, S., Kollegger, H., Berger, T., et al. (2001). Neurology, 57(5):853–857.

Feierman, J. R. (1982). Med Hypotheses, 9(5):455–479.

Feingold, B. F. (1974). Why Your Child Is Hyperactive. New York: Random House.

Feistner, A. T. C., & Price, E. C. (1990). Folia Primatol, 54(1–2):34–45.

Fellows, P. (2000). Food Processing Technology: Principles and Practice, 2nd ed. Cambridge, UK: Woodhead Publishing.

Felsenstein, J. (1990). PHYLIP (Phylogeny Inference Package). Version 3.3. Seattle, WA: University of Washington.

Felthous, A. R., & Robinson, D. B. (1981). J Prev Psychiatry, 1(1):5–14.

Femia, R., Natali, A., L'Abbate, A., & Ferrannini, E. (2006). Arterioscler Thromb Vasc Biol, 26(7):1607–1612.

Fenker, D. B., Schott, B. H., Richardson–Klavehn, A., Heinze, H.–J., et al. (2005). Eur J Neurosci, 21(7):1993–1999.

Ferber, R. (1985). Solve Your Child's Sleep Problems. New York: Simon, & Schuster Books.

Ferketich, A. K., Schwartzbaum, J. A., Frid, D. J., & Moeschberger, M. L. (2000). Arch Intern Med, 160(9):1261–1268.

Ferreira, M. K. L., & Lang, G. C. (2006). Indigenous Peoples and Diabetes: Community Empowerment and Wellness. Durham, NC: Carolina Academic Press.

Feskanich, D., Willett, W. C., Stampfer, M. J., & Colditz, G. A. (1997). Am J Public Health, 87(6):992–997.

Fessler, D. M. T. (2002). Curr Anthropol, 43(1):19–61.

Fessler, D. M. T., & Navarette, C. D. (2003). J Cog Cul, 3:1–40.

Fife, B. (2002). Eat Fat Look Thin: A Safe and Natural Way to Lose Weight Permanently. Colorado Springs, CO: HealthWise.

Fildes, V. (1985). Breasts, Bottles, and Babies: A History of Infant Feeding. Edinburgh, UK: Edinburgh University Press.

Fildes, V. (1995). The culture and biology of breastfeeding: An historical review of western Europe. In: Breastfeeding: Biocultural Perspectives, P. Stuart–Macadam & K. Dettwyler (eds.). New York: Aldine de Gruyter, pp. 101–126.

Finch, C. E., & Sapolsky, R. M. (1999). Neurobiol Aging, 20(4):407–428.

Finkelstein, E. A., Ruhm, C. J., & Kosa, K. M. (2005). Annu Rev Public Health, 26:239–257.

Finn, C. A. (1996). Eur J Obstet Gynecol Reprod Biol, 70(1):3–8.

Firestein, G. S. (2003). Nature, 423(6937):356–361.

Fiscella, K., Kitzman, H. J., Cole, R. E., Sidora, K. J., et al. (1998). Pediatrics, 101(4 [Pt 1]):620–624.

Fisher, B. E., & Rinehart, S. (1990). Pers Individ Dif, 11(5):431–438.

FitzGerald, R. J., Murray, B. A., & Walsh, D. J. (2004). J Nutr, 134(4):980S–988S.

Flatz, G., & Rotthauwe, H. W. (1973). Lancet, 2(7820):76–77.

Flatz, G. (1987). Adv Hum Genet, 16(1–77.

Flaxman, S. M., & Sherman, P. W. (2000). Q Rev Biol, 75(2):113–148.

Flegal, K. M., Carroll, M. D., Kuczmarksi, R. J., & Johnson, C. L. (1998). Intl J Obes Relat Metabol Disord, 22(1):39–37.

Flegal, K. M., Carroll, M. D., Ogden, C. L., & Johnson, C. L. (2002). J Am Med Assoc, 288(14):1723–1727.

Fleming, A. (1945). Penicillin, Nobel Lecture, December 11, 1945.

Fleming, P., Blair, P., & McKenna, J. (2006). Arch Dis Child, 91(10):799–801.

Fleming, P. J. (1994). Curr Opin Pediatr, 6(2):158–162.

Flexner, A., & Pritchett, H. S. (1910). Medical Education in the United States and Canada. New York, Carnegie Foundation for the Advancement of Teaching.

Flinn, M. V., & England, B. G. (1992). Proc Int Soc Psychoneuro, 23:97.

Flinn, M. V., & England, B. G. (1995). Curr Anthropol, 36(5):854–866.

Flinn, M. V., Quinlan, R. J., Decker, S. A., Turner, M. T., et al. (1996). Hum Nat, 7(2):125–162.

Flinn, M. V. (1997). Evol Hum Behav, 18(1):23–67.

Flinn, M. V. (1999). Family environment, stress, and health during childhood. In: Hormones, Health, and Behavior, C. Panter-Brick & C. M. Worthman (eds.). Cambridge, UK: Cambridge University Press, pp. 105–138.

Flinn, M. V., & England, B. G. (2003). Childhood stress: endocrine and immune responses to psychosocial events. In: Social and Cultural Lives of Immune Systems, J. M. Wilce (ed.). London, UK: Routledge Press, pp. 107–147.

Flinn, M. V., & Ward, C. V. (2005). Ontogeny and evolution of the social child. In: Origins of the Social Mind: Evolutionary Psychology and Child Development, B. J. Ellis & D. F. Bjorklund (eds.). New York. Guilford Press, pp. 19–44.

Flinn, M. V. (2006a). Dev Rev, 26(2):138–174.

Flinn, M. V. (2006b). Psychol Inq, 17(2):118–123.

Flinn, M. V., & Leone, D. V. (2006). J Dev Process, 1(1), 31–68.

Flinn, M. V., & Alexander, R. D. (2007). Runaway social selection. In: The Evolution of Mind, S. W. Gangestad & J. A. Simpson (eds.). New York: Guilford Press, pp. 249–255.

Flinn, M.V., & Leone, D.V. (2007). Alloparental care and the ontogeny of glucocorticoid stress response among stepchildren. In: Alloparental Care in Human Societies, G. Bentley & R. Mace (eds.). Oxford, UK: Berghahn Books.

Florencio, T. T., Ferreira, H. S., Cavalcante, J. C., Luciano, S. M., et al. (2003). Eur J Clin Nutr, 57(11):1437–1446.

Fohlman, J., & Friman, G. (1993). Ann Med, 25(6):569–574.

Fontbonne, A. M., & Eschwege, E. M. (1991). Diabetes Care, 14(6):461–469.

Food and Agriculture Organizationof the United Nations , & World Health Organization (1998). Vitamin and Mineral Requirements in Human Nutrition: Report of a Joint FAO/WHO Expert Consultation. Geneva: World Health Organization.

Food and Agriculture Organization of the United Nations (2000). FAOSTAT Nutrition Data. Geneva: Food and Agriculture Organization of the United Nations.

Food and Agriculture Organization of the United Nations (2006), Food Guidelines by Country, http://www.fao.org/ag/agn/nutrition/education_guidelines_country_en.stm

Forbes, L., Jarvis, D., & Burney, P. (1999). Eur Respir J, 14(5):1028–1033.

Ford, E. S., Giles, W. H., & Dietz, W. H. (2002). J Am Med Assoc, 287(3):356–359.

Ford, G. (2001). The Contented Little Baby Book. London: Vermilion.

Ford, R. P. K., Mitchell, E. A., Scragg, R., Stewart, A. W., et al. (1994). J Paediatr Child Health, 30(6):483–489.

Forsdahl, A. (1977). Br J Prevent Soc Med, 31(2):91–95.

Foster, D. L., & Nagatani, S. (1999). Biol Reprod, 60(2):205–215.

Foster, G. D., Wyatt, H. R., Hill, J. O., McGuckin, B. G., et al. (2003). N Engl J Med, 348(21):2082–2090.

Foster-Powell, K., Holt, S. H., & Brand-Miller, J. C. (2002). Am J Clin Nutr, 76(1):5–56.

Fowden, A. L., Giussani, D. A., & Forhead, A. J. (2005). Early Hum Dev, 81(9):723–734.

Francis, G. S., Benedict, C., Johnstone, D. E., Kirlin, P. C., et al. (1990). Circulation, 82(5):1724–1729.

Francis, K., van Beek, J., Canova, C., Neal, J. W., et al. (2003). Expert Rev Mol Med, 5(15):1–19.

Frandson, T. C., Boyd, S. S., & Berger, B. J. (1993). Can J Zool, 71:1799–1803.

Frank, R. T. (1931). Arch Neurol Psychiatry, 26(5):1053–1057.

Frank, S. A. (1996). Q Rev Biol, 71(1):37–78.

Fraser, I. S., & Inceboz, U. S. (2000). Defining disturbances of the menstrual cycle. In: Disorders of the Menstrual Cycle, P. M. S. O'Brien, I. T. Cameron, & A. B. MacLean (eds.). London: RCOG Press, pp. 141–152.

Frassetto, L., Todd, K., Morris, R., & Sebastian, A. (2000). J Gerontol A Biol Sci Med Sci, 55(10):M585–M592.

Freed, D. L. J. (1987). Dietary lectins and disease. In: Food Allergy and Intolerance, J. Brostoff, & S. J. Challacombe (eds.). London: Bailliere Tindall, pp. 375–400.

French, S. A., Fulkerson, J. A., & Story, M. (2000). Prev Med, 31(6):722–731.

Freymuth, F., Vabret, A., Brouard, J., Toutain, F., et al. (1999). J Clin Virol, 13(3):131–139.

Friedman, J. M. (2003). Science, 299(5608):856–858.

Friedman, M. I. (1989). Appetite, 12:70.

Frisch, R. E. (1987). Hum Reprod, 2(6):521–533.

Fritscher, A. M. G., Cherubini, K., Chies, J., & Dias, A. C. O. (2004). J Oral Pathol Med, 33(3):129–132.

Frobisher, C., & Maxwell, S. M. (2003). J Hum Nutr Diet, 16(3):181–188.

Frontini, M. G., Srinivasan, S. R., & Berenson, G. S. (2003). Int J Obes (Lond), 27(11):1398–1404.

Fruth, B., & Hohmann, G. (1996). Nest building in the great apes: the great leap forward? In: Great Ape Societies, W. C. McGrew, L. F. Marchant, & T. Nishida (eds.). Cambridge, UK: Cambridge University Press, pp. 225–240.

Fuchs, E., & Flugge, G. (1995). Psychoneuroendocrinology, 20(1):33–51.

Fuentes, A. (2004). Am Anthropol, 106(4):710–718.

Fukuda, S., Keithley, E. M., & Harris, J. P. (1988). Laryngoscope, 98(4):439–443.

Fuller, F. H., Beghin, J. C., Hu, D., & Rozelle, S. (2004). China's Dairy Market: Consumer Demand Survey and Supply Characteristics. Ames, IA: Center for Agricultural and Rural Development, Iowa State University.

Fullerton, S. M., Clark, A. G., Weiss, K. M., Nickerson, D. A., et al. (2000). Am J Hum Gen, 67(4):881–900.

Fulton, S., Woodside, B., & Shizgal, P. (2000). Science, 287(5450):125–128.

Furneaux, E. C., Langley–Evans, A. J., & Langley–Evans, S. C. (2001). Obstet Gynecol Surv, 56(12):775–782.

Futuyma, D. J. (2005). Evolution. Sunderland, MA: Sinauer Associates.

Gadgil, M., & Bossert, W. H. (1970). Am Nat, 104:1–24.

Galef, B. G. (1989). Appetite, 12:73.

Galef, B. G. (1996). Social influences on food preferences and feeding behaviors of vertebrates. In: Why We Eat What We Eat: The Psychology of Eating, E. D. Capaldi (ed.). Washington, DC: American Psychological Association, pp. 207–231.

Galinsky, E., Kim, S. S., & Bon, J. T. (2001). Feeling Overworked: When Work Becomes Too Much. New York: Families and Work Institute.

Gallagher, S. A., & Hackett, P. H. (2004). Emerg Med Clin North Am, 22(2):329–355.

Galler, J. R., Fox, J. G., Murphy, J. C., & Melanson, D. E. (1979). Br J Nutr, 41(3):611–618.

Gallese, V. (2005). Phenom Cog Sci, 4(1):23–48.

Galli, S. M., & Phillips, M. I. (1996). Proc Soc Exp Biol Med, 213(2):128–137.

Gall-Troselj, K., Mravak-Stipetic, M., Jurak, I., Ragland, W. L., et al. (2001). J Oral Pathol Med, 30(9):560–563.

Garces, C., Benavente, M., Ortega, H., Rubio, R., et al. (2002). Pediatr Res, 52(6):873–878.

Garcia, R. I., Henshaw, M. M., & Krall, E. A. (2001). Periodontology 2000, 25:21–36.

Garcia–Tamayo, J., Castillo, G., & Martinez, A. J. (1982). Acta Cytol, 26(1):7–14.

Gardner, J., & Miller, L. (2005). J Womens Health, 14(1):53–60.

Gardner, J. D. (1983). Ann Hum Biol, 10(1):31–40.

Gardner, J. D., & Valadian, I. (1983). Ann Hum Biol, 10(1):41–55.

Gardner, K. (1995). New Community, 18(4):579–590.

Gardyn, R. (2002). Am Demogr, 24(3):30–33.

Garland, C. F., Garland, F. C., Gorham, E. D., Lipkin, M., et al. (2006). Am J Public Health, 96(2):252–261.

Garn, S. M., LaVelle, M., Rosenberg, K. R., & Hawthorne, V. M. (1986). Am J Clin Nutr, 43(6):879–883.

Garner, J. P., & Mason, G. J. (2002). Behav Brain Res, 136(1):83–92.

Garrett, J. L., & Ruel, M. T. (2005). Food Nutr Bull, 26(2):209–221.

Garty, B. Z., Kanner, D., & Danon, Y. L. (1995). J Pediatr, 127(4):669.

Gasbarrini, A., de Luca, A., Fiore, G., Gambrielli, M., et al. (1998). Hepatogastroenterology, 45(21):765–770.

Gasbarrini, A., Gabrielli, M., Fiore, G., Candelli, M., et al. (2000). Cephalalgia, 20(6):561–565.

Gault, A., O'Dea, K., Rowley, K. G., McLeay, T., et al. (1996). Diabetes Care, 19(11):1269–1273.

Gaydos, C. A., Summersgill, J. T., Sahney, N. N., Ramirez, J. A., et al. (1996). Infect Immun, 64(5):1614–1620.

Ge, R. L., Matsuzawa, Y., Takeoka, M., Kubo, K., et al. (1997). Chest, 111(1):58–64.

Geary, D. C. (2000). Psychol Bull, 126(1):55–77.

Geary, D. C. (2005). The Origin of Mind: Evolution of Brain, Cognition, and General Intelligence. Washington, DC: American Psychological Association.

Gebb, S. A., & Jones, P. L. (2003). Hypoxia and lung branching morphogenesis. In: Hypoxia Through the Lifecycle, R. C. Roach, P. D. Wagner, & P. H. Hackett (eds.). New York: Kluwer Academic/Plenum pp. 117–125.

Geier, A. B., Rozin, P., & Doros, G. (2006). Psychol Sci, 17(6):521–525.

George, L. (2005). The end of menstruation. Maclean's, December 12:41–45.

Georgieff, M. K., Hoffman, J. S., Pereira, G. R., Bernbaum, J., et al. (1985). J Pediatr, 107(4):581–587.

Gerald, M. S., & Higley, J. D. (2002). Addiction, 97(4):415–425.

Gérard, H. C., Wang, G. F., Balin, B. J., Schumacher, H. R., et al. (1999). Microb Pathog, 26(1):35–43.

Gérard, H. C., Wildt, K. L., Whittum-Hudson, J. A., Lai, Z., et al. (2005). Microb Pathog, 39(1–2):19–26.

Gérard, H. C., Whittum-Hudson, J. A., & Hudson, A. P. (2006). *C. pneumoniae utilizes ApoE and the LDL Receptor Family for Host Cell Attachment.* Paper presented at the International Chlamydia Symposium San Francisco, CA.

Gerber, L. M., & Crews, D. E. (1999). Evolutionary perspectives on chronic diseases: Changing environments, life styles, and life expectancy. In: Evolutionary Medicine, W. R. Trevathan, E. O. Smith, & J. J. McKenna (eds.). New York: Oxford University Press, pp. 443–469.

Gerstman, B. B., Piper, J. M., Tomita, D. K., Ferguson, W. J., et al. (1991). Am J Epidemiol, 133(1):32–37.

Ghedin, E., Sengamalay, N. A., Shumway, M., Zaborsky, J., et al. (2005). Nature, 437(7062):1162–1166.

Gheorghiade, M., Orlandi, C., Burnett, J. C., Demets, D., et al. (2005). J Card Fail, 11(4):260–269.

Gibbons, A. (1998). Science, 280(5368):1345–1347.

Gibbins, I. (1994). Comparative anatomy and evolution of the sympathetic nervous system. In: Comparative Physiology and Evolution of the Autonomic Nervous System, S. Nilson, & S. Holmgren (eds.). Chur, Switzerland: Harwood Academic Publishers, pp. 1–67.

Gibbs, N. (2006). The magic of the family meal. Time, 167 (24):50.

Gibbs, R. W. (2006). Embodiment and Cognitive Science. New York: Cambridge University Press.

Gilbert, D. L. (1983). Respir Physiol, 52(3):315–326.

Gilbert, P. (2001). Aust NZ J Psychiatry, 35(1):17–27.

Gilden, D. H. (1999). Ann Neurol, 46(1):4–5.

Gillespie, J. (1977). Am Nat, 111(981):1010–1014.

Giovannucci, E. (2005). Cancer Causes Control, 16(2):83–95.

Glantz, K. (1987). Psychotherapy, 24(1):20–24.

Glantz, K., & Pearce, J. K. (1989). Exiles from Eden: Psychotherapy From an Evolutionary Perspective. New York: Norton.

Glantz, K., & Moehl, M.-B. (2000). Reluctant males: Evolutionary perspectives on male psychology in couples therapy. In: Genes on the Couch: Explorations in Evolutionary Psychotherapy, P. Gilbert & K. G. Baileyl. (eds.). PhiladelphiaBrunner-Routledge, pp. 176–195.

Glasier, A. F., Smith, K. B., van der Spuy, Z. M., Ho, P. C., et al. (2003). Contraception, 67(1):1–8.

Glick, H., Endicott, J., & Nee, J. (1993). Acta Psychiatr Scand, 88(3):149–155.

Glick, I. D., & Stewart, D. (1980). Compr Psychiatry, 21(4):281–287.

Gluckman, P. D., & Pinal, C. S. (2003). J Nutr, 133(5 [Suppl 2]):1741S–1746S.

Gluckman, P. D., & Hanson, M. A. (2004a). Science, 305(5691):1733–1736.

Gluckman, P. D., & Hanson, M. A. (2004b). Trends Endocrinol Metab, 15(4):183–187.

Gluckman, P. D., Cutfield, W., Hofman, P., & Hanson, M. A. (2005). Early Hum Dev, 81(1):51–59.

Gluckman, P. D., & Hanson, M. A. (2005). The Fetal Matrix: Evolution, Development, and Disease. New York: Cambridge University Press.

Gluckman, P. D., Hanson, M. A., Mortan, S. M. B., & Pinal, C. S. (2005). Biol Neonate, 87:127–139.

Gluckman, P. D., Hanson, M. A., & Spencer, H. G. (2005). Trends Ecol Evol, 20(10):527–533.

Gluckman, P. D., & Hanson, M. A. (2006). Trends Endocrinol Metab, 17(1):7–12.

Godwin, S. L., Chambers, E., & Cleveland, L. (2004). J Am Diet Assoc, 104(4):585–594.

Goel, R. M., Thomson, R. B., Sweet, E. M., & Halliday, S. (1981). Scott Med J, 26(4):340–345.

Gokcay, G., Uzel, N., Kayaturk, F., & Neyzi, O. (1997). Child Care Health Dev, 23(2):187–200.

Golay, A., Allaz, A. F., Morel, Y., de Tonnac, N., et al. (1996). Am J Clin Nutr, 63(2):174–178.

Goldberg, J. P., Folta, S. C., & Must, A. (2002). Pediatrics, 110(4):826–832.

Goldin, B. R., Adlercreutz, H., Gorbach, S. L., Warram, J. H., et al. (1982). N Engl J Med, 307(25):1542–1547.

Goldin, B. R., Adlercreutz, H., Gorbach, S. L., Woods, M. N., et al. (1986). Am J Clin Nutr, 44(6):945–953.

Goldman, B. D. (2003). Sci STKE, 2003(192):PE29.

Goldner, E. M., Hsu, L., Waraich, P., Somers, J. M., et al. (2002). Can J Psychiatry, 47(9):833–843.

Goldsby, R. A., Kindt, T. J., Osborne, B. A., & Kuby, J. (2003). Immunology, 5th ed. New York: W. H. Freeman.

Goldsmith, M. F. (1993). J Am Med Assoc, 269(12):1477–1480.

Goldsmith, Z. (1999). Ecologist, 29(3):189–193.

Goldstein, J., Hoff, K., & Hillyard, S. D. (2003). Comp Biochem Physiol A Mol Integr Physiol, 136(3):557–563.

Goldstein Ferber, S., & Makhoul, I. R. (2004). Pediatrics, 113(4):858–865.

Golub, M. S. (2000). Environ Health Perspect, 108(4):355–362.

Good Housekeeping. (1956). Baby Book. London: National Magazine Company.

Goodman, A. H., Dufour, D. L., & Pelto, G. H. (eds.). (2000). Nutritional Anthropology: Biocultural Perspectives on Food and Nutrition. Mountain View, CA: Mayfield Publishing.

Gordeuk, V. R., & Prchal, J. T. (2006). Semin Thromb Hemost, 32(3):289–294.

Gorinstein, S., & Trakhtenberg, S. (2003). Addict Biol, 8(4):445–454.

Gorman, C. (2000). Who needs a period? Time, September, 56.

Goscienski, P. J. (2003). Health Secrets of the Stone Age: What We Can Learn From Deep in Prehistory to Become Leaner, Livelier and Longer Lived. Santa Teresa, NM. New Century Books.

Gosden, R. G., Dunbar, R. I. M., Haig, D., Heyer, E., et al. (1999). Evolutionary interpretations of the diversity of reproductive health and disease. In: Evolution in Health and Disease, S. C. Stearns (ed.). Oxford, UK: Oxford University Press, pp. 108–120.

Gott, P., & Donovan, R. (2006). Dr. Gott's No Flour, No Sugar Diet. Sanger, CA: Quill Driver Books.

Gottlieb, S. S., Dickstein, K., Fleck, E., Kostis, J., et al. (1993). Circulation, 88(4 [Pt 1]):1602–1609.

Gould, S. J., & Lewontin, R. C. (1979). Proc R Soc Lond B Biol Sci, 205(1161):581–589.

Graber, J. A., Lewinsohn, P. M., Seeley, J. R., & Brooks–Gunn, J. (1997). J Am Acad Child Adolesc Psychiatry, 36(12):1768–1776.

Grady, D., Herrington, D., Bittner, V., Blumenthal, R., et al. (2002). J Am Med Assoc, 288(1):49–57.

Graeub, R. (1994). The Petkau Effect. New York: Four Walls Eight Windows.

Graham, J. B., Dudley, R., Aguilar, N. M., & Gans, C. (1995). Nature, 375(6527):117–120.

Grainger, S. (2004). Hum Nat, 15(2):133–145.

Grant, W. B., & Holick, M. F. (2005). Altern Med Rev, 10(2):94–111.

Grassi, G., Seravalle, G., Cattaneo, B. M., Lanfranchi, A., et al. (1995). Circulation, 92(11):3206–3211.

Gray, S., & Olopade, O. I. (2003). J Clin Oncol, 21(17):3191–3193.

Greaves, M. F. (2000). Cancer: The Evolutionary Legacy. Oxford, UK: Oxford University Press.

Greene, R., & Dalton, K. (1953). BMJ, 1(4818):1007–1014.

Greenslade, J. (1995). What's best about breastfeeding. Nursery World, January, 19–21.

Greenspan, F. S., & Gardner, D. G. (2004). Basic and Clinical Endocrinology. New York: Lange Medical Books/McGraw–Hill.

Greenstein, R. J. (2003). Lancet Infect Dis, 3(8):507–514.

Greer, F. R., & Krebs, N. F. (2006). Pediatrics, 117(2):578–585.

Griffin, M. (2004), Issues in the development of school milk, http://www.fao.org/es/ESC/en20953/20999/index.html

Grigoriadis, S., & Seeman, M. V. (2002). Can J Psychiatry, 47(5):437–442.

Grillenberger, M., Neumann, C. G., Murphy, S. P., Bwibo, N. O., et al. (2003). J Nutr, 133(11):3957S–3964S.

Grimes, D. (1999). Network, 19(2):11–13.

Grimes, D. S. (2003). Gut, 52(1):155.

Grimmelikhuijzen, C. J., Dierickx, K., & Boer, G. J. (1982). Neuroscience, 7(12):3191–3199.

Grob, B., Knapp, L. A., Martin, R. D., & Anzenberger, G. (1998). Exp Clin Immunogenet, 15(3):119–129.

Groff, J. L., & Groper, S. S. (2000). Advanced Nutrition and Human Metabolism. Belmont, CA: Wadsworth Publishing Co.

Grohmann, U., Fallarino, F., & Puccetti, P. (2003). Trends Immunol, 24(5):242–248.

Grøon, F. (1984). Om Kostholdet i Norge Indtil aar 1500 [About the Norwegian Diet Until 1500]. Oslo: Kildeforlaget.

Gross, M. R. (2005). Q Rev Biol, 80(1):37–45.

Gross, S. J., Kosmetatos, N., Grimes, C. T., & Williams, M. L. (1978). Am J Dis Child, 132(8):753–756.

Gross, S. J., Oehler, J. M., & Eckerman, C. O. (1983). Pediatrics, 71(1):70–75.

Grossman, C. J. (1985). Science, 227(4684):257–261.

Gudin, R. G. (1952). Bull Soc Anthro (Paris), 3(10):59–87.

Gueguen, L., & Pointillart, A. (2000). J Am Coll Nutr, 19(2):119S–136S.

Guerinot, M. L. (1994). Annu Rev Microbiol, 48:743–772.

Guest, C. S., O'Dea, K., Hopper, J. L., & Larkins, R. G. (1993). Diabetes Res Clin Pract, 20(2):155–164.

Gulledge, C. C., Burow, M. E., & McLachlan, J. A. (2001). Pediatr Clin North Am, 48(5):1223–1240.

Gunnar, M. R., Brodersen, L., Nachmias, M., Buss, K., et al. (1996). Dev Psychobiol, 29(3):191–204.

Gunnar, M. R. (1998). Prev Med, 27(2):208–211.

Gunnar, M. R., & Donzella, B. (2002). Psychoneuroendocrinology, 27(1–2):199–220.

Gunnell, D., Okasha, M., Davey Smith, G., Oliver, S. E., et al. (2001). Epidemiol Rev, 23(2):313–342.

Gupta, S., & Camm, A. J. (1997). BMJ, 314(7097):1778–1779.

Guraya, S. S. (1985). Biology of Ovarian Follicles in Mammals. Berlin, Germany. Springer–Verlag.

Gurkin Rosati, K., & Rosati, R. (2006). The Rice Diet Solution: The World–Famous Low–Sodium, Good–Carb, Detox Diet for Quick and Lasting Weight Loss. New York: Simon, & Schuster.

Gurleyik, G., & Gurleyik, E. (2003). Eur J Emerg Med, 10(3):200–203.

Gurven, M., Hill, K., & Kaplan, H. (2002). J Anthropol Res, 58(1):93–120.

Gutbrod, T., Wolke, D., Woehne, B., Ohrt, B., et al. (2000). Arch Dis Child, 82(3):208–214.

Guthrie, J. F., Lin, B. H., & Frazao, E. (2002). J Nutr Educ Behav, 34(3):140–150.

Guyton, A. C. (1986). Textbook of Medical Physiology, 7th ed. Philadelphia: W.B. Saunders.

Guzman, C., Cabrera, R., Cardenas, M., Larrea, F., et al. (2006). J Physiol, 572(1):97–108.

Haahr, S., Plesner, A. M., Vestergaard, B. F., & Hollsberg, P. (2004). Acta Neurol Scand, 109(4):270–275.

Haan, J., van Broeckhoven, C., van Duijn, C. M., Voorhoeve, E., et al. (1994). Ann Neurol, 36(3):434–437.

Hack, M., Merkatz, I. R., McGrath, S. K., Jones, P. K., et al. (1984). Am J Dis Child, 138(4):370–375.

Hacker, J., & Heesemann, J. (eds.). (2002). Molecular Infection Biology: Interactions Between Microorganisms and Cells. Hoboken, NJ: Wiley–Liss.

Haffajee, A. D., & Socransky, S. S. (2001). J Clin Periodontol, 28(5):377–388.

Haffner, S. M., Miettinen, H., & Stern, M. P. (1997). Diabetes Care, 20(7):1087–1092.

Hagen, T., Taylor, C. T., Lam, F., & Moncada, S. (2003). Science, 302(5652):1975–1978.

Haggerty, C. L., Ness, R. B., Kelsey, S., & Waterer, G. W. (2003). Ann Allergy Asthma Immunol, 90(3):284–291.

Hahnemann, S. (1916). Organon of Medicine, 6thed. Philadelphia: Boericke, & Tafel.

Haig, D. (1993). Q Rev Biol, 68(4):495–532.

Haig, D. (1999). Genetic conflicts in pregnancy and childhood. In: Evolution in Health and Disease, S. C. Stearns (ed.). Oxford, U.K. Oxford University Press, pp. 77–90.

Hairston, I. S., Little, M. T., Scanlon, M. D., Barakat, M. T., et al. (2005). J Neurophysiol, 94(6):4224–4233.

Halaas, J. L., Gajiwala, K. S., Maffei, M., Cohen, S. L., et al. (1995). Science, 269(5223):543–546.

Halász, P., Terzano, M., Parrino, L., & Bódizs, R. (2004). J Sleep Res, 13(1):1–23.

Haldane, J. B. S. (1949). Ric Sci, 19(Suppl):68–76.

Hales, C. N., Barker, D. J. P., Clark, P. M. S., Cox, L. J., et al. (1991). BMJ, 303(6809):1019–1022.

Hales, C. N., & Barker, D. J. P. (1992). Diabetologia, 35(7):595–601.

Hales, C. N., & Barker, D. J. P. (2001). Br Med Bull, 60(5–20.

Hales, D. (2005). What America really eats. Parade Magazine, November 13, p. 4–5.

Hall, M., Bromberger, J., & Matthews, K. A. (1999). Ann NY Acad Sci, 896:427–430.

Hall, R. H. (1976). Food for Nought. The Decline in Nutrition. New York: Random House.

Halliwell, B., & Gutteridge, J. M. C. (1989). Free Radicals in Biology and Medicine. New York: Oxford University Press.

Hallonquist, J. D., Seeman, M. V., Lang, M., & Rector, N. A. (1993). Biol Psychiatry, 33(3):207–209.

Halton, T. L., Willett, W. C., Liu, S., Manson, J. E., et al. (2006). Am J Clin Nutr, 83(2):284–290.

Hamblin, M. T., & Di Rienzo, A. (2000). Am J Hum Gen, 66(5):1669–1679.

Hamelin, B. A., Methot, J., Arsenault, M., Pilote, S., et al. (2003). Am J Med, 114(7):599–602.

Hamilton, J. A., Parry, B. L., Alagna, S., Blumenthal, S., et al. (1984). Psychiatr Ann, 14(6):426–435.

Hamilton, W. D. (1964a). J Theor Biol, 7(1):1–16.

Hamilton, W. D. (1964b). J Theor Biol, 7(1):17–52.

Hamilton, W. D. (1995). The Narrow Paths of Gene Land. New York: W.H. Freeman.

Hamlyn, B., Brooker, S., Oleinikova, K., & Wands, S. (2002). Infant Feeding 2000. London: Department of Health, The Stationary Office.

Hampel, H., Sweet, K., Westman, J. A., Offit, K., et al. (2004). J Med Genet, 41(2):81–91.

Han, Y. W., Shi, W., Huang, G. T. J., Haake, S. K., et al. (2000). Infect Immun, 68(6):3140–3146.

Hanson, R. L., Imperatore, G., Bennett, P. H., & Knowler, W. C. (2002). Diabetes, 51(10):3120–3127.

Haraszthy, V. I., Zambon, J. J., Trevisan, M., Zeid, M., et al. (2000). J Periodontol, 71(10):1554–1560.

Harding, J. E. (2003). Asia Pac J Clin Nutr, 12(Suppl):S28.

Hardy, J. (1995). Am J Med Genet, 60(5):456–460.

Hardyment, C. (1983). Dream Babies: Child Care From Locke to Spock. London: Jonathan Cape Ltd.

Hargens, A. R., Millard, R. W., Pettersson, K., & Johansen, K. (1987). Nature, 329(6134):59–60.

Harlow, B. L., Signorello, L. B., Hall, J. E., Dailey, C., et al. (1998). Am J Med, 105(3A):94S–99S.

Harpending, H., Draper, P., & Pennington, R. (1990). Culture, evolution, parental care, and mortality. In: Disease in Populations in Transition: Anthropological and Epidemiological Perspectives, A. C. Swedlund, & G. J. Armelagos (eds.). South Hadley, MA: Bergin and Garvey, pp. 251–266.

Harris, J. C., Cottrell, S. L., Plummer, S., & Lloyd, D. (2001). Appl Microbiol Biotechnol, 57(3):282–286.

Harris, M. (1978). Hum Nat, 1(2):28–36.

Harris, M. (1986). Good to Eat: Riddles of Food and Culture. New York: Simon, & Schuster.

Harris, M., & Ross, E. B. (eds.). (1987). Food and Evolution: Toward a Theory of Human Food Habits. Philadelphia: Temple University Press.

Harris, M. (1989). Our Kind: Who We Are, Where We Came From, Where We are Going. New York: Harper & Row.

Harris, P. (1983a). Cardiovasc Res, 17(6):313–319.

Harris, P. (1983b). Cardiovasc Res, 17(7):373–378.

Harris, P. (1983c). Cardiovasc Res, 17(8):437–445.

Harris, P. (1985). Adv Myocardiol, 5:1–11.

Harrison, Y., & Horne, J. A. (2000). J Exp Psychol Appl, 6(3):236–249.

Harvey, A. G., Tang, N. K. Y., & Browning, L. M. (2005). Clin Psychol Rev, 25(5):593–611.

Hatalski, C. G., Lewis, A. J., & Lipkin, W. I. (1997). Emerg Infect Dis, 3(2):129–135.

Hauck, F. R., Herman, S. M., Donovan, M., Iyasu, S., et al. (2003). Pediatrics, 111(5):1207–1214.

Hawdon, J. M., Ward-Platt, M. P., & Aynsley-Green, A. (1994). Arch Dis Child, 70(1):F60–64.

Hawkes, C. (2004). Marketing Food to Children: The Global Regulatory Environment. Geneva: World Health Organization.

Hawkes, K. (1992). Sharing and collective action. In: Evolutionary Ecology and Human Behavior, B. Winterhalder, & E. A. Smith (eds.). New York: Aldine, pp. 269–300.

Hawkes, K., O'Connell, J. F., Blurton Jones, N. G., Alvarez, H., et al. (1998). Proc Natl Acad Sci USA, 95(3):1336–1339.

Hawkes, K. (2004). Nature, 428(6979):128–129.

Hayashi, M., Sasaki, S., Tsuganezawa, H., Monkawa, T., et al. (1994). J Clin Invest, 94(5):1778–1783.

Hazon, N., Tierney, M. L., & Takei, Y. (1999). J Exp Zool, 284(5):526–534.

He, J., Vupputuri, T., Allen, K., Prerost, M. R., et al. (1999). N Engl J Med, 340(12):920–926.

Heaney, R. P., McCarron, D. A., Dawson–Hughes, B., Oparil, S., et al. (1999). J Am Diet Assoc, 99(10):1228–1233.

Heaney, R. P. (2000). J Am Coll Nutr, 19(2):83S–99S.

Hediger, M. L., Overpeck, M. D., Maurer, K. R., Kuczmarksi, R. J., et al. (1998). Arch Pediatr Adolesc Med, 152(12):1225–1231.

Hedley, A. A., Ogden, C. L., Johnson, C. L., Carroll, M. D., et al. (2004). J Am Med Assoc, 291(23):2847–2850.

Hegsted, D. M. (2001). Am J Clin Nutr, 74(5):571–573.

Heim, C., Newport, D. J., Heit, S., Graham, Y. P., et al. (2000). J Am Med Assoc, 284(5):592–597.

Heim, C., Newport, D. J., Wagner, D., Wilcox, M. M., et al. (2002). Depress Anxiety, 15(3):117–125.

Heitkemper, M. M., Cain, K. C., Jarrett, M. E., Burr, R. L., et al. (2003). Am J Gastroenterol, 98(2):420–430.

Heller, D. A., de Faire, U., Pedersen, N. L., Dahlen, G., et al. (1993). N Engl J Med, 328(16):1150–1156.

Helsing, E. (1976). Ciba Found Symp, 45:215–230.

Henderson, B. A., & Bernstein, L. (1991). Breast Cancer Res Treat, 18(Suppl 1):11–17.

Henderson, B. E., Ross, R. K., & Pike, M. C. (1993). Science, 259(5095):633–638.

Henderson, S. T. (2004). Med Hypotheses, 62(5):689–700.

Hendrick, V., Altshuler, L. L., & Burt, V. K. (1996). Harv Rev Psychiatry, 4(4):200–207.

Henig, R. M. (2006). Fat factors. New York Times Magazine, August 13, pp. 28–33.

Hetherington, M. M., & Rolls, B. J. (1996). Sensory-specific satiety: Theoretical frameworks and central characteristics. In: Why We Eat What We Eat: The Psychology of Eating, E. D. Capaldi (ed.). Washington, DC: American Psychological Association, pp. 267–290.

Hewlett, B. S., & Lamb, M. E. (2002). Integrating evolution, culture and developmental psychology: Explaining caregiver–infant proximity and responsiveness in central Africa and the USA. In: Between Culture and Biology: Perspectives on Ontogenetic Development H. Keller, Y. H. Poortinga, & A. Scholmerich (eds.). New York: Cambridge University Press, pp. 241–269.

Hewlett, B. S., & Lamb, M. E. (eds.). (2005). Hunter-Gatherer Childhoods: Evolutionary, Developmental, and Cultural Perspectives. New Brunswick, NJ: Aldine Transaction.

Heymsfield, S. B., McManus, C., Smith, J., Stevens, V., et al. (1982). Am J Clin Nutr, 36(4):680–690.

Heymsfield, S. B., Lohman, T. G., Wang, Z., & Going, S. B. (eds.). (2005). Human Body Composition. Champaign, IL: Human Kinetics.

Hilder, A. S. (1994). Early Hum Dev, 38(3):143–149.

Hill, A. J. (2004). Br J Nutr, 92(Suppl 1):S15–S18.

Hill, A. V. S., & Motulsky, A. G. (1999). Genetic variation and human disease: The role of natural selection. In: Evolution in Health and Disease, S. C. Stearns (ed.). Oxford, UK: Oxford University Press, pp. 50–61.

Hill, A. V. S., Sanchez-Mazas, A., Barbujani, G., Dunston, G., et al. (1999). Human genetic variation and its impact on public health and medicine. In: Evolution in Health and Disease, S. C. Stearns (ed.). Oxford, UK: Oxford University Press, pp. 62–74.

Hill, E. M., & Chow, K. (2002). Addiction, 97(4):401–413.

Hill, J. O., & Peters, J. C. (1998). Science, 280(5368):1371–1374.

Hill, K. (1988). Hum Ecol, 16(2):159–197.

Hill, K., & Hurtado, A. M. (1996). Ache Life History. The Ecology and Demography of a Foraging People. New York: Aldine de Gruyter.

Hill, K., & Kaplan, H. (1999). Annu Rev Anthropol, 28:397–430.

Hillis, S. D., Anda, R. F., Dube, S. R., Felitti, V. J., et al. (2004). Pediatrics, 113(2):320–327.

Hinde, R. A. (1974). Biological Bases of Human Social Behaviour. New York: McGraw-Hill.

Hindmarsh, P. C., Matthews, D. R., Di Silvio, L., Kurtz, A. B., et al. (1988). Arch Dis Child, 63:665–666.

Hiraiwa–Hasegawa, M. (1990). Role of food sharing between mother and infant in the ontogeny of feeding behavior. In: The Chimpanzees of the Mahale Mountains, T. Nishida (ed.). Tokyo: University of Tokyo Press, pp. 267–275.

Hirota, K., & Semenza, G. L. (2006). Crit Rev Oncol Hematol, 59(1):15–26.

Hirsch, F. (1976). Social Limits to Economic Growth. Cambridge, MA: Harvard University Press.

Hirschleifer, J. (1966). Q J Econ, 80:252–277.

Hjalmarson, A., & Fagerberg, B. (2000). Basic Res Cardiol, 95(Suppl 1):98–103.

Hobson, J. A., & Pace-Schott, E. F. (2002). Nat Rev Neurosci, 3(9):679–693.

Hoelzel, A. R. (1991). Behav Ecol Sociobiol, 29(3):197–204.

Hoffer, A. (2005). Adventures in Psychiatry.The Scientific Memoirs of Dr. Abram Hoffer. Caledon, Ontario, Canada: Kos Publishing.

Hoffman, H. J., Damus, K., Hillman, L., & Krongrad, E. (1988). Ann NY Acad Sci, 533:13–31.

Hogh, P., Oturai, A., Schreiber, K., Blinkenberg, M., et al. (2000). Mult Scler, 6(4):226–230.

Hohmann, G., & Fruth, B. (1993). Folia Primatol, 60(4):225–229.

Holden, R. J., & Mooney, P. A. (1994). Med Hypotheses, 43(6):420–435.

Holden, R. J. (1995). Med Hypotheses, 44(5):379–391.

Holick, M. F. (2004a). Am J Clin Nutr, 80(Suppl 6):1678S–1688S.

Holick, M. F. (2004b). Am J Clin Nutr, 79(3):362–371.

Holland, J. H. (1992). Daedalus, 121(1):17–30.

Holliday, M. A. (1986). Body composition and energy needs during growth. In: Human Growth: A Comprehensive Treatise, F. Faulkner & J. M. Tanner (eds.). New York: Plenum Press, pp. 101–117.

Hollox, E. J., Poulter, M., Zvarik, M., Ferak, V., et al. (2000). Am J Hum Gen, 68(1):160–172.

Holmes, E. C. (1999). Molecular phylogenies and the genetic structure of viral populations. In: Evolution in Health and Disease, S. C. Stearns (ed.). Oxford, UK: Oxford University Press, pp. 173–182.

Holmes, M. D., Pollak, M. N., Willett, W. C., & Hankinson, S. E. (2002). Cancer Epidemiol Biomarkers Prev, 11(9):852–861.

Holt, S. H., Brand Miller, J. C., & Petocz, P. (1997). Am J Clin Nutr, 66(5):1264–1276.

Holt, R. I. G. (2004). Diabetes Obes Metab, 6(1):83–84.

Holvik, K., & Meyer, H. E. (2005). The Oslo Immigrant Health Study. Oslo: The Norwegian Institute of Public Health.

Hoppe, C., Molgaard, C., Juul, A., & Michaelsen, K. F. (2004). Eur J Clin Nutr, 58(9):1211–1216.

Hoppe, C., Udam, T. R., Lauritzen, L., Molgaard, C., et al. (2004). Am J Clin Nutr, 80(2):447–452.

Hoppe, C., Molgaard, C., & Michaelsen, K. F. (2006). Annu Rev Nutr, 26:131–173.

Hoppeler, H., Vogt, M., Weibel, E. R., & Fluck, M. (2003). Exp Physiol, 88(1):109–119.

Horner, P. J., Crowley, T., Leece, J., Hughes, A., et al. (1998). Lancet, 351(9099):341–342.

Horton, T. H. (1984). Biol Reprod, 31(3):499–504.

Houghton, L. A., Lea, R., Jackson, N., & Whorwell, P. J. (2002). Gut, 50(4):471–474.

Houston, A. I., Welton, N. J., & McNamara, J. M. (1997). Oikos, 78(2):331–340.

Howard, G., & Thun, M. J. (1999). Environ Health Perspect, 107(Suppl 6):S853–858.

Howard, B. V., Van Horn, L., Hsia, J., Manson, J. E., et al. (2006). J Am Med Assoc, 295(6):655–666.

Howell, N. (2000). Demography of the Dobe !Kung. Hawthorne, NY: Aldine de Gruyter.

Howie, P. W., Forsyth, J. S., Ogston, S. A., Clark, A., et al. (1990). BMJ, 300(6716):11–16.

Hoyert, D. L., Heron, M., P., Murphy, S. L., & Kung, H.-C. (2006). Nat Vital Stat Rep, 54(13):1–120.

Hrboticky, N., Leiter, L. A., & Anderson, G. H. (1989). Am J Clin Nutr, 50(1):46–52.

Hrdy, S. B. (1999). Mother Nature: A History of Mothers, Infants, and Natural Selection. New York: Ballantine.

Hrdy, S. B. (2005). Comes the child before Man: How cooperative breeding and prolonged post-weaning dependence shaped human potentials. In: Hunter-Gatherer Childhoods: Evolutionary, Developmental & Cultural Perspectives, B. S. Hewlett & M. E. Lamb (eds.). New Brunswick, NJ: Aldine Transaction, pp. 65–91.

Hruschka, D. J., Lende, D. H., & Worthman, C. M. (2005). Ethos, 33(1):1–19.

Hu, E., Liang, P., & Spiegelman, B. M. (1996). J Biol Chem, 271(18):10697–10703.

Huang, C. Y., & Cheng, S. F. (2006). Hu Li Za Zhi, 53(4):11–16.

Huang, R. C., Burke, V., Newnham, J. P., Stanley, F. J., et al. (2007). Int J Obes (Lond), 31(2):236–244.

Huber, R., Ghilardi, M. F., Massimini, M., & Tononi, G. (2004). Nature, 430(6995):78–81.

Hudson, R., & Distel, H. (1999). Schweiz Med Wochenschr, 129(5):176–181.

Huether, G. (1996). Prog Neurobiol, 48(6):569–612.

Huether, G. (1998). Int J Dev Neurosci, 16(3–4):297–306.

Huey, R. B., & Ward, P. D. (2005). Science, 308(5720):398–401.

Huittinen, T., Leinonen, M., Tenkanen, L., Virkkunen, H., et al. (2003). Circulation, 107(20):2566–2570.

Hulbert, A. (2003). Raising America: Experts, Parents and a Century of Advice About Children. New York: Knopf Publishing.

Hull, J. T., Wright, K. P., & Czeisler, C. A. (2003). J Biol Rhythms, 18(4):329–338.

Humphrey, N. K. (1976). The social function of intellect. In: Growing Points in Ethology, P. P. G. Bateson & R. A. Hinde (eds.). New York: Cambridge University Press, pp. 303–317.

Humphrey, N. K. (1983). Consciousness Regained. Oxford, UK: Oxford University Press.

Hunninghake, R. E. (2005). Basic Health Publications User's Guide to Inflammation, Arthritis, and Aging. Laguna Beach, CA: Basic Health Publications, Inc.

Hunt, S. M., McEwen, J., & McKenna, S. P. (1985). J R Coll Gen Pract, 35(273):185–188.

Hunt, C., Eades, M. R., & Eades, M. D. (1999). Charley Hunt's Diet Evolution: Eat Fat, Get Fit. Beverly Hills, CA: Maximum Human Potential Production.

Hunter, J. M. (1973). Geog Rev, 63(2):170–195.

Hunter, B. T. (1975). Food Additives and Federal Policy: The Mirage of Safety. New York: Charles Scribner's Sons.

Hurtado, A. M., Hurtado, I. A., Sapien, R., & Hill, K. (1999). The evolutionary ecology of child-hood asthma. In: Evolutionary Medicine, W. R. Trevathan, E. O. Smith, & J. J. McKenna (eds.). New York: Oxford University Press, pp. 101–134.

Hussain, R. (1998). Ann Hum Genet, 62(2):147–157.

Hyman, S. E. (2005). Am J Psychiatry, 162(8):1414–1422.

Ibanez, L., Potau, N., Francois, I., & de Zegher, F. (1998). J Clin Endocrinol Metab, 83(10):3558–3562.

Ibanez, L., Ferrer, A., Marcos, M. V., Hierro, F. R., et al. (2000). Pediatrics, 106(5):E72.

Ibanez, L., Potau, N., & de Zegher, F. (2000). J Clin Endocrinol Metab, 85(7):2624–2626.

Ibanez, L., Potau, N., Enriquez, G., & de Zegher, F. (2000). Pediatr Res, 47(5):575–577.

Ibanez, L., Potau, N., Ferrer, A., Rodriguez-Hierro, F., et al. (2002). J Clin Endocrinol Metab, 87(7):3391–3393.

Ibanez, L., Ong, K., Dunger, D. B., & de Zegher, F. (2006). J Clin Endocrinol Metab, 91(6):2153–2158.

Ikeda, J., Amy, N. K., Ernsberger, P., Gaesser, G. A., et al. (2005). J Nutr Educ Behav, 37(4):203–205.

Illius, A. W., Tolkamp, B. J., & Yearsley, J. (2002). Proc Nutr Soc, 61(4):465–472.

Ilveskoski, E., Perola, M., Lehtimaki, T., Laippala, P., et al. (1999). Circulation, 100(6):608–613.

Indravedik, M. S., Skranes, J. S., Torstein, V., Heyerdahl, S., et al. (2005). Pediatr Neurol, 33(4):259–266.

Infante-Rivard, C., Lévy, E., Rivard, G. E., Guiguet, M., et al. (2003). J Med Genet, 40(8):626–629.

Insel, T. R., & Young, L. J. (2001). Nat Rev Neurosci, 2(2):129–136.

Insel, P. M., Turner, R. E., & Ross, D. (2002). Nutrition. Boston: Jones and Bartlett Publishers.

Institute for Systems Biology (2005), Systems biology: The 21st Century Science, http: www.systemsbiology.org/Intro_to_ISB_and_Systems_Biology Systems_Biology_—_the_21st_Century_Science

Institute of Medicine.(1990). Nutrition During Pregnancy. Part I. Weight Gain. Washington, DC: National Academy Press.

International Association for the Study of Obesity (2004), International Obesity Task Force, http://www.iaso.org/contact.asp

International Diabetes Federation. (2001). Diabetes Atlas, 2000. Brussels, Belgium: International Diabetes Federation.

International Diabetes Federation. (2003). Diabetes Atlas, 2nd ed. Brussels, Belgium: International Diabetes Federation.

International Diabetes Federation (2005), The IDF Consensus Worldwide Definition of the Metabolic Syndrome, http://www.idf.org/home/index.cfm?node = 1429

Irwin, M. R., Thompson, J., Miller, C., Gillin, J. C., et al. (1999). J Clin Endocrinol Metab, 84(6):1979–1985.

Isaac, G. L. (1981). Stone age visiting cards: Approaches to the study of early land–use patterns. In: Patterns in the Past I., I. Hodder (ed.). Cambridge, UK: Cambridge University, pp. 37–103.

Ivanov, S. V., Kuzmin, I., Wei, M. H., Pack, S., et al. (1998). Proc Natl Acad Sci USA, 95(21):12596–12601.

Iyer, N. V., Kotch, L. E., Agani, F., Leung, S. W., et al. (1998). Genes Dev, 12(2):149–162.

Jabbour, H. N., Kelly, R. W., Fraser, H. M., & Critchley, H. O. (2006). Endocr Rev, 27(1):17–46.

Jablonka, E., & Lamb, M. J. (1995). Epigenetic Inheritance and Evolution: The Lamarckian Dimension. Oxford, UK: Oxford University Press.

Jablonka, E. (2004). Int J Epidemiol, 33(5):929–935.

Jablonka, E., & Lamb, M. J. (2005). Evolution in Four Dimensions: Genetic, Epigenetic, Behavioral, and Symbolic Variation in the History of Life. Cambridge, MA: MIT Press.

Jabs, J., & Devine, C. M. (2006). Appetite, 47(2):196–204.

Jackson, E. D., Payne, J. D., Nadel, L., & Jacobs, W. J. (2006). Biol Psychiatry, 59(6):516–522.

Jacobs, J. M., Cohen, A., Hammerman-Rozenberg, R., & Stressman, J. (2006). J Am Geriatr Soc, 54(2):325–329.

Jaddoe, V. W. V., & Witteman, J. C. M. (2006). Eur J Epidemiol, 21(2):91–102.

James, W. P. T. (2005). Matern Child Nutr, 1(3):197–203.

Janiger, O., Riffenburgh, R., & Kersh, R. (1972). Psychosomatics, 13(4):226–235.

Janszky, I., Mukamal, K. J., Orth-Gomer, K., Romelsjo, A., et al. (2004). Atherosclerosis, 176(2):311–319.

Jarvis, M. J. (2004). BMJ, 328(7434):277–279.

Jasienska, G., & Ellison, P. T. (1998). Proc R Soc Lond B Biol Sci, 265(1408):1847–1851.

Jasienska, G., Thune, I., & Ellison, P. T. (2000). Eur J Cancer Prev, 9(4):231–239.

Jasienska, G. (2001). Why energy expenditure causes reproductive suppression in women. In: Reproductive Ecology and Human Evolution, P. T. Ellison (ed.). New York: Aldine de Gruyter, pp. 59–84.

Jasienska, G. (2003). Acta Biotheor, 51(1):1–18.

Jasienska, G., & Ellison, P. T. (2004). Am J Hum Biol, 16(5):563–580.

Jasienska, G., Ziomkiewicz, A., Ellison, P. T., Lipson, S. F., et al. (2006). Eur J Cancer Prev, 15(5):439–445.

Jasienska, G., Ziomkiewicz, A., Lipson, S. F., Thune, I., et al. (2006). Am J Hum Biol, 18(1):133–140.

Jeffcoate, W., & Bakker, K. (2005). Lancet, 365(9470):1527.

Jefferson, J. A., Simoni, J., Escudero, E., Hurtado, M. E., et al. (2004). High Alt Med Biol, 5(1):61–69.

Jeffery, R. W., & Utter, J. (2003). Obes Res, 11(Suppl):12S–22S.

Jekanowski, M. D. (1999). Food Rev, 22(1):11–16.

Jelliffe, D. B., & Jelliffe, E. F. P. (1978). Human Milk in the Modern World. London: Oxford University Press.

Jenike, M. R. (2001). Nutritional ecology: Diet, physical activity and body size. In: Hunter-Gatherers: An Interdisciplinary Perspective, C. Panter-Brick, R. Layton, & P. Rowley-Conwy (eds.). Cambridge, UK: Cambridge University Press, pp. 205–238.

Jenkins, D. J. A., Wolever, T. M. S., Taylor, R. H., Barker, H., et al. (1981). Am J Clin Nutr, 34(3):362–366.

Jensen, J., Liljemark, W., & Bloomquist, C. (1981). J Periodontol, 52(10):599–602.

Jeppesen, J., Schaaf, P., Jones, C., Zhou, M. Y., et al. (1997). Am J Clin Nutr, 65(4):1027–1033.

Ji, Y., Urakami, K., Adachi, Y., Maeda, M., et al. (1998). Dement Geriatr Cogn Disord, 9(5):243–245.

Joffe, B. I., Jackson, W. P., Thomas, M. E., Toyer, M. G., et al. (1971). BMJ, 4(781):206–208.

Johansson, P. (2001). Medikament, December, p.72.

Johns, T., & Keen, S. L. (1985). Ecol Food Nutr, 16(3):253–271.

Johns, T. (1990). With Bitter Herbs They Shall Eat It: Chemical Ecology and the Origins of Human Diet and Medicine. Tucson, AZ: University of Arizona Press.

Johnston, J. M., & Amico, J. A. (1986). J Clin Endocrinol Metab, 62(4):653–657.

Johnston-Robledo, I., Ball, M., Lauta, K., & Zekoll, A. (2003). Women Health, 38(3):59–75.

Jolly, A. (1985). The Evolution of Primate Behavior, 2nd ed. New York: Macmillan.

Jones, C. P., LaVeist, T. A., & Lillie-Blanton, M. (1991). Am J Epidemiol, 134(10):1079–1084.

Jones, S., Martin, R. D., & Pilbeam, D. R. (eds.). (1992). The Cambridge Encyclopedia of Human Evolution. Cambridge, UK: Cambridge University Press.

Jones, C. P. (2001). Am J Epidemiol, 154(4):299–304; discussion 305–296.

Jones, J. H. (2005). Am J Hum Biol, 17(1):22–33.

Jongbloet, P. H., Kersemaekers, W. M., Zielhuis, G. A., & Verbeek, A. L. (1994). Ann Hum Biol, 21(6):511–518.

Joslin Diabetes Center. (2002), Why is diabetes more common in Asians and Pacific Islanders?, http://www.joslin.harvard.edu/api/why_common.html

Jotwani, R., & Cutler, C. W. (2004). Infect Immun, 72(3):1725–1732.

Juskevich, J. C., & Guyer, C. G. (1990). Science, 249(4971):875–884.

Juul, A., Bang, P., Hertel, N. T., Main, K., et al. (1994). J Clin Endocrinol Metab, 78(3):744–752.

Kahn, A., Rebuffat, E., Blu, D., Casimir, G., et al. (1987). Sleep, 10(2):116–121.

Kahn, H. S., Narayan, K. M., Williamson, D. F., & Valdez, R. (2000). Int J Obes Relat Metab Disord, 24(6):667–672.

Kahn, J. (2004). Yale J Health Policy Law Ethics, 4(1):1–46.

Kaiser, S., & Sachser, N. (2005). Neurosci Biobehav Rev, 29(2):283–294.

Kaiser Family Foundation. (1999). Kids & Media @ The New Millennium. Menlo Park, CA: Henry J. Kaiser Family Foundation.

Kaiser Family Foundation. (2003). Zero to Six: Electronic Media in the Lives of Infants, Toddlers and Preschoolers. Menlo Park, CA: Henry J. Kaiser Family Foundation.

Kaiser Family Foundation. (2006). It's Child's Play: Advergaming and the Online Marketing of Food to Children. Menlo Park, CA: Henry J. Kaiser Family Foundation.

Kalayoglu, M. V., Miranpuri, G. S., Golenbock, D. T., & Byrne, G. I. (1999). Microbes Infect, 1(6):409–418.

Kalivas , P. W., & Volkow, N. D. (2005). Am J Psychiatry, 162(8):1403–1413.

Kalkwarf, H. J., Khoury, J. C., & Lanphear, B. P. (2003). Am J Clin Nutr, 77(1):257–265.

Kalo-Klein, A., & Witkin, S. S. (1989). Am J Obstet Gynecol, 161(5):1132–1136.

Kalo-Klein, A., & Witkin, S. S. (1990). Infect Immun, 58(1):260–262.

Kalo-Klein, A., & Witkin, S. S. (1991). Am J Obstet Gynecol, 164(5 [Pt 1]):1351–1354.

Kaltiala-Heino, R., Martunnen, M., Rantanen, P., & Rimpelä, M. (2003). Soc Sci Med, 57(6):1055–1064

Kamath, S. K., Murillo, G., Chatterton, R. T., Hussain, E. A., et al. (1999). Nutr Cancer, 35(1):16–26.

Kandel, E. R., Schwartz, J. H., & Jessell, T. M. (2000). Principles of Neural Science, 4th ed. New York: McGraw-Hill.

Kane, S. V., Sable, K., & Hanauer, S. B. (1998). Am J Gastroenterol, 93(10):1867–1872.

Kaperonis, E. A., Liapis, C. D., Kakisis, J. D., Dimitroulis, D., et al. (2006). Eur J Vasc Endovasc Surg, 31(5):509–515.

Kaplan, H., & Hill, K. (1985). Curr Anthropol, 26(2):223–245.

Kaplan, H. (1994). Popul Dev Rev, 20(4):753–791.

Kaplan, H., Hill, K., Lancaster, J., & Hurtado, A. M. (2000). Evol Anthropol, 9(4):156–185.

Kappeler, P. M. (1998). Am J Primatol, 46(1):7–33.

Kaput, J., & Rodriguez, R. L. (2006). Nutritional Genomics: Discovering the Path to Personalized Nutrition. Hoboken, NJ: Wiley-Interscience.

Karlsson, C., Lindell, K., Svensson, E., Bergh, C., et al. (1997). J Clin Endocrinol Metab, 82(12):4144–4148.

Kartoz, C. R. (2004). Am J Matern Child Nurs, 29(1):30–35.

Kasper, H., Thiel, H., & Ehl, M. (1973). Am J Clin Nutr, 26(2):197–204.

Katschinski, M. (2000). Appetite, 34(2):189–196.

Katz, S. H. (1982). Food, behavior, and biocultural evolution. In: The Psychobiology of Human Food Selection, L. M. Barker (ed.). Westport, CT: AVI Publishing Company, Inc, pp. 171–188.

Katz, S. H. (1987). Food and biocultural evolution: A model for the investigation of modern nutritional problems. In: Nutritional Anthropology, F. E. Johnston (ed.). New York: Alan R. Liss, Inc, pp. 41–63.

Katz, S. H. (1990). Hum Nat, 1:233–259.

Katzmarzyk, P. T. (2002). Obes Res, 10(7):666–674.

Kaufman, J. S., & Cooper, R. S. (2001). Am J Epidemiol, 154(4):291–298.

Kawachi, I., & Kennedy, B. P. (2002). The Health of Nations: Why Inequality is Harmful to Your Health. New York: New Press.

Kawakoshi, A., Hyodo, S., Yasuda, A., & Takei, Y. (2003). J Mol Endocrinol, 31(1):209–220.

Kawakoshi, A., Hyodo, S., Inoue, K., Kobayashi, Y., et al. (2004). J Mol Endocrinol, 32(2):547–555.

Keckwick, A., & Pawan, G. L. S. (1956). Lancet, 271(6935):155–161.

Keefe, M. R. (1987). Nurs Res, 36(3):140–144.

Keefe, M. R. (1988). J Obstet Gynecol Neonatal Nurs, 17(2):122–126.

Keeley, L. H. (1996). War Before Civilization: The Myth of the Peaceful Savage. Oxford, UK: Oxford University Press.

Keith, S. W., Redden, D. T., Katzmarzyk, P. T., Boggiano, M. M., et al. (2006). Int J Obes (Lond), 30(11):1585–1594.

Kelada, S. N., Shelton, E., Kaufmann, R. B., & Khoury, M. J. (2001). Am J Epidemiol, 154(1):1–13.

Kelley, A. E., & Berridge, K. C. (2002). J Neurosci, 22(9):3306–3311.

Kelley, T. (2003). New pill fuels debate over benefits of fewer periods. New York: New York Times, October 14.

Kelley, A. E. (2004). Neuron, 44(1):161–179.

Kelly, A. M., Shaw, N. J., Thomas, A. M. C., Pynsent, P. B., et al. (1997). Arch Dis Child, 77(5):401–405.

Kelly, O., Cusack, S., & Cashman, K. D. (2003). Br J Nutr, 90(3):557–564.

Kelly, R. L. (1995). The Foraging Spectrum: Diversity in Hunter-Gatherer Lifeways. Washington, DC: Smithsonian Institution Press.

Kelsey, J. L., Gammon, M. D., & John, E. M. (1993). Epidemiol Rev, 15(1):36–47.

Kelvin, W. T., Tait, P. G., & Darwin, G. H. (1883). Appendix D: On the secular cooling of the earth Appendix E: On the Age of the Sun's heat. In: Treatise on Natural Philosophy. Cambridge, UK: Cambridge University Press, pp. 468–494.

Kemp, J. S., Unger, B., Wilkins, D., Psara, R. M., et al. (2000). Pediatrics, 106(3):e41.

Kendler, K. S., Silberg, J. L., Neale, M. C., Kessler, R. C., et al. (1992). Psychol Med, 22(1):85–100.

Kensara, O. A., Wootton, S. A., Phillips, D. I., Patel, M., et al. (2005). Am J Clin Nutr, 82(5):980–987.

Kermack, W. O., McKendrick, A. G., & L., M. P. (2001). Int J Epidemiol, 30(4):678–683.

Kerr, R. A. (2005). Science, 308(5729):1730–1732.

Keuthen, N. J., O'Sullivan, R. L., Hayday, C. F., Peets, K. E., et al. (1997). Psychother Psychosom, 66(1):33–37.

Key, T. J. A., & Pike, M. C. (1988). Eur J Cancer Clin Oncol, 24(1):29–43.

Key, T. J. A., Chen, J., Wang, D. Y., Pike, M. C., et al. (1990). Br J Cancer, 62(4):631–636.

Keyfitz, N. (1977). Introduction to the Mathematics of Population, with Revisions, 2nd ed. Reading, MA: Addison-Wesley Publishing Co.

Khalili, M., Watson, L. J., Bass, N., Ascher, N. L., et al. (2004). Liver Transpl, 10(3):349–355.

Kiechl, S., Werner, P., Egger, G., Oberhollenzer, F., et al. (2002). Stroke, 33(9):2170–2176.

Kim, J., Peterson, K. E., Scanlon, K. S., Fitzmaurice, G. M., et al. (2006). Obesity, 14(7):1107–1112.

Kim, S. H., Ryu, H., Kang, C. W., Kim, S. Z., et al. (1994). Gen Comp Endocrinol, 94(1):151–156.

Kimpel, D., Dayton, T., Kannan, K., & Wolf, R. E. (2003). Inflammation, 27(2):59–70.

Kingsland, S. (1996). N Engl J Med, 334(16):1067–1068.

Kinjo, K., Sato, H., Sato, H., Ohnishi, Y., et al. (2003). Am Heart J, 146(2):324–330.

Kiple, K. F., & Ornelas, K. C. (eds.). (2000). The Cambridge World History of Food. Cambridge, UK: Cambridge University Press.

Kirchengast, S. (1998). Ann Hum Biol, 25(6):541–551.

Kirchengast, S., Gruber, D., Sator, M., & Huber, J. (1998). Am J Phys Anthropol, 105(1):9–20.

Kirchengast, S., & Hartmann, B. (2000). Soc Biol, 47(1–2):114–126.

Kirschbaum, C., & Hellhammer, D. H. (1994). Psychoneuroendocrinology, 19(4):313–333.

Kitchen, W. H., McDougall, A. B., & Naylor, F. D. (1980). Dev Med Child Neurol, 22(2):163–171.

Kittler, P. G., & Sucher, K. (2004). Food and Culture, 4th ed. Belmont, CA: Thomson Wadsworth.

Kittles, R. A., & Weiss, K. M. (2003). Annu Rev Genomics Hum Genet, 4:33–67.

Klebanoff, M. A., & Yip, R. (1987). J Pediatr, 111(2):287–292.

Klein, R. G. (1999). The Human Career: Human Biological and Cultural Origins, 2nd ed. ChicagoIL: University of Chicago Press.

Kleinman, R. E. (2004). Pediatric Nutrition Handbook. Chicago, : American Academy of Pediatrics.

Kliman, H. J. (2000). Am J Pathol, 157(6):1759–1768.

Kluger, M. J. :(1978). Am Sci, 66:38–43.

Kluger, M. J. (1979). Fever—Its Biology, Evolution, and Function. Princeton, NJ: Princeton University Press.

Kluger, M. J. (1991). The adaptive value of fever. In: Fever: Basic Mechanisms and Management, P. Mackowiak (ed.). New York: Raven Press, pp. 105–124.

Kluger, M. J., Kozak, W., Conn, C. A., Leon, L. R., et al. (1996). Infect Dis Clin North Am, 10(1):1–20.

Kluger, M. J., Kozak, W., Conn, C. A., Leon, L. R., et al. (1998). Ann NY Acad Sci, 856:224–233.

Knapp, L. A. (2002). Evol Anthropol, 11(Suppl 1):140–144.

Knight, D. C., Nguyen, H. T., & Bandettini, P. A. (2005). NeuroImage, 26(4):1193–1200.

Knivsberg, A.-M., Reichelt, K. L., Hoien, T., & Nodland, M. (2002). Nutr Neurosci, 5(4):251–261.

Knowler, W. C., Pettitt, D. J., Savage, P. J., & Bennett, P. H. (1981). Am J Epidemiol, 113(2):144–156.

Knowles, H. J., Raval, R. R., Harris, A. L., & Ratcliffe, P. J. (2003). Cancer Res, 63(8):1764–1768.

Knudtzon, J., Waaler, P. E., Skjærven, R., Solberg, L. K., et al. (1988). Tidsskr Nor Lægeforen, 108(26):2125–2135.

Knudtzon, J., Waaler, P. E., Solberg, L. K., Grieg, E., et al. (1988). Tidsskr Nor Lægeforen, 108(26):2136–2142.

Kobak, R. (1999). The emotional dynamics of disruptions in attachment relationships: Implications for theory, research and clinical interventions. In: Handbook of Attachment : Theory, Research, and Clinical Applications, J. Cassidy, & P. R. Shaver (eds.). New York: Guilford Press, pp. 21–43.

Kochanek, K. D., & Smith, B. L. (2004). Nat Vital Stat Rep, 52(13):1–48.

Koda, Y., Tachida, H., Pang, H., Liu, Y. H., et al. (2001). Genetics, 158(2):747–756.

Koelman, C. A., Coumans, A. B., Nijman, H. W., Doxiadis, II, et al. (2000). J Reprod Immunol, 46(2):155–166.

Koff, E., & Rierdan, J. (1993). J Adolesc Health, 14(6):433–439.

Konner, M. J., & Worthman, C. M. (1980). Science, 207(4432):768–770.

Konner, M. J. (1991). Childhood: A Multicultural View. Boston: Little Brown.

Konno, N., Hyodo, S., Takei, Y., Matsuda, K., et al. (2005). Gen Comp Endocrinol, 140(2):86–93.

Koob, G. F., & Le Moal, M. (2005). Nat Neurosci, 8(11):1442–1444.

Kopp, W. (2006). Prev Med, 42(5):336–342.

Korte, S. M., Koolhaas, J. M., Wingfield, J. C., & McEwen, B. S. (2005). Neurosci Biobehav Rev, 29(1):3–38.

Koshimizu, T. A., Nasa, Y., Tanoue, A., Oikawa, R., et al. (2006). Proc Natl Acad Sci USA, 103(20):7807–7812.

Koutsilieri, E., Sopper, S., Scheller, C., ter Meulen, V., et al. (2002). J Neural Transm, 109(5–6):767–775.

Koziel, S., & Jankowska, E. A. (2002a). J Paediatr Child Health, 38(1):55–58.

Koziel, S., & Jankowska, E. A. (2002b). J Paediatr Child Health, 38(3):268–271.

Kraft, M. (2000). Clin Chest Med, 21(2):301–313.

Kramer, M. S., & Joseph, K. S. (1996). Lancet, 348(9037):1254–1255.

Kramer, M. S. (2000). Cochrane Database Syst Rev, 2:CD000032.

Kreek, M. J., Nielsen, D. A., Butelman, E. R., & LaForge, K. S. (2005). Nat Neurosci, 8(11):1450–1457.

Kringelbach, M. L. (2004). Neurosci Biobehav Rev, 126(4):807–819.

Kripke, D. F., Simons, R. N., Garfinkel, L., & Hammond, E. C. (1979). Arch Gen Psychiatry, 36(1):103–116.

Kripke, D. F., Garfinkel, L., Wingard, D. L., Klauber, M. R., et al. (2002). Arch Gen Psychiatry, 59(2):131–136.

Kroegel, C., & Mock, B. (2001). Chest, 120(3):1035–1036.

Krogman, W. M. (1951). Sci Am, 185:54–57.

Krogman, W. M. (1972). Child Growth. Ann Arbor, MI: University of Michigan Press.

Krueger, G. G., McQuarrie, H. G., & Swinyer, L. J. (1977). Drug Ther, 7(9):46–48.

Krueger, J. M., Majde, J. A., & Obál, F. (2003). Brain Behav Immun, 17(Suppl 1):S41–S47.

Kuczmarski, R. J., Flegal, K. M., Campbell, S. M., & Johnson, C. L. (1994). J Am Med Assoc, 272(3):205–211.

Kunitz, S. J. (1994). Disease and Social Diversity: The European Impact on the Health of Non–Europeans. New York: Oxford University Press.

Kuo, C. C., Shor, A., Campbell, L. A., Fukushi, H., et al. (1993). J Infect Dis, 167(4):841–849.

Kurina, L. M., Goldacre, M. J., Yeates, D., & Seagroatt, V. (2002). J Epidemiol Community Health, 56(7):551–554.

Kuroe, A., Taniguchi, A., Sekiguchi, A., Ogura, M., et al. (2004). Hormones Metab Res, 36(2):116–118.

Kuzawa, C. W. (1998). Am J Phys Anthropol, 107(Suppl 27):177–209.

Kuzawa, C. W. (2001). Maternal Nutrition, Fetal Growth, and Cardiovascular Risk in Filipino Adolescents, Atlanta, GA: Emory University, Department of Anthropology.

Kuzawa, C. W., & Adair, L. S. (2003). Am J Clin Nutr, 77(4):960–966.

Kuzawa, C. W., Adair, L. S., Avila, J. L., Cadungog, J. H., et al. (2003). Am J Hum Biol, 15(5):688–696.

Kuzawa, C. W. (2004). J Nutr, 134(1):194–200.

Kuzawa, C. W. (2005). Am J Hum Biol, 17(1):5–21.

Kuzawa, C. W., Gluckman, P., & Hanson, M. (2007) Developmental perspectives on the origins of obesity. In: Adipose Tissue and Adipokines in Health and Disease, G. Fantuzzi & T. Mazzone (eds.). Totowa, NJ: Humana Press, pp. 207–219.

Kwasniewski, J. (1999). Optimal Nutrition. Warsaw, Poland: Wydawnictwo WGP.

Kwasniewski, J. (2000). Homo Optimus. Warsaw, Poland: Wydawnictwo WGP.

Kwiatkowski, D. P. (2005). Am J Hum Gen, 77(2):171–190.

Labayen, I., Moreno, L. A., Blay, M. G., Blay, V. A., et al. (2006). J Nutr, 136(1):147–152.

Lager, C., & Ellison, P. T. (1990). Am J Hum Biol, 2(3):303–312.

Lahiri, S., Roy, A., Baby, S. M., Hoshi, T., et al. (2006). Prog Biophys Mol Biol, 91(3):249–286.

Lahr, M. M., & Foley, R. A. (1988). Am J Phys Anthropol, 27(Suppl):137–176.

Laitenen, J., Pietilainen, K., Wadsworth, M., Sovio, U., et al. (2004). Eur J Clin Nutr, 58(1):180–190.

Lakoff, G., & Johnson, M. (1999). Philosophy in the Flesh: The Embodied Mind and Its Challenge to Western Thought. New York: Basic Books.

Lamb, M. E., Bornstein, M. H., & Teti, D. M. (2002). Development in Infancy, 4th ed. Mahwah, NJ: Lawrence Erlbaum Associates.

Lamb, M. E. (2005). Hum Dev, 48(1–2):108–112.

Lamont, R. J., Chan, A., Belton, C. M., Izutsu, K. T., et al. (1995). Infect Immun, 63(10): 3878–3885.

Lampl, M., Johnston, F. E., & Malcolm, L. A. (1978). Ann Hum Biol, 5(3):219–227.

Lanari, M., Papa, I., Venturi, V., Lazzarotto, T., et al. (2003). J Med Virol, 70(4):628–632.

Lancaster, J. B., & Lancaster, C. S. (1983). Parental investment: The hominid adaptation. In: How Humans Adapt: A Biocultural Odyssey, D. J. Ortner (ed.). Washington, DC: Smithsonian Institution Press, pp. 33–65.

Landale, N. S., Oropesa, R. S., Llanes, D., & Gorman, B. K. (1999). Soc Forces, 78(2):613–641.

Landrigan, C. P., Rothschild, J. M., Cronin, J. W., Kaushal, R., et al. (2004). N Engl J Med, 351(18):1838–1848.

Lang, T., & Heasman, M. (2004). Food Wars: The Global Battle for Minds, Mouths, and Markets. London: Earthscan.

Langaney, A., & Nadot, R. (1995). Génétique, parenté et prohibition de l'inceste. In: La Frontière des Sexes, A. Ducros & M. Panoff (eds.). Paris: Presses Universitaires de France, pp. 105–126.

Lange, P., Parner, J., Prescott, E., Ulrik, C. S., et al. (2001). Thorax, 56(8):613–616.

Langley-Evans, S. C., Langley-Evans, A. J., & Marchand, M. C. (2003). Arch Physiol Biochem, 111(1):8–16.

Lanou, A. J., Berkow, S. E., & Barnard, N. D. (2005). Pediatrics, 115(3):736–743.

Lappé, M. (1994). Evolutionary Medicine—Rethinking the Origins of Disease. San Francisco,: Sierra Club Books.

Larciprete, G., Valensise, H., Di Pierro, G., Vaspollo, B., et al. (2005). Ultrasound Obstet Gynecol, 26(3):258–262.

Larsen, C. S. (1995). Annu Rev Anthropol, 24:185–213.

Larsen, C. S. (2000). Sci Am, 282(6):62–67.

Larson, S., & Osborn, K. (1997). The Complete Idiot's Guide to Bringing Up Baby. New York: Alpha Books.

Laska, M., Scheuber, H. P., Salazar, L. T. H., & Luna, E.-R. (2003). J Chem Ecol, 29(12):2637–2649.

Lasker, G. W., & Mascie-Taylor, C. G. N. (1988). The framework of migration studies. In: Biological Aspects of Human Migration, C. G. N. Mascie-Taylor & G. W. Lasker (eds.). Cambridge, UK: Cambridge University Press, pp. 1–13.

Lasker, G. W. (1995). The study of migrants as a strategy for understanding human biological plasticity. In: The Study of Migrants as a Strategy for Understanding Human Biological Plasticity, C. G. N. Mascie-Taylor & B. Bogin (eds.). Cambridge, UK: Cambridge University Press, pp. 110–114.

Laszlo, P. (2001). Salt: Grain of Life. New York: Columbia University Press.

Latman, N. S. (1983). Am J Med, 74(6):957–960.

Lau, E. M., Cooper, C., Wickham, C., Donnan, S., et al. (1990). Int J Epidemiol, 19(4):1119–1121.

Laughlin, S. B., de Ruyter van Steveninck, R. R., & Anderson, J. C. (1998). Nat Neurosci, 1(1):36–41.

Law, C. M., Barker, D. J., Osmond, C., Fall, C. H., et al. (1992). J Epidemiol Community Health, 46(3):184–186.

Law, M. (2000). J Cardiovasc Risk, 7(1):5–8.

Lawlor, D. A., Okasha, M., Gunnell, D., Davey Smith, G., et al. (2003). Br J Cancer, 89(1):81–87.

Lawlor, D. A., Riddoch, C. J., Page, A. S., Andersen, L. B., et al. (2005). Arch Dis Child, 90(6):582–588.

Lawrence, R. A., & Lawrence, R. M. (1999). Breastfeeding: A Guide for the Medical Profession, 5th ed. New York: C. V. Mosby.

Le Coutre, J. (2003). Food Technol, 57(8):34–37.

Le Guen, E. (2004). Heart Lung, 33(3):198; author reply 198–199.

Lear, S. A., Toma, M., Birmingham, C. L., & Frohlich, J. J. (2003). Metabolism, 52(10):1295–1301.

Leathwood, P. D., & Ashley, D. V. (1983). Behavioural strategies in the regulation of food choice. In: Nutritional Adequacy, Nutrient Availability and Needs, J. Mauron (ed.). Basel, Switzerland: Birkhauser Verlag, pp. 171–196.

LeBlanc, J. (2000). Appetite, 34(2):214–216.

Lechtig, A., Martorell, R., Delgado, H., Yarbrough, C., et al. (1978). J Trop Pediatr Environ Child Health, 24(5):217–222.

Lecube, A., Hernandez, C., Genesca, J., Esteban, J. I., et al. (2004). Diabetes Care, 27(5):1171–1175.

Ledgerwood, L. G., Ewald, P. W., & Cochran, G. M. (2003). Perspect Biol Med, 46(3):317–348.

Ledikwe, J. H., Blanck, H. M., Kettel Khan, L., Serdula, M. K., et al. (2006). Am J Clin Nutr, 83(6):1362–1368.

LeDoux, J. E. (1995). Annu Rev Psychol, 46:209–235.

LeDoux, J. E. (2000). Annu Rev Neurosci, 23(155–184.

Leduc, D., & Camfield, C. (2006). J Paediatr Child Health, 11(Suppl A):51A–52A.

Lee, M. E., Miller, W. L., Edwards, B. S., & Burnett Jr., J. C. (1989). J Clin Invest, 84(6):1962–1966.

Lee, P. C., Majluf, P., & Gordon, I. J. (1991). J Zool, 225:99–114.

Lee, R. B., & DeVore, I. (eds.). (1969). Man the Hunter. Chicago, : Aldine Publishing Co.

Lee, S. J., & Kanis, J. A. (1994). Bone Miner, 24(2):127–134.

Lee, T. M., Spears, N., Tuthill, C. R., & Zucker, I. (1989). Biol Reprod, 40(3):495–502.

Lee, W. H., & Packer, M. (1986). Circulation, 73(2):257–267.

Lee, W. T. K., Leung, S. S. F., Wang, S.-H., Xu, Y.-C., et al. (1994). Am J Clin Nutr, 60(5):744–750.

Lee, W. T. K., Leung, S. S. F., Leung, D. M. Y., Tsand, H. S. Y., et al. (1995). Br J Nutr, 74(1):125–139.

Lee, Y. L., Cesario, T., Wang, Y., Shanbrom, E., et al. (2003). Nutrition, 19(11–12):994–996.

Lee, Y.-H., & Pratley, R. E. (2005). Curr Diab Rep, 5(1):70–75.

LeGrand, E. K., & Brown, C. C. (2002). Can Vet J, 43(7):556–559.

Lehtonen, A., & Viikari, J. (1978). Acta Physiol Scand, 104(1):121–127.

Leibenluft, E. (1996). Am J Psychiatry, 153(2):163–173.

Leidloff, J. (1975). The Continuum Concept. London: Duckworth Press.

Leidy, L. (1998). Am J Hum Biol, 10(4):451–457.

Leidy, L. (1999). Menopause in evolutionary perspective. In: Evolutionary Medicine, W. R. Trevathan, E. O. Smith, & J. J. McKenna (eds.). New York: Oxford University Press, pp. 407–428.

Leier, C. V., Dei Cas, L., & Metra, M. (1994). Am Heart J, 128(3):564–574.

Leigh, S. R. (2001). Evol Anthropol, 10(6):223–236.

Leighton, G., & Clark, M. L. (1929). Lancet, 213(5520):40–43.

Leinonen, M., & Saikku, P. (1999). Am Heart J, 138(5 [Pt 2]):S504–506.

LeMagnen, J. (1987). Palatability: Concept, terminology, and mechanisms. In: Eating Habits: Food, Physiology and Learned Behaviour, R. A. Boakes, D. A. Popplewell, & M. J. Burton (eds.). Chichester, UK: John Wiley, & Sons, pp. 131–154.

Lende, D. H., & Smith, E. O. (2002). Addiction, 97(4):447–458.

Lende, D. H. (2003). Pattern and Paradox: Adolescent Substance Use and Abuse in Bogotá, Colombia. Atlanta, GA: Emory University, Department of Anthropology.

Lende, D. H. (2005). Ethos, 33(1):100–124.

Lendon, C. L., Martinez, A., Behrens, I. M., Kosik, K. S., et al. (1997). Hum Mutat, 10(3):186–195.

Lenfant, C., & Sullivan, K. (1971). N Engl J Med, 284(23):1298–1309.

Lenz, D. C., Lu, L., Conant, S. B., Wolf, N. A., et al. (2001). J Immunol, 167(3):1803–1808.

Leon, D. A., Lithell, H. O., Vagero, D., Koupilová, I., et al. (1998). BMJ, 317(7153):241–245.

Leonard, H. L., & Swedo, S. E. (2001). Int J Neuropsychopharmacol, 4(2):191–198.

Leonard, W. R., & Robertson, M. L. (1994). Am J Hum Biol, 6(1):77–88.

Leonard, W. R. (2001). Am J Hum Biol, 13(2):159–161.

Leonard, W. R., Robertson, M. L., Snodgrass, J. J., & Kuzawa, C. W. (2003). Comp Biochem Physiol A Mol Integr Physiol, 136(1):5–15.

Leonhardt, M., Lesage, J., Croix, D., Dutriez-Casteloot, I., et al. (2003). Biol Reprod, 68(2):390–400.

Léridon, H. (1993). Demographic and statistical aspects of human fertility. In: Reproduction in Mammals and Man, C. Thibault, M.-C. Levasseur, & R. H. F. Hunter (eds.). Paris: Ellipses, pp. 644–651.

Leshner, A. (1997). Science, 278(5335):45–47.

Lesku, J. A., Rattenborg, N. C., & Amlaner, C. J. (2006). The evolution of sleep: A phylogenetic approach. In: Sleep: A Comprehensive Handbook, T. L. Lee-Chiong (ed.). Hoboken, NJ: John Wiley, pp. 49–61.

Leslie, C. A., & Dubey, D. P. (1994). Prostaglandins, 47(1):41–54.

Lethbridge- Çejku, M., Schiller, J., & Bernadel, L. (2004). Vital Health Stat, 10(222):1–160.

Levene, M. I., & Dubowitz, V. (1985). Le retard de croissance intra-utérin. In: Médecine Néonatale, P. Vert, & L. Stern (eds.). Paris: Masson, pp. 100–126.

Levey, D. J. (2004). Integr Comp Biol, 44(4):284–289.

Levin, B. E., & Dunn–Meynell, A. A. (2002). Am J Physiol Regul Integr Comp Physiol, 283(4):R941–R948.

Levin, B. R., & Bull, J. J. (1994). Trends Microbiol, 2(3):76–81.

Levine, R. A. (1998). Child psychology and anthropology: An environmental view. In: Biosocial Perspectives on Childhood, C. Panter-Brick (ed.). Cambridge, UK: Cambridge University Press, pp. 102–130.

Levine, R. J., Qian, C., Maynard, S. E., Yu, K. F., et al. (2006). Am J Obstet Gynecol, 194(4):1034–1041.

Levine, S. (2005). Psychoneuroendocrinology, 30(10):939–946.

Levins, R. (1968). Evolution in Changing Environments: Some Theoretical Explorations. Princeton, NJ: Princeton University Press.

Levi-Strauss, C. (1969). The Raw and the Cooked. New York: Harper & Row.

Levi-Strauss, C. (1978). The Origin of Table Manners: Introduction of a Science of Mythology. London: Jonathan Cape Ltd.

Levy, D., Kenchaiah, S., Larson, M. G., Benjamin, E. J., et al. (2002). N Engl J Med, 347(18):1397–1402.

Lewontin, R. C., Singh, R. S., & Krimbas, C. B. (2000). Evolutionary Genetics: From Molecules to Morphology. Cambridge, UK: Cambridge University Press.

Ley, R. E., Backhed, F., Turnbaugh, P., Lozupone, C. A., et al. (2005). Proc Natl Acad Sci USA, 102(31):11070–11075.

Li, E. T. S., & Anderson, G. H. (1989). Appetite, 12:70.

Li, J. M., & Mukamal, K. J. (2004). Curr Opin Lipidol, 15(6):673–680.

Li, R., Darling, N., Maurice, E., Barker, L., et al. (2005). Pediatrics, 115(1):31–37.

Li, Z., Bowerman, S., & Heber, D. (2005). Surg Clin North Am, 85(4):681–701.

Lichtenstein, A. H., Appel, L. J., Brands, M., Carnethon, M., et al. (2006). Circulation, 114(1):82–96.

Lieberman, L. S. (2003). Annu Rev Nutr, 23:345–377.

Lieberman, L. S. (2006). Appetite, 47(1):3–9.

Liebman, B. (1999). Nutr Action Healthlett, 26(3):8–9.

Liebman, B., & Schardt, D. (2006). Nutr Action Healthlett, 33(3):8–9.

Liggett, S. B., Mialet–Perez, J., Thaneemit-Chen, S., Weber, S. A., et al. (2006). Proc Natl Acad Sci USA, 103(30):11288–11293.

Lillycrop, K. A., Phillips, E. S., Jackson, A. A., Hanson, M. A., et al. (2005). J Nutr, 135(6):1382–1386.

Lillywhite, H. B. (1995). J Gravit Physiol, 2(1):1–4.

Lillywhite, H. B. (1996). J Exp Zoolog A Comp Exp Biol, 275(2–3):217–225.

Lima, S. L., Rattenborg, N. C., Lesku, J. A., & Amlaner, C. J. (2005). Anim Behav, 70:723–736.

Lin, Y. L., & Lee, C. H. (2003). Pediatr Surg Int, 19(1–2):1–3.

Lindahl, M., Theorell, T., & Lindblad, F. (2005). Acta Paediatr, 94(4):489–495.

Lindamer, L. A., Buse, D. C., Lohr, J. B., & Jeste, D. V. (2001). Biol Psychiatry, 49(1):47–51.

Lindberg, F. A. (2001). Naturlig Slank Med Kost i Balanse [Natural Slimness on a Balanced Diet]. Oslo: Gyldendal Fakta.

Lindberg, F. A. (2002). Kokeboken Naturlig Slank [The Cookbook for Natural Slimness]. Oslo: Gyldendal Fakta.

Lindeberg, S., & Lundh, B. (1993). J Intern Med, 233(3):269–275.

Lindeberg, S. (1994). Apparent Absence of Cerebrocardiovascular Disease in Melanesians: Risk Factors and Nutritional Considerations—The Kitava Study, Department of Community Health Sciences, Lund University. Lund, Sweden: Department of Community Health Sciences, Lund University.

Lindeberg, S., Nilsson-Ehle, P., Terent, A., Vessby, B., et al. (1994). J Intern Med, 236(3):331–340.

Lindeberg, S., & Vessby, B. (1995). Nutr Metab Cardiovasc Dis, 5:45–53.

Lindeberg, S., Nilsson–Ehle, P., & Vessby, B. (1996). Lipids, 31(2):153–158.

Lindeberg, S., Berntorp, E., Carlsson, R., Eliasson, M., et al. (1997). Thromb Haemost, 77(1):94–98.

Lipkin, M., & Newmark, H. L. (1999). J Am Coll Nutr, 18(Suppl 5):392S–397S.

Lipson, S. F., & Ellison, P. T. (1992). J Biosoc Sci, 24(2):233–244.

Lipson, S. F., & Ellison, P. T. (1994). Fertil Steril, 61(3):448–454.

Lipson, S. F. (2001). Metabolism, maturation and ovarian function. In: Reproductive Ecology and Human Evolution, P. T. Ellison (ed.). New York: Aldine de Gruyter, pp. 235–244.

Little, M. A., Galvin, K., & Mugambi, M. (1983). Hum Biol, 55(4):811–830.

Little, M. A., & Johnson, B. R. (1987). Hum Biol, 59(4):695–707.

Littner, M. R., Kushida, C., Wise, M., Davila, D. G., et al. (2005). Sleep, 28(1):113–121.

Liu, J. W. (1982). Md State Med J, 31(2):66–67.

Liu, S., Song, Y., Ford, E. S., Manson, J. E., et al. (2005). Diabetes Care, 28(12):2926–2932.

Liu, X., Liu, L., & Wang, R. (2003). Sleep, 26(7):839–844.

Livingston, C., & Collison, M. (2002). Clin Sci, 102(2):151–166.

Livingstone, F. B. (1958). Am Anthropol, 60(3):533–562.

Livingstone, F. B. (1971). Annu Rev Genet, 5:33–64.

Lobstein, T., Baur, L., Uauy, R., & IASO International Obesity Task Force. (2004). Obes Rev, 5(Suppl 1):4–104.

Long, B., Ungpakorn, G., & Harrison, G. A. (1993). J Biosoc Sci, 25(1):73–78.

Long, K. Z., & Nanthakumar, N. (2004). Am J Hum Biol, 16(5):499–507.

Longstreth, G. F., Hawkey, C. J., Ham, J., Jones, R. H., et al. (2000). Gastroenterology, 118(4):A146.

Loos, R. J., & Rankinen, T. (2005). J Am Diet Assoc, 105(5 [Suppl 1]):S29–34.

Loretz, C. A., & Pollina, C. (2000). Comp Biochem Physiol A Mol Integr Physiol, 125(2):169–187.

Louv, W. C., Austin, H., Perlman, J., & Alexander, W. J. (1989). Am J Obstet Gynecol, 160(2):396–402.

Love, S., Nicoll, J. A., Hughes, A., & Wilcock, G. K. (2003). Neuroreport, 14(11):1535–1536.

Lovegrove, J. M. (2004). J N Z Soc Periodontol, 87:7–21.

Low, B. S. (1978). Am Nat, 112(983):197–213.

Low, B. S. (1996). Hum Nat, 7(4):353–379.

Lucas, A. (1991). Ciba Found Symp, 156:38–50; discussion 50–35.

Ludwig, D. S. (2002). J Am Med Assoc, 287(18):2414–2423.

Lumey, L. H. (1992). Paediatr Perinat Epidemiol, 6(2):240–253.

Lumey, L. H., Stein, A. D., & Ravelli, A. C. (1995). Eur J Obstet Gynecol Reprod Biol, 63(2):197.

Lumey, L. H., & Stein, A. D. (1997). Am J Public Health, 87(12):1962–1966.

Lummaa, V. (2003). Am J Hum Biol, 15(3):370–379.

Lummaa, V., & Temblay, M. (2003). Proc Biol Sci, 270(1531):2355–2361.

Lupien, S. J., King, S., Meaney, M. J., & McEwen, B. S. (2000). Biol Psychiatry, 48(10):976–980.

Lupien, S., Fiocco, A., Wan, N., Maheu, F., et al. (2005). Psychoneuroendocrinology, 30(3):225–242.

Lupton, D. (1994). Sociol Rev, 42(4):664–685.

Lutz, W. (1998). Leben Ohne Brot. Die wissenschaftlichen Grundlagen der Koholhydratarmen Diät. Gräfelfing, Germany: Informed Presse & Werbe GmbH.

Lutz, W. J. (1995). Med Hypotheses, 45(2):115–120.

Ly, A., & Drewnowski, A. (2001). Chem Senses, 26(1):41–47.

Lynch, J., Due, P., Muntaner, C., & Smith, G. D. (2000). J Epidemiol Commun Health, 54(6):404–408.

Ma, H., Bernstein, L., Pike, M. C., & Ursin, G. (2006). Br Cancer Res, 8(4):43.

Ma, J., Giovannucci, E., Pollak, M., Chan, J. M., et al. (2001). J Natl Cancer Inst, 93(17):1330–1336.

Maass, M., Bartels, C., Engel, P. M., Mamat, U., et al. (1998). J Am Coll Cardiol, 31(4):827–832.

MacClancy, J. (1992). Consuming Culture: Why You Eat What You Eat. New York: Henry Holt Publishers.

MacDonald, A. S., Straw, A. D., Dalton, N. M., & Pearce, E. J. (2002). J Immunol, 168(2):537–540.

MacGregor, E. A., Chia, H., Vohrah, R. C., & Wilkinson, M. (1990). Cephalalgia, 10(6):305–310.

MacKarness, R. (1958). Eat Fat and Grow Slim. Garden City, NY: Doubleday and Company.

Mackay, J., & Erikson, M. (2002). The Tobacco Atlas. Geneva: World Health Organization.

Mackay, J., Mensah, G. A., Mendis, S., Greenlund, K., et al. (2004). The Atlas of Heart Disease and Stroke. Geneva: World Health Organization.

Mackay, J., Jemal, A., Lee, N. C., & Parkin, D. M. (2006). The Cancer Atlas. Atlanta, GA: American Cancer Society.

Mackowiak, P. A. (1998). Arch Intern Med, 158(17):1870–1881.

MacMahon, B., Trichopolous, D., Brown, J. B., Andersen, A. P., et al. (1982). Int J Cancer, 30(427–431.

Maddock, J. (2004). Am J Health Promot, 19(2):137–143.

Maes, M., Verkerk, R., Bonaccorso, S., Ombelet, W., et al. (2002). Life Sci, 71(16):1837–1848.

Maestripieri, D., Lindell, S. G., Ayala, A., Gold, P. W., et al. (2005). Neurosci Biobehav Rev, 29(1):51–57.

Magarey, A. M., Daniels, L. A., Boulton, T. J., & Cockington, R. A. (2003). Int J Obes Relat Metabol Disord, 27(4):505–513.

Maggiorini, M., Bartsch, P., & Oelz, O. (1997). BMJ, 315(7105):403–404.

Magnusson, D., Stattin, H., & Allen, V. L. (1985). J Youth Adolesc, 14(4):267–284.

Magos, A., & Studd, J. (1985). Br J Hosp Med, 33(2):68–77.

Mahaney, W. C., Milner, M. W., Mulyono, R., Hancock, G. V., et al. (2000). Int J Environ Health Res, 10(2):93–109.

Mahley, R. W., & Huang, Y. D. (1999). Curr Opin Lipidol, 10(3):207–217.

Maier, S. F., Watkins, L. R., & Fleshner, M. (1994). Am Psychol, 49(12):1004–1017.

Makharia, G. K., Garg, P. K., & Tandon, R. K. (2003). Trop Gastroenterol, 24(4):200–201.

Mäki, M., Mustalahti, K., Kokkonen, J., Kulmala, P., et al. (2003). N Engl J Med, 348(25):2517–2524.

Malina, R. M., Spirduso, W. W., Tate, C., & Baylor, A. M. (1978). Med Sci Sport Excercise, 10(3):218–222.

Malina, R. M., Katzmarzyk, P. T., & Beunen, G. (1996). Obes Res, 4(4):385–390.

Maloyan, A., Eli-Berchoer, L., Semenza, G. L., Gerstenblith, G., et al. (2005). Physiol Genomics, 23(1):79–88.

Manikkam, M., Crespi, E. J., Doop, D. D., Herkimer, C., et al. (2004). Endocrinology, 145(2):790–798.

Mann, G. V., Shaffer, R. D., Anderson, R. S., & Sandstead, H. H. (1964). J Atheroscler Res, 4(289–312.

Mann, G. V., Shaffer, R. D., & Rich, A. (1965). Lancet, 2(7426):1308–1310.

Mann, G. V., & Shaffer, R. D. (1966). J Am Med Assoc, 197(13):1071–1073.

Mann, G. V., Spoerry, A., Gray, M., & Jarashow, D. (1972). Am J Epidemiol, 95:26–37.

Mann, N. J. (2004). Asia Pac J Clin Nutr, 13(Suppl):S17.

Manson, J. E., Hsia, J., Johnson, K. C., Rossouw, J. E., et al. (2003). N Engl J Med, 349(6):523–534.

Mansoor, J. K., Morrissey, B. M., Walby, W. F., Yoneda, K. Y., et al. (2005). High Alt Med Biol, 6(4):289–300.

Marasco, L., & Barger, J. (1999). Breastfeed Abs, 18(4):28–29.

Marchand, L., & Morrow, M. H. (1994). Fam Med, 26(5):319–324.

Marfella, R., Quagliaro, L., Nappo, F., Ceriello, A., et al. (2001). J Clin Invest, 108(4):635–636.

Marinacci, B. (1995). Linus Pauling in His Own Words. Sections From His Writings, Speeches, and Interviews. New York: Simon, & Schuster.

Marinker, M. (1975). J Med Ethics, 1(2):81–84.

Marks, I. M., & Nesse, R. M. (1994). Ethol Sociobiol, 15(5–6):247–261.

Marmot, M. G., Smith, G. D., Stansfeld, S., Patel, C., et al. (1991). Lancet, 337(8754):1387–1393.

Marmot, M. G., & Wilkinson, R. G. (eds.). (1999). Social Determinants of Health. Oxford, UK: Oxford University Press.

Marmot, M. G. (2004). The Status Syndrome: How Social Standing Affects our Health and Longevity. New York: Times Books.

Marouni, M. J., & Sela, S. (2004). J Med Microbiol, 53(Pt 1):1–7.

Marris, P. (1991). The social construction of uncertainty. In: Attachment Across the Life Cycle, C. M. Parkes, J. S. Hinde, & P. Marris (eds.). London: Tavistock/Routledge, pp. 77–90.

Marti, J. J., & Herrmann, U. (1977). Am J Obstet Gynecol, 128(5):489–493.

Marti, H. H. (2004). J Exp Biol, 207(18):3233–3242.

Martin, M. J., Rayner, J. C., Gagneux, P., Barnwell, J. W., et al. (2005). Proc Natl Acad Sci USA, 102(36):12819–12824.

Martin, R. D. (1996). News Physiol Sci, 11:149–156.

Martin, R. M., Smith, G. D., Frankel, S., & Gunnell, D. (2004). Epidemiology, 15(3):308–316.

Martinson, J. J., Hong, L., Karanicolas, R., Moore, J. P., et al. (2000). AIDS, 14(5):483–489.

Martinussen, M., Fischl, B., Larsson, H. B., Skranes, J. S., et al. (2005). Brain, 128(11):2588–2596.

Martorell, R. (1989). Hum Organ, 48(1):15–20.

Martorell, R., Khan, L. K., Hughes, M. L., & Grummer-Strawn, L. M. (2000). Eur J Clin Nutr, 54(3):247–252.

Mason, J. W. (1971). J Psychiatr Res, 8(3):323–333.

Mason, J. W., Buescher, E. L., Belfer, M. L., Artenstein, M. S., et al. (1979). J Human Stress, 5(3):18–28.

Massabuau, J.–C. (2001). Respir Physiol, 128(3):249–261.

Massabuau, J.–C. (2003). Mech Ageing Dev, 124(8–9):857–863.

Massey, L. K. (2001). J Nutr, 131(7):1875–1878.

Massimi, M., Ferrarelli, F., Huber, R., Esser, S. K., et al. (2005). Science, 309(5744):2228–2232.

Mather, H. M., & Keen, H. (1985). BMJ Clin Res Ed, 291(6502):1081–1084.

Mathias, C. J. (2002). Clin Med, 2(3):237–245.

Mattes, R. D. (2000). Appetite, 34(2):177–183.

May, R. M., & Anderson, R. M. (1979). Nature, 280(5722):455–461.

Maynard Smith, J. (1998). Evolutionary Genetics, 2nd ed. Oxford, UK: Oxford University Press.

Maynard Smith, J., Barker, D. J. P., Finch, C. E., Kardia, S. L. R., et al. (1999). The evolution of non-infectious and degenerative disease. In: Evolution in Health and Disease, S. C. Stearns (ed.). Oxford, UK: Oxford University Press, pp. 267–272.

Mayr, E. (1982). The Growth of Biological Thought: Diversity, Evolution, and Inheritance. Cambridge, MA: Harvard University Press.

Mayr, E. (2004). What Makes Biology Unique?: Considerations on the Autonomy of a Scientific Discipline. New York: Cambridge University Press.

McCabe, L. L., & McCabe, E. R. (2004). Genet Med, 6(1):58–59.

McCann, A. L., & Bonci, L. (2001). Dent Clin North Am, 45(3):571–601.

McCarrison, R. (1963). Studies in Deficiency Disease. Milwaukee, WI: Lee Foundation for Nutrition Research.

McClellan, W. S. (1930). J Am Diet Assoc, December:216–228.

McClellan, W. S., & Du Bois, E. F. (1930). J Biol Chem, 87(3):651–658.

McCormick, J., & Elmore-Meegan, M. (1992). Lancet, 340(8826):1042–1043.

McCoy, R. C., Hunt, C. E., Lesko, S. M., Vezina, R., et al. (2004). J Dev Behav Pediatr, 25(3):141–149.

McCracken, R. D. (1971). Curr Anthropol, 12(45):479–517.

McDade, T. W., & Worthman, C. M. (1999). Am J Hum Biol, 11(6):705–711.

McDade, T. W., Beck, M. A., Kuzawa, C. W., & Adair, L. S. (2001). J Nutr, 131(4):1225–1231.

McDevitt, R. M., Bott, S. J., Harding, M., Coward, W. A., et al. (2001). Am J Clin Nutr, 74(6):737–746.

McDonald's (2006), McDonald's Canada FAQs, www.mcdonalds.ca/en/aboutus/faq.aspx

McEwen, B. S. (1995). Stressful experience, brain, and emotions: Developmental, genetic, and hormonal influences. In: The Cognitive Neurosciences, M. S. Gazzaniga (ed.). Cambridge, MA: MIT Press, pp. 1117–1135.

McEwen, B. S. (1998a). Ann NY Acad Sci, 840:33–44.

McEwen, B. S. (1998b). N Engl J Med, 338(3):171–179.

McEwen, B. S., & Seeman, T. (1999). Ann NY Acad Sci, 896:30–47.

McEwen, B. S., & Wingfield, J. C. (2003). Horm Behav, 43(1):2–15.

McEwen, B. S. (2005). J Psychiatry Neurosci, 30(5):315–318.

McGarvey, C., McDonnell, M., Hamilton, K., O'Regan, M., et al. (2006). J Paediatr Child Health, 11(Suppl A):19A–21A.

McGee, E. A., Sawetawan, C., Bird, I., Rainey, W. E., et al. (1996). Fertil Steril, 65(1):87–93.

McGrath, M. F., & de Bold, A. J. (2005). Peptides, 26(6):933–943.

McGrew, W. C., & Feistner, A. T. C. (1992). Two nonhuman primate models for the evolution of human food sharing: Chimpanzees and callitrichids. In: The Adapted Mind: Evolutionary Psychology and the Generation of Culture, J. H. Barkow, & L. Cosmides (eds.). New York: Oxford University Press, pp. 229–243.

McKeigue, P. M., Marmot, M. G., Syndercombe-Court, Y. D., Cottier, D. E., et al. (1988). Br Heart J, 60(5):390–396.

McKeigue, P. M., Shah, B., & Marmot, M. G. (1991). Lancet, 337(8738):382–386.

McKeigue, P. M. (1996). Ciba Found Symp, 201:54–64; discussion 64–57, 188–193.

McKenna, J. J. (1986). Med Anthropol, 10(1):9–53.

McKenna, J. J., Mosko, S., Dungy, C., & McAninch, J. (1990). Am J Phys Anthropol, 83(3):331–347.

McKenna, J. J., Thoman, E. B., Anders, T. F., Sadeh, A., et al. (1993). Sleep, 16(3):263–281.

McKenna, J. J. (1994). Phy Anth News, 13(1):1–4.

McKenna, J. J., Mosko, S. S., & Richard, C. A. (1997). Pediatrics, 100(2 [Pt 1]):214–219.

McKenna, J. J. (2000). Cultural influences on infant and childhood sleep biology, and the science that studies it: Toward a more inclusive paradigm. In: Sleep and Breathing in Children: A Developmental Approach, G. M. Loughlin, J. L. Carroll, & C. L. Marcus (eds.). New York: Marcel Dekker, pp. 199–233.

McKenna, J. J., & Gartner, L. M. (2000). Pediatrics, 105(4 [Pt 1]):917–919.

McKenna, J. J., & Mosko, S. (2001). Mother–infant cosleeping: Toward a new scientific beginning. In: Sudden Infant Death Syndrome: Problems, Progress, & Possibilities, R. Byerd, & H. Krous (eds.). New York: Arnold, pp. 258–272.

McKenna, J. J., & McDade, T. W. (2005). Paediatr Respir Rev, 6(2):134–152.

McKeown, N. M., Meigs, J. B., Liu, S., Saltzman, E., et al. (2004). Diabetes Care, 27(2):538–546.

McKeown, T. (1991). The Origins of Human Diseases. Oxford, UK: Basil Blackwell Ltd.

McKeown, T. (1998). Determinants of health. In: Understanding and Applying Medical Anthropology, P. J. Brown (ed.). Mountain View, CA: Mayfield Publishing Company, pp. 70–76.

McKinnon, S., & Silverman, S. (eds.). (2005). Complexities: Beyond Nature, & Nurture. Chicago: University of Chicago Press.

McLaughlin, T., Abbasi, F., Lamendola, C., Yeni-Komshian, H., et al. (2000). J Clin Endocrinol Metab, 85(9):3085–3088.

McLean, A. (1999). Development and use of vaccines against evolving pathogens: Vaccine design. In: Evolution in Health and Disease, S. C. Stearns (ed.). Oxford, UK: Oxford University Press, pp. 138–151.

McLellan, A. T., Lewis, D. C., O'Brien, C. P., & Kleber, H. D. (2000). J Am Med Assoc, 284(13):1689–1695.

McLoyd, V. C. (1998). Am Psychol, 53(2):185–204.

McMillen, I. C., & Robinson, J. S. (2005). Physiol Rev, 85(2):571–633.

McNamara, P. (2004). An Evolutionary Psychology of Sleep and Dreams. New York: Praeger.

McNeil, W. (1976). Plagues and Peoples. New York: Anchor Press.

McNicholl, B., Egan-Mitchell, B., Stevens, F. M., Phelan, J. J., et al. (1981). History, genetics and natural history of celiac disease: Gluten enteropathy. In: Food, Nutrition and Evolution: Food as an Environmental Factor in the Genesis of Human Variability, D. N. Walcher & N. Kretchmer (eds.). New York: Masson Publishing, pp. 169–177.

Meaney, M. J., Mitchell, J. B., Aitken, D. H., Bhatnagar, S., et al. (1991). Psychoneuroendocrinology, 16(1–3):85–103.

Meaney, M. J. (2001). Annu Rev Neurosci, 24:1161–1192.

Meaney, M. J., & Szyf, M. (2005). Dialog Clin Neurosci, 7(2):103–123.

Medina, E., Goldmann, O., Toppel, A. W., & Chhatwal, G. S. (2003). J Infect Dis, 187(4):597–603.

Mehraein, Y., Lennerz, C., Ehlhardt, S., Remberger, K., et al. (2004). Mod Pathol, 17(7):781–789.

Mehrotra, T. N., Mital, H. S., & Gupta, S. K. (1981). J Assoc Physicians India, 29(6):489–490.

Mehta, S., Brancati, F., Sulkowski, M., Strathdee, S., et al. (2000). Ann Intern Med, 133(8):592–599.

Mela, D. J. (1999). Proc Nutr Soc, 58(3):513–521.

Melanson, K. J. (2004). Nutr Today, 39(5):203–213.

Mellor, A. L., & Munn, D. H. (2004). Nat Rev Immunol, 4(10):762–774.

Mendelson, W. B. (1990). Insomnia: The patient and the pill. In: Sleep and Cognition, R. R. Bootzin, J. F. Kihlstrom, & D. L. Schacter (eds.). Washington, DC: American Psychological Association, pp. 139–147.

Mendez, G. F., & Cowie, M. R. (2001). Int J Cardiol, 80(2–3):213–219.

Meneton, P., Jeunemaitre, X., De Wardener, H. E., & MacGregor, G. A. (2005). Physiol Rev, 85(2):679–715.

Mennella, J. A., & Beauchamp, G. K. (1996). The early development of human flavor preferences. In: Why We Eat What We Eat: The Psychology of Eating, E. D. Capaldi (ed.). Washington, DC: American Psychological Association, pp. 83–112.

Mennella, J. A., & Beauchamp, G. K. (1998). Nutr Rev, 56(7):205–211.

Mercola, J. (2003). The No-Grain Diet: Conquer Carbohydrate Addiction and Stay Slim for Life. New York: Penguin Putman Inc.

Merimee, T. J., Rimoin, D. L., & Cavalli-Sforza, L. L. (1972). J Clin Invest, 51(2):395–401.

Merrilees, M. J., Smart, E. J., Gilchrist, N. L., Frampton, C., et al. (2000). Eur J Nutr, 39(6):256–262.

Mesarovic, M. D., Sreenath, S. N., & Keene, J. D. (2004). Syst Biol, 1(1):19–27.

Messer, E. (1986). Am Anthropol, 88(3):637–647.

Mi, J., Law, C., Zhang, K. L., Osmond, C., et al. (2000). Ann Intern Med, 132(4):253–260.

Mikkelsen, E. (1979). Korn er Liv [Life-Sustaining Grains]. Oslo: Statens Kornforretning.

Milano, M., & Collomp, R. (2005). J Oncol Pharm Pract, 11(4):145–149.

Milk Processor Education Program (2005a), Carson Daly, http://whymilk.org/bios carson_daly.html

Milk Processor Education Program (2005b), Got Milk? Get Tall!, http://www.whymilk.com facts_gotmilk.htm

Milledge, J. S., Thomas, P. S., Beeley, J. M., & English, J. S. C. (1988). Eur Respir J, 1(10):948–951.

Milledge, J. S., Beeley, J. M., Broome, J., Luff, N., et al. (1991). Eur Respir J, 4(8):1000–1003.

Miller, A. D., & Leslie, R. A. (1994). Front Neuroendocrinol, 15(4):301–320.

Miller, B. C., Norton, M. C., Curtis, T., Hill, E., et al. (1997). Youth Soc, 29(1):54–83.

Miller, B. C., Norton, M. C., Fan, X. T., & Christopherson, C. R. (1998). J Early Adolesc, 18(1):27–52.

Miller, B. C., Benson, B., & Galbraith, K. A. (2001). Dev Rev, 21(1):1–38.

Miller, C. L., Llenos, I. C., Dulay, J. R., Barillo, M. M., et al. (2004). Neurobiol Dis, 15(3):618–629.

Miller, J., Rosenbloom, A., & Silverstein, J. (2004). J Clin Endocrinol Metab, 89(9):4211–4218.

Miller, L. (2006), NoPeriod.com, http://www.noperiod.com/

Miller, S. K. (1993). New Sci, 137(1862):10.

Millet, J.–J. (1997). Ontogenèse Crânienne des Chimpanzés et des Gorilles. Vers l'Etude Globale de l'Evolution des Hominidés. Mémoire de Diplôme d'Etudes Approfondies. Paris: Museum National d'Histoire Naturelle de Paris.

Milton, K., & May, M. (1976). Nature, 259:459–462.

Milton, K. (1987). Primate diets and gut morphology: Implications for hominid evolution. In: Food and Evolution: Toward a Theory of Human Food Habits, M. Harris & E. B. Ross (eds.). Philadelphia: Temple University Press, pp. 93–115.

Milton, K. (1999). Nutrition, 15(6):488–498.

Milton, K. (2000). Nutrition, 16(7–8):480–483.

Milton, K. (2003). J Nutr, 133(11 [Suppl 2]):3886S–3892S.

Minehira, K., Bettschart, V., Vidal, H., Di Vetta, V., et al. (2003). Obes Res, 11(9):1096–1103.

Mintz, S. W. (1996). Tasting Food, Tasting Freedom: Excursions into Eating, Culture and the Past. Boston: Beacon Press.

Mirescu, C., Peters, J. D., & Gould, E. (2004). Nat Neurosci, 7(8):841–846.

Misra, A., & Vikram, N. K. (2004). Nutrition, 20(5):482–491.

Mitchell, E. A., & Scragg, R. (1994). Early Hum Dev, 38(3):151–157.

Miyakawa, H., Honma, K., Qi, M., & Kuramitsu, H. K. (2004). J Periodontal Res, 39(1):1–9.

Mizooka, M., Ishikawa, S., & Jichi Medical School Cohort Study Group. (2003). Intern Med, 42(10):960–966.

Mizuno, J., & Takeda, N. (1988). Comp Biochem Physiol A Mol Integr Physiol, 91(4):739–747.

Mjones, S. (1987). Ann Hum Biol, 14(4):337–347.

Moan, J., & Porojnicu, A. (2006). Tidsskr Nor Lægeforen, 126:1048–1052.

Moe, O. W. (2006). Curr Opin Nephrol Hypertens, 15(4):366–373.

Mohammad, A. R., Jones, J. D., & Brunsvold, M. A. (1994). J Calif Dent Assoc, 22(3):69–75.

Mohr, E., Meyerhof, W., & Richter, D. (1995). Vitam Horm, 51:235–266.

Moisan, J., Meyer, F., & Gingras, S. (1990). Cancer Causes Control, 1(2):149–154.

Mokdad, A. H., Ford, E. S., Bowman, B. A., Nelson, D. E., et al. (2000). Diabetes Care, 23(9):1278–1283.

Mokdad, A. H., Bowman, B. A., Ford, E. S., Vinicor, F., et al. (2001). J Am Med Assoc, 286(10):1195–1200.

Molberg, Ø., Uhlen, A. K., Flæte, N. S., Fleckenstein, B., et al. (2005). Gastroenterology, 128(2):393–401.

Molero-Conejo, E., Morales, L. M., Fernandez, V., Raleigh, X., et al. (2003). Arch Latinoam Nutr, 53(4):39–46.

Moll, J., Zahn, R., de Oliveira-Souza, R., Krueger, F., et al. (2005). Nat Rev Neurosci, 6(10):799–809.

Moller, J. K., Andersen, B., Olesen, F., Lignell, T., et al. (1999). Sex Transm Infect, 75(4):228–230.

Monif, G. R. G. (1985). Am J Obstet Gynecol, 152(7 [Pt 2]):935–939.

Montgomery, S. M., Bartley, M. J., & Wilkinson, R. G. (1997). Arch Dis Child, 77(4):326–330.

Moon, U. Y., Park, S. J., Oh, S. T., Kim, W. U., et al. (2004). Arthritis Res Ther, 6(4):R295–R302.

Moore, D. (2004). Contemp Drug Probl, 31(2):181–212.

Moore, K. L. (1988). Essentials of Human Embryology. Toronto, Canada: B.C. Decker.

Moore, P. J., Adler, N. E., Williams, D. R., & Jackson, J. S. (2002). Psychosom Med, 64(2):337–344.

Moore, S. E., Halsall, I., Howarth, D., Poskitt, E. M., et al. (2001). Diabet Med, 18(8):646–653.

Moore, S. E., Jalil, F., Ashraf, R., Szu, S. C., et al. (2004). Am J Clin Nutr, 80(2):453–459.

Moore, S. R., Lima, A. A. M., Conaway, M. R., Schorling, J. B., et al. (2001). Int J Epidemiol, 30(6):1457–1464.

Moore, T., & Ucko, C. (1957). Arch Dis Child, 32(164):333–342.

Moorman, P. G., & Terry, P. D. (2004). Am J Clin Nutr, 80(1):5–14.

Mora, J., de Paredes, B., Wagner, M., de Navarro, L., et al. (1979). Am J Clin Nutr, 32(2):455–462.

Morita, M., Ohneda, O., Yamashita, T., Takahashi, S., et al. (2003). EMBO J, 22(5):1134–1146.

Morrill, A. C., & Chinn, C. D. (2004). J Public Health Policy, 25(3–4):353–366.

Morris, J., & Nilsson, S. (1994). The circulatory system. In: Comparative Physiology and Evolution of the Autonomic Nervous System, S. Nilsson & S. Holmgren (eds.). Chur, Switzerland: Harwood Academic Publishers, pp. 193–246.

Morse, G. G., & House, J. W. (2001). Nurs Res, 50(5):286–292.

Mortola, J. P. (2004). Respir Physiol Neurobiol, 141(3):345–356.

Morton, D. J. (1926). Science, 64(1660):394–396.

Moseng, O. G. (2003). Det Offisielle Helsevesen i Norge 1603–2003. Bind 1: Ansvaret for Undersåttenes Helse 1603–1850 [The Public Health Care System in Norway 1603–2003. Volume 1. The Responsibility for the Subjects Health 1603–1850. Oslo: Universitetsforlaget.

Mosko, S., Richard, C., McKenna, J. J., Drummond, S., et al. (1997). Am J Phys Anthropol, 103(3):315–328.

Mostad, S. B., Kreiss, J. K., Ryncarz, A., Chohan, B., et al. (2000). Am J Obstet Gynecol, 183(4):948–955.

Motulsky, A. G. (1995). Nat Genet, 9(2):99–101.

Mowé, M., Bøhmer, T., & Haug, E. (1998). Tidsskr Nor Lægeforen, 118:3929–3931.

Muchmore, E. A., Diaz, S., & Varki, A. (1998). Am J Phys Anthropol, 107(2):187–198.

Muhlestein, J. B. (2002). Am J Cardiovasc Drugs, 2(2):107–118.

Mukamal, K. J., Muller, J. E., Maclure, M., Sherwood, J. B., et al. (2002). Am J Cardiol, 90(1):49–51.

Muller, H. P., & Heinecke, A. (2004). Clin Oral Investig, 8(2):63–69.

Munck, A., Guyre, P. M., & Holbrook, N. J. (1984). Endocr Rev, 5(1):25–44.

Munger, K. L., Peeling, R. W., Hernan, M. A., Chasan–Taber, L., et al. (2003). Epidemiology, 14(2):141–147.

Munger, K. L., DeLorenze, G. N., Levin, L. I., Rubertone, M. V., et al. (2004). Neurology, 62(10):1799–1803.

Murphy, S. P., Rose, D., Hudes, M., & Viteri, F. E. (1992). J Am Diet Assoc, 92(11):1352–1357.

Murphy, V. E., Smith, R., Giles, W. B., & Clifton, V. L. (2006). Endocr Rev, 27(2):141–169.

Muttalib, M. A., Islam, N., Ghani, J. A., Khan, K., et al. (1975). J Trop Med Hyg, 78(10–11):224–226.

Mysliwska, J., Trzonkowski, P., Bryl, E., Lukaszuk, K., et al. (2000). Eur Cytokine Netw, 11(3):397–406.

Nadel, D., Weiss, E., Simchoni, O., Tastskin, A., et al. (2004). Proc Natl Acad Sci USA, 101(17):6821–6826.

Nakamura, S., Wind, M., & Danello, M. A. (1999). Arch Pediatr Adolesc Med, 153(10):1019–1023.

Narod, S. A., & Offit, K. (2005). J Clin Oncol, 23(8):1656–1663.

Naser, S. A., Ghobrial, G., Romero, C., & Valentine, J. F. (2004). Lancet, 364(9439):1039–1044.

Nasralla, M., Haier, J., & Nicolson, G. L. (1999). Eur J Clin Microbiol Infect Dis, 18(12):859–865.

Nathan, A. T., & Singer, M. (1999). Br Med Bull, 55(1):96–108.

National Center for Health Statistics, & Centers for Disease Control and Prevention (2002), Fast Stats AZ, http://www.cdc.gov/nchs/fastats/Default.htm

National Heart Lung and Blood Institute (1996). Data Fact Sheet: Congestive Heart Failure in the United States: A New Epidemic. Bethesda, MD: National Heart, Lung and Blood Institute.

National Institute of Diabetes and Digestive and Kidney Diseases—Weight-Control Information Network (2001). Understanding Adult Obesity. Washington, DC: National Institute of Diabetes and Digestive and Kidney Diseases.

National Institute of Mental Health (2006). Depression. Washington, DC: National Institute of Mental Health.

National Institute of Population Research and Training, Mitra and Associates, & ORC-Macro. (2001). Bangladesh Demographic and Health Survey 1999–2000. Dhaka, Bangladesh and Calverton, MD: National Institute for Population Research and Training, Mitra and Associates and ORC Macro.

National Institutes of Health. (1994). J Am Med Assoc, 272(24):1942–1948.

National Research Council. (1989). Diet and Health. Washington, DC: National Academy Press.

National Sleep Foundation (2005), Sleep in America Poll, http://www.sleepfoundation.org_content/hottopics/2005_summary_of_findings.pdf

National Women's Health Network (2003). New Version of the Oral Contraceptive Pill. Washington, DC.

Nauck, M. A., Kleine, N., Orskov, C., Holst, J. J., et al. (1993). Diabetologia, 36(8):741–744.

Neal, K. R., Hebden, J., & Spiller, R. (1997). BMJ, 314(7083):779–782.

Neel, J. V. (1962). Am J Hum Gen, 14:352–362.

Neel, J. V., Weder, A. B., & Stevo, J. (1998). Perspect Biol Med, 42(1):44–64.

Neel, J. V. (1999a). Bull WHO, 77(8):694–703.

Neel, J. V. (1999b). Nutr Rev, 57(5 [Pt 2]):S2–S9.

Neel, J. V. (1999c). World Rev Nutr Diet, 84:1–18.

Negus, N. C., & Berger, P. J. (1987). Cohort analysis: Environmental cues and "diapause" in microtine rodents. In: Symposium on Population Biology and Life History Evolution, M. Boyce (ed.). New Haven, CT: Yale University Press, pp. 65–74.

Negus, N. C., Berger, P. J., & Pinter, A. J. (1992). Can J Zool, 70(11):2121–2124.

Nelson, J. L., & Steinberg, A. D. (1987). Sex steroid, autoimmunity and autoimmune diseases. In: Hormones and Immunity, I. Berczi, & K. Kovacs (eds.). Lancaster, UK: MTP Press, pp. 93–119.

Nerheim, P. L., Meier, J. L., Vasef, M. A., Li, W. G., et al. (2004). Am J Pathol, 164(2):589–600.

Nesse, R. M. (1984). Compr Psychiatry, 25(6):575–580.

Nesse, R. M. (1987). Ethol Sociobiol, 8(3, Suppl):73–83.

Nesse, R. M. (1990). Hum Nat, 1(3):261–289.

Nesse, R. M. (1991). Sciences, November/December:30–37.

Nesse, R. M., & Klaas, R. (1994). J Nerv Ment Dis, 182(8):465–470.

Nesse, R. M., & Williams, G. C. (1994). Why We Get Sick—The New Science of Darwinian Medicine. New York: Times Books.

Nesse, R. M., & Berridge, K. C. (1997). Science, 278(5335):63–66.

Nesse, R. M., & Williams, G. C. (1997). Bioscience, 47(10):664–666.

Nesse, R. (1998). Br J Med Psychol, 71(4):397–415.

Nesse, R. M., & Williams, G. C. (1998). Sci Am, 29(5):86–93.

Nesse, R. M. (1999). Neurosci Biobehav Rev, 23(7):895–903.

Nesse, R. M., & Williams, G. C. (1999). Research designs that address evolutionary questions about medical disorders. In: Evolution in Health and Disease, S. C. Stearns (ed.). Oxford, UK: Oxford University Press, pp. 16–26.

Nesse, R. M. (2000). Arch Gen Psychiatry, 57(1):14–20.

Nesse, R. M., & Young, E. A. (2000). Evolutionary origins and functions of the stress response. In: Encyclopedia of Stress, G. Fink (ed.). San Diego, CA: Academic Press, pp. 79–84.

Nesse, R. M. (2001). New Physician, 50(9):8–10.

Nesse, R. M. (2001). The smoke detector principle—Natural selection and the regulation of defensive responses. In: Unity of Knowledge: The Convergence of Natural and Human Science, A. R. Demasio (ed.). New York:New York Academy of Sciences, pp. 75–85.

Nesse, R. M., & Schiffman, J. D. (2003). Bioscience, 53(6):585–587.

Nesse, R. M. (2005). Q Rev Biol, 80(1):62–70.

Nesse, R. M. (2006). Int Congr Ser, 1296:83–94.

Nesse, R. M., Stearns, S. C., & Omenn, G. S. (2006). Science, 311(5764):1071.

Nestle, M., Wing, R., Birch, L., DiSogra, L., et al. (1998). Nutr Rev, 56(5 [Pt 2]):S50–S74.

Nestle, M. (1999). Proc Nutr Soc, 58(2):211–218.

Nestle, M. (2002). Food Politics: How the Food Industry Influences Nutrition and Health. Berkeley, CA: University of California Press.

Neville, M. C., Morton, J., & Umemura, S. (2001). Pediatr Clin North Am, 48(1):35–52.

Newlin, D. B., Miles, D. R., van den Bree, M. B., Gupman, A. E., et al. (2000). Alcohol Clin Exp Res, 24(12):1785–1794.

Newlin, D. B. (2002). Addiction, 97(4):427–445.

Newton, P., & White, N. (1999). Annu Rev Med, 50(1):179–192.

Nicholi, A. M. (1999). History and mental status. In: The Harvard Guide to Psychiatry, A. M. Nicholi (ed.). Cambridge, MA: Harvard University Press, pp. 32–66.

Nicklas, T. A. (2003). J Am Coll Nutr, 22(5):340–356.

Nicolaidis, S., & Rowland, N. (1976). Am J Physiol, 231(3):661–668.

Nielsen, S. J., & Popkin, B. M. (2004). Am J Prev Med, 27(3):205–210.

Nieto, F. J. (1998). Am J Epidemiol, 148(10):937–948.

NIH Consensus Development Panel on Physical Activity and Cardiovascular Health. (1996). J Am Med Assoc, 276(3):241–246.

Nilsson, S. E., Johansson, B., Takkinen, S., Berg, S., et al. (2003). Eur J Clin Pharmacol, 59(4):313–319.

Nishida, T. (1989). Appetite, 12:74–74.

Nishida, T., & Turner, L. A. (1996). Int J Primatol, 17(6):947–968.

Nishida, T., Ohigashi, H., & Koshimizu, K. (2000). Curr Anthropol, 41(3):431–438.

Nishimura, H. (1980). Adv Exp Med Biol, 130:29–77.

Nishimura, H., & Bailey, J. R. (1982). Kidney Int, 22(Suppl 12):S185–S192.

Nishimura, H. (2001). Comp Biochem Physiol A Mol Integr Physiol, 128(1):11–30.

Nonaka, K., Desjardins, B., Legare, J., Charbonneau, H., et al. (1990). Hum Biol, 62(5):701–717.

Norat, T., & Riboli, E. (2003). Eur J Clin Nutr, 57(1):1–17.

Nordenfelt, L. (1997). Talking About Health. Amsterdam: Rodopi.

Nordenfelt, L. (2001). Health, Science, and Ordinary Language. Amsterdam: Rodopi.

Normann, E., Gnarpe, J., Gnarpe, H., & Wettergren, B. (1998). Acta Paediatr, 87(1):23–27.

Northrop-Clewes, C. A., Rousham, E. K., Mascie-Taylor, C. G. N., & Lunn, P. G. (2001). Am J Clin Nutr, 73(1):53–60.

Norwegian Nutrition Council. (2000). Vekt og helse. Rapport nr. 1/2000 [Weight and Health Report No. 1/2000]. Oslo: Statens råd for ernæring og fysisk aktivitet.

Novotny, R., Daida, Y. G., Acharya, S., Grove, J. S., et al. (2004). J Nutr, 134(8):1905–1909.

Null, G., & Null, S. (1978). How to Get Rid of the Poisons in Your Body. New York: Arco Publishing Company, Inc.

Núñez-de la Mora, A. (2005). Developmental Effects on Reproductive Hormone Levels: A Migrant Study, Anthropology. London: University of London, Department of Anthropology.

Núñez-de la Mora, A., Chatterton, R. T., Choudhury, O. A., Napolitano, D. A., et al. (2007a). PLoS Med doi: 10.1371/journal.pmed.0040167.

Núñez-de la Mora, A., Bentley, G. R., Choudhury, O. A., Napolitano, D. A., et al. (2007b). Am J Hum Biol.

Nusche, J. (2002). Can Med Assoc J, 167:675–676.

Nussbaum, M. C. (1995). Human capabilities, female human beings. In: Women, Culture, and Development : A Study of Human Capabilities, M. C. Nussbaum, J. Glover, & World Institute for Development Economics Research (eds.). Oxford, UK: Clarendon Press, pp. 61–104.

O'Conner, T. G., Heron, J., Golding, J., Glover, V., et al. (2003). J Child Psychol Psychiatry, 44(7):1025–1036.

O'Connor, K. A., Brindle, E., Holman, D. J., Klein, N. A., et al. (2003). Clin Chem, 49(7):1139–1148.

O'Dea, K. (1984). Diabetes, 33(6):596–603.

O'Dea, K., Hopper, J. L., Patel, M., Traianedes, K., et al. (1993). Diabetes Care, 16(7):1004–1010.

Offit, K., Groeger, E., Turner, S., Wadsworth, E. A., et al. (2004). J Am Med Assoc, 292(12):1469–1473.

O'Grady, K. (2005). Haven't we learned our lessons yet? Periods are not a curse. Toronto, Canada: The Globe and Mail.

Oh, T. J., Eber, R., & Wang, H. L. (2002). J Clin Periodontol, 29(5):400–410.

O'Hara, M., Harruff, R., Smialek, J. E., & Fowler, D. R. (2000). Pediatrics, 105(4 [Pt 1]):915–917.

Ohayon, M. M. (2002). Sleep Med Rev, 6(2):97–111.

Okasha, M., McCarron, P., Gunnell, D., & Smith, G. D. (2003). Breast Cancer Res Treatm, 78(2):223–276.

O'Keefe Jr., J. H., & Cordain, L. (2004). Mayo Clin Proc, 79(1):101–108.

Oken, E., & Gillman, M. W. (2003). Obes Res, 11(4):496–506.

Okuda, M., Eikichi, M., Nakazawa, T., Minami, K., et al. (2004). Am J Med, 116(3):209–210.

Okuda, M. (2006). Shock, 25(6):557–570.

Olds, J. (1958). Science, 127(3294):315–324.

Olesen, E. S., & Quaade, F. (1960). Lancet, 1:1048–1051.

Oliver, W. J., Cohen, E. L., & Neel, J. V. (1975). Circulation, 52:146–151.

Olmstead, M. C. (2006). Q J Exp Psychol, 59:625–653.

Olson, S. (2002). Science, 298(5597):1324–1325.

Olson, S. (2004). Science, 305:1390–1392.

Omar, H., Kives, S., & Allen, L. (2005). J Pediatr Adolesc Gynecol, 18(4):285–288.

Omran, A. R. (1971). Milbank Mem Fund Q, 49(4):509–538.

Ong, K. K. L., Ahmed, M. L., & Dunger, D. B. (1999). Acta Paediatr Suppl, 88(433):95–98.

Ong, K. K. L. (2006). Horm Res, 65(Suppl 3):65–69.

Opotowsky, A. P., & Bilezikian, J. P. (2003). J Bone Miner Res, 18(11):1978–1988.

Oriel, J. D., Partridge, B. M., & Denny, M. J. (1972). BMJ, 4(843):761–764.

O'Rourke, M. T., & Ellison, P. T. (1993). Endocr J, 1:487–494.

Orr, J. B. (1928). Lancet, 1:202–203.

Ortner, D. J., & Aufderheide, A. C. (eds.). (1991). Human Paleopathology: Current Synthesis and Future Options. Washington, DC: Smithsonian Institution Press.

Ostensen, M., Rugelsjoen, A., & Wigers, S. H. (1997). Scand J Rheumatol, 26(5):355–360.

Ottenhoff, T. H. M., De Boer, T., van Dissel, J. T., & Verreck, F. A. W. (2003). Adv Exp Med Biol, 531:279–294.

Ounsted, M., & Ounsted, C. (1968). Nature, 220(167):599–600.

Ounsted, M., Scott, A., & Ounsted, C. (1986). Ann Hum Biol, 13(2):143–151.

Pace-Schott, E. F., & Hobson, J. A. (2002). Nat Rev Neurosci, 3(8):591–605.

Pachori, A. S., Melo, L. G., Hart, M. L., Noiseux, N., et al. (2004). Proc Natl Acad Sci USA, 101(33):12282–12287.

Packer, M., Bristow, M. R., Cohn, J. N., Colucci, W. S., et al. (1996). N Engl J Med, 334(21):1349–1355.

Packer, M., Fowler, M. B., Roecker, E. B., Coats, A. J., et al. (2002). Circulation, 106(17):2194–2199.

Padoan, A., Rigano, S., Ferrazzi, E., Beaty, B. L., et al. (2004). Am J Obstet Gynecol, 191(4):1459–1464.

Paffenbarger Jr., R. S. (1964). Br J Prevent Soc Med, 18:189–195.

Painter, J. E., Wansink, B., & Hieggelke, J. B. (2002). Appetite, 38(3):237–238.

Paley, W. (1804). Natural Theology, or, Evidences of the Existence and Attributes of the Deity, 12th ed. London: Printed for J. Faulder [Available from University of Michigan Humanities Text Initiative, Ann Arbor, MI, 1998, http://www.hti.umich.edu/cgi/p pd–modeng/pd–modeng–idx?type = header&id = PaleyNatur.].

Palmer, A. E., London, W. T., Sly, D. L., & Rice, J. M. (1979). Lab Anim Sci, 29(1):102–106.

Paneth, N., Ahmed, F., & Stein, A. D. (1996). J Hypertens, 14(Suppl 5):S121–S129.

Pani, L. (2000). Mol Psychiatry, 5(5):467–475.

Panksepp, J. (2000). Evol Cogn, 6(2):108–131.

Panksepp, J., Knutson, B., & Burgdorf, J. (2002). Addiction, 97(4):459–469.

Panter-Brick, C., Lotstein, D. S., & Ellison, P. T. (1993). Hum Reprod, 8(5):684–690.

Panter-Brick, C., Ellison, P. T., Lipson, S. F., & Sukalich, S. (1996). Am J Phys Anthropol, 22(Suppl):182.

Panter-Brick, C. (1998). Biological anthropology and child health: Context, process, and outcome. In: Biosocial Perspectives on Children, C. Panter-Brick (ed.). Cambridge, UK: Cambridge University Press, pp. 66–101.

Panter-Brick, C., Lunn, P. G., Goto, R., & Wright, C. M. (2004). Am J Hum Biol, 16(5):581–587.

Paolisso, G., & Giugliano, D. (1996). Diabetologia, 39(3):357–363.

Paparella, M. M. (1984). Acta Otolaryngol, 406(Suppl):10–25.

Paparella, M. M., & Djalilian, H. R. (2002). Otolaryngol Clin North Am, 35(3):529–545.

Parent, A. S., Teilmann, G., Juul, A., Skakkebaek, N. E., et al. (2003). Endocr Rev, 24(5):668–693.

Park, J. L., & Capps, O. (1997). Am J Agric Econ, 79(3):814–824.

Park, K. S., Kim, S. K., Kim, M. S., Cho, E. Y., et al. (2003). J Nutr, 133(10):3085–3090.

Parker, W. A. (1983). Clin Pharm, 2(1):75–79.

Parmley, W. W. (1992). Clin Cardiol, 15(Suppl 1):5–12.

Parodi, P. W. (1997). J Nutr, 127(6):1055–1060.

Parodi, P. W. (2004). Aust J Dairy Tech, 59(1):3–59.

Parra, E. J., Kittles, R. A., Argyropoulos, G., Pfaff, C. L., et al. (2001). Am J Phys Anthropol, 114(1):18–29.

Parsons, A. A. (2006). Nitric oxide. In: The Headaches, J. Olesen, P. J. Goadsby, N. M. Ramadan, P. Tfelt–Hansen, & K. M. A. Welch (eds.). Philadelphia: Lippincott, Williams, & Wilkins, pp. 151–158.

Pasquali, R., Pelusi, C., Genghini, S., Cacciari, M., et al. (2003). Hum Reprod Update, 9(4):359–372.

Pastor, P., Roe, C. M., Villegas, A., Bedoya, G., et al. (2003). Ann Neurol, 54(2):163–169.

Pate, R. R., Pratt, M., Blair, S. N., Haskell, W. L., et al. (1995). J Am Med Assoc, 273(5):402–407.

Patel, P. D., Lopez, J. F., Lyons, D. M., Burke, S., et al. (2000). J Psychiatr Res, 34(6):383–392.

Patel, S. M., & Nestler, J. E. (2006). Endocrinol Metab Clin North Am, 35(1):137–155.

Patterson, K. D. (2000). Lactose intolerance. In: The Cambridge World History of Foods, K. F. Kiple, & K. C. Ornelas (eds.). Cambridge, UK: Cambridge University Press, pp. 1057–1062.

Patton, S. (2004). Milk: Its Remarkable Contribution to Human Health and Well-Being. New Brunswick, NJ: Transaction Publishers.

Paul, S. A., Simons, J. W., & Mabjeesh, N. J. (2004). J Cell Physiol, 200(1):20–30.

Pauling, L. (1968). Science, 160(825):265–271.

Pauling, L. (1986). How to Live Longer and Feel Better. San Francisco, Freeman.

Pawelczyk, J. A., & Levine, B. D. (2002). J Appl Physiol, 92(5):2105–2113.

Pawlowski, B. (1999). Curr Anthropol, 40(3):257–275.

Peacock, N. (1990). Comparative and cross–cultural approaches to the study of human female reproductive failure. In: Primate Life History and Evolution, C. J. DeRousseau (ed.). New York: Wiley-Liss, pp. 195–220.

Pear, R. (2006). Weight loss surgery comes with risks, Orlando Sentinel. Orlando, FL July 24, A4.

Pechacek, T. F., & Babb, S. (2004). BMJ, 328(7446):980–983.

Pelchat, M. L., & Rozin, P. (1982). Appetite, 3(4):341–351.

Pelchat, M. L. (1997). Appetite, 28(2):103–113.

Pellegrini, A. D., & Archer, J. (2005). Sex differences in competitive and aggressive behavior: A view from sexual selection theory. In: Origins of the Social Mind: Evolutionary Psychology and Child Development, B. J. Ellis & D. F. Bjorklund (eds.). New York: Guilford Press, pp. 219–244.

Pelletier, D. L., Frongillo Jr, E. A., Schroeder, D. G., & Habicht, J. P. (1995). Bull World Health Organ, 73(4):443–448.

Pena, I. C., Teberg, A. J., & Finello, K. M. (1988). J Pediatr, 113(6):1066–1073.

Pender, M. P. (2003). Trends Immunol, 24(11):584–588.

Pénin, X. (1997). Modélisation Tridimensionnelle des Variations Morphologiques du ComplexeCrânio–Facial des Hominoidea. Applications à la Croissance et à l'Évolution. Paris: Université Paris.

Pennington, A. W. (1953a). Am J Clin Nutr, 1(2):100–106.

Pennington, A. W. (1953b). Am J Clin Nutr, 1(5):343–348.

PerezEscamilla, R., Pollitt, E., Lonnerdal, B., & Dewey, K. G. (1994). Am J Public Health, 84(1):89–97.

Perrotta, S., Nobili, B., Ferraro, M., Migliaccio, C., et al. (2006). Blood, 107(2):514–519.

Persky, V. W., Chatterton, R. T., van Horn, L. V., Grant, M. D., et al. (1992). Cancer Res, 52(3):578–583.

Peters, H., & McNatty, K. P. (1980). The Ovary: A Correlation of Structure and Function in Mammals. Berkeley, CA: University of California Press.

Petersen, A. M., & Krogfelt, K. A. (2003). FEMS Immunol Med Microbiol, 36(3):117–126.

Petersen, L., Schnohr, P., & Sorensen, T. I. (2004). Int J Obes Relat Metab Disord, 28(1):105–112.

Petridou, E., Syrigou, E., Toupadaki, N., Zavitsanos, X., et al. (1996). Int J Cancer, 68(2):193–198.

Petterson, F., Fries, H., & Nillius, S. J. (1973). Am J Obstet Gynecol, 117(1):80–86.

Phillips, S. F. (1981). Lactose malabsorption and gastrointestinal function: Effects on gastrointestinal transit and the absorption of other nutrients. In: Lactose Digestion: Clinical and Nutritional Implications, D. M. Paige & T. M. Bayless (eds.). Baltimore, MD: Johns Hopkins University Press, pp. 51–57.

Phillips, S. M., Bandini, L. G., Cyr, H., Colclough–Douglas, S., et al. (2003). Int J Obes Relat Metab Disord, 27(9):1106–1113.

Phillipson, C. (1997). World Rev Nutr Diet, 81:38–48.

Phinney, V. G., Jensen, L. C., Olsen, J. A., & Cundick, B. (1990). Adolescence, 25(98):321–332.

Piazza, P. V., & Le Moal, M. L. (1996). Annu Rev Pharmacol Toxicol, 36:359–378.

Piccinni, M. P., Giudizi, M. G., Biagiotti, R., Beloni, L., et al. (1995). J Immunol, 155(1):128–133.

Pijnenborg, R. (1996). Hypertens Pregnancy, 15(1):7–23.

Pike, I. L. (2000). Hum Nat, 11(3):207–232.

Pike, I. L. (2005). Am J Hum Biol, 17(1):55–65.

Pike, M. C., Spicer, D. V., Dahmoush, L., & Press, M. F. (1993). Epidemiol Rev, 15(1):17–35.

Pimental, M., Chow, E. J., & Lin, H. C. (2003). Am J Gastroenterol, 98(2):412–419.

Pinheiro, S. P., Holmes, M. D., Pollak, M. N., Barbieri, R. L., et al. (2005). Cancer Epidemiol Biomarkers Prev, 14(9):2147–2153.

Pinholt, M., Frederiksen, J. L., & Christiansen, M. (2006). Eur J Neurol, 13(6):573–580.

Pinilla, T., & Birch, L. L. (1993). Pediatrics, 91(2):436–444.

Pinker, S., & Bloom, P. (1990). Brain Behav Sci, 13(4):707–784.

Pirke, K. M., Schweiger, U., Lemmel, W., Krieg, J. C., et al. (1985). J Clin Endocrinol Metab, 60(6):1174–1179.

Pitt, B., Poole–Wilson, P., Segal, R., Martinez, F. A., et al. (1999). J Card Fail, 5(2):146–154.

Pitt, B., Zannad, F., Remme, W. J., Cody, R., et al. (1999). N Engl J Med, 341(10):709–717.

Plinius Secundus Maior, G. (1897). Naturalis Historia. Leipzig, Germany: Teubner.

Plymate, S. R., Moore, D. E., Cheng, C. Y., Bardin, C. W., et al. (1985). J Clin Endocrinol Metab, 61(5):993–996.

Poirier, J., Davignon, J., Boutheillier, D., Kogan, S., et al. (1993). Lancet, 342(8873):697–699.

Polan, H., & Hofer, M. (1999). Psychobiological origins of infant attachment and separation responses. In: Handbook of Attachment : Theory, Research, and Clinical Applications, J. Cassidy, & P. R. Shaver (eds.). New York: Guilford Press, pp. 162–180.

Polan, M. L., Daniele, A., & Kuo, A. (1988). Fertil Steril, 49(6):964–968.

Poleszynski, D. V. (2001). Framveksten av Medisinske Alternativer—Fra Konkurranse til Samarbeid [The Emergence of Medical Alternatives—From Competition to Cooperation]. Kristiansand, Norway. HoyskoleForlaget.

Poleszynski, D. V., & Mysterud, I. (2004). Sukker—En Snikende Fare [Sugar—Lurking Danger]. Oslo: Gyldendal Akademisk.

Polivy, J., & Herman, C. P. (2006). Appetite, 47(1):30–35.

Pollard, A. J., Niermeyer, S., Barry, P., Bartsch, P., et al. (2001). High Alt Med Biol, 2(3):389–403.

Pollard, T. M., Unwin, N. C., Fischbacher, C. M., & Chamley, J. K. (2006). Am J Hum Biol, 18(6):741–747.

Polnay, L., Blair, M., Horn, N., & Nathan, D. (1996). Manual of Community Paediatrics, 2nd ed. London, UK: Churchill Livingstone.

Polson, D. W., Wadsworth, J., Adams, J., & Franks, S. (1988). Lancet, 1 (8590):870–872.

Pomerleau, C. S. (1997). Addiction, 92(4):397–408.

Ponzio, G., Debant, A., Contreres, J. O., & Rossi, B. (1990). Cell Signal, 4(4):377–386.

Popkin, B. M. (1994). Nutr Rev, 52(9):285–298.

Popkin, B. M., Richards, M. K., & Montiero, C. A. (1996). J Nutr, 126(12):3009–3016.

Popkin, B. M. (1999). World Dev, 27(11):1905–1916.

Popkin, B. M. (2001). J Nutr, 131(3):871–873.

Popkin, B. M. (2004). Nutr Rev, 62(7 [Pt 2]):140–143.

Popkin, B. M., & Gordon-Larsen, P. (2004). Int J Obes Relat Metab Disord, 28(Suppl 3):S2–S9.

Poretsky, L., Grigorescu, F., Seibel, M., Moses, A. C., et al. (1985). J Clin Endocrinol Metab, 61(4):728–734.

Poretsky, L., Cataldo, N. A., Rosenwaks, Z., & Guidice, L. C. (1999). Endocr Rev, 20(4):535–582.

Porte Jr., D., Baskin, D. G., & Schwartz, M. W. (2002). Nutr Rev, 60(10 [Pt 2]):S20–S29.

Porter, R. (1997). The Greatest Benefit to Mankind. London: Fontana Press.

Poser, S., Raun, N. E., Wikstrom, J., & Poser, W. (1979). Acta Neurol Scand, 59(2–3):108–118.

Post, R. H. (1962). Eugen Q, 9:131–146.

Potts, R. (1998). Evol Anthropol, 7(3):81–96.

Powell, B. L., Frey, C. L., & Drutz, D. J. (1983). Estrogen Receptor in Candida albicans. A Possible Explanation for Hormonal Influences in Vaginal Candidiasis. Twenty-third Interscience Conference on Antimicrobial Agents and Chemotherapy. Las Vegas, NV, p. 222.

Power, M. L., & Tardif, S. D. (2005). Maternal nutrition and metabolic control of pregnancy. In: Birth, Distress and Disease: Placental-Brain Interactions, M. L. Power & J. Schulkin (eds.). Cambridge, UK: Cambridge University Press, pp. 88–112.

Prentice, A. M., & Moore, S. E. (2005). Arch Dis Child, 90(4):429–432.

Price, E. C., & Feistner, A. T. C. (1993). Am J Primatol, 31(3):211–221.

Price, J., Sloman, L., Gardner, R., Gilbert, P., et al. (1994). Br J Psychiatry, 164(309–315.

Price, K. C., Hyde, J. S., & Coe, C. L. (1999). Obstet Gynecol, 94(1):128–134.

Price, K. C., & Coe, C. L. (2000). Hum Reprod, 15(2):452–457.

Price, W. A. (1970). Nutrition and Physical Degeneration. La Mesa, CA: Price-Pottenger Nutrition Foundation.

Prior, I. A., Davidson, F., Salmond, C. E., & Czochanska, Z. (1981). Am J Hum Nutrition, 34(8):1552–1561.

Profet, M. (1992). Pregnancy sickness as adaptation: A deterrent to maternal ingestion of teratogens. In: The Adapted Mind: Evolutionary Psychology and the Generation of Culture, J. E. Barkow, L. Cosmides, & J. Tooby (eds.). New York: Oxford University Press, pp. 327–365.

Profet, M. (1993). Q Rev Biol, 68(3):335–386.

Promislow, D. E. L., & Harvey, P. H. (1990). J Zool (Lond), 220(Pt 3):417–437.

Promislow, D. E. L., & Harvey, P. H. (1991). Acta Oecol, 12(1):119–137.

Proos, L., Hofvander, Y., & Tuvemo, T. (1991a). Acta Paediatr Scand, 80(9):825–858.

Proos, L., Hofvander, Y., & Tuvemo, T. (1991b). Indian J Pediatr, 58(1):105–114.

Pugh, M. B. (ed.) (2000). Stedman's Medical Dictionary. Baltimore, MD: Lippincott, Williams, & Wilkins.

Pulec, J. L. (1977). Laryngoscope, 87(4 [Pt 1]):542–556.

Putnam, R. D. (2000). Bowling Alone: The Collapse and Revival of American Community. New York: Simon & Schuster.

Pyorala, M., Miettinen, H., Laakso, M., & Pyorala, K. (2000). Diabetes Care, 23(8):1097–1102.

Qiu, H., Yang, J., Bai, H., Fan, Y., et al. (2004). Immunology, 111(4):453–461.

Quartz, S., & Sejnowski, T. (2000). Behav Brain Sci, 23(5):785–792.

Quas, J. A., Bauer, A., & Boyce, W. T. (2004). Child Dev, 75(3):797–814.

Queller, D. C. (1995). Q Rev Biol, 70(4):485–489.

Quillin, S. I., & Glenn, L. (2004). J Obstet Gynecol Neonatal Nurs, 33(5):580–588.

Quinlan, R. J., & Flinn, M. V. (2005). Hum Nat, 16(1):32–57.

Quinn, N. P., & Marsden, C. D. (1986). Mov Disord, 1(1):85–87.

Quintero, G., & Davis, P. (2002). Med Anthropol Q, 16(4):439–457.

Quistorff, B., & Grunnet, N. (2003). Ugeskrift for Læger, 165:1552–1553.

Rabin, R. (2004). The new pill in town: Controversial form of birth control delays monthly cycle. Newsday, January 25.

Rachagan, S. S. (2004). The Junk Food Generation: A Multicountry Survey of the Influence of Television Advertisements on Children. London: Consumers International Asian Pacific Office.

Ragonese, P., Salemi, G., D'Amelio, M., Gammino, M., et al. (2004). Neuroepidemiology, 23(6):306–309.

Rahman, K. (2001). J Nutr, 131(Suppl 3):977S–979S.

Rako, S. (2003). No More Periods?: The Risks of Menstrual Suppression and Other Cutting-Edge Issues About Hormones and Women's Health. New York: Harmony Books.

Rama, A. N., Cho, S. C., & Kushida, C. A. (2006). Normal human sleep. In: Sleep: A Comprehensive Handbook, T. L. Lee-Chiong (ed.). Hoboken, NJ: John Wiley, pp. 3–9.

Ramakrishnan, U., Martorell, R., Schroeder, D. G., & Flores, R. (1999). J Nutr, 129(Suppl 2):S544–S549.

Ramsay, D. S., Seeley, R. J., Bolles, R. C., & Woods, S. C. (1996). Ingestive homeostasis: The primacy of learning. In: Why We Eat What We Eat: The Psychology of Eating, E. D. Capaldi (ed.). Washington, DC: American Psychological Association, pp. 11–27.

Raphael, D. (1976). J Pediatr, 88(1):169–170.

Rapp, D. J. (2004). Our Toxic World: A Wake Up Call. Buffalo, NY. Environmental Medical Research Foundation.

Rasgon, N., Bauer, M., Glenn, T., Elman, S., et al. (2003). Bipolar Disorder, 5(1):48–52.

Ratledge, C., & Dover, L. G. (2000). Annu Rev Microbiol, 54:881–941.

Ravelli, G., Stein, Z. A., & Susser, M. W. (1976). N Engl J Med, 295(7):349–353.

Ravnskov, U. (2000). The Cholesterol Myths. Exposing the Fallacy That Saturated Fat and Cholesterol Cause Heart Disease. Washington, DC: New Trends Publishing.

Ravnskov, U. (2002). Q J Med, 95(6):397–403.

Ravussin, E. (1995). Int J Obes Relat Metab Disord, 19(Suppl 7):S8–S9.

Ravussin, E., & Bogardus, C. (2000). Br J Nutr, 83(Suppl 1):S17–S20.

Rayco–Solon, P., Fulford, A. J., & Prentice, A. M. (2005). Am J Obstet Gynecol, 192(4):1133–1136.

Raymond, J., & Segrè, D. (2006). Science, 311(5768):1764–1767.

Raynor, H. A., & Epstein, L. H. (2001). Psychol Bull, 127(3):325–341.

Rea, T., Russo, J., Katon, W., Ashley, R., et al. (1999). Arch Intern Med, 159(8):865–870.

Read, A. F., Aaby, P., Antia, R., Ebert, D., et al. (1999). What can evolutionary biology contribute to understanding virulence? In: Evolution in Health and Disease, S. C. Stearns (ed.). Oxford, UK: Oxford University Press, pp. 205–215.

Reaven, G. M. (1988). Diabetes, 37(12):1595–1607.

Reaven, G. (1998). J Basic Clin Physiol Pharmacol, 9(2–4):387–406.

Reaven, G. M. (2005). Endocrinol Metab Clin North Am, 34(1):49–62.

Rebuffe-Scrive, M., Enk, L., Crona, N., Lonnroth, P., et al. (1985). J Clin Invest, 75(6):1973–1976.

Rebuffe-Scrive, M., Bronnegard, M., Nilsson, A., Eldh, J., et al. (1990). J Clin Endocrinol Metab, 71(5):1215–1219.

Rechtschaffen, A. (1998). Perspect Biol Med, 41(3):359–390.

Reddy, S., & Sanders, T. A. B. (1992). Atherosclerosis, 95(2–3):223–229.

Reddy, K. S. (2004). N Engl J Med, 350(24):2438–2440.

Redgrave, P., Prescott, T. J., & Gurney, K. (1999). Trends Neurosci, 22(4):146–151.

Redish, A. D. (2004). Science, 306(5703):1944–1947.

Redman, C. W., & Sargent, I. L. (2005). Science, 308(5728):1592–1594.

Reed, B. D. (1992). Obstet Gynecol Surv, 47(8):551–560.

Reed, E. S. (1996). Encountering the World: Towards an Ecological Psychology. New York: Oxford University Press.

Reed, M. J., Dunkley, S. A., Singh, A., Thomas, B. S., et al. (1993). Prostaglandins Leukot Essent Fatty Acids, 48(1):111–116.

Reeve, H. K., & Sherman, P. W. (1993). Q Rev Biol, 68(1):1–32.

Reeve, J. R., Gull, S. E., Johnson, M. H., Hunter, S., et al. (2004). Eur J Obstet Gynecol Reprod Biol, 113(2):199–203.

Reichelderfer, P. S., Kovacs, A., Wright, D. J., Landay, A., et al. (2000). AIDS, 14(14):2101–2107.

Reichelt, K.-L., & Knivsberg, A.–M. (2003). Nutr Neurosci, 6(1):19–28.

Reichelt, K.-L., & Jensen, D. (2004). Acta Neurol Scand, 110(4):239–241.

Reilly, S. M., Wiley, E. O., & Meinhardt, D. J. (1997). Biol J Linn Soc Lond, 60(1):119–143.

Reimão, R., Souza, J. C. R. P. D., Medeiros, M. M., & Almirao, R. I. (1998). Arq Neuropsiquiatr, 56(4):703–707.

Reimão, R., Souza, J. C., Gaudioso, C. E. V., Guerra, H. D. C., et al. (2000a). Arq Neuropsiquiatr, 58(2A):233–238.

Reimão, R., Souza, J. C., Gaudioso, C. E. V., Guerra, H. D. C., et al. (2000b). Arq Neuropsiquiatr, 58(1):39–44.

Rhind, S. M., Rae, M. T., & Brooks, A. N. (2001). Reprod, 122(2):205–214.

Rhodes, J. S., Garland Jr. , T., & Gammie, S. C. (2003). Behav Neurosci, 117(6):1243–1256.

Rice, P. L. (2000). J Reprod Infant Psychol, 18(1):21–32.

Richard, C., Mosko, S., McKenna, J. J., & Drummond, S. (1996). Sleep, 19(9):685–690.

Richards, A. (1932). Hunger and Work in a Savage Society. London: Routledge.

Richards, M. (1998). The meeting of nature and nurture and the development of children: Some conclusions. In: Biosocial Perspectives on Children, C. Panter-Brick (ed.). Cambridge, UK: Cambridge University Press, pp. 131–146.

Richards, R. J. (1987). Darwin and the Emergence of Evolutionary Theories of Mind and Behavior. Chicago: University of Chicago Press.

Richardson, G. S. (2005). J Clin Psychiatry, 66(Suppl 9):3–9.

Richerson, P. J., & Boyd, R. (2005). Not By Genes Alone: How Culture Transformed Human Evolution. Chicago: University of Chicago Press.

Rickenlund, A., Carlstrom, K., Ekblom, B., Brismar, T. B., et al. (2004). J Clin Endocrinol Metab, 89(9):4364–4370.

Rideout, V., Roberts, D., & Ulla, G. (2005). Generation M: Media in the Lives of 8–18 Year-Olds. Menlo Park, CA: Henry J. Kaiser Foundation.

Ridker, P. M., Cushman, M., Stampfer, M. J., Tracy, R. P., et al. (1997). N Engl J Med, 336(14):973–979.

Ridker, P. M., Hennekens, C. H., Buring, J. E., & Rifai, N. (2000). N Engl J Med, 342(12):836–843.

Ridley, M. (1996). The Origins of Virtue: Human Instincts and the Evolution of Cooperation. New York: Viking.

Ridley, M. (2004). Evolution. Oxford, UK: Blackwell Scientific.

Rigda, R. S., McMillen, I. C., & Buckley, P. (2000). J Paediatr Child Health, 36(2):117–121.

Righard, L., & Alade, M. O. (1990). Lancet, 336(8723):1105–1107.

Rilling, J. K. (2006). Evol Anthropol, 15(2):65–77.

Rimestad, A. H., Borgejordet, Å., Vesterhus, K. N., Sygnestveit, K., et al. (2001). Den store matvaretabellen [The Comprehensive Food and Nutrients Guide]. Oslo: Gyldendal Undervisning.

Riordan, J., & Auerbach, K. G. (eds.). (1993). Breastfeeding and Human Lactation. Boston: Jones and Bartlett.

Risch, N., Burchard, E., Ziv, E., & Tang, H. (2002). Genome Biol, 3(7):1–12.

Risdon, T. (2003). Many infants who die are sleeping with a parent. London, UK: The Guardian, January 16.

Ritenbaugh, C., Teufel-Shone, N. I., Aickin, M. G., Joe, J. R., et al. (2003). Prev Med, 36(3):309–319.

Roach, R. C., Bartsch, P., Hackett, P. H., Oelz, O., et al. (1993). The Lake Louise Acute Mountain Sickness Scoring System. In: Hypoxia and Molecular Medicine, J. R. Sutton, & C. S. Houston (eds.). Burlington, VT: Queen City Printers, Inc, pp. 272–274.

Roach, R. C., & Hackett, P. H. (2001). J Exp Biol, 204(18):3161–3170.

Roberts, A. C., Butterfield, G. E., Cymerman, A., Reeves, J. T., et al. (1996). J Appl Physiol, 81(4):1762–1771.

Roberts, A. C., Reeves, J. T., Butterfield, G. E., Mazzeo, R. S., et al. (1996). J Appl Physiol, 80(2):605–615.

Roberts, J. M., Taylor, R. N., Musci, T. J., Rodgers, G. M., et al. (1989). Am J Obstet Gynecol, 161(5):1200–1204.

Robertson, S. A., Bromfield, J. J., & Tremellen, K. P. (2003). J Reprod Immunol, 59(2):253–265.

Robillard, P.-Y., Hulsey, T. C., Périanin, J., Janky, E., et al. (1994). Lancet, 344(8928):973–975.

Robillard, P.-Y., & Hulsey, T. C. (1996). Lancet, 347(9001):619.

Robillard, P.-Y., Dekker, G. A., & Hulsey, T. C. (1999). Eur J Obstet Gynecol Reprod Biol, 84(1):37–41.

Robillard, P.-Y., Dekker, G. A., & Hulsey, T. C. (2002). Am J Reprod Immunol, 47(2):104–111.

Robillard, P.-Y., Chaline, J., Chaouat, G., & Hulsey, T. C. (2003). Curr Anthropol, 44(1):130–135.

Robillard, P.-Y., Hulsey, T. C., Dekker, G. A., & Chaouat, G. (2003). J Reprod Immunol, 59(2):93–100.

Robinson, T. E., & Berridge, K. C. (1993). Brain Res Brain Res Rev, 18(3):247–291.

Robinson, T. E., & Berridge, K. C. (2001). Addiction, 96(1):103–114.

Robinson, T. E., & Berridge, K. C. (2003). Annu Rev Psychol, 54:25–53.

Robson, C. (1993). Real World Research: A Resource for Social Scientists and Practitioner-Researchers. Oxford, UK: Blackwell.

Rodin, D. A., Bano, G., Bland, J. M., Taylor, K., et al. (1998). Clin Endocrinol, 49(1):91–99.

Rodin, J. (1989). Appetite, 12:76–77.

Rodin, M. (1992). Soc Sci Med, 35(1):49–56.

Rodman, P. S. (2002). Plants of the apes: Is there a hominoid model for the origins of the hominid diet? In: Human Diet: Its Origin and Evolution, P. S. Ungar, & M. F. Teaford (eds.). Westport, CT: Bergin & Covey, pp. 77–109.

Rodriguez, L. G. A., & Ruigomez, A. (1999). BMJ, 318(7183):565–566.

Rodway, G. W., Hoffman, L. A., & Sanders, M. H. (2003). Heart Lung, 32(6):353–359.

Rogers, I., Emmett, P., Gunnell, D., Dunger, D., et al. (2006). Public Health Nutr, 9(3):359–363.

Rogers, P. J. (1999). Proc Nutr Soc, 58(1):59–67.

Rogers, R. G. (1992). Demography, 29(2):287–303.

Rogers, T. J., & Balish, E. (1980). Microbiol Rev, 44(4):660–682.

Rohlf, F. J., & Bookstein, F. L. (1990). Proceedings of the Michigan Morphometrics Workshop. Ann Arbor, MI: University of Michigan Museum of Zoology.

Rolls, B. J., Rowe, E. A., Rolls, E. T., Kingston, B., et al. (1981). Physiol Behav, 26(2):215–221.

Rolls, B. J. (1986). Nutr Rev, 44(3):93–101.

Rolls, B. J. (2003). Nutr Today, 38(2):42–53.

Romani, L. (2004). Nat Rev Immunol, 4:1–23.

Rombauer, I., Becker, M. R., Becker, E., & Guarnaschelli, M. (1997). Joy of Cooking. New York: Scribner.

Romero, I., Jorgensen, P., Bolwig, G., Fraser, P. E., et al. (1999). Neuroreport, 10(11):2255–2260.

Rona, R. J., & Chinn, S. (1989). J Epidemiol Community Health, 43(1):66–71.

Ronald, J., & Akey, J. M. (2005). Hum Genomics, 2(2):113–125.

Rosch, E. (1996). The environment of minds: Towards a noetic and hedonic ecology. In: Cognitive Ecology, M. P. Friedman, & E. C. Carterette (eds.). San Diego, CA: Academic Press, pp. 1–23.

Rose, H., & Rose, S. P. R. (eds.). (2000). Alas, Poor Darwin: Arguments Against Evolutionary Psychology. London: Jonathan Cape Ltd.

Rosenberg, K. (1992). Yearb Phys Anthropol, 35:89–124.

Rosenberg, K., & Trevathan, W. R. (1996). Evol Anthropol, 4:161–168.

Rosenberg, K., & Trevathan, W. R. (2002). Br J Obstet Gynaecol, 109(11):1199–1206.

Rosenberg, M. (1990). Am Anthropol, 92(2):399–415.

Rosenberg, M. J., & Waugh, M. S. (1998). Am J Obstet Gynecol, 179(3 [Part 1]):577–582.

Rosenberg, N. A., Pritchard, J. K., Weber, J. L., Cann, H. M., et al. (2002). Science, 298(5602):2381–2385.

Rosenthal, G. E., & Landefeld, C. S. (1990). J Clin Epidemiol, 43(1):15–20.

Rosenthal, L. (2006). Physiologic processes during sleep. In: Sleep: A Comprehensive Handbook, T. L. Lee-Chiong (ed.). Hoboken, NJ: John Wiley, pp. 19–23.

Rossouw, J. E., Anderson, G. L., Prentice, R. L., LaCroix, A. Z., et al. (2002). J Am Med Assoc, 288(3):321–333.

Roth, T. (2004). J Clin Psychiatry, 65(Suppl 16):8–11.

Rottenberg, M. E., Gigliotti Rothfuchs, A., Gigliotti, D., Ceausu, M., et al. (2000). J Immunol, 164(9):4812–4818.

Roumain, J., Charles, M. A., de Courten, M. P., Hanson, R. L., et al. (1998). Diabetes Care, 21(3):346–349.

Rowe, J. (2003). Nurs Inq, 10(3):184–192.

Rowland, N. E., Li, B. H., & Morien, A. (1996). Brain mechanisms and the psychology of feeding. In: Why We Eat What We Eat: The Psychology of Eating, E. D. Capaldi (ed.). Washington, DC: American Psychological Association, pp. 173–204.

Roy, K., Valentine, J. W., Jablonski, D., & Kidwell, S. M. (1996). Trends Ecol Evol, 11(11):458–463.

Royal College of Midwives. (2002). Successful Breastfeeding, 3rd ed. London: Churchill Livingstone.

Rozemond, M. (1998). Descarte's Dualism. Cambridge, MA: Harvard University Press.

Rozin, E. (1982). The structure of cuisine. In: The Psychobiology of Human Food Selection, L. M. Barker (ed.). Westport, CT: AVI Publishing Company, Inc, pp. 189–203.

Rozin, P. (1976). Psychobiological and cultural determinants of food choice. In: Appetite and Food Intake, T. Silverstone (ed.). New York: VCH Publishers, pp. 285–312.

Rozin, P., & Rozin, E. (1981). Nat Hist, 90(2):6–14.

Rozin, P. (1982). Human food selection: The interaction of biology, culture and individual experience. In: The Psychobiology of Human Food Selection, L. M. Baker (ed.). Westport, CT: AVI Publishing Company, Inc, pp. 225–254.

Rozin, P., Ebert, L., & Schull, J. (1982). Appetite, 3(1):13–22.

Rozin, P., & Kennel, K. (1983). Appetite, 4(2):69–77.

Rozin, P., & Millman, L. (1987). Appetite, 8(2):125–134.

Rozin, P. (1996). Sociocultural influences on human food selection. In: Why We Eat What We Eat: The Psychology of Eating, E. D. Capaldi (ed.). Washington, DC: American Psychological Association, pp. 233–263.

Rozin, P. (2000). The psychology of food and food choices. In: The Cambridge History of Food, K. Kiple & K. Ornelas (eds.). Cambridge, UK: Cambridge University Press, pp. 1476–1486.

Rozin, P. (2005). J Nutr Educ Behav, 37(Suppl 2):S107–S112.

Rudge, S. R., Kowanko, I. C., & Drury, P. L. (1983). Ann Rheum Dis, 42(4):425–430.

Ruidavets, J. B., Bongard, V., Simon, C., Dallongeville, J., et al. (2006). J Hypertens, 24(4):633–634.

Ruislova, Z. (1998). Stud Psychol, 40(4):277–281.

Rundqvist, B., Elam, M., Bergmann-Sverrisdottir, Y., Eisenhofer, G., et al. (1997). Circulation, 95(1):169–175.

Rupert, J. L., & Koehle, M. S. (2006). High Alt Med Biol, 7(2):150–167.

Rutter, M., O'Connor, T. G., & English and Romanian Adoptees Study Team. (2004). Dev Psychol, 40(1):81–94.

Ryan, D. H. (2003). Int J Clin Pract, 134(Suppl):28–35.

Saah, T. (2005). Harm Reduct J, 2:8–15.

Sabeti, P. C., Schaffner, S. F., Fry, B., Lohmueller, J., et al. (2006). Science, 312(5780):1614–1620.

Sachdev, H. S., Fall, C. H., Osmond, C., Lakshmy, R., et al. (2005). Am J Clin Nutr, 82(2):456–466.

Sadegh-Zadeh, K. (2000). J Med Philos, 25(5):605–638.

Sahi, T. (1994a). Scand J Gastroenterol, 29(Suppl 202):7–20.

Sahi, T. (1994b). Scand J Gastroenterol, 29(Suppl 202):1–6.

Sahlins, M. D. (1976). Cultural and Practical Reason. Chicago: University of Chicago Press.

Saikku, P. (1993). Eur Heart J, 14(Suppl K):62–65.

Saikku, P. (1995). Chronic Chlamydia pneumoniae infections. In: Chlamydia pneumoniae Infection, L. Allegra, & F. Blasi (eds.). Milan, Itlay: Springer, pp. 96–113.

Saikku, P., Laitinen, K., & Leinonen, M. (1998). Atherosclerosis, 140(Suppl 1):S17–S19.

Sakai, K. L. (2005). Science, 310(5749):815–819.

Salamone, J. D., Correal, M., Mingote, S., & Weber, S. M. (2003). J Pharmacol Exp Ther, 305(1):1–8.

Salariya, E. M., Easton, P. M., & Cater, J. I. (1978). Lancet, 2(8100):1141–1143.

Salem, M. L. (2004). Curr Drug Targets Inflamm Allergy, 3(1):97–104.

Salmeron, J., Ascherio, A., Rimm, E. B., Colditz, G. A., et al. (1997). Diabetes Care, 20(4):545–550.

Salmeron, J., Manson, J. E., Stampfer, M. J., Colditz, G. A., et al. (1997). J Am Med Assoc, 277(6):472–477.

Salminen, K. K., Vuorinen, T., Oikarinen, S., Helminen, M., et al. (2004). Diabet Med, 21(2):156–164.

Salter, M., Hazelwood, R., Pogson, C. I., Iyer, R., et al. (1995). Biochem Pharmacol, 49(10):1435–1442.

Samaha, F. F., Iqbal, N., Seshadri, P., Chicano, K. L., et al. (2003). N Engl J Med, 348(21):2074–2081.

Samoto, T., Maruo, T., Ladines–Llave, C. A., Matsuo, H., et al. (1993). Endocr J, 40(6):715–726.

Sampson, J. B., Cymerman, A., Burse, R. L., Maher, J. T., et al. (1983). Aviat Space Environ Med, 54(12 [Pt 1]):1063–1073.

Samson, M., Libert, F., Doranz, B. J., Rucker, J., et al. (1996). Nature, 382(6593):722–725.

Sanchez, A., Kissinger, D. G., & Phillips, R. I. (1981). Med Hypotheses, 7(11):1339–1345.

Sanchez, M. M., Young, L. J., Plotsky, P. M., & Insel, T. R. (2000). J Neurosci, 20(12):4657–4668.

Sanchez del Rio, M., & Moskowitz, M. A. (1999). Adv Exp Med Biol, 474:145–153.

Sanderson, J. E. (2004). Hong Kong Med J, 10(2):64–76.

Sandler, D. P., Wilcox, A. J., & Horney, L. F. (1984). Am J Epidemiol, 119(5):765–774.

Sandler, R. B., Slemenda, C. W., LaPorte, R. E., Cauley, J. A., et al. (1985). Am J Clin Nutr, 42(2):270–274.

Sandros, J., Papapanou, P. N., & Dahlen, G. (1993). J Periodontal Res, 28(3):219–226.

Sandyk, R. (1995). Int J Neurosci, 83(3–4):187–198.

Santarelli, L., Saxe, M., Gross, C., Surget, A., et al. (2003). Science, 301(5634):805–809.

Saper, C. B., Cano, G., & Scammell, T. E. (2005). J Comp Neurol, 493(1):92–98.

Sapolsky, R. M. (1994). Why Zebras Don't Get Ulcers: A Guide to Stress, Stress Related Diseases, and Coping. New York: W.H. Freeman.

Sapolsky, R. M. (1996). Science, 273(5276):749–750.

Sapolsky, R. M. (1998). Why Zebras Don't Get Ulcers: An Updated Guide to Stress, Stress-Related Diseases, and Coping, 2nd ed. New York: W.H. Freeman.

Sapolsky, R. M., Romero, L. M., & Munck, A. U. (2000). Endocr Rev, 21(1):55–89.

Sapolsky, R. M. (2005). Science, 308(5722):648–652.

Sargent, R. C., & Gross, M. R. (1985). Behav Ecol Sociobiol, 17(1):43–45.

Sarich, V., & Miele, F. (2004). Race: The Reality of Human Differences. Boulder, CO: Westview Press.

Saunders, A. M., Strittmatter, W. J., Schmechel, D., St. George-Hyslop, P. H., et al. (1993). Neurology, 43(8):1467–1472.

Sawada, S., & Takei, M. (2005). Autoimmun Rev, 4(2):106–110.

Sawaya, A. L., Grillo, L. P., Verreschi, I., da Silva, A. C., et al. (1998). J Nutr, 128(Suppl 2):S415–S420.

Saydah, S. H., Miret, M., Sung, J., Varas, C., et al. (2001). Diabetes Care, 24(8):1397–1402.

Scarpellini, F., Scarpellini, L., Dino, N., & Benvenuto, P. (1993). Clin Exp Obstet Gynecol, 20(3):182–188.

Schaal, B., Marlier, L., & Soussignan, R. (2000). Chem Senses, 25(6):729–737.

Schachter, S., & Rodin, J. (1974). Obese Humans and Rats. Potomac, MD: L. Erlbaum Associates.

Schachter, D., Cartier, L., & Borzutzky, A. (2003). Bone, 33(2):192–196.

Schafe, G. E., & Bernstein, I. L. (1996). Taste aversion learning. In: Why We Eat What We Eat: The Psychology of Eating, E. D. Capaldi (ed.). Washington, DC: American Psychological Association, pp. 31–51.

Schaffer, W. M. (1974). Ecology, 55(2):291–303.

Schaffer, W. M. (1983). Am Nat, 121(3):418–431.

Scheers, N. J., Rutherford, G. W., & Kemp, J. S. (2003). Pediatrics, 112(4):883–889.

Scheper–Hughes, N. (1991). Lancet, 337(8750):1144–1147.

Schiøotz, A. (2003). Det Offisielle Helsevesen i Norge 1603–2003. Bind 2: Folkets Helse—Landets Styrke 1850–2003 [The Public Health Care System in Norway 1603–2003. Volume 2: The Population's Health—The Strength of the Country 1850–2002]. Oslo: Universitetsforlaget.

Schlichting, C. D., & Pigliucci, M. (1998). Phenotypic Evolution: A Reaction Norm Perspective. Sunderland, MA: Sinauer.

Schlosser, E. (2001). Fast Food Nation: The Dark Side of the All-American Meal. Boston, MA: Houghton Mifflin.

Schluep Campo, I., & Beghin, J. C. (2006). Food Policy, 31(3):228–237.

Schmalhausen, I. I., & Dobzhansky, T. (1949). Factors of Evolution: The Theory of Stabilizing Selection. Philadelphia: Blakiston.

Schmedtje Jr., J. F., & Yan–Shan, J. I. (1998). Trends Cardiovasc Med, 8(1):24–33.

Schmid, D. A., Held, K., Ising, M., Uhr, M., et al. (2005). Neuropsychopharmacology, 30(6):1187–1192.

Schmidt–Nielsen, K. (1990). Animal Physiology: Adaptation and Environment. Cambridge, UK: Cambridge University Press.

Schnatz, P. T. (1985). Adv Psychosom Med, 12:4–24.

Schneider, M., Bernasch, D., Weymann, J., Holle, R., et al. (2002). Med Sci Sports Exerc, 34(12):1886–1891.

Scholes, D., LaCroix, A. Z., Ichikawa, L. E., Barlow, W. E., et al. (2002). Epidemiology, 13(5):581–587.

Scholl, T. O., Hediger, M. L., Vasilenko 3rd, P., Ances, I. G., et al. (1989). Ann Hum Biol, 16(4):335–345.

Schroeder, D. G., Martorell, R., & Flores, R. (1999). Am J Epidemiol, 149(2):177–185.

Schultz, A. H. (1926). Q Rev Biol, 1:465–521.

Schultz, A. H. (1936). Q Rev Biol, 11:259–283, 425–455.

Schultz, A. H. (1955). Am J Phys Anthropol, 13:97–120.

Schultz, A. H. (1960). Age changes in primates and their modifications in man. In: Human Growth, J. M. Tanner (ed.). Oxford, UK: Pergamon Press, pp. 1–20.

Schultz, A. H. (1969). The Life of Primates. London, Weidenfeld & Nicolson.

Schultz, W. (2000). Nat Rev Neurosci, 1(3):199–207.

Schulz, R., Hummel, C., Heinemann, S., Seeger, W., et al. (2002). Am J Respir Crit Care Med, 165(1):67–70.

Schumacher, L. B., Pawsoni, G., & Kretchener, N. (1987). Pediatrics, 80(6):861–868.

Schwabe, M. J., & Konkol, R. J. (1992). Pediatr Neurol, 8(1):43–46.

Schwartz, S. M., Petitti, D. B., Siscovick, D. S., Longstreth Jr., W. T., et al. (1998). Stroke, 29(11):2277–2284.

Schwarz, J. M., Linfoot, P., Dare, D., & Aghajanian, K. (2003). Am J Clin Nutr, 77(1):43–50.

Schweiger, U., Laessle, R. G., Pfister, H., Hoehl, C., et al. (1987). Fertil Steril, 48(5):746–751.

Scientific Advisory Committee on Nutrition, & Department of Health (2001). An Update on Child Nutrition: Optimal Duration of Exclusive Breastfeeding. London: Department of Health.

Scientific Committee on Food. (2000). Guidelines of the Scientific Committee on Food for the Development of Tolerable Upper Intake Levels for Vitamins and Minerals. Brussels, Belgium: European Commission.

Sciubba, J. J. (2003). Gen Dent, 51(6):510–516.

Scrimshaw, N. S., & Béhar, M. (1965). N Engl J Med, 272(193–198.

Sears, B., & Lawren, B. (1995). The Zone: A Dietary Road Map. New York: Regan Books.

Sears, B. (1997). Mastering the Zone: The Next Step in Achieving Superhealth and Permanent Fat Loss. New York: Regan Books.

Sears, B. (1999). The Anti-Aging Zone. New York: Regan Books.

Sears, B., & Lawren, B. (2000). Finn Din Sone [Find Your Zone]. Oslo: Hilt, & Hansteen.

Sears, B. (2001). Hold Deg Ung i Sonen: Forebygg for Tidlig Aldring [Keep Young in the Zone: Prevent Too Early Aging]. Oslo: Hilt, & Hansteen.

Sears, B. (2002). The Omega Rx Zone: The Miracle of the New High-Dose Fish Oil. New York: Regan Books.

Sears, B. (2003). Omega–Sonen [The Omega Zone]. Oslo: Hilt, & Hansteen.

Seckl, J. R., & Meaney, M. J. (2004). Ann NY Acad Sci, 1032:63–84.

Seckler, D. (1982). Small but healthy? A basic hypothesis in the theory, measurement and policy of malnutrition. In: Newer Concepts in Nutrition and Their Implications for Policy, P. V. Sukhatme (ed.). Pune, India: Maharashtra Association for the Cultivation of Science Research Institute, pp. 127–137.

Seeman, M. (1996). J Psychiatry Neurosci, 21(2):123–127.

Seger, J., & Brockmann, J. (1987). What is bet-hedging? In: Oxford Surveys in Evolutionary Biology, P. Harvey & L. Partridge (eds.). Oxford, UK: Oxford University Press, pp. 182–211.

Segerstråle, U. C. O. (2000). Defenders of the Truth: The Battle for Science in the Sociobiology Debate and Beyond. New York: Oxford University Press.

Seidman, D. S., Ever–Hadani, P., Stevenson, D. K., & Gale, R. (1989). Eur J Obstet Gynecol Reprod Biol, 33(2):109–114.

Sekine, M., Yamagami, T., Handa, K., Saito, T., et al. (2002). Child Care Health Dev, 28(2):163–170.

Sekine, M., Chandola, T., Martikainen, A., McGeoghegan, D., et al. (2005). J Public Health (Bangkok), 28(1):63–70.

Semendeferi, K., Armstrong, E., Schleicher, A., Zilles, K., et al. (2001). Am J Phys Anthropol, 114(3):224–241.

Semenza, G. L. (2000). Genes Dev, 14(16):1983–1991.

Semenza, G. L. (2001). Cell, 107(1):1–3.

Semenza, G. L. (2002a). Sci Med (Phila), 8(6):338–347.

Semenza, G. L. (2002b). Biochem Pharmacol, 64(5–6):993–998.

Semenza, G. L. (2004). Physiology, 19:176–182.

Semler, C. N., & Harvey, A. G. (2004). Psychosom Med, 66(2):242–250.

Sen, A. K. (1992). Inequality Reexamined. New York: Russell Sage Foundation.

Sen, A. K. (1993). Capability and well-being. In: The Quality of Life, M. C. Nussbaum, A. K. Sen, & World Institute for Development Economics Research. (eds.). Oxford, UK: Clarendon Press, pp. 30–53.

Sennett, R., & Cobb, J. (1973). The Hidden Injuries of Class. New York: Vintage Books.

Sept, J. (1998). Am J Primatol, 46(1):85–101.

Serre, D., & Pääbo, S. (2004). Genome Res, 14(9):1679–1685.

Servan-Schreiber, D., Printz, H., & Cohen, J. D. (1990). Science, 249(4971):892–895.

Seta, N., Shimizu, T., Nawata, M., Wada, R., et al. (2002). Rheumatology, 41(9):1072–1073.

Severinghaus, J. W., Chiodi, H., Eger II, E. I., Brandstater, B., et al. (1966). Circ Res, 19(2):274–282.

Sewell, D. D. (1996). Schizophr Bull, 22(3):465–473.

Seymour, R. M., Allan, M. J., Pomiankowski, A., & Gustafsson, K. (2003). Proc R Soc Lond B Biol Sci, 271(1543):1065–1072.

Shams, M., & Williams, R. (1997). J Biosoc Sci, 29(1):101–109.

Shangold, M. M., Freeman, R., Thyssen, B., & Gatz, M. (1979). Fertil Steril, 31(2):699–702.

Shangold, M. M., Kelly, M., Berkeley, A. S., Freedman, K. S., et al. (1989). South Med J, 82(4):443–445.

Shannon, S. (1987). Diet for the Atomic Age. How to Protect Yourself From Low Level Radiation. Wayne, NJ: Avery Publishing Group.

Shaper, A. G. (1962). Am Heart J, 63:437–442.

Sharman, M. J., Kraemer, W. J., Love, D. M., Avery, N. G., et al. (2002). J Nutr, 132(7):1879–1885.

Shaw, A. (2000). Kinship and Continuity: Pakistani Families in Britain. Amsterdam: Harwood Academic.

Sheline, Y. I., Gado, M. H., & Kraemer, H. C. (2003). Am J Psychiatry, 160(8):1516–1518.

Shell-Duncan, B. (1993). Am J Hum Biol, 5:225–235.

Shermer, M. (1997). Skeptic, 5(1):72–79.

Sherwin, C. M. (1998). Anim Behav, 56(1):11–27.

Shibasaki, M., Takeda, K., Sumazaki, R., Nogami, T., et al. (1992). Ann Allergy, 68(4):315–318.

Shimizu, H., Ross, R. K., Bernstein, L., Yatani, R., et al. (1991). Br J Cancer, 63(6):963–966.

Shintani, Y., Fujie, H., Miyoshi, H., Tsutumi, T., et al. (2004). Gastroenterology, 126(3):840–848.

Shor, A., Kuo, C. C., & Patton, D. L. (1992). S Afr Med J, 82(3):158–161.

Shor, A., Libby, P., Ridker, P. M., & Maseri, A. (2002). Circulation, 106(18):e135–136.

Shorris, E. (1997). New American Blues: A Journey Through Poverty to Democracy. New York: W.W. Norton.

Short, R. V. (1976). Proc R Soc Lond B Biol Sci, 195(118):3–24.

Shröcksnadel, H., Baier–Bitterlich, G., Dapunt, O., Wachter, H., et al. (1996). Obstet Gynecol, 88(1):47–50.

Siegel, J. M. (2005). Nature, 437(7063):1264–1271.

Siegler, J. (1977). BMJ, 2(6099):1416.

Signore, C., Mills, J. L., Qian, C., Yu, K., et al. (2006). Obstet Gynecol, 108(2):338–344.

Silk, J. B. (1978). Folia Primatol, 29(2):129–141.

Silverman, W. A. (2004). Pediatrics, 113(2):394–396.

Simon, M. C. (2006). Cell Metab, 3(3):150–151.

Simoons, F. J. (1969). Am J Dig Dis, 14(12):819–836.

Simoons, F. J. (1978). Am J Dig Dis, 23(11):963–980.

Simoons, F. J. (1981a). Geographic patterns of primary adult lactose malabsorption: A further interpretation of evidence for the Old World. In: Lactose Digestion: Clinical and Nutritional Implications, D. M. Paige & T. M. Bayless (eds.). Baltimore, MD: Johns Hopkins University Press, pp. 23–48.

Simoons, F. J. (1981b). Celiac disease as a geographic problem. In: Food, Nutrition, and Evolution, D. Walacher & N. Kretcher (eds.). New York: Masson Publishing Company, pp. 179–199.

Simoons, F. J. (1982). Geography and genetics as factors in the psychobiology of human food selection. In: The Psychobiology of Human Food Selection, L. M. Barker (ed.). Westport, CT: AVI Publishing Company, Inc, pp. 205–224.

Simoons, F. J. (1994). Introduction. In: Eat Not This Flesh: Food Avoidances from Prehistory to the Present, F. J. Simoons (ed.). Madison, WI: University of Wisconsin Press, pp. 3–12.

Simoons, F. J. (2001). Ecol Food Nutr, 40(5):397–469.

Simopoulos, A. P. (1999). Prostaglandins Leukot Essent Fatty Acids, 60(5–6):421–429.

Simor, A. E., Poon, R., & Borczyk, A. (1989). J Clin Microbiol, 27(2):353–355.

Sinervo, B. (2006), Optimal Foraging Theory, http://bio.research.ucsc.edu/~barrylab/classes animal_behavior/FORAGING.HTM

Singer, D. (1999). Comp Biochem Physiol A Mol Integr Physiol, 123(3):221–234.

Singer, P. (2000). A Darwinian Left: Politics, Evolution, and Cooperation. New Haven, CT: Yale University Press.

Singer, D. (2004). Respir Physiol Neurobiol, 141(3):215–228.

Singer, L. T., Linares, T. J., Ntiri, S., Henry, R., et al. (2004). Drug Alcohol Depend, 74(3):245–252.

Singh, B., Mortensen, N. J. M., Jewell, D. P., & George, B. (2004). Br J Surg, 91(7):801–814.

Singh, D. (1993). J Pers Soc Psychol, 65(2):293–307.

Singh, R. B., Sharma, J. P., Rastogi, V., Raghuvanshi, R. S., et al. (1997). Eur Heart J, 18(11):1728–1735.

Singhal, A., Wells, J., Cole, T. J., Fewtrell, M., et al. (2003). Am J Clin Nutr, 77(3):726–730.

Sinnathuray, T. A. (1988). Malays J Reprod Health, 6(2):70–82.

Skaldeman, S. S. (2005). Ät Dig Ner i Vikt: Praktisk Viktminskning för Feta Män och Runda Kvinnor [Eating for Weight Loss: Practical Weight Reduction for Fat Men and Chubby Women]. Stockholm, Sweden. Prisma.

Skjervold, H. (1992). Lifestyle Diseases and the Human Diet: How Should the New Discoveries Influence Future Food Production. Lillestrøm, Norway: Media Øst Trykk.

Sloane, E. (2002). Biology of Women, 4th ed. Albany, NY: Delmar Thomson Learning.

Small, M. F. (1998). Our Babies Ourselves—How Biology and Culture Shape the Way We Parent. New York: Doubleday Dell Publishing Group Inc.

Smith, B. H. (1991). Am J Phys Anthropol, 86(2):157–174.

Smith, B. H., Watt, G. C., Campbell, H., & Sheikh, A. (2006). Br J Gen Pract, 56(524):214–221.

Smith, C. P., Dunger, D. B., Williams, A. J. K., Taylor, A. M., et al. (1989). J Clin Endocrinol Metab, 68(5):932–937.

Smith, D. J. (2006). Science, 312(5772):392–394.

Smith, E. A., Udry, J. R., & Morris, N. M. (1985). J Health Soc Behav, 26(3):183–192.

Smith, E. A., Borgerhoff Mulder, M., & Hill, K. (2000). Anim Behav, 60(4):F21–F26.

Smith, E. O. (1999). Evolution, substance abuse, and addiction. In: Evolutionary Medicine, W. R. Trevathan, E. O. Smith, & J. J. McKenna (eds.). New York: Oxford University Press, pp. 375–405.

Smith, R., & Studd, J. W. W. (1992). J R Soc Med, 85(10):612–613.

Smith, T. G., Brooks, J. T., Balanos, G. M., Lappin, T. R., et al. (2006). PLoS Med, 3(7):e290.

Smits, L. J., Van Poppel, F. W., Verduin, J. A., Jongbloet, P. H., et al. (1997). Hum Reprod, 12(11):2572–2578.

Sneath, P. H. A. (1967). J Zool, 151(Pt 1):65–122.

Snowden, R., Christian, B., & World Health Organization. (1983). Patterns and Perceptions of Menstruation: A World Health Organization International Collaborative Study in Egypt, India, Indonesia, Jamaica, Mexico, Pakistan, Philippines, Republic of Korea, United Kingdom and Yugoslavia. New York: St. Martin's Press.

Sobel, J. D. (1985). Am J Obstet Gynecol, 152(7 [Pt 2]):924–935.

Society for Menstrual Cycle Research (2003). Menstrual Supression. Pittsburgh: Society for Menstrual Cycle Research

Solomon, C. G., & Manson, J. E. (1997). Am J Clin Nutr, 66(Suppl 4):1044S–1050S.

Solomon, C. G. (1999). Endocrinol Metab Clin North Am, 28(2):247–263.

Solomons, N. W., Mazariegos, M., Brown, K. H., & Klasing, K. (1997). Nutr Rev, 51(11):327–332.

Solomons, N. W. (2003). J Nutr, 133(5):1237–1237.

Solvoll, K., Lund-Larsen, K., Søyland, E., Sandstad, B., et al. (1993). Scand J Nutr, 37(150–155.

Somer, E. (2001). The Origin Diet: How Eating Like a Stone Age Ancestor Will Maximize Your Health. New York: Henry Holt and Company.

Sopori, M. (2002). Nature Reviews. Immunology, 2(5):372–327.

Sorbi, S., Nacmias, B., Forleo, P., Piacentini, S., et al. (1995). Ann Neurol, 38(1):124–127.

Southam, A. L., & Gonzaga, F. P. (1965). Am J Obstet Gynecol, 91(1):142–165.

Sözmen, M. (1992). Biol Neonate, 62:67–68.

Spangler, G., & Grossmann, K. E. (1993). Child Dev, 64(5):1439–1450.

Speakman, J. R. (2004). J Nutr, 134(Suppl 8):2090S–2105S.

Speroff, L., Glass, R. H., & Kase, N. G. (1999). Clinical Gynecologic Endocrinology and Infertility, 6th ed. Philadelphia: Lippincott Williams, & Wilkins.

Speth, J. D., & Spielman, K. A. (1983). J Anthro Arch, 2(1):1–31.

Speth, J. D. (1991). Philos Trans R Soc Lond B Biol Sci, 334(1270):265–269; discussion 269–270.

Spiegel, A. M., & Nabel, E. G. (2006). Nat Med, 12(1):67–69.

Spiegel, K., Leproult, R., & van Cauter, E. (1999). Lancet, 354(9188):1435–1439.

Spiegel, K., Leproult, R., L'Hermite-Baleriaux, M., Copinschi, G., et al. (2004). J Clin Endocrinol Metab, 89(11):5762–5771.

Spiegel, K., Tasali, E., Penev, P., & van Cauter, E. (2004). Ann Intern Med, 141(11):846–850.

Spiegel, K., Knutson, K., Leproult, R., Tasali, E., et al. (2005). J Appl Physiol, 99(5):2008–2019.

Spiller, R. C. (2003). Hosp Med, 64(5):270–274.

Spinella, M. (2003). Int J Neurosci, 113(4):503–512.

Spinillo, A., Capuzzo, E., Nicola, S., Baltaro, F., et al. (1995). Contraception, 51(5):293–297.

Spock, B. (1946). The Common Sense Book of Baby and Child Care. New York: Duell.

Spock, B., & Parker, S. (1998). Dr. Spock's Baby and Child Care: A Handbook for Parents of the Developing Child from Birth Through Adolescence, 7th ed. New York: Dutton.

Spock, B., & Needlman, R. (2004). Dr. Spock's Baby and Child Care: A Handbook for Parents of Developing Children From Birth Through Adolescence, 8th ed. New York: Simon & Schuster, Inc.

Spurlock, M. (2005). Don't Eat This Book: Fast Food and the Supersizing of America. New York: G. P. Putnam's Sons.

Srebrnik, A., & Segal, E. (1990). Acta Derm Venereol, 70(6):459–462.

Sriram, S., Mitchell, W., & Stratton, C. (1998). Neurology, 50(2):571–572.

St. Geme, J. W. (2002). Cell Microbiol, 4(4):191–200.

Stamler, J. (1997). Am J Clin Nutr, 65(Suppl 2):626S–642S.

Stanley, O. H., & Speidel, B. D. (1985). J Perinat Med, 13(5):253–255.

Stearns, S. C. (1982). The role of development in the evolution of life histories. In: Evolution and Development, J. T. Bonner (ed.). Berlin: Springer-Verlag, pp. 237–258.

Stearns, S. C. (1992). The Evolution of Life Histories. Oxford, UK: Oxford University Press.

Stearns, S. C. (ed.) (1999). Evolution in Health and Disease. Oxford, UK: Oxford University Press.

Stearns, S. C., & Ebert, D. (2001). Q Rev Biol, 76(4):417–432.

Stearns, S. C., & Hoekstra, R. F. (2005). Evolution: An Introduction, 2nd ed. Oxford, UK: Oxford University Press.

Steckler, T., Wang, J. R., Bartol, F. F., Roy, S. K., et al. (2005). Endocrinology, 146(7):3185–3193.

Stefansson, V. (1937). J Am Diet Assoc, 13:102–119.

Stefansson, V. (1946). Not By Bread Alone. New York: Macmillan Company.

Stefansson, V. (1960). Cancer: Disease of Civilization. An Anthropological and Historical Study. New York: Hill and Wang.

Steiger, A. (2003). Front Biosci, 8:S358–S376.

Stein, A. D., & Lumey, L. H. (2000). Hum Biol, 72(4):641–654.

Stein, C. J., & Colditz, G. A. (2004). J Clin Endocrinol Metab, 89(6):2522–2525.

Steinberg, A. D., & Steinberg, B. J. (1985). J Rheumatol, 12(4):816–817.

Steiner, A. A., & Branco, L. G. (2002). Annu Rev Physiol, 64:263–288.

Stempsey, W. E. (2000). Theor Med Bioeth, 21(4):321–330.

Stephan, F. K. (2002). J Biol Rhythms, 17(4):284–292.

Stephens, D. W., & Krebs, J. R. (1986). Foraging Theory. Princeton, NJ: Princeton University Press.

Stephensen, C. B. (1999). J Nutr, 129(2):534S–538S.

Steppan, C. M., Bailey, S. T., Bhat, S., Brown, E. J., et al. (2001). Nature, 409(6818):307–312.

Sternglass, E. J., & Bell, S. (1983). Phi Delta Kappan, April:539–545.

Sternglass, E. J., & Bell, S. (1984). Phi Delta Kappan, January:372–373.

Stevens, A., & Price, J. (1996). Evolutionary Psychiatry: A New Beginning. London, UK: Routledge.

Steyn, K., Bourne, L., Jooste, P., Fourie, J. M., et al. (1998). East Afr Med J, 75(1):35–40.

Stiner, M. C., Munro, N. D., Survovell, T. A., Tchernov, E., et al. (1999). Science, 283(5399):190–194.

Stiner, M. C., Munro, N. D., & Surovell, T. A. (2000). Curr Anthropol, 41(1):39–73.

Stiner, M. C. (2001). J Arch Res, 10(1):1–63.

Stiner, M. C., & Munro, N. D. (2002). J Arch Meth Theo, 9(2):181–214.

Stinson, S. (1992). Annu Rev Anthropol, 21(143–170.

Stirbu, I., Kunst, A. E., Bos, V., & Mackenbach, J. P. (2006). BMC Public Health, 6:78.

Stobo, J. D., Paul, S., Van Scoy, R. E., & Hermans, P. E. (1976). J Clin Invest, 57(2):319–328.

Stocker, R., Yamamoto, Y., McDonagh, A. F., Glazer, A. N., et al. (1987). Science, 235(4792):1043–1046.

Stoltenberg, J. L., Osborn, J. B., Pihlstrom, B. L., Herzberg, M. C., et al. (1993). J Periodontol, 64(12):1225–1230.

Størmer, F. C. (1993). Tidsskr Nor Lægeforen, 113:1061–1063.

Story, M., & French, S. (2004). Int J Behav Nutr Phys Act, 1:3.

Stradling, J. R., & Davies, R. J. O. (2004). Thorax, 59(1):73–78.

Strassmann, B. I. (1996). Q Rev Biol, 71(2):181–220.

Strassmann, B. I. (1997). Curr Anthropol, 38(1):123–129.

Strassmann, B. I. (1999). J Womens Health, 8(2):193–202.

Strassmann, B. I., & Dunbar, R. I. M. (1999). Human evolution and disease: Putting the stone age in perspective. In: Evolution in Health & Disease, S. C. Stearns (ed.). Oxford, UK: Oxford University Press, pp. 91–101.

Streeten, D. (1993). J Clin Endocrinol Metab, 77(2):339–340.

Striedter, G. F. (2006). Behav Brain Sci, 29(1):1–36.

Strine, T. W., & Chapman, D. P. (2005). Sleep Med, 6(1):23–27.

Stroebele, N., & de Castro, J. M. (2004). Appetite, 42(1):111–113.

Strohman, R. C. (1993). Perspect Biol Med, 37(1):112–145.

Struthers, A. D. (1996). J Card Fail, 2(1):47–54.

Stuart-Macadam, P. (1995). Biocultural perspectives on breastfeeding. In: Breastfeeding: Biocultural Perspectives, P. Stuart-Macadam & K. Dettwyler (eds.). New York: Aldine de Gruyter, pp. 1–37.

Suarez, F. L., Adshead, J., Furne, J. K., & Levitt, M. D. (1998). Am J Clin Nutr, 68(5):1118–1122.

Sullivan, J. L. (1989). Am Heart J, 117(5):1177–1188.

Sullivan, J. L. (1996). J Clin Epidemiol, 49(12):1345–1352.

Sullivan, J. L., & Weinberg, E. D. (1999). Emerg Infect Dis, 5(5):724–726.

Sullivan, R. J., & Hagen, E. H. (2002). Addiction, 97(4):389–400.

Sumaya, C. V., Myers, L. W., Ellison, G. W., & Ench, Y. (1985). Ann Neurol, 17(4):371–377.

Suomi, S. J. (1997). Long-term effects of differential early experiences on social, emotional, and physiological development in nonhuman primates. In: Neurodevelopmental Models of Adult Psychopathology, M. S. Keshevan & R. M. Murra (eds.). Cambridge, UK: Cambridge University Press, pp. 104–116.

Sureender, S., Prabakaran, B., & Khan, A. G. (1998). Soc Biol, 45(3–4):289–301.

Susman, E., & Pajer, K. (2004). Biology-behavior integration and antisocial behavior in girls. In: Aggression, Antisocial Behavior, and Violence Among Girls: A Developmental Perspective, M. Putallaz & K. L. Bierman (eds.). New York: Guilford Press, pp. 23–47.

Svensson, K., Matthiesen, A.-S., & Widstrom, A.-M. (2005). Birth, 32(2):99–106.

Swagerty, D. L., Walling, A. D., & Klein, R. M. (2002). Am Fam Physician, 65(9):1845–1850.

Swallow, D. M. (2003). Annu Rev Genet, 37(197–219).

Swanborg, R. H., Whittum-Hudson, J. A., & Hudson, A. P. (2003). J Neuroimmunol, 136(1–8.

Swanton, A., & Child, T. (2005). J Br Menopause Soc, 11(4):126–131.

Swedberg, K., Eneroth, P., Kjekshus, J., & Wilhelmsen, L. (1990). Circulation, 82(5):1730–1736.

Swedo, S. E. (1994). J Am Med Assoc, 272(22):1788–1791.

Swedo, S. E., Leonard, H. L., Garvey, M., Mittleman, B., et al. (1998). Am J Psychiatry, 155(2):264–271.

Sweet, J. B., & Butler, D. P. (1977). Am J Obstet Gynecol, 127(5):518–519.

Sweet, K. M., Bradley, T. L., & Westman, J. A. (2002). J Clin Oncol, 20(2):528–537.

Symonds, M. E., Mostyn, A., Pearce, S., Budge, H., et al. (2003). J Endocrinol, 179(3):293–299.

Symons, D. (1978). Play and Aggression: A Study of Rhesus Monkeys. New York: Columbia University Press.

Szathmáry, E. J. E. (1994). Annu Rev Anthropol, 23(1):457–482.

Taheri, S., Lin, L., Austin, D., Young, T., et al. (2004). PLoS Med, 1(3):e62.

Taieb, O., Baleyte, J. M., Mazet, P., & Fillet, A. M. (2001). Eur Psychiatry, 16(1):3–10.

Takahashi, E. (1966). Hum Biol, 38(2):112–130.

Takahashi, E. (1971). Jinruigaku Zasshi, 79(3):259–285.

Takahashi, E. (1984). Hum Biol, 56(3):427–437.

Takahashi, L. K. (1992). Clin Neuropharmacol, 15(Suppl 1 [Pt A]):153A–154A.

Takahashi, M., & Yamada, T. (2001). Adv Neurol, 86:91–104.

Takala, A. K., & Clements, D. A. (1992). J Infect Dis, 165(Suppl 1):S11–S15.

Takei, Y. (2001). Comp Biochem Physiol B Biochem Mol Biol, 129(2–3):559–573.

Takei, Y., & Hirose, S. (2002). Am J Physiol Regul Integr Comp Physiol, 282(4):R940–R951.

Talpade, M., & Talpade, S. (2001). Adolescence, 36(144):789–794.

Tamer, E., Ikizoglu, G., Toy, G. G., & Alli, N. (2003). Int J Dermatol, 42(6):455–458.

Tan, K. S. (2001). Drugs, 61(14):2079–2086.

Tanasescu, C., Parvu, M., Antohi, I., & Lazar, S. (1999). Rom J Intern Med, 37(1):53–64.

Tang, N. K., Schmidt, D. A., & Harvey, A. G. (2007) J Behav Ther Exp Psychiatry, 38(1)40–55.

Tangpricha, V., Turner, A., Spina, C., Decastro, S., et al. (2004). Am J Clin Nutr, 80(6):1645–1649.

Tanner, J. M. (1962). Growth at Adolescence, With a General Consideration of the Effects of Hereditary and Environmental Factors Upon Growth and Maturation From Birth to Maturity, 2nd ed. Oxford, UK: Blackwell Scientific Publications.

Tanner, J. M., & Taylor, G. R. (1965). Growth. New York: Time.

Tanner, J. M., Whitehouse, R. H., & Takaishi, M. (1966). Arch Dis Child, 41(219):454–471.

Tanner, J. M. (1990). Fetus Into Man: Physical Growth from Conception to Maturity. Cambridge, MA: Harvard University Press.

Tanner, J. M. (1992). Horm Res, 38(Suppl 1):106–115.

Targum, S. D., Caputo, K. P., & Ball, S. K. (1991). J Affect Disord, 22(1–2):49–53.

Tasaki, N., Nakajima, M., Yamamoto, H., Imazu, M., et al. (2003). Atherosclerosis, 171(1):117–122.

Tattersall, G. J., Blank, J. L., & Wood, S. C. (2002). J Appl Physiol, 92(1):202–210.

Tattersall, I. (1998). Becoming Human: Evolution and Human Uniqueness. New York: Harcourt Brace & Company.

Taubes, G. (2001). Science, 291(5513):2536–2545.

Tavassoli, M. (1987). Bull Adler Mus Hist Med, 13(2):48–49.

Taylor, A. L., Ziesche, S., Yancy, C., Carson, P., et al. (2004). N Engl J Med, 351(20):2049–2057.

Taylor, F. K. (1980). Psychol Med, 10(3):419–424. Taylor, M. W., & Feng, G. (1991). FASEB J, 5(11):2516–2522.

te Velde, S. J., van Rossum, E. F., Voorhoeve, P. G., Twisk, J. W., et al. (2005). BMC Endocr Disord, 5:5.

Teegarden, D., Lyle, R. M., Proulx, W. R., Johnston, C. C., et al. (1999). Am J Clin Nutr, 69(5):1014–1017.

Teicher, M. H., Andersen, S. L., Polcari, A., Anderson, C. M., et al. (2003). Neurosci Biobehav Rev, 27(1–2):33–44.

Tell, G. S., & Vellar, O. D. (1988). Prev Med, 17(1):12–14.

Ten Have, H. (1995). Theor Med, 16(1):3–14.

Tennekoon, K. H., Arulambalam, P. D., Karunanayake, E. H., & Seneviratne, H. R. (1994). Asia Oceania J Obstet Gynaecol, 20(3):311–319.

Terayama, H., Nishino, Y., Kishi, M., Ikuta, K., et al. (2003). Psychiatry Res, 120(2):201–206.

Teruya, H., Yamazato, M., Muratani, H., Sakima, A., et al. (1997). J Clin Invest, 99(11):2791–2798.

Tesali, E., & van Cauter, E. (2002). Am J Respir Crit Care Med, 165(5):562–563.

Tesch, P. A., & Karlsson, J. (1985). J Appl Physiol, 59(6):1716–1720.

Thom, D. H., Nelson, L. M., & Vaughan, T. L. (1992). Am J Obstet Gynecol, 166(1 [Pt 1]):111–116.

Thom, T., Haase, N., Rosamond, W., Howard, V. J., et al. (2006). Circulation, 113(6):e85–151.

Thomas, D. B., & Karagas, M. R. (1987). Cancer Res, 47(21):5771–5776.

Thys–Jacobs, S., Silverton, M., Alvir, J., Paddison, P. L., et al. (1995). J Womens Health, 4(2):161–168.

Tinbergen, N. (1963). Z Tierpsychol, 20:410–433.

Tissot van Patot, M. C., Leadbetter, G., Keyes, L. E., Bendrick-Peart, J., et al. (2005). J Appl Physiol, 98(5):1626–1629.

Tobler, I. (2000). Phylogeny of sleep regulation. In: Principles and Practice of Sleep Medicine, M. H. Kryger, T. Roth, & W. C. Dement (eds.). Philadelphia: W.B. Saunders, pp. 72–81.

Tolstoi, E. (1929). J Biol Chem, 83(3):753–758.

Tononi, G. (2005). Sleep Med, 6(Suppl 1):S8–S12.

Toop, T., & Donald, J. A. (2004). J Comp Physiol [B], 174(3):189–204.

Toppari, J. (2002). Sem Reprod Med, 20(3):305–311.

Tordoff, M. G. (1989). Appetite, 12:74.

Torrey, E. F., & Yolken, R. H. (2003). Emerg Infect Dis, 9(11):1375–1380.

Torrey, E. F., & Yolken, R. H. (2005). Beasts of the Earth. New Brunswick, NJ: Rutgers University Press.

Toth, A., Lesser, M. L., Naus, G., Brooks, C., et al. (1988). J Int Med Res, 16(4):270–279.

Travis, J. (1994). Ecological genetics of life-history traits: Variation and its evolutionary significance. In: Ecological Genetics, L. Real (ed.). Princeton, NJ: Princeton University Press, pp. 171–204.

Treloar, A. E., Boynton, R. E., Behn, B. G., & Brown, B. W. (1967). Int J Fertil, 12(1 [Part 2]):77–126.

Treloar, S. A., Heath, A. C., & Martin, N. G. (2002). Psychol Med, 32(1):25–38.

Trevathan, W. (1987). Human Birth: An Evolutionary Perspective. New York: Aldine de Gruyer.

Trevathan, W. R., & McKenna, J. J. (1994). Child Envir, 11(2):88–104.

Trevathan, W. R. (1999). Evolutionary obstetrics. In: Evolutionary Medicine, W. R. Trevathan, E. O. Smith, & J. J. McKenna (eds.). New York: Oxford University Press, pp. 407–427.

Trevathan, W. R., Smith, E. O., & McKenna, J. J. (eds.). (1999). Evolutionary Medicine. New York: Oxford University Press.

Trichopolous, D., Yen, S., Brown, J. P., Cole, P., et al. (1984). Cancer, 53(1):187–192.

Trivers, R. L. (1972). Parental investment and sexual selection. In: Sexual Selection and the Descent of Man, B. G. Campbell (ed.). Chicago: Aldine, pp. 136–179.

Trivers, R. L. (1974). Am Zool, 14:249–264.

Trivers, R. (2002). Natural Selection and Social Theory: Selected Papers of Robert Trivers. Oxford, UK: Oxford University Press.

Trussell, J., & Kost, K. (1987). Stud Fam Plann, 18(5):237–283.

Trzonkowski, P., Mysliwska, J., Lukaszuk, K., Szmit, E., et al. (2001). Horm Metab Res, 33:348–353.

Tubman, J. G., Windle, M., & Windle, R. C. (1996). Child Dev, 67(2):327–343.

Tuffaha, A., Gern, J. E., & Lemanske, R. F. (2000). Clin Chest Med, 21(2):289–300.

Tunca, S., Turkay, C., Tekin, O., Kargili, A., et al. (2004). Acta Neurol Belg, 104(4):161–164.

Turini, G. A., Brunner, H. R., Gribic, M., Waeber, B., et al. (1979). Lancet, 313(8128):1213–1215.

Turner, P., Runtz, M., & Galambos, N. (1999). J Reprod Infant Psychol, 17(2):111–118.

Tverdal, A. (1996). Tidsskr Nor Lægeforen, 116(18):2152–2156.

Twaddle, A., & Nordenfeldt, L. (1993). Disease, Illness and Sickness: Three Central Concepts in the Theory of Health. Linköping, Sweden. Linköping University. Department of Health and Society.

Tworoger, S. S., Davis, S., Vitiello, M. V., Lentz, M. J., et al. (2005). J Psychosom Res, 59(1):11–19.

Tyner, R., & Turett, G. (2004). South Med J, 97(4):393–394.

Tzourio, C., Tehindrazanarivelo, A., Iglesias, S., Alperovitch, A., et al. (1995). BMJ, 310(6983):830–833.

Udry, J. R. (1979). J Biosoc Sci, 11(4):433–441.

Udry, J. R., & Cliquet, R. L. (1982). Demography, 19(1):53–63.

Ulijaszek, S. J., & Strickland, S. S. (1993). Nutritional Anthropology: Prospects and Perspectives. London: Smith-Gordon.

Ulijaszek, S. J. (2002). Proc Nutr Soc, 61(4):517–526.

Ungar, P. S., & Teaford, M. F. (2002). Perspectives on the evolution of human diet. In: Human Diet: Its Origin and Evolution, P. S. Ungar & M. F. Teaford (eds.). Westport, CT: Bergin & Garvey, pp. 1–6.

United Nations International Children's Emergency Fund (2006). The State of the World's Children: 2006. Information by Country, http://www.unicef.org/infobycountry bangladesh_bangladesh_statistics.html

United Nations International Children's Emergency Fund United Kingdom Baby Friendly Initiative (2000). Implementing the Baby Friendly Best Practice Standards. London, UK: United Kingdon Committee on UNICEF.

United States Census Bureau (2006). Table 596. Persons on shift schedules: 2004, http://www.census.gov/compendia/statab/labor_force_employment_earnings employed_persons/

United States Department of Agriculture (1990). Fluid Milk Promotion Act of 1990, http://www.ams.usda.gov/dairy/fldact.htm

United States Department of Agriculture (1998). US Government Agriculture Fact Book, http:// www.usda.gov/news/pubs/fbook98/ch1a.htm

United States Department of Agriculture (2003). The National School Lunch Program: History and Development, http://www.fns.usda.gov/cnd/lunch/AboutLunch/ProgramHistory.htm

United States Department of Agriculture (2004). Report to Congress on the National Dairy Promotion and Research Program and the National Fluid Milk Processor Promotion Program. Washington, DC: United States Department of Agriculture.

United States Department of Agriculture (2005). Nutrient Database for Standard Reference, Release 18, http://www.nal.usda.gov/fnic/foodcomp

United States Department of Agriculture (2006). Production, Supply and Distribution Online, http://www.fas.usda.gov/psdonline/psdHome.aspx

United States Department of Health and Human Services (2003). National Sleep Disorders Research Plan, L. National Institutes of Health. National Heart, and Blood Institute. National Center on Sleep Disorders Research (ed.). Washington, DC: National Institutes of Health.

United States Department of Health and Human Services, & United States Department of Agriculture (2005). Dietary Guidelines for Americans 2005, http://www.health.gov dietaryguidelines/dga2005/document/pdf/DGA2005.pdf

United States Food and Drug Administration (2003). FDA Approves Seasonale Oral Contraceptive. Washington, DC.

Urakami, K., Adachi, Y., Wakutani, Y., Isoe, K., et al. (1998). Dement Geriatr Cogn Disord, 9(5):294–298.

Uvnas-Moberg, K., Widstrom, A.-M., Werner, S., Matthiesen, A.-S., et al. (1990). Acta Obstet Gynecol Scand, 69(4):301–306.

Vaag, A., Jensen, C. B., Poulsen, P., Brons, C., et al. (2006). Horm Res, 65(Suppl 3):137–143.

Vadheim, C. M., Greenberg, D. P., Bordenave, N., Ziontz, L., et al. (1992). Am J Epidemiol, 136(2):221–235.

Valdez, R., Athens, M. A., Thompson, G. H., Bradshaw, B. S., et al. (1994). Diabetologia, 37(6):624–631.

Valentin, S. R. (2005). Pediatrics, 115(1):269–271.

Valentino, R., Savastano, S., Tommaselli, A. P., Riccio, A., et al. (1993). J Endocrinol Invest, 16(8):619–624.

Valentin-Weigand, P. (2004). Berl Munch Tierarztl Wochenschr, 117(11–12):459–463.

Valenzuela, M. (1997). Dev Psychol, 33(5):845–855.

Valkonen, M., & Kuusi, T. (1998). Circulation, 97(20):2012–2016.

van Broeckhoven, C., Backhovens, H., Cruts, M., Martin, J. J., et al. (1994). Neurosci Lett, 169(1–2):179–180.

van Cauter, E., & Spiegel, K. (1999). Ann NY Acad Sci, 896:254–261.

van der Heijden, I. M., Wilbrink, B., Tchetverikov, I., Schrijver, I. A., et al. (2000). Arthritis Rheum, 43(3):593–598.

van der Spuy, Z. M., & Dyer, S. J. (2004). Best Pract Res Clin Obstet Gynaecol, 18(5):755–771.

van der Wielen, R. P. J., Lowik, M. R. H., van den Berg, H., de Groot, L., et al. (1995). Lancet, 346(8969):207–210.

van Hooff, M. H. A., Voorhorst, F. J., Kaptein, M. B. H., Hirasing, R. A., et al. (2004). Hum Reprod, 19(2):383–392.

van Mil, A. H., Spilt, A., Van Buchem, M. A., Bollen, E. L., et al. (2002). J Appl Physiol, 92(3):962–966.

van Schilfgaarde, M., Eijk, P., Regelink, A., van Ulsen, P., et al. (1999). Microb Pathog, 26(5):249–262.

van Weissenbruch, M. M., Engelbregt, M. J., Veening, M. A., & Delemarre–van de Waal, H. A. (2005). Endocr Dev, 8:15–33.

VandenBergh, M. F. Q., DeMan, S. A., Witteman, J. C. M., Hofman, A., et al. (1995). J Epidemiol Community Health, 49(3):299–304.

Vanhaereny, M., d'Errico, F., Stringer, C., James, S. L., et al. (2006). Science, 312(5781):1785–1788.

Varki, A. (2001). Yearb Phys Anthropol, 44:54–69.

Venkatesha, S., Toporsian, M., Lam, C., Hanai, J., et al. (2006). Nat Med, 12(6):642–649.

Venturoli, S., Porcu, E., Fabbri, R., Magrini, O., et al. (1987). Fertil Steril, 48(1):78–85.

Verhoef, C. M., van Roon, J. A. G., Vianen, M. E., Bruijnzeel-Koomen, C. A. F. M., et al. (1998). Ann Rheum Dis, 57(5):275–280.

Verrett, J. (1974). Eating May Be Hazardous to Your Health. The Case Against Food Additives. New York: Simon & Schuster.

Vessey, M., & Painter, R. (2001). Contraception, 63(2):61–63.

Vessey, M., Painter, R., & Yeates, D. (2002). Contraception, 66(2):77–79.

Via, S. (1994). The evolution of phenotypic plasticity: What do we really know? In: Ecological Genetics, L. Real (ed.). Princeton, NJ: Princeton University Press, pp. 35–57.

Vieth, R. (1999). Am J Clin Nutr, 69(5):842–856.

Vieth, R. (2001). J Nutr Environ Med, 11:275–291.

Vihko, R., & Apter, D. (1984). J Steroid Biochem, 20(1):231–236.

Vioque, J., Torres, A., & Quiles, J. (2000). Int J Obes Relat Metab Disord, 24(12):1683–1688.

Vitzhum, V. (2001). Why not so great is still good enough. In: Reproductive Ecology and Human Evolution, P. T. Ellison (ed.). New York: Aldine de Gruyter, pp. 179–202.

Vitzthum, V. J., Bentley, G. R., Spielvogel, H., Caceres, E., et al. (2002). Reprod, 17(7):1906–1913.

Vitzthum, V. J., Spielvogel, H., & Thornburg, J. (2004). Proc Natl Acad Sci USA, 101(6):1443–1448.

Vogel, F., & Motulsky, A. G. (1997). Human Genetics, 3rd ed. Berlin. Springer-Verlag.

Vohr, B. R., & Oh, W. (1983). J Pediatr, 103(6):941–945.

von Bertalanffy, L. (1950a). Br J Philos Sci, 1:134–165.

von Bertalanffy, L. (1950b). Science, 111(2872):23–29.

von Bertalanffy, L. (1969). General System Theory. New York: George Braziller.

von Hertzen, L. C. (1998). Ann Med, 30(1):27–37.

von Hertzen, L. C. (2002). Eur Respir J, 19(3):546–556.

Vorobyev, M. (2004). Clin Exp Optom, 87(4–5):230–238.

References

Vorster, H. H., Venter, C. S., Wissing, M. P., & Margetts, B. M. (2005). Public Health Nutr, 8(5):480–490.

Vu–Hong, T. A., Durand, E., Deghmoun, S., Boutin, P., et al. (2006). J Clin Endocrinol Metab, 91(6):2437–2440.

Waagstein, F., Hjalmarson, A., Varnauskas, E., & Wallentin, I. (1975). Br Heart J, 37(10):1022–1036.

Waaler, P. E. (1983). Acta Paediatr Scand, 308(Suppl.):1–41.

Wade, D. T., & Halligan, P. W. (2004). BMJ, 329(7479):1398–1401.

Wagner, J. D., Flinn, M. V., & England, B. G. (2002). Evol Hum Behav, 23(6):437–442.

Wagner, K. D. (1996). J Clin Psychiatry, 57(4):152–157.

Waldenstrom, U., & Swenson, A. (1991). Midwifery, 7(2):82–89.

Walker, J. J. (2000). Lancet, 356(9237):1260–1265.

Walker, M. P., & Stickgold, R. (2006). Annu Rev Psychol, 57:139–166.

Walker, R., Gurven, M., Hill, K., Migliano, A., et al. (2006). Am J Hum Biol, 18(3):295–311.

Wallace, D. C. (2005). Annu Rev Genet, 39:359–407.

Wamala, S. P., Wolk, A., & Orth-Gomer, K. (1997). Prev Med, 26(5 [Pt 1]):734–744.

Wang, C., Fortin, P. R., Li, Y., Panaritis, T., et al. (1999). J Rheumatol, 26(4):808–815.

Wang, C. C., McClelland, R. S., Overbaugh, J., Reilly, M., et al. (2004). AIDS, 18(2):205–209.

Wang, G. J., Volkow, N. D., Thanos, P. K., & Fowler, J. S. (2004). J Addict Dis, 23(3):39–53.

Wang, Y., Campbell, H. D., & Young, I. G. (1993). J Steroid Biochem Mol Biol, 44(3):203–210.

Wang, Y., Harvey, C. B., Hollox, E. J., Phillips, A. D., et al. (1998). Gastroenterology, 114(6):1230–1236.

Wang, Y., Jiang, J. D., Xu, D., Li, Y., et al. (2004). Cancer Res, 64(12):4105–4111.

Wansink, B. (1996). J Mark, 60(3):1–14.

Wansink, B., & van Ittersum, K. (2003). J Consum Res, 30(3):455–463.

Wansink, B. (2004). Annu Rev Nutr, 24:455–479.

Wansink, B., & Liebman, B. (2004). Nutr Action Healthlett, 31(2):1, 3–6.

Wansink, B. (2005). Marketing Nutrition: Soy, Functional Foods, Biotechnology, and Obesity. Urbana, IL: University of Illinois Press.

Wansink, B., van Ittersum, K., & Painter, J. E. (2006). Am J Prev Med, 31(3):240–243.

Ward, M. P., Milledge, J. S., & West, J. B. (2000). High Altitude Medicine and Physiology. London: Oxford University Press.

Warren, M. P. (1980). J Clin Endocrinol Metab, 51(5):1150–1157.

Warren, M. P., & Goodman, L. R. (2003). J Endocrinol Invest, 26(9):873–878.

Wassertheil–Smoller, S., Hendrix, S. L., Limacher, M., Heiss, G., et al. (2003). J Am Med Assoc, 289(20):2673–2684.

Waterlow, J. C. (1972). BMJ, 3(826):566–568.

Waterlow, J. C. (1981). The Energy Cost of Growth, Joint FAO/WHO/UNU Expert Consultation on Energy and Protein Requirements. Geneva: Food and Agriculture Organization of the United Nations, World Health Organization, The United Nations University.

Watkins, E. S. (1998). On the Pill: A Social History of Oral Contraceptives 1950–1970. Baltimore, MD: Johns Hopkins University Press.

Watkins, L. R., & Maier, S. F. (2000). Annu Rev Psychol, 51:29–57.

Watnick, A. S., & Russo, R. A. (1968). Proc Soc Exp Biol Med, 128(1):1–4.

Watson, J. B. (1928). Psychological Care of the Infant and Child. New York: W. W. Norton, & Co.

Weale, S. (2003). Too close for comfort?, London: The Guardian.

Weatherall, D. J. (1995). J Nutr Environ Med, 5:63–76.

Weatherall, D. J. (1997). Ann Trop Med Parasitol, 91(7):885–890.

Weatherby, S. J., Mann, C. L., Fryer, A. A., Strange, R. C., et al. (2000). J Neurol Neurosurg Psychiatry, 68(4):532–541.

Weaver, D. R., & Reppert, S. M. (1986). Endocrinology, 119(6):2861–2863.

517

.voni, N., Champagne, F. A., D'Alessio, A. C., et al. (2004). Nat Neurosci, 4.

(2003). J Exp Biol, 206(17):2911–2922.

.mmings, G. P. (2005). Med Hypotheses, 64(3):547–552.

Weil, 1993). Evolution and Congestive Heart Failure, Annual Meeting American Association for the Advancement of Science, Boston.

Weinberg, E. D. (1978). Microbiol Rev, 42(1):45–66.

Weinberg, G. A., Friis, H., Boelaert, J. R., & Weinberg, E. D. (2001). Clin Infect Dis, 33(12):2098–2100.

Weiner, H. (1992). Perturbing the Organism: The Biology of Stressful Experience. Chicago: University of Chicago Press.

Weinsier, R. L., & Krumdieck, C. L. (2000). Am J Clin Nutr, 72:681–689).

Weiss, D. J., Charles, M. A., Dunaif, A., Prior, D. E., et al. (1994). Metab Clin Exp, 43(7):803–807.

Weiss, F. (2005). Curr Opin Pharmacol, 5(1):9–19.

Weiss, K. M., Ferrell, R. E., & Hanis, C. L. (1984). Yearb Phys Anthropol, 27:153–178.

Wellens, R., Malina, R. M., Roche, A. F., Chumlea, W. C., et al. (1992). Am J Hum Biol, 4(6):783–787.

Wells, J. C. (2003). J Theor Biol, 221(1):143–161.

Wells, J. C., Hallal, P. C., Wright, A., Singhal, A., et al. (2005). Int J Obes (Lond), 29(10):1192–1198.

West, J. B. (2004). Ann Intern Med, 141(10):789–800.

West, K. M., Bailey, C. P., Coniglione, T. C., Smith, W. O., et al. (1974). Diabetes, 23(Suppl 1):385.

West–Eberhard, M. J. (2003). Developmental Plasticity and Evolution. New York: Oxford University Press.

Westman, E. C., Yancy, W. S., Edman, J. S., Tomlin, K. F., et al. (2002). Am J Med, 113(1):30–36.

Westman, E. C., Mavropoulos, J., Yancy, W. S., & Volek, J. S. (2003). Curr Atheroscler Rep, 5(6):476–483.

Westman, E. C., Yancy, W. S., & Humphreys, M. (2006). Perspect Biol Med, 49(1):77–83.

Wexler, R., & Feldman, D. (2006). J Fam Pract, 55(4):291–298.

Wharton, C. H. (2001). Metabolic Man: Ten Thousand Years from Eden. Orlando, FL: Winmark Publishers.

Whitacre, C. C., Reingold, S. C., & O'Looney, P. A. (1999). Science, 283(5406):1277–1278.

White, H. D., Crassi, K. M., Givan, A. L., Stern, J. E., et al. (1997). J Immunol, 158(6):3017–3027.

Wichers, M. C., & Maies, M. (2004). J Psychiatry Neurosci, 29(1):11–17.

Wiedenmayer, C. P. (2004). Neurosci Biobehav Rev, 28(1):1–12.

Wieseler–Frank, J., Maier, S. F., & Watkins, L. R. (2005). Neurosignals, 14(4):166–174.

Wikipedia (2006a), Hormones, http//en.wikipedia.org/wiki/Hormone

Wikipedia (2006b), Kentucky Fried Chicken (KFC), http://en.wikipedia.org/wiki/KFC

Wikipedia (2006c), Neuropeptides, http//en.wikipedia.org/wiki/Neuropeptide

Wikipedia (2006d), Pizza Hut, http://en.wikipedia.org/wiki/Pizza_hut

Wild, S., Roglic, G., Green, A., Sicree, R., et al. (2004). Diabetes Care, 27(5):1047–1053.

Wiley, A. S. (2004). Am Anthropol, 106(3):506–517.

Wiley, A. S. (2005). Am J Hum Biol, 17(4):425–441.

Wiley, A. S. 46 (3–4): 281–312. Ecol Food Nutr.

Wilkinson, G. S. (1984). Nature, 308(5955):181–184.

Wilkinson, R. G. (1996). Unhealthy Societies: The Afflictions of Inequality. London: Routledge.

Wilkinson, R. G. (2001). Mind the Gap: Hierarchies, Health and Human Evolution. New Haven, CT: Yale University Press.

Wilkinson, R. G. (2005). The Impact of Inequality: How to Make Sick Societies Healthier. New York: New Press.

Willerson, J. T., & Ridker, P. M. (2004). Circulation, 109(21 [Suppl 1]):II–2–II–10.

Willett, W. C. (1998a). Am J Clin Nutr, 68(6):1149–1150.

Willett, W. C. (1998b). Am J Clin Nutr, 67(Suppl 3):556S–562S.

Willett, W. C., Skerrett, P. J., Giovannucci, E. L., & Callahan, M. (2001). Eat, Drink and Be Healthy: The Harvard Medical School Guide to Healthy Eating. New York: Simon & Schuster.

Willett, W. C., & Stampfer, M. J. (2003). Sci Am, 288(1):52–59.

Willett, W. C. (2006). Public Health Nutr, 9(1A):105–110.

Williams, G. C. (1957). Evolution, 11(4):398–411.

Williams, G. C. (1966). Adaptation and Natural Selection: A Critique of Some Current Evolutionary Thought. Princeton, NJ: Princeton University Press.

Williams, G. C., & Nesse, R. M. (1991). Q Rev Biol, 66(1):1–22.

Williams, G. C. (1992). Natural Selection: Domains, Levels, and Challenges. New York: Oxford University Press.

Williams, G. C. (2000). Am J Hum Biol, 12(1):10–16.

Williams, K. E., & Koran, L. M. (1997). J Clin Psychiatry, 58(7):330–334.

Williams, L. L., Lowery, H. W., & Shannon, B. T. (1987). Arch Otolaryngol Head Neck Surg, 113(4):397–400.

Williams, R. J. (1987). The Wonderful World Within You. Wichita, KS: Bio-Communications Press.

Williams, R. J. (1998). Biochemical Individuality: The Basis for the Genetotrophic Concept. New Canaan, CT: Keats Publishing.

Willis, D., Mason, H., Gilling-Smith, C., & Franks, S. (1996). J Clin Endocrinol Metab, 81(1):302–309.

Wilmore, J. H., & Costill, D. L. (2004). Physiology of Sport and Exercise. Champaign, IL: Human Kinetics.

Wilson, E. E. (2003). Ethn Dis, 13(2 [Suppl 2]):S164–S166.

Wilson, E. O. (1998). Consilience: The Unity of Knowledge. New York: Knopf.

Wilson, M. E. (1998). J Endocrinol, 158(2):247–257.

Wilson, W. J. (1996). When Work Disappears: The World of the New Urban Poor. New York: Knopf.

Wingfield, J. C., & Sapolsky, R. M. (2003). J Neuroendocrinol, 15(8):711–724.

Winterhalder, B., & Smith, E. A. (eds.). (1981). Hunter-Gatherer Foraging Strategies: Ethnographic and Archeological Analyses. Chicago: University of Chicago Press.

Winterhalder, B., Lu, F., & Tucker, B. (1999). J Arch Res, 7(4):301–340.

Winterhalder, B., & Smith, E. A. (2000). Evol Anthropol, 9(2):51–72.

Wirleitner, B., Neurauter, G., Schroksnadel, K., Frick, B., et al. (2003). Curr Med Chem, 10(16):1581–1591.

Wise, R. A. (2002). Neuron, 36:229–240.

Witkin, S. S., Yu, I. R., & Ledger, W. J. (1983). Am J Obstet Gynecol, 147(7):809–811.

Wolf, F. W., & Heberlein, U. (2003). J Neurobiol, 54(1):161–178.

Wolf, K. (2002). Curr Biol, 12(7):R253–255.

Wong, M. D., Shapiro, M. F., Boscardin, W. J., & Ettner, S. L. (2002). N Engl J Med, 347(20):1585–1592.

Wood, J. W. (1994). Dynamics of Human Reproduction: Biology, Biometry, Demography. New York: Aldine.

Woolridge, M. W. (1995). Baby-controlled breastfeeding. In: Breastfeeding: Biocultural Perspectives, P. Stuart-Macadam & K. Dettwyler (eds.). New York: Aldine de Gruyter, pp. 217–242.

World Health Organization. (1999a). Birth, 26(4):255–258.

World Health Organization. (1999b). Reduction of Maternal Mortality: A Joint WHO/UNFPA UNICEF/World Bank Statement. Geneva: World Health Organization.

World Health Organization (2000a). Obesity: Preventing and Managing the Global Epidemic. Geneva: World Health Organization, pp. 1–253.

World Health Organization. (2000b). The Asia-Pacific Perspective: Redefining Obesity and Its Treatment. Geneva: World Health Organization.

World Health Organization (2001a), The optimal duration of exclusive breastfeeding: Results of a WHO systematic review, http://www.who.int/inf-pr-2001/en/note2001–07.html

World Health Organization (2001b), Mental and Neurological Disorders, http://www.who.int mediacentre/factsheets/fs265/en/

World Health Organization (2002), Obesity and environmental fact sheet 02, http: www.who.int/hpr/NPH/doc/gs_obesity.pdf

World Health Organization. (2003). Report of the World Health Organization and International Diabetes Federation Meeting. Geneva: World Health Organization.

World Health Organization (2004). Development of Food-based Dietary Guidelines for the Western Pacific Region. Geneva: World Health Organization.

World Health Organization (2005a). The World Health Report 2005. Geneva: World Health Organization.

World Health Organization (2005b), Tobacco Free Initiative, http://www.who.int/tobacco

World Health Organization (2006). 2005 Obesity and Overweight. Fact Sheet No 311, http://www.who.int/mediacentre/factsheets/fs311/en/index.html.

Worthman, C. M., Smith, E. O., & Weil, E. J. (1992). Why Do Women Menstruate? Annual Meeting American Anthropological Association, San Francisco, CA.

Worthman, C. M. (1998). Adolescence in the Pacific: A biosocial view. In: Adolescence in Pacific Island Societies, G. Herdt & S. C. Leavitt (eds.). Pittsburgh: University of Pittsburgh Press, pp. 27–52.

Worthman, C. M. (1999a). Epidemiology of human development. In: Hormones, Health, and Behaviour: A Socio-ecological and Lifespan Perspective, C. Panter-Brick & C. M. Worthman (eds.). Cambridge, UK: Cambridge University Press, pp. 47–104.

Worthman, C. M. (1999b). Evolutionary perspectives on the onset of puberty. In: Evolutionary Medicine, W. R. Trevathan, E. O. Smith, & J. J. McKenna (eds.). New York. Oxford University Press, pp. 135–164.

Worthman, C. M., & Melby, M. (2002). Toward a comparative developmental ecology of human sleep. In: Adolescent Sleep Patterns: Biological, Social, and Psychological Influences, M. A. Carskadon (ed.). New York: Cambridge University Press, pp. 69–117.

Worthman, C. M., & Kuzara, J. (2005). Am J Hum Biol, 17(1):95–112.

Worthman, C. M., & Brown, R. A. (2007). J Fam Psychol, 21(1):124–135.

Wrangham, R., McGrew, W. C., de Waal, F. B. M., & Heltne, P. (eds.). (1994). Chimpanzee Cultures. Cambridge, MA: Harvard University Press.

Wrangham, R. W., Jones, J. H., Laden, G., Pilbeam, D., et al. (1999). Curr Anthropol, 40(5):567–594.

Wray, C., & Gnanou, J. C. (2000). Int J Antimicrob Agents, 14(4):291–294.

Wright, P., MacCleod, H., & Cooper, M. J. (1983). Child Care Health Dev, 9(6):309–319.

Wright, P. (1987). Hunger, satiety, and feeding behavior in early infancy. In: Eating Habits: Food, Physiology and Learned Behaviour, R. A. Boakes, D. A. Popplewell, & M. J. Burton (eds.). Chichester, UK: John Wiley, & Sons, pp. 75–106.

Wright, K. P., Hull, J. T., Hughes, R. J., Ronda, J. M., et al. (2006). J Cogn Neurosci, 18(4):508–521.

Wu, H. M., Huang, C. C., Chen, S. H., Liang, Y. C., et al. (2003). Eur J Neurosci, 18(12):3294–3304.

Wurbel, H. (2001). Trends Neurosci, 24(4):207–211.

Wyatt, G., Durvasula, R. S., Guthrie, D., LeFranc, E., et al. (1999). Arch Sex Behav, 28(2):139–157.

Wyatt, H. R., Peters, J. C., Reed, G. W., Barry, M., et al. (2005). Med Sci Sports Exerc, 37(5):724–730.

Wykoff, C. C., Beasley, N. J., Watson, P. H., Turner, K. J., et al. (2000). Cancer Res, 60(24):7075–7083.

Wynne, K., Stanley, S., McGowan, B., & Bloom, S. (2005). J Endocrinol, 184(2):291–318.

Wysocki, C. J., & Pelchat, M. L. (1993). Crit Rev Food Sci Nutr, 33(1):63–82.

Xiao, B. G., Liu, X., & Link, H. (2004). Steroids, 69(10):653–659.

Yackinous, C., & Guinard, J. X. (2001). Physiol Behav, 72(3):427–437.

Yajnik, C. S., Fall, C. H., Vaidya, U., Pandit, A. N., et al. (1995). Diabet Med, 12(4):330–336.

Yajnik, C. S. (2000). Proc Nutr Soc, 59(2):257–265.

Yajnik, C. S. (2004). J Nutr, 134(1):205–210.

Yakova, M., Lezin, A., Dantin, F., Lagathu, G., et al. (2005). Retrovirology, 2(1):4–12.

Yamaguchi, S., & Ninomiya, K. (2000). J Nutr, 130(Suppl 4):921S–926S.

Yamauchi, Y., & Yamanouchi, I. (1990). Acta Paediatr Scand, 79(11):1017–1022.

Yanagawa, B., Spiller, O. B., Proctor, D. G., Choy, J., et al. (2004). J Infect Dis, 189(8):1431–1439.

Yancy, W. S., Foy, M., Chalecki, A. M., Vernon, M. C., et al. (2005). Nutr Metab, 2(34). http://www.nutritionandmetabolism.com/content/2/1/34

Yang, X., Schadt, E. E., Wang, S., Wang, H., et al. (2006). Genome Res, 16(8):995–1004.

Yavlovich, A., Tarshis, M., & Rottem, S. (2004). FEMS Microbiol Lett, 233(2):241–246.

Yehuda, R., Engel, S. M., Brand, S. R., Seckl, J., et al. (2005). J Clin Endocrinol Metab, 90(7):4115–4118.

Yell, J. A., & Burge, S. M. (1993). Br J Dermatol, 129(1):18–22.

Yip, R., Scanlon, K., & Trowbridge, F. (1992). J Am Med Assoc, 267(7):937–940.

Yip, R., Scanlon, K., & Trowbridge, F. (1993). Crit Rev Food Sci Nutrition, 33(4–5):409–421.

Ylitalo, N., Sorensen, P., Josefsson, A., Frisch, M., et al. (1999). Int J Cancer, 81(3):357–365.

Yolken, R. H., Bachmann, S., Ruslanova, I., Lillehoj, E., et al. (2001). Clin Infect Dis, 32(5):842–844.

Yoon, P. W., Scheuner, M. T., & Khoury, M. J. (2003). Am J Prev Med, 24(2):128–135.

Young, A. J., Young, P. M., McCullugh, R. E., Moore, L. G., et al. (1991). Eur J Appl Physiol Occup Physiol, 63(5):315–322.

Young, D. (2005). Birth, 32(3):161–163.

Young, J., Fleming, P., Blair, P., & Pollard, K. (2002). Night-time infant care practices: A longitudinal study of the importance of close contact between mothers and their babies. In: Stillmanagement und Laktation. Leipzig: Leipziger Universitätsverlag, pp. 179–209.

Young, J. B. (2004). Med Clin North Am, 88(5):1135–1143.

Young, J. H., Chang, Y. P., Kim, J. D., Chretien, J. P., et al. (2005). PLoS Genet, 1(6):e82.

Young, L. R., & Nestle, M. S. (1995). Nutr Rev, 53(6):149–158.

Young, L. R., & Nestle, M. S. (2002). Am J Public Health, 92(2):246–249.

Young, L. R., & Nestle, M. S. (2003). J Am Diet Assoc, 103(2):231–234.

Young, R. S., & Rosenbloom, A. L. (1998). Clin Pediatr (Phila), 37(2):63–65.

Young, S. E., Rhee, S. H., Stallings, M. C., Corley, R. P., et al. (2006). Behav Genet, 36(4):603–615.

Young, T. B., Peppard, P. E., & Gottlieb, D. J. (2002). Am J Respir Crit Care Med, 165(9):1217–1239.

Young, T. B. (2004). J Clin Psychiatry, 65(Suppl 16):12–16.

Young, T. K., Reading, J., Elias, B., & O'Neil, J. D. (2000). Can Med Assoc J, 163(5):561–566.

Yuen, M. F., Chan, T. M., Hui, C. K., On–On Chan, A., et al. (2001). J Viral Hepat, 8(6):459–464.

Zabin, L. S., Smith, E. A., Hirsch, M. B., & Hardy, J. B. (1986). Demography, 23(4):595–605.

Zambrano, E., Martinez-Samayoa, P. M., Bautista, C. J., Deas, M., et al. (2005). J Physiol, 566 (Pt 1):225–236.

Zampieri, F. (2006). Dal Darwinismo Medico Ottocentesco alla Medicina Darwiniana Contemporanea. Selezione Naturale, Disadattamento e Predisposizione Nell'Origine e nella Causalità delle Malattie [From 19th Century Medical Darwinism to Contemporary Darwinian Medicine, Natural Selection, Maladaptation and Predisposition in the Origin and Causality of Diseases], History. Parma, Italy: Department of History, University of Parma.

Zemel, B., Worthman, C., & Jenkins, C. (1993). Differences in endocrine status associated with urban-rural patterns of growth and maturation in Bundi (Gende-speaking) adolescents in Papua New Guinea. In: Urban Health and Ecology in the Third World, L. M. Schell, M. T. Smith, & A. Bilsborough (eds.). Cambridge, UK: Cambridge University Press, pp. 38–60.

Zentilin, P., Seriolo, B., Dulbecco, P., Caratto, E., et al. (2002). Aliment Pharmacol Ther, 16(7):1291–1299.

Zepelin, H. (2000). Mammalian sleep. In: Principles and Practice of Sleep Medicine, M. H. Kryger, T. Roth, & W. C. Dement (eds.). Philadelphia: W.B. Saunders, pp. 82–92.

Zera, A. J., & Harshman, L. G. (2001). Annu Rev Ecol Syst, 32:95–126.

Zhou, Y., Damsky, C. H., & Fisher, S. J. (1997). J Clin Invest, 99(9):2152–2164.

Zhu, M. J., Ford, S. P., Means, W. J., Hess, B. W., et al. (2006). J Physiol, 575(1):241–250.

Ziegler, R. G., Hoover, R. N., Pike, M. C., Hildesheim, A., et al. (1993). J Natl Cancer Inst, 85(22):1819–1827.

Zieske, A. W., Takei, H., Fallon, K. B., & Strong, J. P. (1999). Atherosclerosis, 144(2):403–408.

Zimmet, P., Taft, P., Guinea, A., Guthrie, W., et al. (1977). Diabetologia, 13(2):111–115.

Zimmet, P., Alberti, K. G., & Shaw, J. (2001). Nature, 414(6865):782–787.

Zlotogora, J. (1997). Am J Med Genet, 68(4):472–475.

Zorgdrager, A., & De Keyser, J. (1997). J Neurol Sci, 149(1):95–97.

INDEX

A amylase, 19, 76
ABO blood type, 68–69
ABN, 144
Accidents, 3, 30, 45, 53, 98, 292, 301, 303
Acclimatization, 138, 259, 270–72, 275
ACE, 387
ACE inhibitor, 384
Acetazolamide, 276
Acne, 104, 171, 194, 201, 417
ACTH, 304
Acute mountain sickness, 259–76
Acute phase reaction, 273
Adaptation, 2, 11, 116, 196, 259, 264, 279,
    285, 291, 306, 308–9, 313, 325, 375, 400,
    426, 428, 432, 439n; and attachment, 141;
    biopsychosocial, 49, 246, 285; dietary, 58, 64,
    66, 70, 102–3, 117, 131–32; and developmental
    plasticity, 162, 317, 329, 342, 345, 348; disease,
    6, 40, 279, 324, 401, 421; cardiovascular, 383,
    386, 388–89, 395, 397; environmental extremes,
    6, 11, 372; and hypoxia, 264; to malaria, 6–7;
    and pregnancy, 139, 199, 222–23; Paleolithic,
    61, 53, 106, 335; maximizing reproductive
    success, 136–37, 143–44, 146; mechanistic,
    138, 421; and reproduction, 165, 182, 197–98;
    for rest, 306, 309; tradeoffs, 147, 308
Adaptationist approach, 138–39, 141, 143–44, 146,
    197, 305, 309, 313, 401; and ultimate
    explanations, 138, 146,
Adaptive functions, 247, 417, 433; responses, 284,
    312, 314, 317, 319
ADD, 34
Addiction, 45–46, 48, 51–52, 277–90, 437
ADHD, 34
Adiponectin, 77
Adipose tissue, 77, 79, 82, 94. See also Fat
Adopted girls, 142, 143, 166
Adrenal gland, 247, 319, 387–88, 394
Adrenocorticotrophic hormone, 304
Adolescence, 36, 164, 245, 253, 321; adoption,
    166; exercise, 168; growth, 36, 127, 322, 336,
    402; mental health problems, 35; ovulation,
    161; sleep, 294, 303
Aerobic, 153, 260–62, 267–69, 274–75
Aetiology, 400
Africa, 7, 15–16, 26, 32, 36, 58, 68, 75, 84, 103,
    117–20, 130, 149, 192–93, 223, 250, 299,
    346–47, 356, 369, 371, 376–77, 380, 391, 427
African American, 81, 84, 118, 128, 130, 346–47,
    371, 374–75, 380; birth weight, 347;
    bone mass, 130; lactase persistence, 118; milk
    consumption, 128, 130; obesity, 84; thrifty
    genotype, 81

Agriculture, 3, 7, 12, 15, 17, 19, 56, 64–66, 70, 99,
    101–5, 120–24, 182, 344, 360, 364, 391, 396;
    dietary adaptations (genetic), 87, 100–103, 105,
    355–57; rise of, 65
Agricultural revolution, 64–65, 97–99; human
    health prior to, 97, 104
AIM. See Ancestral informative markers
Alcohol, 20, 36, 48, 51, 62, 88, 145, 160, 199, 280–81,
    285, 287, 352, 363–64, 366, 390–91, 395–97
Aldosterone, 382–83, 387–88, 394–95
Aleut, 81, 369
Allostatic load, 146–47, 308
Alu inserts, 369
Alzheimer's disease, 350, 353–54, 356, 357–59,
    366, 425
Amenorrhea. See Menstruation, amenorrhea
American Heart Association, 391, 397
American Indian, 85, 121, 369
Amphibian, 296, 330, 331, 383–84, 386, 389–90
AMS. See Acute mountain sickness
Anadromy, 389
Anaerobic, 261, 267–68, 274–75
Ancestral informative markers, 369, 371–72, 374
Ancestry: continental, 369; geographic, 368,
    370–71, 375–77, 379–80
Androgens, 169, 171–72, 174, 178–79
Anemia, hemolytic, 379
Angiogenesis, 271
Angiotensin, 382–83, 387, 394; angiotensin
    converting enzyme, 387; angiotensin converting
    enzyme inhibitor, 384
Animal protein, 58, 104, 114, 128, 130
Anopheles spp., 6–7
Anovulation, 171
ANP, 389
Antibiotic resistance, 1, 8, 12, 15, 414, 417, 421,
    424–25
Antiobesity drugs, 78, 94
Antioxidants, 105, 111, 262, 266, 269–70, 361
Anthropology, 5, 56, 179, 300, 423; applied, 227;
    biocultural, 278, 282–83, 290;
    biological/physical, 6, 179, 402; medical, 278;
    public health and, 425; sociocultural, 279
Appetite, hormonal control of, 76
Arthritis, 19, 37, 102, 104, 207, 357, 412
Ashkenazi, 369, 371–72, 378
Asian, 41, 42, 82, 91, 103, 118, 121, 163, 173, 175,
    178, 369, 376, 380, 435
Asian American, 380
Assortative mating, 81, 370
Asthma, 7, 34, 102, 208–9, 213, 274
Atherosclerotic coronary artery disease, 383
ATP, 268
Atrial natriuretic peptide, 129, 389

Attachment, 139, 141, 145, 257; parent-infant, 26, 248; theory, 139
Attention deficit disorder, 34
Attention deficit-hyperactivity disorder, 34
Australian aborigines, 3, 171, 173

Bantu, 369
Barker, David, 81–82, 327, 329
Baroreceptors, 385, 386, 388–89, 392, 393
Basal metabolic rate, 58, 273, 275, 335
Behavioral ecology, 91, 278–79, 286, 288–89, 300, 437
bGH, 123
Bilirubin, 269, 374, 424, 426
Bioassay, 138, 141, 151, 158
Bio-ethnocentrism, 116–17, 350
Biological predispositions, 373
Biologie, 438
Biology: as a basic science for medicine, 403; history of, 402, 437n; modern synthesis, 401; and the "normal," 412
Biomass index, 74–75, 80, 83, 153, 175–78, 244, 303, 321, 326, 396
Biostatistical theory, 438
Bipedalism, 2, 24, 220, 298
Birth weight, 30–31, 327–28, 336–39; and adult size, 335; African American, 346–48; age at menarche and, 127; diabesity and, 94; diabetes and, 345; genetic contribution, 336; insulin resistence and, 346; interuterine nutrition and, 328; low birth weight offspring (*see* Low birth weight offspring); macaques, 339; maternal consumption, 327, 337; maternal growth, 337, 338; milk intake, 127; mortality and, 53, 327; obesity and, 82; ponderal index, 160–61; public health and, 53; sleep, 297; time of conception, 337
Blastocyst, 184, 186, 437
Blood-brain barrier, 266–68, 271
Blood letting, 272, 402
Blood pressure, 19, 27, 40, 82, 97, 104–5, 114, 131, 216–17, 270, 294, 325–26, 328, 335–46, 363, 370, 376, 382–83, 385–90, 392–93, 395–97, 426
Blood vessels, 208, 266, 270–72, 274, 383–90, 429
Blood volume, 383–90, 392–94, 397
Blumenbach, J. F., 380
BMI. *See* Biomass index
BMR. *See* Basal metabolic rate
BNP, 389, 394
Body, as a machine, 428
Body composition, 74, 82, 113, 165, 176, 314–15, 317, 319–22, 324, 373
Body mass index. *See* Biomass index
Bone density, 128–30, 205, 213; and aging, 129; and milk consumption, 128, 130; and physical activity, 129
Bone fracture: and milk intake, 128–130
Bone growth, 123–24, 129
Boorse, Christopher, 438
Bovine growth hormone, 123
Bovine milk, 99, 101–3, 105–8, 116–17, 119, 121–25, 127–29, 131–33, 228, 230; age at menarche, 128; allergenic properties of, 132; child growth and, 122–23, 127–28, 132; consumption, 116–17, 120–22; chronic disease and, 130, 132; evolutionary perspective, 117,

132; IGF levels and, 124–25, 131; lactase activity, 118; lactase impersistence, 121; life history and, 132; nutritional advantages, 119; osteoporosis, 128–30, 132
Brain development, 24, 26, 31, 296–97, 318–21
Brain encephalization, 57, 58, 59
Brain natriuretic peptide, 389, 394
Brain optimization rule, 315, 318–22
BRCA. *See* Breast cancer, promoting genes
Breast cancer, 21, 22, 42, 131, 149, 151, 158, 168, 179–80, 185, 188–89, 371–72, 381; BRCA mutations, 372; promoting genes, 371–72, 378
Breastfeeding, 226–41; bed sharing, 231; birth interval, 29; breast cancer, 42; 158; and breathing, 433n; duration, 233, 241; evolution of, 29–30; initiation of, 229, 232, 234; learning to, 27, 229; and mother infant sleep, 227, 232, 238–39; perinatal mortality, 27; SIDS, 7, 227; termination of, 132, 234
Breast milk, 124, 228–32, 234–35; benefits, 232; composition, 231
British Pakistanis, 175

C-type natriuretic peptide, 389
Calcium, 17, 19, 56, 66–67, 119, 123–25, 128–33, 384, 390, 437n; paradox, 130, 132
Callitrichidae, 140
Cancer, 3, 7, 17, 19, 21–22, 28, 35, 37–38, 41–46, 48, 53, 56, 97, 102, 104–5, 108, 114, 128–32, 146, 149, 151, 158, 168, 171, 179–80, 185, 188–89, 194, 228, 255, 258, 274, 315, 366, 369–72, 378–81, 401, 415, 426, 430; bovine milk consumption and, 128, 130–32, 228; breast cancer (*see* Breast cancer); chronic disease, 37–38; colon, IGF-1, 131; developed vs. developing countries, rates, 44; estrogen and, 185; ethnicity and, 42; evolution of, 41, 43, 426, 430; genetics, 369–70, 380–81; HIF1, 274; lung cancer, 43; and nutrition, 17, 19, 56; obesity, 315; oral contraceptives and, 188, 194; prostate cancer, 43–44, 171; reproductive organs, 146, 158, 168, 180, 188; sex differences, 41, 43; and smoking, 45; social milieu, 258; stomach cancer, 42
Candida albicans, 202, 209, 211
Cardiac output, 385, 390, 392
Cardiovascular disease, 7, 10, 19, 37, 40–41, 46, 48, 56, 74, 97, 104, 108–9, 110, 111, 114, 128, 130–32, 170–71, 174–75, 208, 255, 274, 308, 325, 360, 361–62, 363, 365, 383, 397
Carvedilol, 394
Caseomorphin, 106
Catadromy, 389
Catch-up growth, *See* Growth, catch-up
Causation, 11, 12, 366–67; and evolutionary medicine, 53; and chronic disease, 198, 350–52, 360, 362, 365; and premenstrual syndrome, 209, 212, 215,
CCK, 76, 78
Celiac disease, 19, 51, 103, 436
Cereal grain: composition, 19, 105, 111; consumption, 19, 106–7, 113; disease and, 102; influence on human genetics, 102, 105; Paleolithic diet and, 101; population size and, 20; problems, 107–8; tolerance, 103

CF. *See* Cystic fibrosis
Cheese, 70, 88, 119, 120, 122, 131
Childbirth, 24, 48, 161, 197, 210, 225, 428; pelvic
    inlet size, 25
Child development, 28, 33–34, 243, 423, 427
Child health, 31–32, 36, 139, 146, 163, 258
Chlamydia spp.: *C. trachomatis,* 200–201, 211,
    357, 366; *C. pneumonia,* 208, 352, 357, 366
Cholecystokinin, 76, 78
Cholesterol, 17, 18, 40, 56, 110–11, 113, 326,
    328–29, 332, 346, 353, 355–56, 359–60, 365,
    376, 390, 396, 434
CHF. *See* Congestive heart failure
Chronic degenerative conditions, 100–101, 325,
    368–69, 372–73
Chronic diseases, 13, 17, 32, 36, 37, 38, 40, 42, 43, 46,
    48, 74, 82, 97, 98, 101, 102, 104, 107, 111, 115,
    130, 132, 167, 196, 198, 202, 215, 313, 315, 317
Clarke, John, 187, 248
CNP, 389
Comfort foods, 140
The Common Sense Book of Baby and Child Care, 28
Congestive heart failure, 40, 371, 382–83, 385, 387,
    389–93, 395, 397
Coronary artery disease, 40, 367, 370, 381, 383
Coronary heart disease, 82, 110, 131, 145, 175
Corticosterone, 144
Corticotrophin-releasing factor, 331
Corticotrophin-releasing hormone, 248, 253, 331
Cow's milk consumption, 116–17, 120–22
CRH, 248, 253, 331
CRF, 331
Critical periods, developmental, 62, 317–18, 343
Cortisol, 27, 32, 80, 82, 105, 145, 242–43, 244,
    245, 247–49, 251–58, 303–4, 308
Coughing, 358, 409–10
Cow's milk. *See* Bovine milk
Cross-tolerance, 275
Crying, 28, 227–28, 236, 252, 427
Cuisines, 63–64, 69
Culture, 2–4, 7, 12, 14–15, 17, 19, 25, 27–30, 33,
    36, 40, 43, 45, 48, 50, 56, 64–66, 70, 83, 99,
    100–105, 117, 120–24, 152, 182, 191, 196, 199,
    218, 223–25, 228, 245, 250, 268, 277, 282–83,
    288, 298, 300–301, 313, 344, 354–57, 360, 364,
    368, 372, 375, 379–80, 391, 396, 406, 416, 433
Cutaneous lupus. *See* Systemic lupus
    erythematosus
CVD. *See* Cardiovascular disease
Cystic fibrosis, 214, 351, 353, 367, 376, 413
Cytokines, interleukin, 79, 273, 306; tumor
    necrosis factor-α, 79, 273, 306

Dairy products, 56, 68, 86, 122–23, 126, 129–32
Dairying, 116, 119
Darwin, Charles, 5, 401, 420
Darwin, Erasmus, 5, 419–20
Darwinian evolution assumptions, 10
Darwinian medicine, 5, 7, 72–73, 75, 77, 79, 81,
    83, 85, 87, 89, 91, 93, 95, 383, 400–401, 411,
    416, 418–19, 420, 423, 430, 438
*De Sedibus Et Causis Morborum Per Anatomen
    Indagatis,* 438
Defenses, 6, 13–5, 26, 47, 52, 273, 275, 363,
    409–10, 417, 423–24, 432

Definitions: adolescence, 36; CHF, 40; diabetes,
    73; disease, 406–7; health, 405; illness, 407;
    PMS, 198; race, 369, 374, 380; sickness, 406
Delinquency, 146
Depression, 7, 46–49, 79, 139, 145–46, 198, 200,
    203, 206, 210, 212, 215, 253, 307, 417, 427
Descartes, René, 428
Development, 36, 70, 90, 144, 151, 157, 163, 167–68,
    227, 229, 237, 247,248, 249, 257–58, 281, 288,
    325, 334, 339, 341–42, 344–45, 348, 397;
    adaptability/plasticity, 162, 166, 249, 314, 316,
    323, 239, 330, 331, 333, 343; attachment, 141;
    brain, 57, 58, 211, 246, 296, 297, 318, 319, 320,
    321; child, 28, 33, 127, 128, 132, 142, 243, 245,
    292, 338, 423, 427; critical periods, 317; cultural,
    225; diet, 56, 62, 112; disease, 203, 327, 329,
    332, 336, 346, 355, 358, 361, 363; disorders of,
    34; drug, 14–16, 378–79; evolutionary medicine,
    402, 422; fetal, 22, 24, 26, 43, 160–61, 198, 218,
    220, 253, 274, 319; follicular, 187–88; infant, 27,
    94, 157, 229–30, 232, 240, 254, 328; learning,
    63; malnutrition and, 31; nonhuman primates,
    30; obesity, 315; policy, 36; process, 14, 135,
    158–59; reproductive strategies, 138, 139, 143,
    147, 165, 167; theory, 28
Dexamethasone, 276, 340
Diabetes, 12, 17, 23–24, 37–38, 46, 68, 71–75, 77,
    79–85, 95–97, 145, 219, 228, 303, 308, 315,
    318, 325–29, 332, 335–36, 345–48, 355, 366,
    373–74, 377, 390–91, 396–98, 417, 430, 434;
    type 1, 19, 73, 102, 205; type 2, 14, 19, 56,
    72–74, 79, 81–85, 93, 95, 97, 101–2, 104, 112,
    114, 131, 166, 170–75, 205, 370, 396,
    worldwide prevalence, 84
Diarrhea, 30–32, 49, 120, 204, 345, 386, 397, 409–10
Dietary breadth, 70–72
Dietary recommendations, 68, 96, 98, 106–7, 113–14
Diet composition comparisons, 18
Dieting, 80, 93, 95, 151, 153
Digitalis, 395
Discordance hypothesis, 290
"Dis-ease," 408–9
Disease and Evolution, 400
Disease etiology, 371
Diuretics, 394
DNA predictive testing, 378
Dogon of Mali, 185
DOHaD, 327–30
Domestication, 3, 17, 19; animal, 3, 34, 119;
    plant, 3, 103. *See also* Agriculture; Dairying
Dominica, 242–43, 245, 250, 253, 258
Dopamine, 76–77, 248, 280, 285–87, 437
Drapetomania, 406–7
Drugs, 1, 9, 11, 13, 15, 26, 45, 48, 50–52, 78,
    80–81, 94, 97, 114, 146, 276, 279–89, 373, 376,
    380, 394–95, 397, 417, 426
Duffy antigen, 427
Duffy null allele, 371, 377
Dutch famine winter, 143, 322, 338
Dutch, 143, 161, 322, 338, 371, 436
Dysaesthesia Æthiopsis, 406

E%. *See* Total dietary energy
Early family trauma, 253–55, 257
Eat Right 4 Your Type, 68–69

Eclampsia, 22–24, 216–17, 222, 224
Ecology, 3, 24, 63, 72, 91, 151, 154–55, 166,
    278–79, 286, 288–89, 291–93, 295, 297,
    299–301, 303, 305, 307, 309, 311, 313, 329–30,
    332, 334–35, 337–38, 343–45, 437
Edema, 40, 218, 260, 276, 390, 394
EEA, 285
Efé (Democratic Republic of the Congo), 3, 26
Encephalization, 57–59
Endometritis, 187
Endometrium, 151, 184–88, 218
Endothelin, 271
Endothelin receptor, 271
Energy balance, 29, 75, 83, 139–40, 153–56, 326,
    344–45
Environment of evolutionary adaptedness, 285
Environment, feast/famine, 73, 81–82, 89, 318
Environmental risk, 136–40, 360, 367
Epidemiology, 13, 167, 260, 289, 317, 323–24,
    346, 360, 370, 372, 374, 379–80, 391, 400, 417,
    424–25, 427
Epidemiological transitions, 3
Epigenetic, 340–43, 346, 348
Erythropoietin, 269
Estabrooks, George H., 400, 403
    Estradiol, 22, 149, 151–55, 158, 160, 163,
        169–71, 175, 179, 189, 436
Estrogen, 21, 44, 90, 171, 179, 180, 183, 184, 185,
    188, 189, 190, 195, 199, 200, 209, 210, 211,
    212, 213, 214, 215, 436
ET-1, 271
ET. See Trauma, early family
ETH, 58
Ethnography, 250, 288–89
Ethnoracial, 368, 370–72, 375–76, 379–80
ETR. See Endothelin receptor
Eugenics, 403
Evidence-based medicine, 323, 404
Evolution and healing, 409, 438
Evolutionary epidemiology, 370
Evolutionary explanation, 275, 407–9, 413,
    420, 422, 426, 428, 429–30, 432–33;
    AMS, 260; disease in general, 400, 407–9,
    422, 426, 430, 432–33; inequality and ill
    health, 146; menstruation, 186; obesity, 12,
    81; PMS, 198; pregnancy sickness, 22; prostate
    cancer, 44; schizophrenia, 289; type 2
    diabetes, 81
Evolutionary health science, 412
Evolutionary medicine, 1, 4–8, 10, 12–13, 15, 17,
    22, 24, 26, 29, 33, 36–38, 40–42, 45, 52–54, 57,
    64–65, 68–69, 71, 167–68, 180, 182, 197, 227,
    232–33, 241, 243, 246, 257–58, 260, 266, 275,
    279, 286, 290, 314–316, 323–25, 351, 353, 367,
    368–72, 376, 378–81, 400–419, 421, 422–27,
    430, 439 n
Evolutionary Medicine: Rethinking the Origins of
    Disease, 401
Evolutionary psychology, 278–79, 286, 288–89
Exercise. See Physical activity
Expensive Tissue hypothesis, 58

Fat, 11–12, 17, 19, 20, 22, 50, 60–61, 66, 67, 69–70,
    82–83, 88, 91, 99, 101, 103–5, 108, 113–14,

127–28, 173, 315, 317, 319–20, 326, 344–45,
    352, 360, 362–63, 396, 436n; abdominal, 80,
    170, 315, 320–23, 328, 374; body, 65, 73, 74;
    metabolism, 77, 81; Norwegian diet, 107, 108,
    109, 110, 112; Paleolithic diet and, 18, 65, 86,
    100, 326, 395; saturated, 3, 56, 131, bovine
    milk, 108, 123, 131, 133, 228; storage, 12, 75,
    78–79, 82, 85, 94, 318, 335–37, 353, 355, 370;
    South Pacific islanders diet, 111; trans, 94
Fatfold. See Skinfold thickness
Fatigue, 59, 64, 80, 198, 206, 261, 409–10, 423
Favism, 70
Fetal growth, 338; reduced, 314–15, 319–22,
    324, 328; restriction of, 147, 160, 323, 328,
    337, 347
Fetal nutrition, 219, 221, 329, 334, 336–40, 344
Fetal origins of adult disease, 139, 142, 146
Fetus, 22–24, 53, 60, 62, 134, 139, 143–44, 147,
    159–60, 197, 203, 216–20, 225, 315, 322, 325,
    327, 329–40, 342–45
Fever, 11, 201, 244, 249, 273, 275, 409–10, 412,
    417, 423–24, 426, 432
Finn, Colin A., 186
Fish: bony, 384; cartilaginous, 386; dipnoan, 386
Fitness, evolutionary, 10, 23, 27, 47–50, 52, 57, 59,
    81, 119, 135–138, 146, 157, 168, 197, 246, 279,
    283–84, 286, 316–17, 354, 360, 432–33;
    physical, 39, 261
Flavor principles, 63–64
Flexner, Abraham, 421
Folklore, 230
Follicle-stimulating hormone, 160–61, 183, 188
Food, biochemical effects, 56
Food choice, 56–62, 69–71, 284
Food guide, 56
Food processing: enhancing nutrient content, 64;
    genetic adaptations in, 102; health effects, 19;
    health policy and, 99; milk, 123; Paleolithic
    diet, 65, 86; toxin removal, 64
Formula feeding: digestion, 10; evolutionary
    context, 227–28; effects of, 239; mother-infant
    separation and, 229; prevalence, 28; sleep, 28,
    239; Western society, 228
Forager, 3, 60, 65–66, 90, 99, 170–71, 326, 355–58,
    396; female reproductive history, 21
Franklin, Benjamin, 423
FSH. See Follicle-stimulating hormone
Future reproduction, 135–37, 148, 158
Fusobacterium nucleatum, 201

G6PD, 13, 379
Gene analysis, candidate, 376
Gene corporations, 370
Gene expression, 144, 267, 340–41
Gene frequencies, 326, 335, 341, 346–48, 425
Gene pool, 404
General life history problem, 135–36
Genetic clusters, 372
Genetic drift, 17, 119–20, 370, 375, 377
Genetic polymorphism, 13, 106, 427
Genetic predisposition, 174, 198, 219, 366, 368
Genetics, 17, 118, 281, 283, 287–88, 290, 337,
    346, 369–70, 374, 378–80, 401, 417, 421,
    424–25, 427

Genomics, 370, 380
Geographic origin, 372, 377
German, 61, 89, 153, 201, 369, 408, 436
Gestation, 10, 23, 24, 26, 30, 73, 143, 149, 156, 158, 160–61, 172, 216–17, 297, 317, 329, 333, 338–39, 342, 344–45, 347
Gestational diabetes, 23–24, 73, 172, 345
GFR. *See* Glomerular filtration rate
Gliadin intolerance, 106, 434n
Global milk production, 121
Glomerular filtration rate, 387, 388, 392
Glucocorticoid, 144, 243, 247–49, 253, 256, 341
Glucose, 13, 23–24, 50, 73–74, 77–79, 81–83, 85–86, 108, 112, 118, 120, 170, 173, 176, 205, 261, 266, 268, 272, 303–4, 318, 329, 335–36, 340–41, 345, 379
Glossitis, 201
Gluten intolerance, 19, 103, 434n
Glycemic foods, 105, 114; index, 86, 99, 170; load, 86, 99, 108, 110, 114, 120
Glycolysis, 268, 271–72, 274
GnRH. *See* Gonadotropin releasing hormone
Gonadotropin-releasing hormone, 160, 183, 188, 212
Gravity, 4, 382, 384–86, 397
Greek, 45, 49, 356, 374
Growth: catch up, 147, 166, 295, 348; in utero, 315, 318, 322
Growth hormone: synthetic bovine, 123–24, 435n, 436n

Hahnemann, Samuel, 418
Haldane, J. B. S., 400
Haplotypes, 376
HDP (hypertensive disorders of pregnancy). *See* Hypertension, pregnancy
Health and disease: developmental origins, 327–30
Health care system: Norway, 97
Health policy: breastfeeding and, 9, 29; eating and physical activity, 94; future survivorship, 33; infant care, 241; and the "normal," 36; sleep, 29; "small but healthy" hypothesis, 32;
Health inequalities, 134–35, 147, 312
Heart, 3, 15, 19, 38–40, 50, 56, 68, 82, 104–5, 109–11, 131, 145, 175, 192, 194, 243, 268, 273–74, 287, 293–94, 299, 304, 310, 315, 325, 347–48, 353–54, 362, 371, 376, 382–97, 417, 429
Heart failure: left, 390–91; right, 391
Helicobacter pylori, 201
Hematocrit, 265–66
Hemolytic anemia, 379
Hemophilus influenza, 200, 208
Hierarchy, 33, 49, 140, 145
HIF1, 267–76
High blood pressure. *See* Hypertension
High-carbohydrate and low-fat diet, 108
Hispanic: diabetes, 85; lactase persistence, 118; obesity, 84
HGP, 13
HHSV, 201, 203, 206, 211
HIV, 12–13
HLA. *See* Human leukocyte antigen
HTLV-1. *See* T-cell lymphotrophic virus type 1
Homeopathy, 417

Homeostasis, 50, 77–78, 82, 176, 260, 262, 267, 342, 348, 385
Homeotherms, 412
Hominid family tree, 2
Hominin evolution, 17, 79, 259
Homology, 331
Hormonal effects of foods, 98, 105
Hormone therapy, 437
Hormones, 21–22, 76–80, 82, 93–94, 146, 150–51, 156, 158–60, 162–63, 166, 168–69, 171, 179, 182–83, 188, 192, 194, 209–14, 236, 243, 247–50, 256, 262, 272, 304, 319, 332, 336, 347–48, 388–89, 392, 397
How to test an evolutionary hypothesis, 430, 432
HPA. *See* Hypothalamic-pituitary-adrenal axis
HPO, 159–60
Human biology, 26, 73, 152, 250, 274, 283, 347, 374, 402, 412
Human evolution, 1–2, 5, 6, 11, 19, 25–26, 30, 33–34, 47, 50–51, 55, 60, 68, 70, 170, 225, 245, 246, 259, 274, 283, 285, 298–99, 313, 316, 318, 325, 353, 355, 362, 396
Human family, evolution of, 33, 245
Human Genome Project, 13
Human herpes simplex virus, 201, 203, 206, 211
Human immunodeficiency virus, 12–13
Human leukocyte antigen, 13, 103, 224, 376
Humors, 434n
Hunter-gatherers. *See* Forager
HVR, 264–66, 272
Hydrogéologie, 438
Hyperandrogenism, 172, 179
Hypercholesterolemia, 111, 376
Hyperinsulinemia, 160, 169–71, 174, 179–80, 374
Hyperlactasia, 121
Hyperlipidemia, 373, 390–91, 397
Hypertension, 41, 110, 114, 131, 172, 225, 302, 304, 326–27, 347–48, 373, 417, 425–26, 435n; African American, 346; breast feeding, 228, 328; cardiovascular disease, 40; congestive heart failure, 390–91, 397; diet, 56, 68; environment, 376; evolution of, 17, 287, 326, 374–75, 425; foraging people, 3; genetics, 377; gestational, 216; lifestyle, 376; low birth weight, 82, 327; metabolic syndrome X, 433n; mortality, 37–38; obesity, 315; preeclampsia and, 24, 219; pregnancy, 216–219, 222–23, 225; sleep restriction, 303
Hypolactasia, 121
Hypothalamic peptide pro-opimelanocortin, 77
Hypothalamic-pituitary-adrenal axis, 134, 139–40, 142–45, 247–48, 251, 253–54
Hypothalamic-pituitary-ovarian axis, 159–60
Hypothalamus, 59, 77–78, 93–94, 183, 294, 319, 388
Hypoxemia, 264, 266
Hypoxia, 259–276, 294, 390, 437; hypoxia inducible factor 1, 267–76, hypoxia inducible factor 1α, 267, 269, 271, 274, hypoxia inducible factor 1β, 267; hypoxic ventilatory response, 264–66, 272

IBS, 213
Icelandic, 369, 371
IGA. *See* Ancestry, geographic

IGF. *See* Insulin-like growth factor
IL. *See* Interleukin
[IL]-1, 273, 306
[IL]-6, 273
Immunoglobins, 12, 34, 244; IgA, 12–13, 224,
    257; IgD, 12–13; IgE, 12,-3, 34; IgG, 12,-13,
    359; IgM, 12–13
Impaired glucose tolerance, 74, 77, 85, 340,
Immigration/migration studies. *See* Migrant studies.
Immune function, 14, 145, 167, 199, 247–48,
    256–57, 361, 365
Implantation, 22, 151, 184, 186–87, 196, 216, 218,
    220–21, 223, 225
Inbreeding, 369, 372, 379
Incest, 24, 223–25
Individual variation, 120, 131, 160, 285, 433
Indigenous/traditional people: diabetes type 2, 173;
    health care, 80, 104; health experience, 98
Inequality, 65, 135, 144–48, 290, 313
Infant care: breastfeeding, 226, 227; cultural
    knowledge, 23, 228; cultural variation, 33, 227,
    229; evolution of, 240–41; health policy and,
    241; industrialization and, 229; pediatric
    medicine, 28, 227; Western practices, 228, 231
Infertility, 172, 178, 187
Inheritance, epigenetic, 340–41
Insulin, 23, 59, 76, 86, 90, 94, 100, 105, 107, 113,
    159–160, 175, 205, 272, 304, 329, 335, 345, 346,
    374; resistance, 51, 74, 77–79, 82–83, 110, 114,
    169–74, 176, 178–80, 318–19, 327–28,
    336, 346
Insulin-like growth factor, 43, 123–27, 131–32,
    159, 168, 171, 336; beneficial effects, 132;
    overall growth, 127, 129, 168; milk
    consumption, 125, 132;and ovarian function,
    159, 171; and prostate cancer, 43
Intercourse, 222; age at first, 141
Intergenerational phenotypic inertia, 143
Intergenerational variance in number of offspring,
    136–37
Interleukin, 79, 273, 306
Intolerance: gliadin, 106, 434n; glucose, 205, 341;
    gluten, 19, 103, 434n; lactose, 116, 120–22
Intrauterine growth retardation, 23, 31, 142, 218
Irritable bowel syndrome, 213
Irish, 369
Italian, 356, 369, 374
IUGR. *See* intrauterine growth retardation

Kelvin, Lord, 421
Kidney disease, 217, 265, 274, 276, 386–89,
    392–95, 398; cancer, 42–44; CHF and, 40;
    diabetes, 74; fetal growth, 147; mortality and,
    38; obesity, 74; preeclampsia, 225; pregnancy,
    24; smoking and, 45
!Kung (Botswana and Namibia), 23, 9, 104, 355, 396

Lactase, 103, 116–22, 130–33, 436; persistence,
    118–21, 131–33; distribution, 118, 120;
    evolution, 119; population variation, 132;
    impersistence, 116, 118, 120–21, 130;
    deficiency, 121
Lactational amenorrhea, 21, 189

Lactogenesis II, 234
Lactose, 10, 70, 103, 106, 116–22, 133, 436;
    intolerance, 116, 120–22; malabsorption, 121;
    tolerance, 121
Lamarck, Jean-Baptiste, 438
Lappé, Marc, 401
LBW. *See* Low birth weight offspring
Learning, 27, 30, 33–34, 57–58, 61–63, 69–70,
    245, 247, 249, 253, 275, 280, 282, 286, 295,
    298, 307, 316, 341–42, 399, 423, 428, 433
Lectin, 90, 107, 436 n
Le Gros Clark, W. E., 5
Leptin, 76–78, 80, 82, 94, 159, 171, 303–4
Lese (Democratic Republic of the Congo), 150–52,
    154–55, 157
LG. *See* Rodents, maternal behavior
LH. *See* Luteinizing hormone
Life cycle, 10, 35–36, 132, 135, 138, 149, 157, 162,
    329–30, 340, 342, 347
Life expectancy, 52, 67, 97–98, 104, 222, 326, 334, 343
Life history theory, 10, 12, 23, 36, 58, 135, 138,
    148, 157, 167, 278
Life history traits, 10, 58, 135, 138, 157, 162, 185,
    297, 429
Lineage extinction, 136–37, 143, 146–48
Linkage disequilibrium, 371
Livingstone, Frank, 6–7
Longevity, 145–47, 157, 197, 355, 423
Low birth weight offspring, 31, 82, 94, 142–43,
    146, 161, 297, 348
Luteinizing hormone, 99, 160–67, 172, 183–84,
    188, 243, 248–50, 317, 392
Lybrel, 436

Major histocompatibility complex proteins, 13
Maladaptation, 383, 400
Malaria, 6, 7, 13, 15, 17, 30, 31, 119, 427, 432
Mammal, 2, 7, 17, 25, 29–30, 35, 44, 55, 57, 61,
    116–20, 122–23, 135, 144, 159–60, 217–22,
    261, 267, 273, 296–97, 300, 316, 330–32, 341,
    343–44, 382, 384, 386, 388–90
Man, The Mechanical Misfit, 400
Material resources, 138–40, 145
Maximin/minimax strategy, 136–37, 143, 148
Meats, wild and domestic compared, 20
Menarche: age, 21, 35, 128, 131, 140–42, 146–47,
    161–62, 164–65, 167, 185. secular trend, 35,
    158, 330, milk consumption, 128
Medical: schools, 6, 405, 418, 428; textbooks, 382,
    400; curriculum, 417, 427
Melatonin, 333, 343
Menarche, 21, 35–36, 42, 60, 128, 131, 134,
    140–43, 146–47, 158, 160–62, 164–68, 171,
    185, 330; age at, 128, 166, 330; early, 42,
    141–43, 146–47, 158, 161, 171
Menstrual cycle, 164–65, 172–73, 175–76, 178,
    205, 207–10, 212–14; adolescent sterility, 35;
    characteristics, 182–83; depression and, 48;
    duration, 435n; endometrium, 184; estradiol,
    175; estrogen, 185, 190; European and British
    Pakastani women, 176; evolution, 21, 181–82,
    186; follicle growth, 172; follicular phase,
    183–84; hyperinsulinemia, 179; IBS, 212–13;
    immune function, 199, 210, 214; infection,

209, 213; luteal phase, 179, 183–84, 197–202, 204, 206–8, 210–12, 214, 437n; migraine headaches and, 205; oral contraceptives, 181–82, 194; ovarian function, 151–52, 160; PMS and, 197; SLE, 207; suppression, 182, 186–87, 189–91, 193–95, 437n, 438n
Menstrual-suppressing oral contraceptives, 181–82, 194
Menstruation: amenorrhea, 21, 171, 188–89, 191, 193; cultural perceptions, 182, 188, 191–93; diabetes, 205; evolution, 22, 181–82, 185, 197, 436n; hypotheses, defective embryo removal, 186–87, evolutionary byproduct, 186, pathogen removal, 186–88, postnatal fecundability, 186–88; hormonal control of, 184–85; hypoxia, 436n; immunosupression, 200–202, 214; MSOC, 18–82, 186–90, 193–95 (see also Menstrual cycle, suppression); oligomenorrhea, 171; Parkinson's disease, 202
Menstruation hypotheses: defective embryo removal, 186–87; evolutionary byproduct, 186; pathogen removal, 186–87; postnatal fecundability, 187–88
Mental problems, categories of, 48
Metabolic syndrome, 35, 74, 82, 304, 374, 390, 434
Metabolism, 53, 72, 76–81, 83, 124, 155, 170, 246, 260–62, 267, 268–71, 274–75, 297, 303–4, 325–27, 329–30, 334–35, 337, 340, 344–46, 361, 363–64, 370, 376, 381, 394
Methylation, 340–41
Metoprolol, 394
MHC, 13
Microsatellites, 369
Microtus montanus, 332–34, 326, 343–44
Migrant studies, 151, 158, 162–66, 173–6, 346, 347
Milk consumption, 116–25, 127–33; and bone density, 128; in childhood, 129; and growth, 122
Mind, 12, 54, 113, 245, 247, 258, 277, 399–400, 402, 409–10, 420, 428, 430, 435, 437–38
Miscarriage, 23, 172, 219, 222–24
Mismatch hypothesis, 345, 383,
Mitochondria, 83, 261–63, 266, 268–69, 272, 336
Modern American diet, 56, 67, 70
Molecular oncology, 370
Molecular revolution, 368, 370, 379
Mongoloid, 380
Montane vole. See Microtus montanus
Morbidity, 3, 25–26, 47, 97, 100, 104, 145, 167, 245, 253–54, 257, 272, 375, 380, 383, 394
Morgagni, Giovanni Battista, 408
Morphogenesis, 220, 331
Mortality rates, 31, 33, 136, 138–40, 144–46, 163, 167, 327, 392
Mortality risk, 134, 138–40, 305
Morten, Dudley J., 5, 6
Mother fetal conflict, 23; vascular exchange, 217; communication, 334, 339, 341–42
Mouthsense, 55, 59
M. pneumonia, 200, 208,
MSOC, 18–82, 186–90, 193–95
Multiple founder mutations, 369, 371
Multiple sclerosis, 19, 102, 206–7, 211, 214, 353–56, 358–59
Muscle mass, 74, 314–15, 317–21, 323, 325, 335
Museum of Menstruation, 191

Mutation, 43, 50, 51, 77, 117–19, 271, 353–54, 358, 369–72, 377–79, 421, 425, 427, 432–33
Mycoplasma spp., 206
Myopia, 171

National Health and Nutrition Examination Survey, 56, 83, 127
Native American, 45, 80–82, 118, 121, 173–74, 326–27, 345, 380
Natriuretic peptides, 389–90, 393, 397
Natural selection, 14, 17, 40, 47, 57, 188, 243, 262, 269–70, 274, 276, 316, 324, 326, 332, 335, 342–43, 348, 355, 362, 367, 370, 413, 419–25, 428–29, 431–33, 438n; blood types, 69; brains, 209, 270; by-product, 221; cheating, 11; defenses, 409; handicap, 214; host/pathogen, 323; infancy/childhood, 26–27, 32, 236, 258; mental disorder, 47, 50, 278; obesity, 75; sickle cell, 6; suboptimal, 353,
Nauru, 173
Nausea, 22, 49, 62, 120, 197–98, 204, 260–61, 266, 409–10, 423
Neel, J. V., 81, 355
Neisseria gonorrheae, 211
Nesse, Randolph, 4, 5, 400
Neocortex, 57–58
Neo-Darwinian medicine, 401, 438
Neolithic. See Agricultural revolution
Neonatal hyperbilirubinemia, 374
Neophobia, 59, 61, 63
Neoplasm, 369, 380
Nesiritide, 394
Neural mechanisms, 59
Neuroendocrine, 134, 139, 141–42, 144–45, 160, 247, 249
Neurohormonal activation, 392–93, 395, 397
Neuronal cell death, 145
Neuropeptides, 76–79; neuropeptide Y, 59, 76
NHANES. See National Health and Nutrition Examination Survey
Nicotiana tabacum. See Tobacco
Nitric oxide synthase, 270–71
Nomenclature, 418, 419
Nonorganic failure to thrive, 140
Norepinephrine, 59, 385–86, 392
Norway, 35, 96–101, 103–8, 111–15, 435; dietary recommendations, 98; health care system, 97
NOS, 270–71
NPY, 59, 76
NREM. See Sleep, non rapid eye movement
Null model, 319–20
Nutrition, 32, 37, 55–57, 59–60, 65, 69, 82,89, 119–20, 143, 167, 284, 331, 346, 372, 381, 417; cultural influences on, 63, 373; development, 35, 127, 132,140, 142, 159, 160, 166, 168, 232, 319, 338, 341; disease and, 30, 33, 40–41, 93, 139, 345, 351, 353; ecology, 155, 330, 343; evolutionary perspective, 99; flavor principle, 64; learning and, 90; maternal, 29, 53, 143, 219, 332, 337; mortality and, 31, 138, 146; nutritional transition, 172–73; Paleolithic, 17–20, 66, 68, 383; pregnancy and, 22–24, 219–221, 327–39, 332, 334–35, 339–40, 342, 347–49
Nutrogenetics, 370

ω-3 fatty acid, 101, 103, 108, 111, 114, 436 n
ω-6: ω-3 ratio, 101, 108, 111, 114, 436 n
Obesity, 7, 19, 36–37, 56, 66, 68, 71,-85, 87, 92–96,
    101, 105, 108–12, 140, 146, 160, 169–71, 173,
    179, 219, 290, 302–5, 307–8, 314–26, 328,
    344–45, 373–77, 390–91, 396–97, 434;
    abdominal, 170, 317, 319, 374; adolescence and,
    36; bacteria in gut, 79; biocultural model of, 71;
    brains, 318; breastfeeding and, 328; CHF and,
    390; chronic disease, 37, 315; "comfort foods"
    and, 140; cross-cultural comparison, 75, 76, 83,
    172, 326, 396; diagnostic criteria for, 74;
    distribution of, 74, 374; early menarche and, 146;
    early onset, 77; epidemic of, 7, 19, 56, 93, 315,
    evolutionary models, 320; fast food, 92. 101; fetal
    growth and, 315, 322; genetics and, 370, 376,
    377; immune function and, 79; lifestyles, 81, 82,
    110, 326; low birth weight and, 81, 82, 317–18;
    McDonald's® and, 87; menstrual cycle effects,
    171; in Norway, 96, 111–12; Paleolithic and, 68;
    prevalence, 83; psychosocial stress and, 80; sex
    differences in, 74; sleep and, 303–305, 307–8;
    television viewing and, 93; tolerant ethnic groups,
    81; type 2 diabetes, 72, 73
Obsessive-compulsive disorder, 47–48, 50, 203,
    212, 286
OCD. See Obsessive compulsive disorder
Oligomenorrhea, 171
Omnivory, 70
Oncogenes, 369, 378–79
Optimal nutrient intake, 98, 106, 115
Oral contraceptives, 22, 181–83, 185, 187–91,
    193–96, 210–13, 436, 437
Origin of Species, 402, 416, 420
Orthomolecular medicine, 106
Osmoreceptors, 389
Osteoporosis, 17, 56, 68, 97, 102, 104, 128–30,
    132, 204–5, 213
Ovarian function, 29, 149, 150–53, 156, 158–59,
    162, 165–72, 174, 178–79, 196, 426
Ovulation, 22, 24, 29, 150–51, 155, 161, 163,
    171–72, 181, 184–85, 188, 222–23, 225, 437
oxytocin, 27, 144, 232, 248

Pain, 8, 13, 26, 37, 89, 139–40, 144, 191, 198, 206,
    212, 214, 236–37, 266, 270–71, 276, 282, 307,
    409–10, 423, 432, 435
Paleolithic diet, 19, 65–66, 68–69, 85, 86, 100, 102,
    106–7, 115, 395
Paleopathology, 104, 106
Paley, William, 426
Pancreas, 42, 44, 45, 76, 77, 78, 170
Pancreatic peptide, 76, 78
PAR. See Predictive adaptive response
Parenting, 22, 33, 228–30
Pathogenesis, 207, 364, 366, 372
Pathology, 6, 7, 47, 104, 106, 147, 156, 170, 200,
    207, 212, 214–15, 248, 258, 274, 278, 291, 319,
    324, 365, 406–7, 412
Pathophysiology, 260, 400, 412
PCOS. See Polycystic ovarian syndrome
Peptostreptococcus micros, 201
Pharmacogenetics, 370
Pharmacological therapeutics, 373

Phenotype, 34, 73, 81, 94, 138, 174, 314–16,
    323–24, 329–30, 340–41, 368, 377, 379–80,
    428, 439n
Phenotypic inertia, 143, 339
Phenotypic plasticity, 138, 141, 157, 247, 249, 316
Phenylketonuria, 34, 376, 377, 378
Phenylthiocarbamide 6, 10, 60
Philippines, 3, 91, 121, 326, 328
Photoperiod, 333–34, 343
Phylogeny, 243, 354, 356, 422
Physical activity, 38–40, 67, 75, 82–83, 94, 110,
    112, 129–30, 132–33, 154, 159, 165, 170–71,
    173–74, 250, 254, 276, 308, 326, 328, 337
Phytoestrogens, 179
Pima (Native American), 174, 345
PKU. See Phenylketonuria
Placenta, 24, 76, 82, 216–17, 223, 225, 274,
    331–34, 336–38, 345, 347, 437
Plasmodium, 6–7, 207
PMOC, 77
PMS. See Premenstrual syndrome
Poikilotherms, 412
Polish, 150, 154, 371
Polycystic ovarian syndrome, 160, 172, 173, 178, 179
Polycythemia, Chuvash, 271–72
Polymorphism, 13, 106, 369, 371, 376, 427
POMC, 77
Ponderal index, 160–61
Populations in transition, 173–74, 178, 180
PCOS. See Polycystic ovary syndrome
Postagricultural, 383, 396–97
Postindustrial, 227, 232, 241, 310, 383, 396, 397
Potawatomi, 374
Potatoes, ingestion of, 108–10
PP, 76, 78
Prediabetes. See Impaired glucose tolerance
Predictive adaptive response, 315, 317–22, 329
Preeclampsia: animal models of, 24; characteristics
    of, 24; complications of pregnancy, 22–24,
    216, 219, 222–24; condom use, 220; couples'
    disease, 219; eclampsia, 217–18; evolution,
    24, 197, 221, 225; HDP (see Hypertension,
    pregnancy); HLA compatibility, 224; incest
    avoidance, 223–24; mate fidelity, 220, 222–23;
    oral sex, 220; paternal antigens, 220, 223;
    PCOS (see Polycystic ovary syndrome);
    premature birth, 24
Pregnancy, 21–24, 29, 36, 48, 53, 63, 73, 75, 81,
    94, 132, 151, 156, 182, 186–87, 189, 194–95,
    197, 203, 210–14, 216–20, 222–25, 328–29,
    331, 333–34, 336–38, 347
Premenstrual Syndrome, 197–99, 202, 204, 206,
    208, 209–10, 213, 215
Preparation for reproduction, 147
Prevotella spp., 201, 211
Priority rules, 317
Profet, Margie, 186–87, 194, 197, 438 n
Progesterone, 21, 29, 149–58, 163–65, 169–71,
    179, 183–84, 186, 188–90, 199–201, 209–10,
    213–14
Prolactin, 234, 241
Pro-opiomelanocortin (POMC) hypothalamic
    peptide, 77
PROP, 60
Propionibacterium acnes. See Acne

Prostate cancer, 43–44, 171
Proteomics, 370
Proximate cause, 5, 11–12, 37, 144, 260, 263, 265–67, 270, 273–75
Proximate Explanations, 138, 422, 432
Psychoactive substances, 51–52, 279
Psychosocial stress. *See* Stress, social
PTC, 6, 10, 60
Public health, 23, 35–36, 53, 74, 83, 97–99, 227, 237, 243, 258, 304, 316, 324, 366, 370, 372, 374–75, 383, 391, 424–25; policy, 9, 29, 33, 36, 241, 292, 315,

RA. *See* Rheumatoid arthritis
RAAS. *See* Renin-angiotensin-aldosterone system
Race: genetics of, 346, 368–69, 372, 375
Race-based medicine/therapeutics, 369–70, 372–74, 376, 379–80
Random process, 317, 319
REM. *See* Sleep, rapid eye movement
rbGH. *See* Growth hormone, synthetic bovine
Reification of disease, 407
The Relation of Evolution to Medicine, 5
Renin-angiotensin-aldosterone system, 382–83, 385–89, 392–95, 397
Reproduction, 10, 11, 35, 42, 100, 135–140, 144, 146–47, 156–59, 167–68, 185, 197, 216–17, 223–25, 246, 282, 284, 316–17, 332, 335–36, 344, 354–55, 397, 404, 423, 426, 428, 432; age at first, 135, 140, 144, 147, 148
Reproductive cancers, 28, 35, 42, 131–32, 146, 158, 168, 189. *See also* Breast cancer; Cancer, reproductive organs
Reproductive suppression, 140–41. *See also* Menstrual cycle, suppression
Reptile, 296, 331, 383–84, 386, 389–90
Resistin, 77
Rheumatoid arthritis, 19, 37, 102, 104, 207, 211, 357
Risk and uncertainty, 134, 136–40, 147
Risk factors: activity, 37; Alzheimer's, 358; AMS, 261, 268; bed sharing, 237; breast cancer, 185; cardiovascular disease, 174–75; categories of, 352; CHF, 390, 396–97; developmental, 167; diabetes, type 2, 174–75; environmental, 360, 367; extrinsic, 41; genetic inheritance, 43; hypertension, 40; intrinsic, 41; lifestyle, modifiable, 43, 380; mood disorders, 48; neonatal hyperbilirubinemia, 374; nutrition, 37, 353; postnatal mortality, 227; poverty, 42; serum cholesterol, 40; sleep apnea, 302; smoking, 205; substance abuse, 288
Risk-taking behavior, 36, 45, 282, 285, 287, 298
Ritual, 33, 57, 72, 280, 283, 288, 299, 307, 311
Rodents, 78; appetite controlling drugs, 94; arched back nursing, 144; HPA stress response, 253–54; intergenerational signaling, 332; licking and grooming, 144; maternal behavior, 144; wheel running, 286;

Salt, 60, 62, 66, 91, 101, 200, 287, 326, 387, 389, 393, 395–97
Sapolsky, Robert, 49
Scaphiopus hammondii, 330

Scars of Evolution, 400
Schizophrenia, 47, 48, 50, 51, 203, 204, 209, 212, 351, 352, 366, 436 n
School milk programs, 120, 122
Seasonale®, 182, 188, 193–95, 435 n1, 436 n9–10
Seasonality, 60, 160
Secular trend, 35, 158, 163, 167, 330
Self-medication, 145
Senescence, 372, 402, 426
Sensory-specific satiety, 59, 61, 63
Serotonin, 59, 77, 200, 215
17 β-estradiol, 29. *See also* Estradiol
Sex hormone-binding globulin, 169, 171–72, 174–79
Sexual behavior, 144, 282, 285
sFLT-1, 269, 271
SGA, 23, 160, 217
SHBG. *See* Sex hormone-binding globulin
Short, Roger, 21, 158, 168
Sialic acid, 17
Sickle cell, 6, 7, 13, 376, 413, 427, 432
Sickness response, 273
SIDS. *See* Sudden infant death syndrome
Signaling molecules, 59
Single nucleotide polymorphisms, 369
Sioux, 374
6–n-propylthiouracil, 60
6–phosphate dehydrogenase, 13, 379
Skinfold thickness, 62, 74, 176, 321, 328
SLE, 207–8
Sleep, 227, 229, 237, 292–93, 296, 298, 300–301, 305–6, 308–9, 312; AMS, 261, 274; apnea, 80, 274, 302; breastfeeding and, 231–232, 235; comparative animal patterns, 296; cross cultural comparisons, 300–301; cultural differences, 26–28; depression, 48; difficulties with, 201–2, 207; dreaming and, 293; duration of, 80, 94; ecology of, 299; EEG, 293, 295; evolution of, 237, 292, 312–13; functions of, 296–98; health and, 292–93, 297–98; health disparities and, 312; homeostatic model of, 294–95; human evolution and, 298–300, 309–10; infant safety, 237; insomnic, 302; location experiment, 233–36; loss of, 302–3; mortality and, 304–5; mother-infant proximity during, 29, 226–27, 231–32, 234–35, 237–41; non rapid eye movement, 293–95, 297–98, 307; obesity and, 304; oxygen desaturation during, 29; paradoxes of, 305; physiological components of, 293–94; as risky behavior, 298; rapid eye movement, 230, 293–94, 295, 297–8, 301, 307, 210; restriction of, 304, 311; SIDS, 29; "sleep debt", 295, 308; solitary infant, 28–29, 230; stages of, 293, 309; stress, 80, 255–56, 305–6; uninterrupted infant, 230; wakefulness and, 310–11
Small size at birth, 315, 317–19, 321–22
Small for gestational age, 23, 160, 217
Social capital, 141, 144–45
Social learning, 57–58, 62
Socioassay, 141
Sociocultural, construction, 369; environment, 372; factors, 287, 372; settings, 374, 375; variables, 375, 377
Socioeconomic status, 145, 162, 163, 312, 327, 346, 377, 381; transition, 169–70

INDEX

SES. *See* Socioeconomic status
SNS. *See* Sympathetic nervous system
Sodium, 17–18, 20, 40, 56, 61, 67, 384, 386–90, 393–97
South Pacific, 83, 110, 369
Spironolactone, 394
Spock, Benjamin, 28
Staphylococcus, 1
Stearns, Steven. C., 135, 188, 402, 405, 422,
Strassman, Beverly, 185–86,
Stress hormones, 146, 243, 248, 250, 256, 347–48
Stress, 199, 242–45, 247–59, 264–65, 268, 272–73, 275, 280–82, 287–90, 293, 295, 297, 304–8, 310, 312–13, 325, 327, 329, 331, 337, 340–42, 347–48, 350, 366, 372–73, 385, 386, 418, 426; social, 32, 79, 94, 134–35, 137, 139–47, 166, 247–50, 252, 254–55, 257, 281, 287, 348
Stress response: evolution of, 243, 247–49, 258
Sudden infant death syndrome, 7, 9, 17, 29, 227, 231, 227, 237
Sympathetic nervous system, 148, 382–83, 385–87, 389, 392–95, 397
Symptom oriented medicine, 99
Systemic lupus erythematosus, 207–8

T-cell receptors, 12, 13, 205
T-cell lymphotrophic virus type 1, 205, 207
Taste papillae, 60
Taste properties, 60–61
Tay-Sachs, 377–78
Testing evolutionary hypotheses, 429, 433
Testosterone, 44, 171–72, 174–79, 247, 335
Tetrapod vertebrates, 385–88
Theory, 3, 4; attachment, 139, 141; behaviorism, 28; Darwin on heredity, 421; evolutionary, 9, 13, 15, 17, 24, 34, 46–47, 50–51, 68, 135, 151, 173, 194, 278–79, 283–84, 289, 323, 400–403, 409, 411, 413, 419–21, 424, 432, 436 n2; foraging, 91; forward/backward looking, 330, 334; game, 136, 137; of humors, 402; life history, 10, 12, 23, 36, 58, 135, 138, 148, 157, 167, 278; microeconomic, 318; of mind, 247, 258; natural selection, 421; nutritional crisis, 65; of the organism as a unified whole, 404; optimality, 279, 436 n1; spoiling (theory of development), 28
Thirst, 73, 387, 389
Thrifty genotype hypothesis, 81, 355
Thrifty phenotype hypothesis, 174
Tinbergen, Niko, 243, 422; four questions, 422
TNF, 79, 273, 306
TNF α, 79, 273, 306
Tobacco, 41, 45–46, 80, 94, 199, 360, 390–91, 395–97; deaths, 46
Tolvaptan, 394
Tongan, 374
Total dietary energy, 99, 100, 109, 111, 112
Toxoplasma gondii, 203, 366,

Tradeoff, 135, 146, 298, 423; current reproduction, 135–36, 137, 144, 147; physiological, 316–18
Trauma, early family, 251, 252, 253, 254, 257; life threatening, 97; psychosocial, 80; sleep disruption and, 256
Treviranus, Gottfried, 438
Trophoblastic implantation, 220, 221, 223

Ultimate cause, 11, 275
United States Department of Agriculture, 56, 67, 70, 88, 105, 435
Uric acid, 424, 426, 434
USDA. *See* United States Department of Agriculture
UVB radiation, 103, 119, 130, 133

Vaccine, 13, 14, 16, 425, 427
Vaginal opening, 144
Vascular endothelial growth factor, 269, 271, 274
Vascular endothelial growth factor receptor, 269, 271
Vasoconstriction, 270–72, 274, 392
Vasodilation, 270–72
Vasopressin, 248, 382–83, 385, 388–89, 393–95, 397
VEGF. *See* vascular endothelial growth factor
Vertebrates, evolution, 385, 388–89; terrestrial, 385, 388
Virchow, Rudolf, 408
Visceral fat, 74, 170
Vision, 2, 73, 79, 89, 90, 233, 294, 423, 429,
Vitamins, A, 19, 111, 123; B, 123; C, 17, 108, 269, 272, 436 n D, 103, 106, 111, 119, 123–24, 130–33, 436 n
Vomiting, 22, 62, 261, 386, 397, 409–10, 423
Vulnerability, 199, 209, 211, 298, 309–10, 312–13; to disease, 185, 198–99, 256, 322–23, 332, 353–60, 362, 367, 422–23, 425–427, 432–33; to drugs, 51, 281–82, 287,

Weaning, 35, 101, 116–18, 120, 122, 133, 333, 340, 343; age, 10, 29–30, 117–18; food supplementation and, 20, 229; lactase production and, 117; Paleolithic, 395
Western spadefoot toad, 330
WHO. *See* World Health Organization
WHO/UNICEF Baby-Friendly Hospital, 232, 241
Why We Get Sick, 400–401, 404, 409, 417
Williams, George, 4, 116, 400, 419
World Health Organization, 9, 83, 112, 193, 217, 232, 241, 396, 410, 437n12

Yogurt, 10, 119–20, 122
Yoruba, 369, 374

Zoonomia, 5, 4, 19